# Diagnostic Medical Sonography

A GUIDE TO CLINICAL PRACTICE

VOLUME II
**Echocardiography**

VOLUME I **Obstetrics and Gynecology**

Edited by
Mimi C. Berman, Ph.D., R.D.M.S.
Associate Professor, Diagnostic Medical Imaging Program
College of Health Related Professions
State University of New York
Health Science Center at Brooklyn
Brooklyn, New York

VOLUME II **Echocardiography**

Edited by
Marveen Craig, R.D.M.S.
Founder
International Ultrasound Institute
Dallas, Texas

VOLUME III **Abdomen**

Edited by
Diane M. Kawamura, M.Ed., R.T.(R), R.D.M.S.
Professor, Radiological Sciences
Weber State College
Ogden, Utah

# Diagnostic Medical Sonography

## A GUIDE TO CLINICAL PRACTICE

VOLUME II   **Echocardiography**

Edited by
MARVEEN CRAIG, R.D.M.S.

**J. B. Lippincott Company**

PHILADELPHIA      NEW YORK
LONDON      HAGERSTOWN

Acquisitions Editor: Charles McCormick, Jr.
Developmental Editor: Kimberly Cox
Production Manager: Janet Greenwood
Production: Editorial Services of New England, Inc.
Compositor: University Graphics
Printer/Binder: Halliday Lithograph

1 3 5 6 4 2

**Library of Congress Cataloging-in-Publication Data**

Echocardiography / edited by Marveen Craig.
    p.    cm. — (Diagnostic medical sonography ; v. 2)
    Includes bibliographical references.
    Includes index.
    1. Echocardiography.  I. Craig, Marveen.  II. Series.
    [DNLM  1. Echocardiography.  2. Heart Diseases—diagnosis.  WB 289 D5355 v. 2]
    RC78.7.U4D48  vol. 2
    [RC683.5.U5]
    616.07'543 s—dc20
    [616.1'207543]
    DNLM/DLC
    for Library of Congress                      90-6559
                                              CIP

ISBN 0-397-50953-7
ISBN 0-397-50954-5 (set)

The authors and publisher have exerted every effort to ensure that drug selection and dosage set forth in this text are in accord with current recommendations and practice at the time of publication. However, in view of ongoing research, changes in government regulations, and the constant flow of information relating to drug therapy and drug reactions, the reader is urged to check the package insert for each drug for any change in indications and dosage and for added warnings and precautions. This is particularly important when the recommended agent is a new or infrequently employed drug.

TO ALL THE EARLY PIONEERS who shared their knowledge of diagnostic ultrasound and their experiences with us.

"The whole art of teaching is only the art of awakening the natural curiosity of young minds for the purpose of satisfying it afterwards."
*Anatole France, 1844–1924*

# Contributors

David Adams, R.C.P.T., R.D.M.S.
Chief Cardiac Sonographer,
Duke University Medical Center,
Durham, North Carolina

Kathleen R. Baker, B.A., M.A.S., R.D.M.S.
Clinical Instructor of Pediatrics,
Division of Pediatric Cardiology,
University of Maryland Medical School;
Instructor in Echocardiography,
Maryland Institute of Ultrasound Technology,
Baltimore, Maryland

Ramesh C. Bansal, M.D.
Associate Professor of Medicine,
Director, Echocardiography Laboratory,
Loma Linda University Medical Center,
Loma Linda, California

Louis L. Battey, M.D., F.A.C.P.
Cardiovascular Associates of Augusta;
Clinical Professor of Medicine,
Medical College of Georgia,
Augusta, Georgia

Mimi C. Berman, Ph.D., R.D.M.S.
Associate Professor, Diagnostic Medical
Imaging Program,
College of Health Related Professions,
State University of New York,
Health Science Center at Brooklyn,
Brooklyn, New York

Rita M. Carriere, Ph.D.
Assistant Professor of Anatomy and Cell Biology,
State University of New York,
Health Science Center at Brooklyn,
Brooklyn, New York

Judah A. Charnoff, M.D.
Assistant Cardiologist,
Maimonides Medical Center,
Brooklyn, New York

Marveen Craig, R.D.M.S.
Founder,
International Ultrasound Institute,
Dallas, Texas

Marie De Lange, B.S., R.D.M.S., R.D.C.S.
Program Director,
School of Allied Health Radiation Sciences,
Diagnostic Medical Sonography Program;
Chief Sonographer,
Loma Linda University Medical Center,
Loma Linda, California

Evalie DuMars, B.S., R.D.C.S.
Adjunct Faculty,
Long Beach State University,
Orange Coast College,
Costa Mesa, California;
Senior Cardiac Sonographer,
Hoag Memorial Hospital-Presbyterian,
Newport Beach, California

**Sue A. George, Sc.D., Ph.D., R.D.M.S.**
Chief, Echocardiography,
Self Memorial Hospital,
Greenwood, South Carolina

**Alvin Greengart, M.D.**
Director,
Noninvasive Cardiology,
Maimonides Medical Center,
Brooklyn, New York

**Pamela Harrigan, R.D.C.S.**
Technical Director, Outpatient Cardiac
Ultrasound Laboratory,
Massachusetts General Hospital,
Boston, Massachusetts

**Diane M. Kawamura, M.Ed., R.T.(R), R.D.M.S.**
Professor, Radiological Sciences,
Weber State University,
Ogden, Utah

**Gerson S. Lichtenberg, B.S., R.D.C.S., R.T.**
Assistant in Medicine,
University of Rochester School of Medicine
and Dentistry,
Rochester, New York

**Paula K. Logan, R.D.C.S.**
Clinical Instructor, Department of Radiologic
Technology,
The University of Oklahoma Health Sciences
Center;
Cardiac Sonographer,
Oklahoma Medical Center,
Oklahoma City, Oklahoma

**Sally Moos, R.D.M.S.**
Technical Director, Heart Station,
University of Alabama Hospital,
Birmingham, Alabama

**Barbara A. Nichols, B.S., R.N., R.D.C.S.**
Supervisor, Echocardiographic Laboratory,
Mayo Clinic,
Rochester, Minnesota

**John C. Pope, B.S., P.A.C., R.D.C.S., R.D.M.S.**
Affiliate Clinical Instructor,
Medical College of Georgia;
Director, Echocardiography Laboratory,
Cardiovascular Associates of Augusta,
Augusta, Georgia

**Holly Racker, R.T., R.D.M.S.**
Sonographer,
Kelseyville, California

**Andrea C. Skelly, B.S., R.D.C.S., R.D.M.S.**
Assistant Professor
Chair, Diagnostic Ultrasound,
Seattle University,
Seattle, Washington

**Barbara Sternlight, B.A., R.D.M.S.**
Manager of Ultrasound Education,
Toshiba America Medical Systems,
Tustin, California

**Lore Tenckhoff, M.D**
Clinical Professor of Pediatrics,
University of Washington School of Medicine;
Pediatric Cardiologist,
Children's Hospital and Medical Center,
Seattle, Washington

**Henny J. Wasser, B.S., R.D.M.S.**
Adjunct Lecturer, College of Health Related
Professions,
State University of New York,
Health Science Center at Brooklyn;
Supervisor of Echocardiography,
Maimonides Medical Center,
Brooklyn, New York

**Diana Kawai Yankowitz, B.S., R.D.M.S.**
Program Director,
Maryland Institute of Ultrasound Technology,
Baltimore, Maryland

# Preface

Knowledge of the structure and function of the human body as well as common disease processes affecting the various organ systems of the body is essential for students of diagnostic ultrasound.

While in previous educational experiences students may have been required to *memorize* many facts, in the pursuit of diagnostic ultrasound they are encouraged to discard this habit. It is more important to *understand* how the bodily functions are accomplished in order to appreciate the many symptoms of malfunction of particular organs or systems. This is because the body functions as a whole, not as individual parts or systems, and it is the interdependency of the different organ systems that helps the body compensate for specific disabilities.

These were the basic reasons that we felt it necessary to provide a text that went beyond the fundamentals of cardiac imaging. In this text, the chapters on physical principles, equipment, and echocardiographic measurements and techniques form the basic foundation necessary to produce diagnostic quality images. The chapters dealing with cardiac and cardiovascular anatomy, physiology, pathology and pathophysiology also include important information: the clinical signs of cardiac disease and abnormalities, their appropriate treatment and usual prognosis, as well as other pertinent diagnostic imaging techniques.

By understanding these clinical principles as well as general imaging concepts, cardiac sonographers will be better able to deal with the many unpredictable situations that echocardiography often presents.

MARVEEN CRAIG, R.D.M.S.
DIANE M. KAWAMURA, M.ED., R.T.(R), R.D.M.S.
MIMI C. BERMAN, PH.D., R.D.M.S.

# Acknowledgments

It has been said that the hardest form of writing is collaboration. Trying to get three editors and over sixty contributors, separated by thousands of miles, to agree on everything for the year and a half it takes to produce a manuscript should be next to impossible. Happily, it is not only possible, but—in retrospect—enjoyable!

My first thanks go to Mimi Berman and Diane Kawamura, who understood my dream and were willing to work to make it happen. From there, the three of us learned the important lesson that the finished product would represent the combined ideas and efforts of dozens of people. Thus, thanks also go to the numerous contributors to all three volumes of *Diagnostic Medical Sonography.*

Thanks must also go to the J. B. Lippincott Company for their belief in this project: to Lisa Biello and De Lois Patterson, who fought for the project; to Jay Lippincott, who believed in it enough to approve it; to Charles McCormick and Kim Cox, who signed on in mid-stream and kept us all on track; and to the many able assistants we have never even met, who paid meticulous attention to editing, illustration, production, promotion, and delivery.

Last, but by no means least, my thanks go to the members of our families for all of their encouragement, patience, and faith.

M.C.

# Contents

PART IV     **Special Echocardiographic Techniques**

PART V     **Pediatric Echocardiography**

PART VI     **The Profession of Diagnostic Cardiac Sonography**

# List of Color Plates

*The following figures appear in a full-color insert beginning after page 352. They also appear in context as black-and-white reproductions.*

# PART ONE

# Structure and Function of the Heart

# CHAPTER 1

# Anatomy of the Pericardial and Thoracic Cavities

DIANE M. KAWAMURA

## Anatomic Relationships

Surrounded by the rib cage and separated from the abdominal cavity by the muscular diaphragm, the thoracic cavity contains several divisions. It is divided into two pleural cavities, each containing a lung, and the pericardial cavity located in the mediastinum.[1] Serving as a partition between the lungs, the mediastinum is a mass of tissue extending from the sternum to the vertebral column that contains almost all of the contents of the thoracic cavity except the lungs (Fig. 1-1).[6]

Although detailed knowledge of the anatomy of the skeletal framework is not essential to performing a diagnostic echocardiographic examination, a brief presentation of skeletal anatomy may help the reader understand correlative imaging procedures such as chest radiography, computed tomography, and magnetic resonance imaging.

## Skeletal Framework

A bony and muscular framework creates the thoracic wall, which protects the vital organs in the thorax and prevents collapse of the thorax during respiration.[7] The sternum, thoracic vertebrae, and ribs with their associated costal cartilages comprise the skeletal framework.[9] (Costal is the adjectival form of the Latin word for ribs.)

### STERNUM

The sternum, or breastbone, is flat, narrow, and about 15 cm long. Shaped like a sword, it is divided into three parts: (1) the manubrium, the triangular superior portion shaped like the handle of a sword; (2) the body, the middle and largest portion resembling the sword's blade (the old term for it was *gladiolus,* Latin for sword); and (3) the xiphoid process, the inferior, smallest portion comparable to the sword tip.[7]

At the base of the neck, an important bony landmark, the suprasternal (jugular) notch, is palpable as a depression on the superior surface of the manubrium. On each side of the notch are clavicular notches that articulate with the medial ends of the clavicle. The manubrium also articulates with the costal cartilage of the first rib.[4]

The sternal angle on the anterior thorax locates the point at which the manubrium joins the body of the sternum. The palpable sternal angle is important clinically. Its lateral borders serve as the attachment points for the cartilage of the second rib. This provides a starting point for counting the ribs when they are used as landmarks for other thoracic structures, such as areas of the heart.[4,9]

The cartilage of the third through the seventh ribs attaches to the body of the sternum and the eighth, ninth, and tenth ribs attach indirectly to the body of the sternum. No ribs attach to the xiphoid process, but some abdominal muscles do (Fig. 1-2).[4,7]

### THORACIC VERTEBRAE

The vertebral column has four distinct regions: (1) the cervical, (2) the thoracic, (3) the lumbar, and

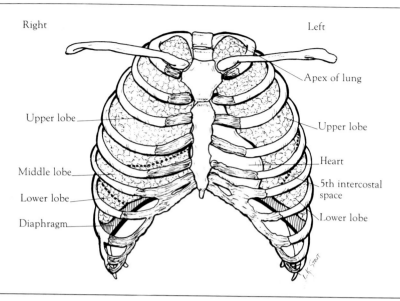

Right                                                  Left

Apex of lung

Upper lobe                                    Upper lobe

Heart

Middle lobe                                  5th intercostal space

Lower lobe                                   Lower lobe

Diaphragm

FIGURE 1-1. Anterior aspect of the thoracic cavity with the outline of the heart and lungs superimposed.

(4) the sacral and coccygeal. Each region has specific characteristics that tend to blend at the boundaries. Long transverse processes and long, thin spinous processes directed inferiorly characterize the 12 thoracic vertebrae.[7,9]

The first 10 thoracic vertebrae (T1–T10) have facets on their transverse processes for articulating with the tubercles of the ribs. The tubercles on the eleventh and twelfth ribs do not articulate with their respective vertebrae.[4,6]

### RIBS AND COSTAL CARTILAGES

Twelve pairs of ribs comprise the sides and a portion of the posterior and anterior thoracic cavity. The first through the seventh ribs increase in length. These seven are referred to as true or vertebrosternal ribs, because they articulate with the thoracic vertebrae posteriorly and attach directly to the sternum anteriorly through their costal cartilage. Rib length decreases from the eighth to the twelfth. Because these five inferior ribs attach to the vertebrae posteriorly but do not directly attach to the sternum they are called false ribs. False ribs are subdivided into two groups. The vertebrochondral ribs (eighth, ninth, and tenth) are joined an-

teriorly to a common cartilage, which in turn attaches to the sternum. The floating or vertebral ribs (eleventh and twelfth) have no attachment to the sternum (Fig. 1-3).[1,3,4,6,7,9]

At the posterior end of the rib is a projection, the head. The heads of the first, tenth, eleventh, and twelfth ribs have only one facet and articulate with their respective thoracic vertebra. The second through ninth ribs have a wedge-shaped head and two facets that articulate with the bodies of two adjacent thoracic vertebrae.[1,3,4,6,7,9]

Lateral to the head is a short constricted portion called the neck of the rib. The neck has a knoblike structure called the tubercle on the posterior surface where it joins the body. The tubercle consists of a nonarticular part, where ligaments attach, and an articular part. The articular part of the first to the tenth ribs joins the facet on the transverse process of the lower of the two vertebrae, to which the head of the rib is connected. The tubercles on the eleventh and twelfth ribs do not articulate with the transverse process (Fig. 1-4).[1,3,4,6,7,9]

The next portion of the rib is the body or shaft. A short distance from the tubercle, the shaft has a sharp curve, the costal angle. Each rib body has a

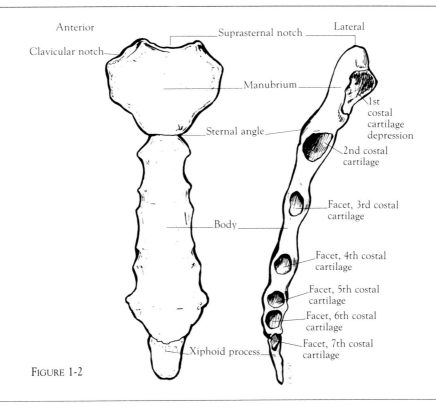

FIGURE 1-2

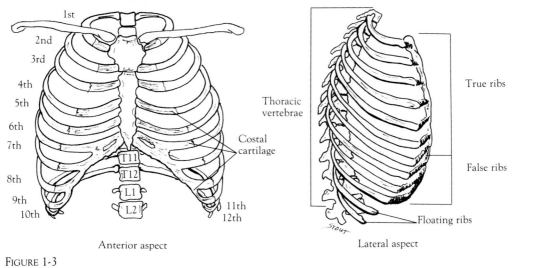

FIGURE 1-3

FIGURE 1-2. Structure, shape, articulating surfaces, and landmarks of the anterior and lateral sternum.

FIGURE 1-3. Anterior and lateral aspect of the bony thorax demonstrating the difference between the true and false ribs.

Superior view                 Oblique view

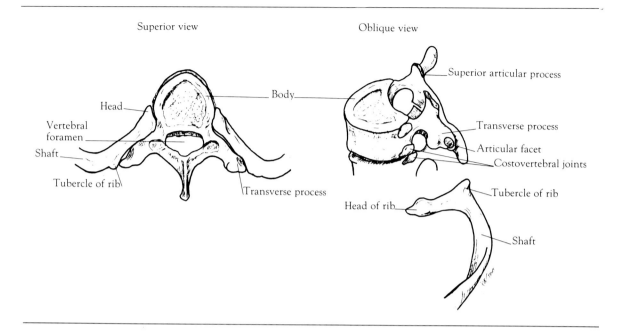

FIGURE 1-4. Superior and oblique views of the articulation of a rib with a thoracic vertebra.

groove on its inner surface that protects blood vessels and a small nerve.[4,7,9]

Spaces between ribs, called intercostal spaces, are occupied by intercostal muscles, blood vessels, and nerves.[1,4,7,9] The second to sixth intercostal spaces may serve as acoustic windows for echocardiographic examinations. The standard interspace describes the intercostal space where the mitral valve leaflet can be visualized with the transducer directed posteriorly and slightly medially. This standard interspace may vary with body habitus, pathology, or chest wall deformities.

The ribs curve inward laterally from the vertebrae to the sternum. Each rib has its own range and variety of movements. In the respiratory excursions of the thorax, the movement of all the ribs is combined. The costal cartilages are composed of hyaline cartilage, which allows lateral rib movement and lateral expansion of the thoracic cavity. Elevating the ribs can increase the anteroposterior dimension of the thoracic cavity, and depressing the diaphragm increases the superoinferior dimension.[4,7,9]

## Muscles of Respiration

The primary function of the deep muscles of the thorax is the movements of respiration. Contraction of the muscles of inspiration expands the thorax to accommodate inspired air. When the muscles of inspiration relax, the elastic properties of the thorax and lungs cause a passive decrease in thoracic volume and expiration occurs. During labored breathing, the inspiratory muscles contract more forcefully, causing a greater increase in thoracic volume. The muscles of respiration, in addition to the passive recoil of the thorax and lungs, can contract, producing a more rapid and greater decrease in thoracic volume (Fig. 1-5).[1,4,6,7,9]

Four major groups of muscles are associated with the respiratory movement of the rib cage: the scalene, the external intercostal muscles, the internal intercostal muscles, and the diaphragm. The anterolateral walls of the thoracic cavity are formed by, from outermost to innermost, the external intercostals, the internal intercostals, and the transverse thoracic muscles. The tripartite transverse thoracic muscle, which consists of many slips, orig-

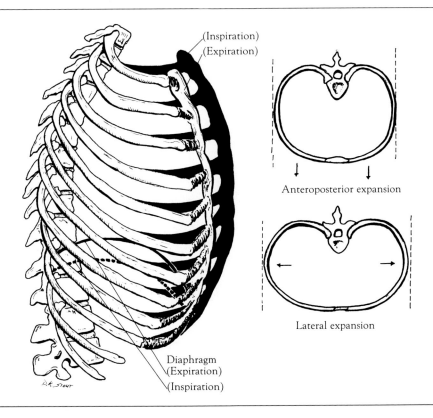

(Inspiration)
(Expiration)

Anteroposterior expansion

Lateral expansion

Diaphragm
(Expiration)
(Inspiration)

D.K. STOUT

FIGURE 1-5. Demonstration of thoracic volume changes during inspiration and expiration.

inates at the sternum and inserts in the second to sixth costal cartilages. Its function is still controversial; it is theorized that it narrows the chest.[4,6,7,9]

SCALENE MUSCLES

Originating on the transverse processes of the cervical vertebrae and inserting posterolaterally on the first two ribs, the anterior, middle, and posterior scalene muscles aid in inspiration by elevating the first two ribs. They are innervated by the cervical nerves (Fig. 1-6).[4]

EXTERNAL INTERCOSTAL MUSCLES

From their point of origin on the inferior border of the rib above to their insertion in the superior border of the rib below, the fibers of the 11 pairs of external intercostal muscles course obliquely downward and forward. In the lower intercostal spaces, the fibers are continuous with the external oblique muscles, forming part of the abdominal wall. These muscles elevate the ribs during inspiration to increase the lateral and anteroposterior dimensions of the thorax. They are innervated by the intercostal nerves.[4,6,7,9]

INTERNAL INTERCOSTAL MUSCLES

The 11 pairs of internal intercostals serve as antagonists to the external intercostals. These muscle fibers run deep and at right angles to those of the external intercostals. Originating in the costal groove of the rib above and inserting in the superior border of the rib below, these muscles course downward and posteriorly. The lower internal intercostal muscles are continuous with the fibers of the internal oblique muscle of the abdominal wall. They decrease the lateral and anteroposterior di-

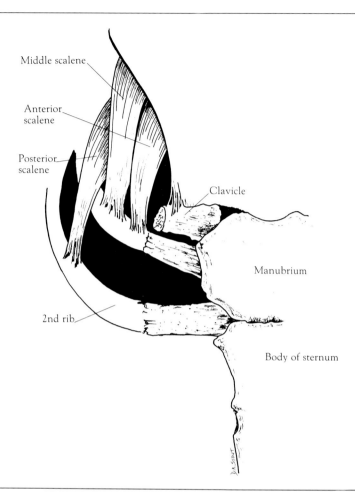

FIGURE 1-6. Anterior view of the anterior, middle, and posterior scalene muscles.

mensions of the thoracic cavity by drawing adjacent ribs together during forced expiration. They are also innervated by the intercostal nerves (Fig. 1-7).[4,6,7,9]

DIAPHRAGM
The major movement during quiet breathing is produced by the diaphragm, the most important muscle of respiration and the boundary between the thoracic and the abdominopelvic cavity. If this wall of muscle or the phrenic nerve supplying it is severely damaged, air exchange in the lungs may be so compromised as to cause death.

The diaphragm is a broad skeletal muscle. The fibers converge from the inferior border of the rib cage, the sternum, the costal cartilages of the last six ribs, and the lumbar spine and course toward a boomerang-shaped central tendon. During relaxation it is dome-shaped but when the diaphragm contracts, it flattens, increasing the vertical dimension of the thorax. If the muscle contraction is strong enough, intra-abdominal pressure may be increased dramatically (Fig. 1-7).[1,3,4,6,7,9]

## Vascular Supply
The heart serves as a double pump for two distinct circulations, each with its own route through arteries, arterioles, capillaries, venules, and veins. The

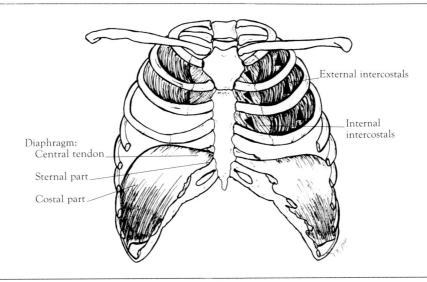

FIGURE 1-7. Anterior view showing the antagonistic relationship of the internal intercostal (*down arrow*) and the external intercostal (*up arrow*) muscles. An anterior view of the diaphragm is also demonstrated.

pulmonary circulation is the short route. Oxygen-poor blood goes from the right ventricle through the pulmonary arteries to the alveolar capillaries in the lungs where it is oxygenated and returns through the pulmonary veins to the left atrium. In the systemic circulation oxygenated blood from the left ventricle goes to the body and oxygen-poor blood returns to the right atrium.[4,5,7,9]

In the thoracic cavity, systemic circulation supplies the bronchi with oxygenated blood through the bronchial arteries, which branch off the thoracic aorta. Oxygen-poor blood from the proximal part of the major bronchi returns to the heart through the bronchial veins and azygous system; more distally, the venous drainage from the bronchi enters the pulmonary veins. Oxygenated blood returning from the alveoli in the pulmonary veins is mixed with a small amount of oxygen-poor blood returning from the bronchi.[1,3,4,9]

The systemic circulation has two other subdivisions: the coronary (cardiac) circulation and the hepatic portal circulation.[4,7,9]

### PULMONARY CIRCULATION

Oxygen-poor blood from the right ventricle is pumped into the pulmonary trunk. This 5-cm-long vessel bifurcates into the right and left pulmonary arteries, which transport blood to each lung. These branches each serve one lung lobe by dividing into three lobar arteries to the right lung and two lobar arteries to the left lung. The lobar arteries parallel the main bronchi into the lungs and then subdivide into arterioles and continue branching until they form networks of pulmonary capillaries surrounding and clinging to the alveoli in the lungs. Carbon dioxide is passed from the blood into the alveoli and is exhaled from the lungs. Inspired oxygen passes from the alveoli into the blood. The pulmonary capillary beds then unite and drain into venules, which continue to unite, forming the two pulmonary veins exiting from each lung. The four pulmonary veins complete the pulmonary circulation by returning oxygen-rich blood to the left atrium. The pulmonary veins are the only veins that carry oxygenated blood. When the left ventricle contracts, the oxygenated blood is sent into the systemic circulation (Fig. 1-8).[1,3-7,9]

### SYSTEMIC ARTERIAL CIRCULATION

Oxygenated blood that has entered the heart from the pulmonary veins passes through the left atrium into the left ventricle. From the left ventricle the

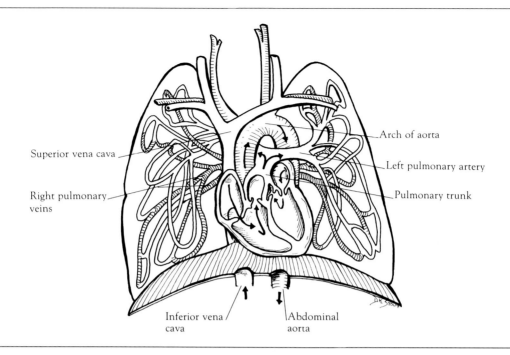

Superior vena cava

Right pulmonary veins

Arch of aorta

Left pulmonary artery

Pulmonary trunk

Inferior vena cava

Abdominal aorta

FIGURE 1-8. A sectional view demonstrates the path of the pulmonary circulation.

blood is pumped into the aorta and thence to all portions of the body.[4,7,9]

*Aorta.* All arteries of the systemic circulation originate either directly or indirectly from the aorta, which is divided into three general portions, the ascending aorta, the aortic arch, and the descending aorta, which further divides into a thoracic and an abdominal aorta.[4,7,9]

The aorta is about 2.8 cm in diameter at its origin from the left ventricle. Where it passes superiorly from the heart it is called the ascending aorta. It is approximately 5 cm long, and the right and left coronary arteries, which supply blood to the cardiac muscle, branch from it.[5-7,9]

The aorta then arches posteriorly and curves to the left, forming the aortic arch. Blood is supplied to the head and upper limbs by three branches originating from the aortic arch: the brachiocephalic (innominate) artery, the left common carotid artery, and the left subclavian artery (Fig. 1-9).[1,4-7,9]

*Thoracic aorta and its branches.* The descending aorta, the next and longest portion, extends

through the thorax in the left side of the mediastinum and through the abdomen to the superior margin of the pelvis. Branches of thoracic descending aorta can be divided into two groups: the visceral arteries supplying the thoracic organs and the parietal arteries supplying the thoracic wall. Even though the lungs have a large quantity of blood flowing through them, the visceral branches are required as a separate oxygenated blood supply for the lungs, esophagus, and pericardial sac.[1,3,5-7,9]

The walls of the thorax are supplied with blood by the anterior and posterior intercostal arteries. The internal thoracic arteries branch off of the subclavian arteries and are located on the inner surface of the anterior chest wall. The anterior intercostals are tributaries of the internal thoracic artery. The posterior intercostals originate as bilateral branches directly from the descending aorta. The anterior and posterior intercostal arteries course along the inferior margin of each rib and form anastomoses with each other approximately midway between the anterior midline and the dorsal aorta (Fig. 1-10).[4,7,9]

Also branching off the descending thoracic aorta

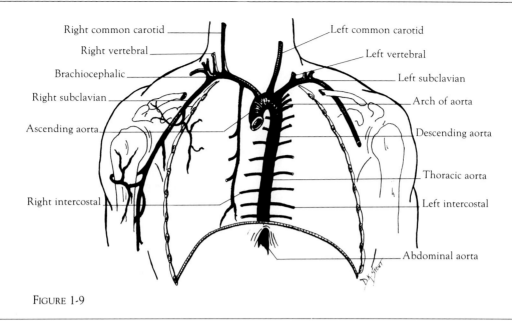

FIGURE 1-9

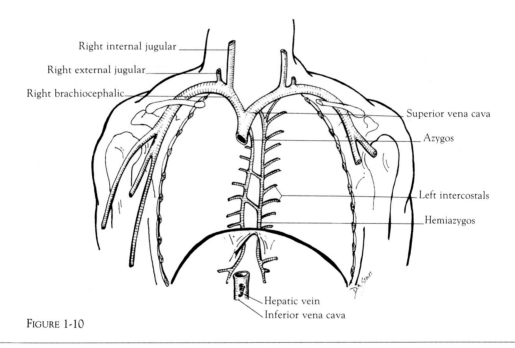

FIGURE 1-10

FIGURE 1-9. A sectional view of systemic arterial circulation.

FIGURE 1-10. A sectional view of systemic venous circulation.

are the superior phrenic arteries, which supply blood to the diaphragm.[3,4,7,9]

### Systemic Venous Circulation

The three major veins that return blood from the body to the right atrium are (1) the coronary sinus returning blood from the walls of the heart, (2) the superior vena cava returning blood from the head, neck, thorax, and upper limbs, and (3) the inferior vena cava returning blood from the abdomen, pelvis, and lower limbs.[4,7,9]

Veins are more numerous and more variable than arteries. Generally, the smaller veins follow the same course as the arteries and often have the same name; whereas, larger veins usually have different names and follow a different course than large arteries.[1,4,7,9]

Veins are of three types: superficial, deep, and sinuses. In the limbs, the superficial veins generally are larger than the deep veins, but in the trunk, the superficial veins are smaller. The venous sinuses are located primarily in the cranial vault and the heart.[4,7,9]

*Veins of the Thorax.* The right and left brachiocephalic veins and the azygos vein are the three major veins that return blood from the thorax to the superior vena cava.[2,4,7,9] The brachiocephalic vein is formed by the union of the internal jugular and the subclavian vein on both right and left sides. They drain blood from the head, neck, upper extremities, mammary glands, and the first two to three intercostal spaces. The right and left brachiocephalics join to form the superior vena cava.[2,4,7,9]

The vast majority of blood in the thoracic tissues and the thoracic wall is drained by a complex network of veins called the azygos system. The azygos vein, hemiazygos vein, and the accessory hemiazygos vein make up the system. The azygos vein is the continuation of the right ascending lumbar vein. Blood from the posterior thoracic wall is collected by posterior intercostal veins and drains into the azygos vein on the right and the hemiazygos or accessory hemiazygos vein on the left. The hemiazygos and accessory hemiazygos veins empty into the azygos, which drains into the superior vena cava (Fig. 1-10).[2,4,7] The coronary veins transport blood from the walls of the heart and return it to the right atrium.[1,4,7,9]

## Thoracic Viscera

### Mediastinum

The mediastinum or *mediastinal* septum is situated between the right and left pleural sacs, posterior to the sternum, and anterior to the thoracic vertebrae. It extends from the inlet of the thorax down to the diaphragm. The mediastinum is divided into four parts that are related to the position of the pericardial sac, superior, anterior, middle, and posterior (Fig. 1-11).[3,5,6]

The superior portion of the mediastinum lies above a plane drawn from the sternal angle to the inferior border of the fourth thoracic vertebra. Inferior to this plane, the mediastinum is subdivided into the anterior portion (in front of the pericardial sac); the middle portion (containing the pericardial sac); and the posterior portion (behind the pericardial sac).[3,6]

The superior mediastinum contains the aortic arch, the brachiocephalic artery, the origins of the left common carotid and left subclavian arteries, the right and left brachiocephalic veins as they join to form the superior vena cava, the trachea, the esophagus, the thoracic duct, the thymus gland remnant, and a few lymph nodes and nerves.[3,6]

Only a small amount of fascia, a few lymph nodes, and vessels lie in the anterior mediastinum.[3,6] The middle mediastinum contains the pericardium and heart, the origin of the ascending aorta, the terminal part of the superior vena cava with the azygos vein draining into it, the pulmonary artery dividing into the right and left branches, the terminal parts of the right and left pulmonary veins, and the right and left phrenic nerves.[3,6]

The posterior mediastinum contains the thoracic descending aorta; the bifurcation of the trachea and the right and left main bronchi; the esophagus; the azygos and hemiazygos veins; the right and left vagus nerves; the splanchnic nerves; and the thoracic lymphatic duct with many additional lymph nodes.[3,6]

### Organs of Respiration in the Thoracic Cavity

*Trachea.* The trachea, or windpipe, functions as an air passage and it filters, warms, and moistens incoming air. It begins in the neck and descends into the thoracic cavity in front of the esophagus to enter the mediastinum and measures approxi-

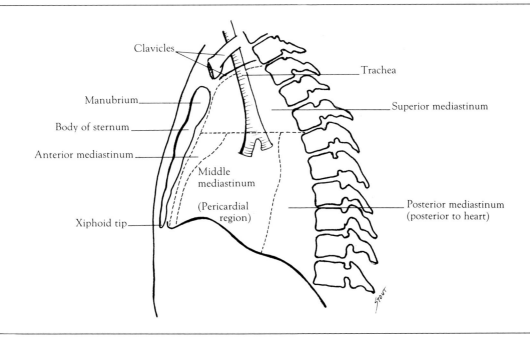

FIGURE 1-11. A sectional view showing the four divisions of the mediastinum.

mately 15 cm long and 1.5 to 2.5 cm in diameter. The trachea divides into the right and left primary bronchi at the level of the fifth thoracic vertebra. It is a very mobile structure that can be moved from side to side by probing fingers and that stretches and descends during inspiration and recoils during expiration.[4,7,9]

Fifteen to twenty **C**-shaped pieces of hyaline cartilage reinforce the regular connective tissue and smooth muscle, protect the trachea, allow flexible twisting and elongation, and keep the airway open. The cartilage forms the anterior and lateral sides of the trachea and abuts the esophagus posteriorly. The posterior wall consists of a ligamentous membrane and smooth muscle, which can alter the diameter of the trachea during respiration and allows the esophagus to expand anteriorly during swallowing.[1,3,4,7,9]

Pseudostratified ciliated columnar epithelium containing numerous seromucous glands that secrete thick mucus lines the trachea. The cilia propel mucus laden with foreign particles toward the larynx, where it can be swallowed or expelled.[1,3,4,7,9]

*Bronchial Tree.* The bronchial tree serves as an air passage connecting the trachea with the alveoli and warms and moistens incoming air. The right and left primary bronchi, the secondary and tertiary bronchi, and the bronchioles make up the tree.[1,3,4,6,7,9]

At the level of the sternal angle, the right and left primary bronchi are formed by the division of the trachea. Each bronchus extends obliquely in the mediastinum before entering the medial depression (hilus) of its respective lung. The right primary bronchus is shorter, wider, and more vertical than the left one. Inside the lungs, the primary bronchi divide into the secondary (lobar) bronchi. Three secondary bronchi in the right lung and two in the left lung conduct air to each lobe.[3,4,6,7,9]

The secondary bronchi branch into the tertiary (segmental) bronchi, which extend into the lobules. The bronchial tree continues to branch repeatedly, dividing into smaller and smaller bronchioles with an end diameter of 0.5 mm.[3,4,7,9]

Primary bronchi are similar to the trachea in structure. They are lined with pseudostratified cil-

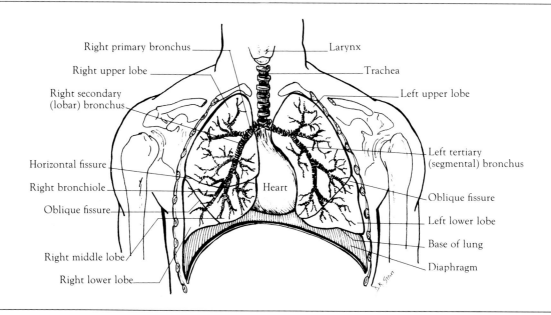

FIGURE 1-12. A sectional view demonstrates the lobes of the lung, bronchial tree, and other thoracic structures.

iated columnar epithelium and are supported by **C**-shaped cartilage bands up to the point where they enter the lungs. When the bronchus enters the lungs, the cartilage plates come together to form a complete circle that is smaller and more irregular. The cartilage appears as a separate layer of interlacing bundles and rather than being internal to the muscle, it assumes an external position, no longer offering supportive cartilage in the tube walls. This allows the airway lumen to become occluded by a contraction of the muscle. Farther into the respiratory tree, the cartilage becomes smaller and more sparse, and smooth muscle becomes more abundant. The bronchioles are devoid of cartilage. They are lined with mucosal epithelium, which becomes thinner and changes progressively from pseudostratified ciliated columnar epithelium to ciliated columnar epithelium in the terminal bronchioles (Fig. 1-12).[1,4,7,9]

*Alveoli.* The bronchioles also subdivide numerous times to become terminal bronchioles, which divide into the respiratory bronchioles, which divide again to form alveolar ducts that end as clusters of air sacs called the alveoli. An alveolar sac is composed of two or more alveoli that share a common outpouching into the alveolar ducts. The chambers of the alveoli are the main sites of gas exchange.[1,3,4,6,7,9]

Alveoli are the termination of the bronchial tree. They are microscopic chambers clustered densely together. The walls of the alveolar ducts and the alveoli are composed of simple squamous epithelium that facilitates diffusion of gas through the epithelial layer underlined with basement membrane. The external surfaces are associated with pulmonary capillaries. Secretory cells are also present on the alveolar wall which produces surfactant, a substance that reduces surface tension and helps prevent the lungs from collapsing. Macrophages on the surface of the alveolar epithelium remove debris that has passed below the terminal bronchioles (Fig. 1-13).[6,7,9]

*Lungs.* The lungs are the principal organs of respiration and occupy all of the thoracic cavity except the mediastinum. They house the respiratory passageways smaller than the primary bronchi. By vol-

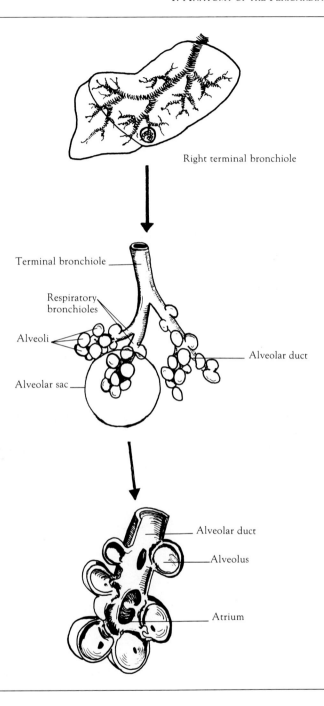

FIGURE 1-13. Diagram of the alveoli, alveolar duct, and alveolar sac in relationship to the terminal bronchiole.

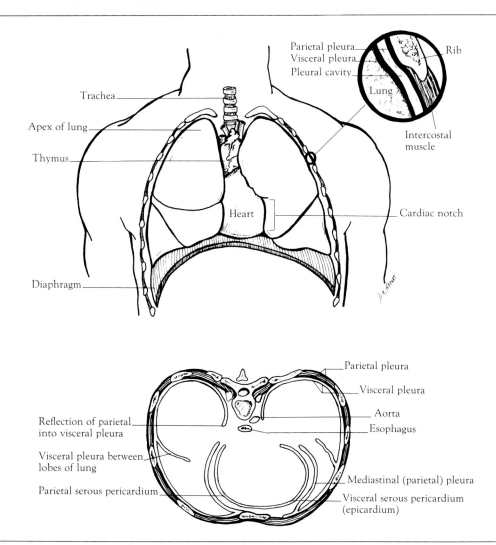

FIGURE 1-14. Anterior and sectional view of the pleural cavities.

ume, the lungs are among the largest organs of the body. On the medial (mediastinal) surface, each lung is indented with the hilus, which provides entry into the lung for blood vessels of the pulmonary and systemic circulation and the primary bronchi. The vascular and bronchiolar attachments—collectively called the lung root—suspend each lung in its own pleural cavity.[3,4,6,7,9]

The costal surfaces are located anterior, lateral, and posterior as the lungs and lie in close contact with the ribs. Each lung is conical. Its base rests on the diaphragm and its apex extends superiorly to a point about 2.5 cm superior to each clavicle.[1,3,4,6,7,9]

The two lungs are somewhat different in shape because the heart is located slightly to the left of the thoracic midline. The right lung is larger (average 620 g) and has superior, middle, and inferior lobes. The left lung (560 g) has two lobes, superior and inferior. The cardiac notch, a concavity in the medial aspect of the left lung, is molded to and accommodates the heart.[4–7]

Prominent fissures on the surface of the lung separate each lobe. Each lobe further divides into lobules separated from each other by connective tissue. These separations are not visible as surface fissures. Because major blood vessels and bronchi do not cross the connective tissues individual diseased lobules can be surgically removed, leaving the rest of the lung relatively intact. There are nine lobules in the left lung and ten in the right lung (Fig. 1-12).[4,6,7,9]

COVERINGS OF THE LUNGS AND PLEURA

The lungs are contained in the thoracic cavity and each lies in a separate pleural cavity. The pleural cavities are lined with an exceedingly thin, double-layered serous membrane (serosa).[1,3,4,7−9]

The names of the serous membranes reflect the cavity and organs with which they are associated. For example, the parietal and visceral peritoneum refers to the abdominopelvic cavity; the parietal and visceral pericardia are associated with the pericardial cavity and the heart; and the parietal and visceral pleura covers the thorax walls and lungs respectively. The two pleural (lung) cavities and the pericardial (heart) cavity are the three serous membrane–lined cavities of the thorax.[1,3,4,7,9]

The outer layer of the membrane (parietal pleura or serosa) adheres to the thoracic wall, diaphragm, and mediastinum. The parietal pleura continues around the heart and between the lungs, forming the mediastinal enclosure. A cufflike extension on each side (the pulmonary ligament) supports the lung and snugly encloses its root. At the root, the parietal pleura becomes continuous with the visceral pleura (the portion of the serous membrane in contact with the external lung surface), dipping into and lining its fissures.[4,6,7,9]

A potential space between the visceral and parietal membranes is normally filled with a thin lubricating film of serous (pleural) fluid produced by the membranes. Pleural fluid has two functions: it acts as a lubricant to reduce friction which allows the pleural membranes to slide past each other as the lungs and thorax change shape during respiration, and it helps to hold the pleural membranes tightly together (Fig. 1-14).[4,7−9]

## References

1. Anthony CP, Thibodeau GA. Textbook of Anatomy and Physiology. 10th ed. St Louis: CV Mosby; 1979.
2. Goodwin D, Chen JT. Pictorial essay: Thoracic venous anatomy. AJR. 1986; 147:674–684.
3. Goss CM (ed). Gray's Anatomy: Anatomy of the Human Body. 29th ed. Philadelphia: Lea & Febiger; 1973.
4. Marieb EN. Human Anatomy and Physiology. Redwood City, CA: Benjamin/Cummings; 1989.
5. Netter FH. The CIBA Collection of Medical Illustrations: Heart. Rochester, NY: Case-Hoyt Corporation; 1978; 5.
6. Netter FH. The CIBA Collection of Medical Illustrations: Respiratory System. Rochester, NY: Case-Hoyt Corporation; 1979; 7.
7. Seeley RR, Stephens TD, Tate P. Anatomy and Physiology. St Louis: Times Mirror/Mosby College Publishing; 1989.
8. Thomas CL (ed). Taber's Cyclopedic Medical Dictionary. 15th ed. Philadelphia: FA Davis; 1985.
9. Tortora GJ, Anagnastakos NP. Principles of Anatomy and Physiology. 5th ed. New York: Harper & Row; 1987.

# CHAPTER 2

# Anatomy of the Heart

MIMI C. BERMAN, RITA M. CARRIERE

Although the structure of the heart is well-understood, attempts to build a fully functioning implantable artificial heart have been unsuccessful. However, replacement valves, coronary by-pass surgery, angioplasty, and pacemakers are a few of the technologically derived repairs that can extend its ability to function. The role of diagnostic ultrasound in the ongoing attempts to extend the life of the heart has been to delineate anatomic anomalies and dynamic malfunctions so that appropriate treatment can be provided.

As in every area of diagnostic ultrasound, a thorough knowledge of the anatomy is a prerequisite to performing and interpreting echocardiograms. Because the heart's anatomical structure is designed for motion, it lends itself particularly well to examination by real-time imaging. Keeping in mind that the unique features of each part of the heart are related to its function, a study of the anatomy of the heart is a fascinating endeavor.

## Location

Located in the middle mediastinum, the heart is surrounded by the lungs laterally and posteriorly, by the manubrium and second through sixth costal cartilages and thymus anteriorly, and by the diaphragm inferiorly. Also in contact with the heart posteriorly are the esophagus and the descending aorta (Figs. 2-1, 2-5).

The pleural sacs and lungs cover the lateral mar-

gins and the anterior surface of the heart, leaving bare only a small triangular area on the lower left side of the anterior surface. This open area, located at the caudal part of the body of the sternum and at the medial edges of the fourth and fifth costal cartilages, is important to echocardiographers because it provides the acoustic window often needed to visualize the heart. It is referred to clinically as the "bare area" of the heart or pericardium.

## Pericardium

The term pericardium, as used clinically, denotes the saclike structure surrounding the heart. It is composed of two layers: a thick, fibrous outer layer, or fibrous pericardium, and a thin serous membrane called the parietal pericardium (Fig. 2-2A).

At the sites where the great vessels enter or leave the heart, the serous membrane is reflected and continues onto the surface of the heart, where it forms the outermost covering of the heart itself, facing the pericardial cavity. This is called the visceral pericardium (see Fig. 2-2A). It is part of the epicardial layer of the heart (see below). Since the visceral and parietal pericardium are in continuity at the attachments of the great vessels, together they constitute a collapsed sphere or bubble, with a potential cavity between them, the pericardial cavity. The cavity is narrow, following the contours of the heart, and it contains the pericardial fluid, a filtrate of the serous membrane, which al-

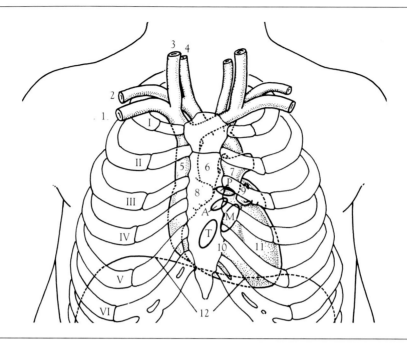

Figure 2-1. Anterior view of the heart shows its relation to the ribs, diaphragm, and manubrium. The location of the tricuspid (T) pulmonary (P), mitral (M), and aortic (A) valves is indicated. I through VI identify the ribs. 1, right subclavian vein; 2, right subclavian artery; 3, right jugular vein; 4, right carotid artery; 5, superior vena cava; 6, aorta; 7, pulmonary artery; 8, right auricle and atrium; 9, left auricle and atrium; 10, right ventricle; 11, left ventricle; 12, diaphragm.

lows the adjacent serous membranes to move freely and to accommodate the changes in the heart's shape during systole and diastole.

There are two recesses or sinuses within the pericardial cavity (Fig. 2-2B) partially walled off by the lines of reflection of the serous membrane around the great vessels. The transverse sinus lies posterior to the aorta and pulmonary artery and anterior to the superior vena cava, forming a passage between these vessels. The oblique sinus is between the left atrium and the posterior wall of the pericardium, and it is bounded by the inferior vena cava, the right pulmonary veins, and the superior vena cava on the right and by the left pulmonary veins on the left. The oblique sinus accommodates the pulsations of the left atrium. Both sinuses may contain pericardial fluid, as they are merely recesses of the pericardial cavity.

The inferior part of the fibrous pericardium is firmly attached to the central tendon of the diaphragm and it follows the diaphragmatic respiratory excursions. The superior part of the fibrous pericardium blends with the connective tissues of the mediastinum and of the great vessels as the latter enter the heart.

## Measurements

The size of a person's heart depends on body size, age, and lifestyle. Larger people have bigger hearts, as do those who exercise regularly. A given person's heart is roughly the size of his or her fist.[3] Specific dimensions have been reported: length, 12 cm; width, 8 to 9 cm; anteroposterior diameter, 6 cm. A woman's heart weighs 230 to 280 g, a man's, 280 to 340 g.

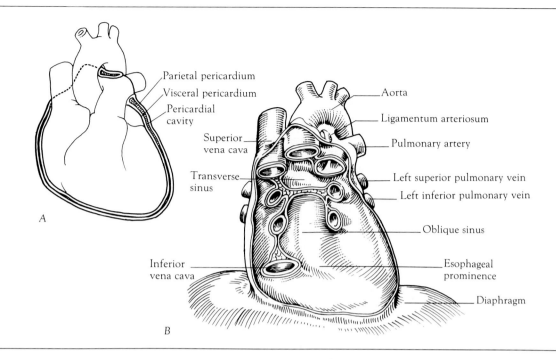

FIGURE 2-2. (A) The heart is shown surrounded by the pericardium, the outermost layer of which, the fibrous pericardium, is lined by the parietal pericardium. Intimately connected with the epicardium, the outermost layer of the heart, is the visceral pericardium. Between the parietal and visceral pericardium is a potential space called the pericardial cavity. A dotted line indicates the extent of the pericardium around the great vessels. (B) A view of the pericardial cavity with the heart removed shows the posterior wall of the pericardial cavity, the transverse sinus, and the oblique sinus.

## Structure of the Heart Wall

The heart wall is composed of three layers, each in turn made up of several tissues (Fig. 2-3C). The endocardium is the innermost layer of the heart wall. Its most important component is the endothelium, a single layer of flattened cells lying on connective tissue. The endothelial cell surface has the property of preventing blood from clotting. Blood in contact with any other tissue, except the placental trophoblast, clots.

Like the entire vascular system, the heart is lined with endothelium. The heart valves are flaps or folds made up of two layers of endocardium, providing endothelial coverage on both surfaces of the fibrous core. The myocardium, the middle layer of the heart wall, consists primarily of a specialized muscle unique to the heart: cardiac muscle. This is involuntary muscle, as it is regulated by the autonomic nervous system. The myocardial layer also contains connective tissue, with abundant blood capillaries to supply the muscle tissue. In the atria, the myocardium is very thin. It is thickest in the left ventricle, which must pump blood into the systemic circulation (Fig. 2-3).

The outer layer of the heart wall, the epicardium, consists of fat and connective tissue covered by a thin epithelial membrane, the serous pericardium described above. In this layer are the coronary blood vessels, autonomic nerves, and lymphatics, all ramifying to supply the myocardium.

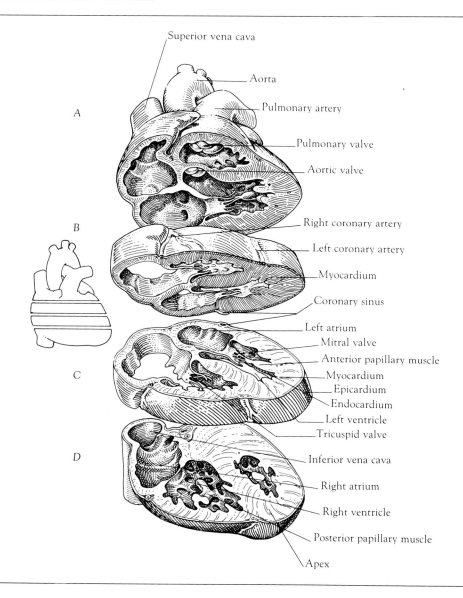

Superior vena cava

Aorta

Pulmonary artery

*A*

Pulmonary valve

Aortic valve

Right coronary artery

*B*

Left coronary artery

Myocardium

Coronary sinus

Left atrium

Mitral valve

Anterior papillary muscle

*C*

Myocardium

Epicardium

Endocardium

Left ventricle

Tricuspid valve

*D*

Inferior vena cava

Right atrium

Right ventricle

Posterior papillary muscle

Apex

FIGURE 2-3. The heart is sliced into four sections to show the relationship of the heart chambers, the location of the papillary muscles and chordae tendinae, and the changes in thickness of the muscle wall and interventricular and interatrial septa. (A) The base of the heart is sectioned and viewed from below. Note the thinning of the interventricular septum adjacent to the atria. (B) A more inferior section is viewed from below. (C) A section through the middle of the heart is seen from above. (D) A section through the apex of the heart is composed mainly of the left ventricular wall.

## Heart Skeleton

Areas of the heart wall that are strengthened by a fibrous tissue resembling cartilage (chondroid connective tissue) constitute the heart's "skeleton." The most important parts are two rings that completely surround the atrioventricular openings and two short collars that surround the bases of the aorta and pulmonary trunk at the level of the semilunar valves. When the valves are closed, blood exerts a strong pressure against them and if the tissue around the base, or attachment, of the valves were soft and elastic, the valves would splay open under pressure. In other words, the diameter of the atrioventricular opening or the arterial diameter would increase and the valve leaflets would no longer meet in the center. For a valve to function effectively—to close tightly—its base must not expand. The rings and collars of connective tissue provide a rigid base for the leaflets (Fig. 2-4). Another function of the atrioventricular rings is to provide attachment for the bundles of cardiac muscle so that they have something to pull against when they contract. Both ends of a muscle bundle are attached to the ring.

## Impulse-Conducting System

The autonomic nervous system regulates the rate of contraction via the impulse-conducting system of the heart, which contains several forms of modified cardiac muscle cells. The sinoatrial node (SA node) is a group of specialized small cells that receive autonomic fibers from the vagus nerve. This node is located just below the opening of the superior vena cava in the wall of the right atrium, and it is the original site of control, the pacemaker. The impulse is passed on to atrial muscle fibers and they contract, but it is also passed on to specialized conducting atrial fibers, which transmit the impulse more rapidly to the atrioventricular (AV) node in the septal wall of the right atrium, near the opening of the coronary sinus.[3] Here another group of small specialized cells comparable to those of the SA node receives impulses from nerve fibers and from the atrial conducting bundles. Large conducting fibers, Purkinje fibers, emanate from the AV node, forming the bundle of His, or atrioventricular bundle, which courses down the interventricular septum to spread out in the ventricles and

regulate the contraction of ventricular muscle fibers. The SA node is the pacemaker, but in the event of pathology in the atria, the AV node, with its autonomic nerve supply, can take over the regulation of ventricular contraction.[9]

## Shape and Position

Differences in physique and shape of the chest are reflected in variations in the shape and position of the heart. The hearts of adolescents and slender persons lie more vertically, whereas those of elderly and heavier persons lie more horizontally.[7] The general shape of the heart is a cone with the tip (apex) formed by the left ventricle pointing inferiorly and anteriorly at the 5th intercostal space (see Figs. 2-1, 2-3C, D).[8] At the cranial end of the heart and angled to the right and dorsally, the base of the heart is formed by the left atrium, part of the right atrium, the proximal sections of the aorta and venae cavae and the bifurcation of the pulmonary trunk.

The four chambers of the heart are called the right atrium and ventricle and the left atrium and ventricle, but in actuality both ventricles lie on the left and the atria on the right. The relative position of the chambers can be appreciated by studying cross sections (see Figs. 2-3, 2-5).

## Right Atrium

Probably because the superior and inferior venae cavae empty into the right atrium, it lies almost vertically, about 1.25 cm to the right of the sternal edge at the right edge of the heart (Fig. 2-6).[3] The superior vena cava empties into the cranial posterior part; the inferior vena cava empties inferiorly, forming almost its entire lower end. In adults near the orifice of the inferior vena cava a rudimentary form of the fetal eustachian valve may persist. Its function in fetal life is to direct the blood from the inferior vena cava into the foramen ovale. With the closing of the foramen ovale, it has no significant function but persists as a single crescent-shaped fold attached along the left anterior margin of the orifice of the inferior vena cava.[3,4] The coronary sinus draining the veins of the coronary circulation opens into the right atrium between the inferior vena cava and the tricuspid valve. Coro-

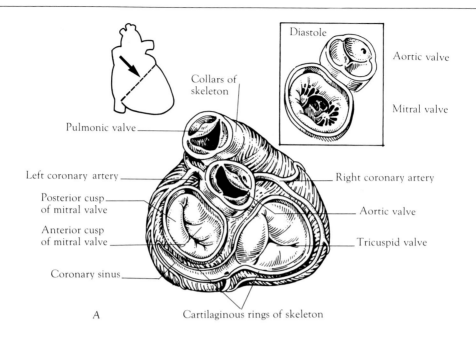

Diastole

Aortic valve

Mitral valve

Collars of skeleton

Pulmonic valve

Left coronary artery

Posterior cusp of mitral valve

Anterior cusp of mitral valve

Coronary sinus

Right coronary artery

Aortic valve

Tricuspid valve

Cartilaginous rings of skeleton

A

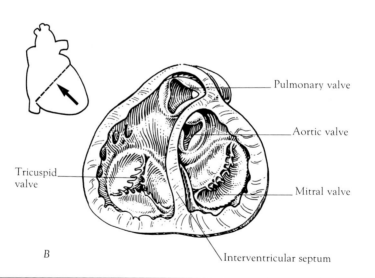

Pulmonary valve

Aortic valve

Tricuspid valve

Mitral valve

Interventricular septum

B

FIGURE 2-4. (A) A superior view of the valves during systole. The aortic and pulmonary valves are open to permit outflow from the ventricles while the atrioventricular valves are closed to prevent back flow from the ventricles to the atria. The inset illustrates closing of the aortic valve and opening of the mitral valve during diastole. Note the thick rings of the heart skeleton surrounding the mitral and tricuspid valves. The areas where the collars surround the aortic and pulmonic valves are indicated. (B) Heart valves during systole viewed from below. This is the orientation usually seen in echocardiographic studies.

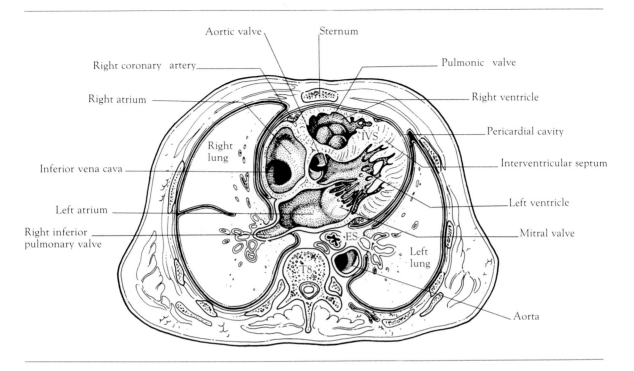

FIGURE 2-5. A cross section through the heart as seen from below (IVS, interventricular septum; MV, mitral valve). The left and right ventricles are located to the left of the midline, whereas the left and right atria are mainly to the right of the vertebra (T8). This section also illustrates the relation of the heart to the lungs, esophagus (Es), aorta (Ao), and sternum.

nary veins called thebesian veins also empty directly into this chamber. Extending from the right atrium is a blind pouch, called the atrial appendage, or auricle. It lies between the superior vena cava and the right ventricle.

The interatrial septum forms the dorsal wall of the right atrium; the left atrium lies posterior to it. In a triangle formed by the venae cavae and the coronary sinus, the closed foramen ovale of the fetal heart can be seen as a depression in the wall, now called the fossa ovalis.[3,6]

The tricuspid, or atrioventricular, valve is located in the inferior anterior section of the right atrium.[1] Three triangular cusps of fibrous tissue project into the (approximately) 4-cm opening between the atrium and ventricle. The anatomic position of each is described in relationship to the right ventricle. The largest cusp (ventral, anterior, or infundibular), located ventrally, is attached to

the ventral wall in the area of the infundibulum; the smallest cusp (dorsal, marginal, or posterior) is attached to the diaphragmatic surface of the ventricle and the medial or septal cusp is connected to the septal wall. At their bases the cusps are continuous with each other; the lines of fusion are the commissures (Fig. 2-4).[5]

## Right Ventricle

The right ventricle constitutes most of the ventral surface of the heart and lies to the left of the right atrium. Between the two is the atrioventricular groove, which runs vertically on the surface and anteroposteriorly on the inferior border. The right coronary artery courses in this groove. Superiorly, the right ventricle tapers, forming an inverted funnel called the conus arteriosus, or infundibulum, which ends as the pulmonary trunk or artery. In-

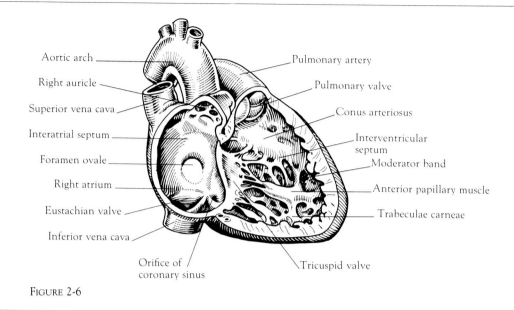

Aortic arch

Right auricle

Superior vena cava

Interatrial septum

Foramen ovale

Right atrium

Eustachian valve

Inferior vena cava

Orifice of
coronary sinus

Pulmonary artery

Pulmonary valve

Conus arteriosus

Interventricular
septum

Moderator band

Anterior papillary muscle

Trabeculae carneae

Tricuspid valve

FIGURE 2-6

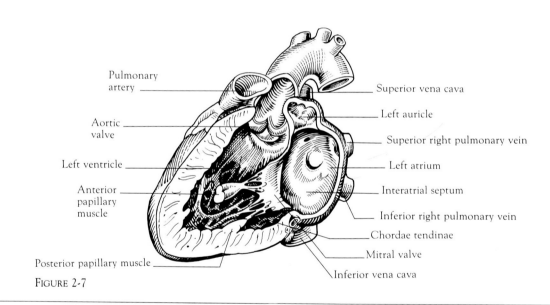

Pulmonary
artery

Aortic
valve

Left ventricle

Anterior
papillary
muscle

Posterior papillary muscle

Superior vena cava

Left auricle

Superior right pulmonary vein

Left atrium

Interatrial septum

Inferior right pulmonary vein

Chordae tendinae

Mitral valve

Inferior vena cava

FIGURE 2-7

FIGURE 2-6. Lateral wall of the heart is removed to show the interior of the right atrium and right ventricle and the interatrial and interventricular septa.

FIGURE 2-7. Wall of the heart is removed to show the interior of the left atrium and left ventricle.

feriorly, the right ventricle forms the right inferior border of the heart, resting on the diaphragm (Fig. 2-6). The interior surface of the right ventricle, except the area of the conus arteriosus, has bands of muscles and ridges (trabeculae carneae) projecting into it.

There are also conical projections of muscle tissue called papillary muscles. In the right ventricle are two main papillary muscles, anterior and posterior. They vary in size and location; the larger and more stable anterior one is located near or on the moderator band. Owing to their location, the papillary muscles of the right ventricle cannot be demonstrated sonographically. The chordae tendinae—strong fibrous cords covered with endothelium—extend from the papillary muscles and attach to the free edges of the tricuspid leaflets, holding them in place so that they cannot open into the atrium during ventricular systole.

One thick band of muscle, the moderator band, traverses the inferior cavity of the right ventricle from the anterior wall to the septal wall, carrying in it fibers of the heart's impulse-conducting system. Because it can be visualized sonographically, it has become a right ventricular landmark (Fig. 2-6).[3,6]

Owing to the greater size of the left ventricle, the interventricular septum projects into the right ventricle, causing the right ventricular cavity to be somewhat crescent shaped.

## Pulmonary Valve and Trunk

At the cranial end of the conus arteriosus lies the pulmonary orifice with the pulmonary valve. This valve lies cranial and to the left of the tricuspid and cranially to the aortic valve. The pulmonary valve has three semilunar cusps (right, left, and anterior). They are cup-shaped, with the convexity extending into the ventricle. The points in the vessel wall where the attachments of the different cusps meet are called commissures (Fig. 2-4). At the center of the free edge of each cusp is a thickening, the nodule. When the valve is closed, the 3 nodules fit closely together to ensure complete closure.

The pulmonary trunk has its origin at the pulmonary valve. Thus it begins superior and posterior to the aortic valve and then runs posteriorly

and to the left of the ascending aorta, until it reaches the bottom of the aortic arch. Here it bifurcates into the right and left pulmonary arteries. The right pulmonary artery runs horizontally posterior to the ascending aorta and superior vena cava while the left pulmonary artery, the shorter and smaller one, courses horizontally in front of the left bronchus and descending aorta. Both end in lobes of the adjacent lungs (Fig. 2-6).[4]

## Left Atrium

After the blood is oxygenated, it is carried from the lungs by two pulmonary veins from each lung (or often three from the left). These empty into the dorsal wall of the left atrium, two on each side, or two on the right and three on the left.

The left atrium is located posterior and slightly superior to the right atrium. Like the right atrium, it has an appendage, called the left auricle. The left atrium is smaller than the right and has thicker walls (~3 mm; see Figs. 2-3, 2-7).[3]

## Mitral or Bicuspid Valve

The left atrioventricular valve, the mitral valve, is composed of two leaflets, a large anterior one and a smaller posterior one. Occasionally, there are small cusps between them. The anterior cusp is adjacent to the aortic opening (Fig. 2-4).

## Left Ventricle

Located posterior to the right ventricle, the left ventricle is longer, more conical, and has much thicker walls (Figs. 2-3, 2-7). It forms the left margin and about half of the diaphragmatic surface of the heart. Because the interventricular septum bulges into the right ventricle, a cross section of the left ventricular cavity appears round. More trabeculae carneae can be found than in the right ventricular cavity, but they are less coarse and are not found in the basal third. Only two papillary muscles are attached to the ventral and dorsal walls. These are large and quite prominent, providing an excellent sonographic landmark of the left ventricle. Chordae tendinae from the papillary muscles attach to both mitral valve cusps.

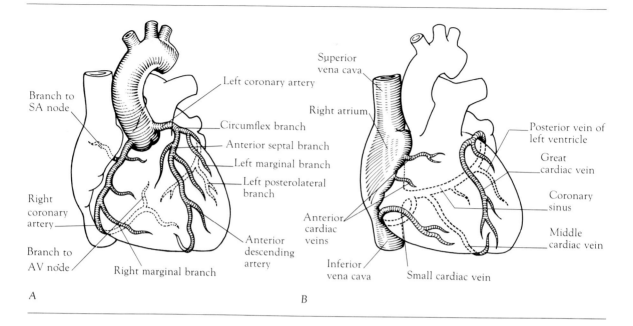

FIGURE 2-8. Coronary circulation. (A) An anterior view of the heart with its arterial circulation. The vessels drawn with dotted lines represent the arteries on the posterior surface of the heart. (B) Anterior view of the venous drainage of the heart. The veins of the posterior wall are drawn in dotted lines.

## Aortic Valve and Aorta

The aortic valve is located to the right and ventral to the mitral valve. It is similar to the pulmonary valve in having three cup-shaped cusps or semilunar cusps—right, left, and posterior (noncoronary) cusps (Fig. 2-4)[8], but its cusps are stronger and thicker. There are three sinuses or dilations of the aortic wall, one immediately above each valve cusp. The left and right coronary arteries originate from the aorta at sinuses caused by dilatation of the aortic wall above the right and left cusps, respectively.

## Interventricular Septum

Most of the interventricular septum is as thick as the wall of the left ventricle, but it thins out in the area where it attaches to the fibrous skeleton and the atrial septum. This area, called the membranous interventricular septum, is devoid of muscle tissue and is often the site of septal defects.

## Coronary Arteries

The blood vessels of the epicardial layer of the heart constitute the larger channels of the coronary circulation, which supply and drain the smaller channels, the microcirculation of the myocardium. The coronary arteries lie within the epicardial layer, surrounded by fatty tissue, and they subdivide into smaller branches penetrating the myocardial layer, eventually providing the capillaries of the myocardium. The capillaries collect into veins, which return to the epicardial layer, and the final major vein is the coronary sinus, which empties directly into the right atrium (Fig. 2-8). The right and left coronary arteries travel within the grooves separating the atria from the ventricles (coronary sulcus) and the ventricles from each other (interventricular sulcus). The right coronary artery arises from the right aortic sinus and travels in the coronary sulcus to reach the posterior surface of the heart. It supplies branches to the atria and ventri-

TABLE 2-1. The blood supply of the heart

| AREA | CIRCULATION |
| --- | --- |
| Right ventricle | |
|   Anterior wall | Marginal branch of RCA and RCA |
|   Left part of anterior wall | Interventricular branch of LCA |
| Left ventricle | LCA |
|   Right part of posterior wall | RCA |
| Interventricular septum | |
|   Anterior two thirds | LCA |
|   Posterior one third | RCA |
| Conducting system | |
|   SA node | RCA |
|   AV node | RCA |
|   AV bundle | RCA |
|   Bundle branches | LCA, except posterior limb of left bundle branch, LCA and RCA |
| Right atrium | RCA |
| Left atrium | LCA |

Adapted from Anderson JE. Grant's Atlas of Anatomy. 8th ed. Baltimore: Williams & Wilkins; 1983.

cles. Eventually it anastomoses with the circumflex branch of the left coronary artery. Its major branches are the marginal, atrioventricular, and nodal arteries and the posterior descending artery which travels down the posterior interventricular sulcus.

The left coronary artery originates from the left posterior aortic sinus. It divides into the circumflex branch, which passes posteriorly in the coronary sulcus to join the right coronary artery and the anterior descending artery, which passes from the coronary sulcus into the anterior interventricular sulcus.

There are variations in the areas supplied by the different branches of the coronary arteries. Knowing which arterial branch supplies each segment of the heart is particularly important when examining the heart for ischemia. In the majority of persons the right and left coronary arteries supply the heart equally; in 15%, the left vessel is dominant.[1] The most common distribution is summarized in Table 2-1.

## Cardiac Veins

Cardiac veins accompany the coronary arteries. Sixty percent of the blood returns to the right atrium via the coronary sinus. Four main veins drain into the coronary sinus: the great, middle, and small cardiac veins and the posterior vein of the left ventricle.[2] The other 40% of venous return drains through veins which open directly into the extent of the right atrium, especially its anterior wall near the antrioventricular groove (Fig. 2-8).

## References

1. Anderson JE. Grant's Atlas of Anatomy. 8th ed. Baltimore: Williams & Wilkins; 1983.
2. Anson BJ (ed). Morris' Human Anatomy. 12th ed. New York: McGraw-Hill; 1966.
3. Goss CM (ed). Gray's Anatomy: Anatomy of the Human Body. 29th ed. Philadelphia; Lea & Febiger; 1973.
4. Gray H. Anatomy: Descriptive and Surgical. 15th ed. New York: Bounty Books; 1977.
5. Hollinshead WH. Textbook of Anatomy. 2d ed. New York: Harper & Row; 1967.
6. Last RJ. Anatomy Regional and Applied. 6th ed. New York: Churchill-Livingstone; 1978.
7. Leonhardt H. Color Atlas and Textbook of Human Anatomy. 2d ed. Stuttgart: Georg Thieme Verlag; 1984; 2.
8. Philo R, Bosner MS, LeMaistre A, et al. Guide to Human Anatomy. Philadelphia: WB Saunders; 1985.
9. Tortora GJ, Anagnastakos NP. Principles of Anatomy and Physiology. 5th ed. New York: Harper & Row; 1987.

# CHAPTER 3

# Normal Cardiac Physiology

EVALIE DUMARS

**K**nowledge of cardiac anatomy and the echocardiographic appearances of pathology are important to producing and recognizing diagnostic images, but the full value of such studies can be derived only by those with a sound understanding of cardiac function and hemodynamics. In this chapter, we explain the double circulation of the heart, the events of the cardiac cycle, and the normal hemodynamic pressures.

The heart is a muscular pump that is responsible for pumping blood to the body. In order for blood to be adequately distributed, blood pressure must be maintained. Both pressure and flow are governed by a complex control mechanism that responds to metabolic requirements of various parts of the body and their functional interrelationships.

The human heart consists of two fluid pumps that are presented side by side anatomically but functionally are connected in series. The right side of the heart supplies the pulmonary (lung) circulation. The normal pressure in the right ventricle is about 22 mm Hg. From the lungs, the blood returns to the left side of the heart, which supplies blood to the body via the systemic circulation. The pressure in the left ventricle is about 120 mm Hg. The volume pumped by the two sides of the heart is the same to ensure the normal circuit of flow. This equality is balanced even when the volume pumped is increased as much as five times by exercise demand. The blood is pumped from the ventricles during systole and the ventricles receive blood during the relaxation phase, diastole.

## Right Heart Circulation

Venous blood returns from the body to the right atrium via the superior and inferior venae cavae. During atrial systole, blood travels through the tricuspid valve into the right ventricle, which is in diastole (Fig. 3-1). The blood returning from the body has a lower oxygen saturation (75%) than that pumped from the left side (95 to 100%).

The tricuspid valve is closed during right ventricular systole, and the blood contained in the right ventricle is propelled out of the right ventricular outflow tract (the conus arteriosus or infundibulum) through the open semilunar pulmonic valve to the pulmonic circulation.

## Left Heart Circulation

The left atrium receives blood from the lungs through four pulmonary veins located in the back of the left atrial cavity. As left atrial systole occurs, the mitral valve (left atrioventricular {AV} valve) is in the open position, allowing the blood in the left atrium to be propelled down into the left ventricular cavity. The left atrium acts as a reservoir

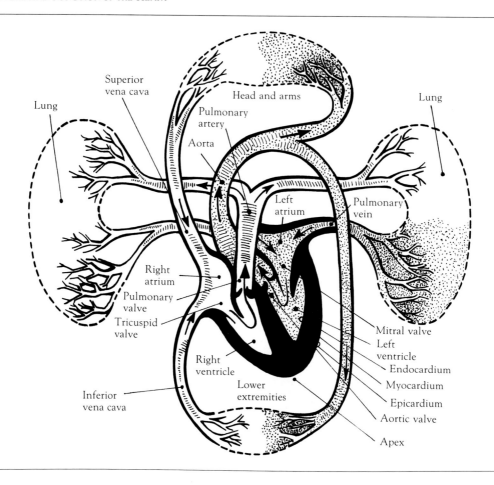

Figure 3-1. Plan of circulation.

during ventricular systole and as a conduit during ventricular diastole. As ventricular systole occurs, the mitral valve is closed and the blood is propelled out of the left ventricular outflow tract through the open semilunar aortic valve to the systemic circulation.

## Blood Supply of the Heart

Two major arteries, the left and right coronary arteries, supply blood to the heart muscle and to the proximal portions of the great vessels. The coronary arteries arise from the base of the aorta, just above the valve leaflets at the sinus of Valsalva (see Chapter 1). The aortic valve cusps are named according to their specific arterial system origin: right coronary cusp, left coronary cusp, and noncoronary cusp.

### Right Coronary Artery

The right coronary artery courses in the coronary sulcus along the diaphragmatic surface of the heart before descending to the apex. Branches arise from this artery that supply the right atrium, the free wall of the right ventricle, and in approximately 70% of hearts, the posterior third of the ventricular septum and posterior wall of the left ventricle.[4,17,24] An ascending coronary artery arises from the right coronary sinus approximately 50% of the time. This short vessel, the conus artery, supplies the outflow tract of the right ventricle at or near the level of the pulmonic valve.[24]

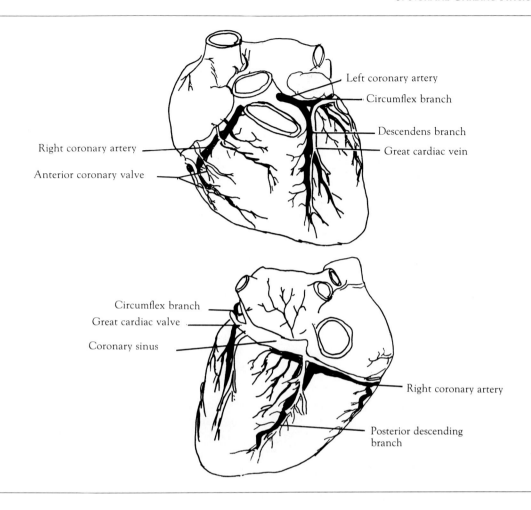

FIGURE 3-2. Coronary arterial and venous blood supply.

### LEFT CORONARY ARTERY

The left coronary artery bifurcates into two major branches at or just beyond its origin. The left circumflex artery arises at right angles to the major vessel and courses through the AV sulcus before turning down to the apex. The left atrium and lateral wall of the left ventricle receive blood from this vessel. Both the right coronary artery and the circumflex artery supply blood to the posterior left ventricular wall (Fig. 3-2).[24]

The left anterior descending artery continues as an extension of the main vessel before coursing downward in the interventricular groove toward the cardiac apex. The left ventricular free wall, ventricular septum, and to a limited extent, the anterior wall of the right ventricle receive their blood supply from this artery.[24,26]

Approximately 50 to 60% of the time, a special branch of the right coronary artery supplies blood to the sinoatrial (SA) node. This artery is also the main source of blood for the atrial myocardium and the atrial septum. The AV node receives its blood supply from a branch of the right coronary artery in about 90% of persons and from the left circumflex artery in the remainder.[24,26] Some variations in vascular patterns exist and are not thought to be significant of coronary insufficiency or as a predictor of the total amount of myocardium sup-

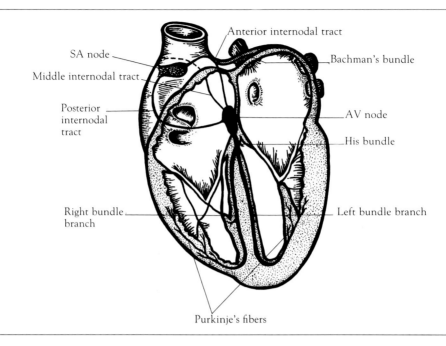

SA node

Middle internodal tract

Posterior internodal tract

Right bundle branch

Anterior internodal tract

Bachman's bundle

AV node

His bundle

Left bundle branch

Purkinje's fibers

Figure 3-3. Intrinsic conduction system of the heart.

plied by the right or the left coronary artery system.[13,17,24,26]

VENOUS DRAINAGE

The coronary sinus, which lies in the posterior part of the AV groove, drains most of the blood from the heart walls into the right atrium to the left of the inferior vena cava. The coronary sinus is a continuation of the great cardiac vein, and the small and middle cardiac veins are tributaries of the coronary sinus. The anterior vein and some small cardiac veins return the remainder of the blood to the right atrium and cardiac chambers via direct openings.[17,26]

## Intrinsic Innervation of the Heart

CONDUCTION SYSTEM OF THE HEART

To ensure that the chambers of the heart act in an orderly way, the heart possesses specialized conductive tissue responsible for the initiation, propagation, and coordination of the heartbeat. This conduction system consists of (1) the SA node, (2) the atrial internodal pathways, (3) the AV node, (4) the common AV bundle (bundle of His), (5) the

right and left bundle branches, and (6) the Purkinje system (Fig. 3-3).

The SA node lies in the sulcus between the superior vena cava and the right atrium. It is referred to as the pacemaker of the heart because it is the source of bursts of electrical nerve impulses that spread through the walls of the heart. Because the SA node is located high in the atria, the first structures to contract in the normal activation sequence are the two atria. Once initiated, the impulse spreads throughout the atrial myocardium to the level of the AV node. The AV node is located in the lower part of the atrial septum just above the attachment of the septal cusp of the tricuspid valve. The electrical impulse coming from the atria slows somewhat at the AV node and a delay occurs.[2,5,17,19]

From the AV node, the impulse is conducted to the ventricles by specialized conducting tissue, the AV bundle (or bundle of His) and its divisions, the right and left bundle branches. These structures ramify and become continuous with the fibers of the Purkinje network. At this time, the ventricles contract and the blood is ejected to the pulmonic and systemic circulations.

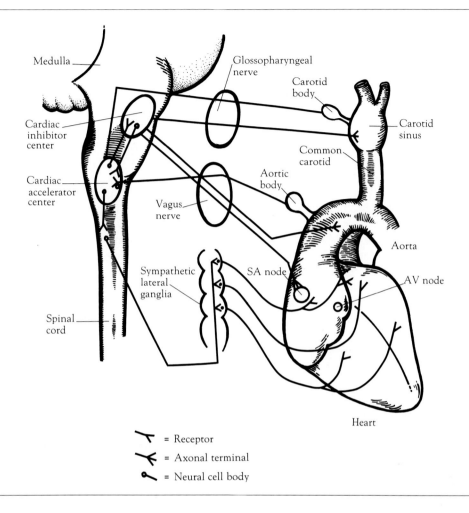

FIGURE 3-4. Extrinsic innervation of the heart.

## Extrinsic Innervation of the Heart

Although the heart possesses its own intrinsic rhythmicity (conduction system), its rate is modified by the autonomic nervous system. Fibers from both the sympathetic and the parasympathetic nervous systems (which are divisions of the autonomic nervous system) are received by the heart (Fig. 3-4).

The *sympathetic nervous system* sends its fibers mainly to the atria via the right and left vagus nerves, thereby contributing to the control of the SA and the AV nodes. These sympathetic fibers are derived from the upper thoracic sympathetic ganglia (and cord segments). They pass superiorly in the sympathetic trunk to the cervical region where they are given off as the cervical sympathetic cardiac nerves, which then pass down through the neck to reach the cardiac plexus around the coils of the great vessels.[8,9,23,27,28,36] From here they are distributed to the atria (SA node) and to the ventricular musculature. Stimulation of the sympathetic nervous system fibers to the heart causes four effects: it increases heart rate, increases transmission between the atria and the ventricles, increases force of contraction, and increases conduction rate of nodes and atria.

The *parasympathetic* nerves are derived from the vagus and are given off in the neck as the vagal cardiac nerves.[9,15,23] They enter the cardiac plexus and there connect to the SA node.

Stimulation of the parasympathetic nervous system fibers to the heart also causes four effects: it decreases heart rate, retards transmission between the atria and ventricles, decreases force of contraction, and decreases conduction rate of nodes and atria.

It is now obvious that the sympathetic and the parasympathetic nervous systems have basically opposite effects on the heart.[23,24] These two systems are reciprocally innervated, so increased activity in one is usually accompanied by decreased activity in the other. The reflex centers for both are in the medulla oblongata (Fig. 3-4).

Figure 3-4 shows the neural connections between the heart and various receptors via the central nervous system (CNS). Located in the medulla, the paired centers that influence heart rate are the cardioaccelerator center (CAC) and the cardioinhibitor center (CIC). The CAC sends efferent (conducting away from the CNS) fibers to the heart by way of the sympathetic nervous system and the CIC sends efferent fibers to the heart via the parasympathetic system. These two centers receive afferent (conducting toward the CNS) fibers from receptors located in one of four places: the carotid sinus, the aortic arch, the aortic bodies, and the carotid bodies. The cardioinhibitor and cardioaccelerator centers are also reciprocally innervated so that when the activity in one increases, the activity in the other decreases.[8,9,15,16,23,27,31]

## Events of the Cardiac Cycle

The cardiac cycle includes all of the electrical and mechanical events that occur during the cycle of one heartbeat. With each cardiac cycle or heartbeat there are two phases of passage of oxygenated and deoxygenated blood through the heart.

Cardiac contraction is preceded by electrical stimulation, which leads in turn to a series of events that are associated with the heart's function as a pump. These electrical and mechanical events are presented schematically in Figure 3-5. Representative pressure pulses from the left atrium, left ventricle, and aorta are shown along with the scalar electrocardiogram (ECG). Heart sounds are presented below the ECG. Note also, the timing of the echocardiographic representation of mitral valve (AV) and aortic valve (SL) patterns.

Our discussion of the cardiac cycle will begin with ventricular systole. The onset of ventricular systole commences with the peak of the R wave of the electrocardiogram and the initial vibration of the first heart sound (lub; see Fig. 3-5).

The first phase of ventricular systole is *isovolumic contraction*, which begins with the start of ventricular contraction and ends with the opening of the semilunar valves (aortic and pulmonic). At the onset of ventricular contraction there is a rapid increase in ventricular pressure, which squeezes the blood inside the ventricle against the closed valves. During this time the circumference of the left ventricle increases, the apex-to-base length decreases, and the left ventricle becomes more spherical.[7,20,26,29] These changes are well-demonstrated in the normal left ventricular echocardiographic comparing the apical and short axis views.[14,25]

The semilunar valves open when the pressure within the respective ventricles exceeds the diastolic pressure of its great artery, i.e., the aortic valve opens when left ventricular pressure exceeds diastolic aortic pressure.[22] Under normal circumstances, this rise in ventricular pressure (to exceed the aortic diastolic pressure) occurs within approximately 0.06 to 0.08 seconds after the onset of contraction.[13,17,19,20,24,32] Ventricular pressure continues to increase, and as it rises above aortic pressure, the aortic valve cusps are forced open and the period of *rapid ejection* begins, lasting until peak ventricular and aortic pressures are achieved. During this time (approximately 0.10 to 0.11 seconds from the onset of ejection), 80 to 85% of stroke volume leaves the heart and the blood quickly reaches its maximal velocity (approximately 150 cm/sec or 1.5 m/sec).[14]

Near the end of the period of rapid cardiac ejection, ventricular pressure peaks and begins to fall with *reduced ejection* occurring when aortic and left ventricular pressure closely approximate one another. The reduced ejection phase continues until the aortic valve closes (after approximately 0.17 sec). The reduced ejection phase represents the period during which runoff of blood from the aorta into the peripheral vessels exceeds the ventricular output. Normally about 50% of the blood contained in the ventricle before contraction is ejected.

Ventricular diastole commences with the closure of the aortic valve. This is indicated by the *incisura*

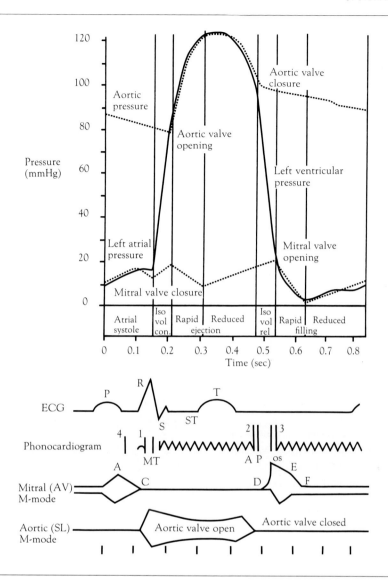

FIGURE 3-5. Events of the cardiac cycle. (Adapted from Netter FH. The CIBA Collection of Medical Illustrations. 1974; Little RC. Physiology of the Heart and Circulation. 1977; Rushmer RF. Cardiovascular Dynamics. 1961.)

(notch) on the aortic pressure tracing (see Fig. 3-5). This notch occurs as a result of the rapid deceleration of the fluid column and closure of the aortic valve producing a sharp oscillation in the aortic pressure.

The second heart sound (dub) is now heard. It represents closure of the aortic and pulmonic valves. At this time blood pours into the two atria from the inferior vena cava and the pulmonary veins.

The first phase of diastole, the *isovolumic relaxation* phase, commences with the closing of the semilunar valves (aortic and pulmonic) and continues until the opening of the atrioventricular valves (mitral and tricuspid). This period is characterized by a precipitous fall in ventricular pressure without a change in ventricular volume. As the ventricular pressure drops below the left atrial pressure, generating an AV pressure gradient, the AV valve cusps are forced open.[13,17,19,24]

The next phase in diastole is the *rapid filling phase* which commences with the opening of the AV valves and with the release of atrial blood into the ventricles, which are now in a relaxed state. The period of rapid filling lasts approximately 0.06 seconds after the opening of the mitral valve, or until the left ventricular pressure reaches its lowest level and begins a rapid upward swing.

The rapid filling phase is followed by the *reduced filling* phase, during which blood returning from the periphery flows into the right ventricle and blood from the lungs flows into the left ventricle.

The final phase of ventricular diastole, *atrial systole,* occurs at the peak of the P wave on an ECG. This transfer of atrial blood to the ventricles by atrial contraction completes ventricular filling. The mitral and tricuspid valves close as a result of reduced blood flow against the atrial surface of these valves and to increased eddy current forces upon the ventricular surface of the valves. This marks the end of atrial systole and of ventricular diastole.[13,17,19,24]

The electrical events in the heart are visible on an ECG. The *P wave* represents atrial depolarization, or contraction. The *QRS complex* represents ventricular contraction. The time between the P wave and the QRS complex, the *PR interval,* represents slowing of the conduction through the AV node. The *T wave* represents repolarization of the ventricles. The isoelectric period between the S and the T wave is the *ST segment,* during which the heart is refractory to electrical stimulation.[5,17,26]

## References

1. Arvidsson H. Angiocardiograph determination of left ventricular volume. Acta Radiol 1961; 56:321.
2. Badeer HS. "Contractility" of the non-failing hypertrophied heart. Am Heart J. 1967; 73:693.
3. Berglund E. Ventricular function. VI. Balance of left and right ventricular output: Relation between left and right atrial pressure. Am J Physiol. 1954; 178:381.
4. Berglund E. The function of the ventricles of the heart. Acta Physiol Scand. 1955; 33(suppl 119):1.
5. Bernreiter M. Electrocardiography. 2d ed. Philadelphia: JB Lippincott; 1963; Chap. 1.
6. Blair HA, Wedd AM. The action of cardiac ejection on venous return. Am J Physiol. 1946; 145:528.
7. Bowe AA. Radiographic evaluation of dynamic geometry of the left ventricle. J Appl Physiol 1971; 31:227.
8. Bronk DW, Ferguson LK, Margaria R, et al. The activity of the cardiac sympathetic centers. Am J Physiol. 1936; 111:237.
9. Bruce TA, Chapman CB, Baker O, et al. The role of autonomic and myocardial factors in cardiac control. J Clin Invest 1963; 42:721.
10. De Geest H, Levy MN, Zieske H, et al. Depression of ventricular contractility by stimulation of the vagus nerves. Circ Res. 1965; 17:222.
11. Gebber G, Snyder DW. Hypothalamic control of the baroreceptor reflexes. Am J Physiol. 1969; 218:124.
12. Guyton AC, Langston JB, Carrier O. Decrease in venous return caused by right atrial pulsation. Circ Res. 1962; 10:188.
13. Guyton AG, Jones CE, Coleman TG. Circulatory Physiology: Cardiac Output and Its Regulation. Philadelphia: WB Saunders; 1973.
14. Hatle L, Angelsel B. Doppler Ultrasound in Cardiology: Physical Principles and Clinical Applications. 2nd ed. Philadelphia: Lea & Febiger; 1985.
15. Higgins CB, Vatner SF, Braunwald E. Parasympathetic control of the heart. Pharmacol Rev. 1973; 25:119.
16. Hockman CH, Taliesnic J, Livingston KE. Central nervous system modulation of baroreceptor reflexes. Am J Physiol. 1969; 217:1681.
17. Hurst JW, Logue RB, Schlant RD, et al. The Heart. New York: McGraw-Hill; 1978.
18. James TN. The connecting pathways between the sinus node and the AV node and between the right and left atrium of the human heart. Am Heart J. 1963; 66:498.
19. Katz AM. Physiology of the Heart. New York: Raven Press; 1977.
20. Katz LN. Relation of initial volume and initial pressure to dynamics of the ventricular contraction. Am J Physiol. 1928; 87:348.
21. Kircheim HR. Systemic arterial baroreceptor reflexes. Physiol Rev. 1976; 56:100.
22. Laniado S, Yellin E, Terdiman R, et al. Hemodynamic correlates of the normal aortic valve echogram: A study of sound, flow and motion. Circulation. 1976; 54:729.
23. Levy MN, Ng M, Martin P, et al. Sympathetic and parasympathetic interactions upon the left ventricle of the dog. Circ Res. 1966; 19:5.
24. Little RC. Physiology of the Heart and Circulation. Chicago: Year Book Medical Publishers; 1977; 32–41.

25. Nanda NC, Gramiak R. Clinical Echocardiography. St Louis: CV Mosby; 1978.

26. Netter FH. The CIBA Collection of Medical Illustrations. Rochester, NY: Case-Hoyt Corporation; 1974; 5.

27. Randall WC, McNally H. Augmentor action of the sympathetic cardiac nerves in man. J Appl Physiol. 1960; 15:629.

28. Robinson BF, Epstein SE, Beiser GD, et al. Control of heart rate by the autonomic nervous system: Studies in man on the interrelationship between baroreceptor mechanisms and exercise. Circ Res 1966; 19:400.

29. Rushmer RF. Length-circumference relations of the left ventricle. Circ Res. 1955; 3:639.

30. Rushmer RF. Pressure-circumference relations of the left ventricle. Am J Physiol. 1956; 186:115.

31. Rushmer RF. Autonomic balance in cardiac control. Am J Physiol. 1958; 192:631.

32. Rushmer RF. Cardiovascular Dynamics. Philadelphia: WB Saunders; 1961; 75–96.

33. Sonnenblick EH, Ross J Jr, Covell JW, et al. The ultrastructure of the heart in systole and diastole: Changes in sarcomere length. Circ Res. 1967; 21:423.

34. Spencer MP, Greiss FC. Dynamics of ventricular ejection. Circ Res. 1962; 10:274.

35. Titus JL. Normal anatomy of the human cardiac conduction system. Mayo Clin Proc. 1973; 48:24.

36. Zimmerman BG. Separation of responses of arteries and veins to sympathetic stimulation. Circ Res. 1966; 18:429.

# PART TWO

# Principles and Practical Applications of Echocardiography

# CHAPTER 4

# Echocardiography Instruments and Principles

GERSON S. LICHTENBERG

## The Interactive Approach

All sonographic examinations represent an interaction among a patient, an ultrasound source, a processing and display system, and a brain. As a pianist must know the effect of each piano key, singly and in combination, the sonographer must understand the tools and technique of diagnostic sonography to produce the equivalent of an ultrasonic symphony. Application of ultrasound to the heart (echocardiography) may utilize six display modes, each with specific requirements, limits, and benefits. When the roles and needs of each part of the interaction are well-understood, the applications of echocardiography can be approached logically and the technical expertise and reasoning process can develop.

Subtle transducer (sound source) manipulation in the small spaces between the ribs and lungs that allow access to the heart is a key to success. It can be practiced best by sorting out the motions: moving the transducer to a different spot, rotating the transducer, and angulating the transducer. Each small motion may have a major impact on the information obtained. Combinations of these motions provide infinite opportunities for obtaining useful information or creating total confusion for the echocardiographer (cardiac sonographer) and the reviewing physicians. In order to make the ultrasound source perform well, it must be handled in a logical, methodical, slow, search pattern, as

one would use a flashlight to search a dark room thoroughly. Sonographers must recognize patterns of structure and motion, so they must allow enough time to recognize the motion before moving on.

Echocardiographic information is relative data. It is dependent on transducer placement, control settings, and recording of relevant information. To do this properly, it is essential to understand what happens to ultrasound as it passes into and through the patient. Otherwise, sonographers will be unable to control the examination technique sufficiently to provide interpretable, unambiguous recordings.

Once proper data is located, the examiner must assemble his or her impression into a meaningful sequence and store it in an appropriate format to convince those who review the recordings of that impression. The brain plays the decision-making role: What data is valid? What other determinations are needed to make sense out of what is found (i.e., What other questions will be asked)? What other explanations or suggestions for further investigation can be proposed?

With six available modes of presentation, many decisions must be made along the way. An echocardiogram must be efficient, intelligently designed, and built on understanding rather than just repetition. To integrate all of the available clinical knowledge, technique, and equipment manipula-

43

tion the echocardiographer must have a strong understanding of the physical principles and instrumentation used in echocardiography.

## Transducers, The Source

A transducer is anything that transforms one form of energy into another form. This is accomplished in ultrasound with a piezoelectric crystal, which responds to any change in voltage by changing shape. The resulting changes in pressure when applied to surrounding material causes a pressure wave or vibration. A piezoelectric transducer also functions as a receiver by responding to incoming sounds or pressure waves with a change in electrical potential across opposite crystal faces.[40]

The natural operating frequency of a transducer depends on its thickness. Thinner wafers vibrate at higher frequencies but are more difficult to produce because of the delicacy of thin crystals. Although a higher frequency offers better image quality, its ability to penetrate tissue is decreased. Frequencies above 2.0 to 3.0 MHz possess suboptimal characteristics for quantitative Doppler echocardiography. In most adults, good image quality is obtainable at 3.5 MHz, whereas pediatric studies require 5.0 MHz. Actual operating frequencies and usefulness vary greatly.[7,40]

### Two-Dimensional Transducers

Two-dimensional (2-D) echocardiography units automatically angle an ultrasound beam along one plane at rates of 10 to 30 times per second. The information obtained in such a sweep can be compiled into a planar or cross-sectional image with up to an 80- or 90-degree arc, representing the relative positions of structures during that period. The two basic methods for steering the ultrasound beam in different directions are (1) automatically moving a single large (13- to 19-mm diameter) crystal in different directions and (2) electronically sequencing voltage pulses to an array of 32 to 128 small crystals, 13- to 19-mm in length (phased array). Comparison of these approaches and the options for applying them needs to be done on an individual basis by examining the type of patient, expense, sonographer experience and comfort, resolution, frequency requirements, focusing, space, mobility, Doppler and upgradability needs, and service sup-

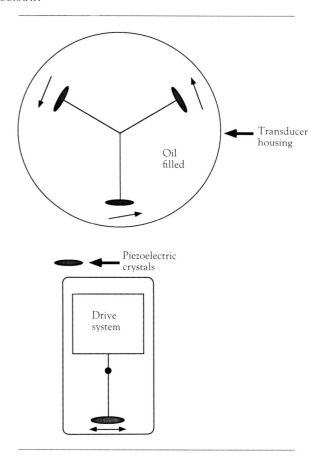

FIGURE 4-1. Mechanically steered transducers. *(Top)* In a three-crystal rotating system only the crystal facing the patient is active. When it moves away from the patient, the next crystal is activated. *(Bottom)* This single-crystal "wobbler" is driven by a motor or an electromagnet system. It slows slightly at the end of each movement, creating lines of information slightly closer at the sides of the image than those in the center.

port of the facility. It is interesting that more than a decade after 2-D echocardiography became clinically available, both mechanical and electronic (phased-array) steering equipment are still in production.

*Mechanically Steered Transducers.* These consist of one to three crystals within a housing filled with sonolucent oil. A single crystal can be "wobbled" back and forth by either a motor or an electromagnet system (Fig. 4-1, bottom). Early motors were

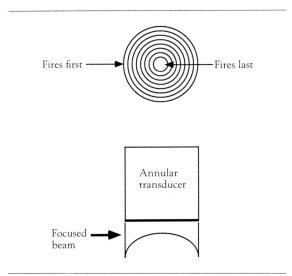

FIGURE 4-2. Annular focusing of mechanical transducers. *(Top)* An annular transducer crystal consists of a series of concentric rings that are fired in rapid sequence, causing the effective beam to be concentrated in the center. The location of the main focus can be altered by changing the firing sequence. *(Bottom)* Curved, focused wavefronts result from the phasing of the annular transducer. The beam is then focused in all directions.

bulky, but current models are much smaller and lighter. Another design uses three crystals mounted around an axle at 120-degree intervals (Fig. 4-1, top). As the axle spins, the machine activates the crystal that faces the patient.

The ultrasound beam can be focused three ways: through a concave acoustic lens on the crystal; through curved crystals; and through an annular array. The acoustic lens, or curved crystal, provides a fixed focus over a small range. The annular array consists of a round crystal cut into concentric rings (Fig. 4-2).[20] By firing the outer rings first, a converging beam is created with the focal range electronically controlled. Because the crystals are round, focusing occurs in all directions perpendicular to the beam's axis. In this instance, the electronics control only the focus, not the steering. It must still be steered mechanically. Dynamic (rapidly changing) focusing can be done to increase the effective length of the focal zone.

*Phased-Array Transducers.* Early attempts to image the heart with large linear-array transducers met with limited success. The large transducer face had to overlie ribs and lungs, giving little access to the heart. Smaller-faced transducers have since been developed that fit the available space better (Fig. 4-3A).[37] They consist of a line of narrow rectangular crystals. If all of the crystals are fired at once, the sum of the spherical waves from the many small sources forms a large, flat wavefront travelling perpendicular to the face of the transducer. If we stagger or slightly delay the firing of adjacent crystals, a large flat wavefront occurs, but it is no longer perpendicular to the face (Fig. 4-3B). Altering the time delay between crystals changes the angle of beam travel. Thus beam direction can be changed while further alterations can focus the beam in one plane, as in the annular-array design.

The returning signal also provides directional information, because it will activate the nearer crystals before the farther crystals. This factor allows directional focusing in the receiver and offers the opportunity to process multidirectional echoes if the unit has multiple or parallel processors.[30]

Thus, with no moving transducer parts, the beam can be steered by manufacturer-determined programs. Electronic focusing occurs only in one plane; that is, the thickness of the cross-sectional slice is not decreased by focusing a linear phased-array transducer. As a result, only the side-to-side definition within the plane is improved.

## MOTION-MODE (M-MODE) TRANSDUCERS

Echocardiographs that perform only M-mode examinations are no longer marketed. Since M-mode looks along only one line through the heart at a time, the transducer initially consisted of one round crystal in a cylindrical housing that was long enough to be grasped comfortably. Operating frequencies varied from 2.0 to 3.5 MHz for adults and 5.0 to 7.5 MHz for neonates.

Focusing was achieved with either a concave acoustic lens adherent to the flat crystal or a curved piezoelectric crystal. Some work was done with annular-array transducers, but they failed to receive clinical acceptance.[6]

M-mode examinations are currently performed by using mechanical transducers frozen at one interrogation angle or phased-array transducers in

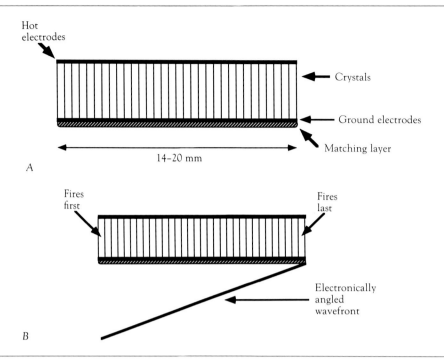

Figure 4-3. Linear phased-array transducers. (A) Between 32 and 128 small, adjacent, rectangular crystals are activated by a separate electronic connection. A single, small crystal with a very short near field produces a spherical rather than a flat wavefront. The sum of many such neighboring waves results in a large, flat wavefront. (B) The direction of the large wavefront is determined by the timing of crystal activation. Changing the timing of this sequence varies the angle up to 45 degrees. Reversing the sequence, so that the right-side crystal fires first, permits another 45 degrees of angulation capability, for a total arc of 90 degrees. Sensing the order of crystal activation by the returning signal allows the machine to reject incoming signals from inappropriate directions.

which the center crystals are selected to operate in M-mode. Currently available machines no longer have ports for M-mode–only transducers.

### DOPPLER TRANSDUCERS

Continuous-mode Doppler (often called continuous-wave or CW) requires two crystals, one operating constantly as transmitter, the other constantly as receiver. Usually, one round crystal is split in half for this purpose (Fig. 4-4).[17] Continuous-mode Doppler transducers further differ from imaging transducers because the housing behind the crystal is hollow, allowing the crystal to ring freely. The handle of the transducer arises at an angle from the crystal head to allow easy access to

the suprasternal notch or the cardiac apex with the patient lying on the left side.[12]

Phased-array transducers may be used for continuous-mode operation; crystals in the 2.0-MHz range give the best Doppler signals. A phased-array housing with both 2.0-MHz crystals and higher-frequency imaging crystals has also been marketed in an attempt to optimize both CW and high-resolution two-dimensional functions in one transducer.

Pulsed-mode operation can be performed with any single or multiple crystal probe that is stationary. Higher frequencies, however, tend to severely limit velocity measurement capability and signal sensitivity. When the pulsed method is achieved with the split-crystal continuous-wave probe, both

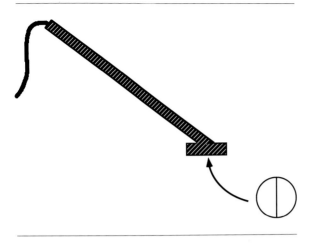

FIGURE 4-4. Doppler transducer with a split crystal. In continuous-mode Doppler, one semicircular crystal is always sending while the other is always receiving. Because they are meant to ring continuously rather than giving short pulses, there is no backing material on the crystals. If a transducer rattles when shaken, one of the crystals is floating free within the housing. In the pulsed mode, the crystals are fired simultaneously, as if they were one crystal. The transducer is often equipped with a movable crossbar, to aid in steady manipulation of the beam. The angled handle optimizes maneuverability when placed in the suprasternal notch or apex of a patient turned on the left side.

halves are fired for transmission and then act as receivers.

Color flow doppler is most often performed through phased-array transducers, but it has also been accomplished via an annular-array transducer. Precise advantages and disadvantages are not yet well enough established through clinical application to formulate any definite rules. Again, 2.0-MHz frequencies usually provide the most sensitive, unambiguous color data; however, the quality of the 2-D images is often suboptimal.

### Transesophageal Transducers

Commercially available transducers for examining the heart through the esophagus operate on the phased-array principle. One company is trying to market a mechanical design.[28] The phased array is mounted on a flexible gastroscope long enough to be advanced down the esophagus. It travels behind the left atrium and is positioned behind the posterior wall of the left ventricle. The entire apparatus can be rotated or moved up or down to find an echocardiographic window. Lateral or anteroposterior angulation can be achieved through manipulation of two control knobs or rings at the operator's end. These controls can often be locked in position to obtain continuous monitoring of a particular area.

The optimal frequency of these transducers is usually 5.0 MHz, since greater resolution is more desirable and less penetration is needed. The cost of such probes is usually 5 to 6 times the cost of a standard 2-D probe. Such probes are capable of operating in all modes except continuous-mode Doppler. In the United States their most common use is in intraoperative examinations, but European and Eastern investigators also describe them as being useful in conscious patients. Some U.S. centers are now compiling data on transesophageal echocardiography in conscious patients.[29]

### Experimental Transducers

Other designs are currently being developed with the objective of providing multiple simultaneous cross sections of the heart. They may take time to develop, but prototypes such as Duke University's O-mode transducer show promise.[33] These not only enhance the possibilities of three-dimensional demonstration of cardiac anatomy but may provide interesting dimensions in Doppler flow demonstration. Modifications of the O-mode design are already under way.

## Tissue Interactions

After the piezoelectric crystal produces an ultrasonic signal, the signal passes through a coupling gel and into the human body. Many interactions occur between the ultrasonic waves and the tissues, but this discussion will be limited to those likely to have an impact on cardiac diagnosis. Ultrasound users must always remember that these interactions are complex and not all are completely understood. We must refrain from calling every signal we don't understand or can't identify, an artifact. Artifacts are signals that are displayed in such a way that they inaccurately represent the anatomy or flow characteristics of the subject.

While all sound with a frequency above 20,000

Hz (cycles per second) is considered ultrasound, only that in the 2.0- to 12.0-MHz range is used for cardiac investigation. In the high-frequency range, sound travelling through human soft tissue is found to have a fairly constant range of velocity and energy loss.[10] The influence of mechanical waves as they travel through the body is better appreciated and understood by reviewing a model of the basic interactions (transmission, reflection, and absorption; Fig. 4-5).

*Transmission* is the movement of the energy through a material. Since the source of the vibration is large compared to the particles of the tissue, the energy is transmitted into the body as a column as wide as the transducer face. For most applications, short bursts or pulses of ultrasound are produced. Each particle in a stable material is held in place by the balancing forces of surrounding particles but is able to vibrate around its resting position if sufficient pressure is applied. When the transducer's vibrations pass into the body, each tissue particle pushes against the particle in front of it. Energy travels quickly, in fact faster than the motion of any one particle, because as soon as one starts to move, it exerts influence on the balancing, or restoring, forces of its neighbors, thus pushing without actually reaching the next particle. A good demonstration of the speed of energy travel can be seen in the common desk toy made of several steel balls suspended on strings (Fig. 4-6). An end ball pulled away and allowed to swing back hits the next one. The ball at the opposite end appears to move immediately. While you can see the ball swing through the air, the time it takes for the energy to travel through the rigid balls is not discernible. This demonstrates that speed of energy transmission is much greater than the velocity of particle motion.

The velocity of high-frequency sound in human soft tissues falls into the range of 1500 to 1600 m per second, and an average of 1540 m per second is used to calibrate echocardiographic imaging systems. This represents the speed of the main or longitudinal ultrasound wave travelling out from the face of the transducer housing.

Now look at what happens to our model when the wave reaches a second material with different acoustic properties (usually representing a difference in density and transmission velocity). The

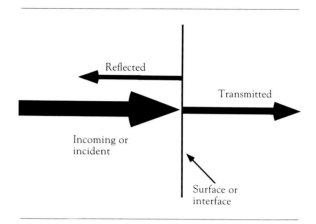

FIGURE 4-5. Transmission and reflection characteristics. The incoming sound beam approaches an interface between two tissues with different acoustic properties. The particles in the material on the far side of the interface do not line up in the same way as they do in the first material, causing some disruption in the forward progress of the beam. The amount of *acoustic impedance mismatch* (the difference between the materials) determines the percentage of sound reflected from an interface of a particular size.

mismatch of particle alignment and velocity in adjacent material forms a partial boundary that some of the energy will not cross. In effect, this boundary vibrates. The major portion of the wave continues in its original direction if the boundary or interface does not have an extreme mismatch, while a small portion of the wave bounds away from the new material, becoming reflected energy. It is the *difference* between the density of the *two* materials, the *acoustic impedance mismatch,* and not simply the density of one material, that affects the percentage of energy reflected.

The fraction of the beam that encounters the interface determines the amount of energy *reflected.* Specular interfaces are large and smooth with respect to the wavelength of the sound beam (Fig. 4-7). Surfaces such as the anterior mitral leaflet-to-blood interface or the pericardium-to-lung interface are good examples. They are wider than the ultrasound beam and are usually smooth. They reflect a great deal of the sound, just as a solid wall inevitably reflects a tennis ball thrown at it. The reader should remember that the transducer crystal acts as both sender and receiver of the reflected sig-

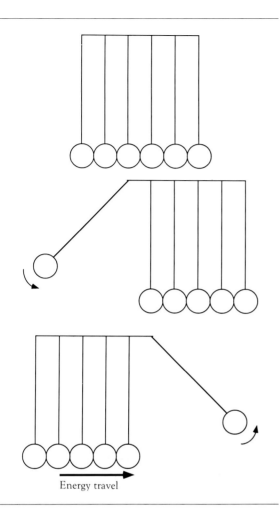

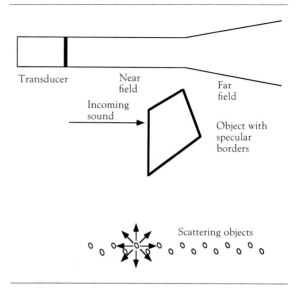

FIGURE 4-7. Specular and scattering reflection. There are many different types of surfaces within the human body. For simplification, we can look at the extreme examples of large flat surfaces (specular) and very small structures (scatterers). The specular interfaces reflect a large percentage of the sound beam at an angle equal to its approach angle. Scatterers reflect a smaller percentage of the sound beam and send it out over a wide range of angles. Reception at the transducer of strong echoes from specular reflectors is very dependent on the angle between the transducer and the interface; reception of the weak echoes from the scatterers does not depend on the approach angle.

FIGURE 4-6. Propagation velocity. The speed of sound or mechanical energy traveling through a row of balls (representing the particles that make up an acoustic medium) is much faster than the speed of the ball. When the ball swings down and hits its neighbor, the ball at the other end takes off. Sound travels rapidly through soft tissue (approximately 1540 m per second) without producing any net motion in the tissue. The individual tissue particles transmit the energy by jiggling around their resting location, just as the balls in the middle of the model shown above did not actually move.

nal, similar to a lone ball player. If the ball strikes the wall at an angle, it bounces away from the player. Reception of the strong signals returning from a specular interface is very dependent on the beam striking the interface at a 90-degree angle.

There are a few degrees of leeway in angulation, but beyond this, angulation causes echo strength to drop off dramatically.

Scattering reflectors are structures smaller than the ultrasound beam's wavelength. Myocardial fibers usually act as scatterers, as do the internal surfaces of a thrombus or of an atrial myxoma. Essentially, the entire reflector vibrates and acts as a source of energy. This could be demonstrated by attaching a string to a submerged rock, bringing the other end above the surface and holding it taut (Fig. 4-8A). Plucking the string to set it in motion would cause surface waves to spread in all directions. So scatterers reflect sound in a spherical pattern (Fig. 4-8B). The reflector receives less energy than a specular interface because it intercepts only a small fraction of the beam, and it spreads that small amount in all directions. The intensity of the signal returning to the transducer is extremely low, but it does not depend on careful angulation.

Some structures, like the endocardial surface, are large but not very smooth and may exhibit some of the features of specular and scattering reflectors. The endocardium usually returns a low-amplitude signal but this is fairly dependent on proper angulation.

Additionally, in most patients all of these interfaces are moving continually. Most ultrasound units must receive a signal over more than one pulse or sampling cycle to establish and display it. The angle between the wave front and the reflector is likely to change as a structure such as the mitral valve moves. Reflection strength and the amount reflected toward the sensor often changes dramatically, creating a great challenge for the display and interpretation of ultrasound reflections from the heart.

In 1968, the ability to introduce artificial (not artifactual) reflectors into the heart was described.[13,14] *Contrast agents* were introduced and they are of increasing interest and use in today's practice. The reflectors consist of microscopic gas bubbles approximately 10 to 200 $\mu$m in diameter before they are injected. Because of the great acoustic impedance mismatch between a gas and the surrounding blood, nearly all of the intercepted ultrasound is reflected. Since the bubbles are small, they interfere with a small portion of the beam and usually not with overall transmission of energy through the heart. The reflections are strong enough to be displayed as relatively high-intensity signals on most systems. Specially prepared 3- to 10-$\mu$m bubbles approximate the size of red blood cells and can enter small blood vessels to demonstrate blood flow to the myocardium (Fig. 4-9). Much larger bubbles are trapped in the larger vessels and are detected only in larger blood pool areas such as the cardiac chambers.

As sound passes through any material some of its energy is *absorbed*,[11] because energy is required to overcome the inertia of the nonmoving particles and the resistance of the forces holding the particles in their original positions. The absorbed energy, which appears as heat, has been demonstrated and measured in vitro.

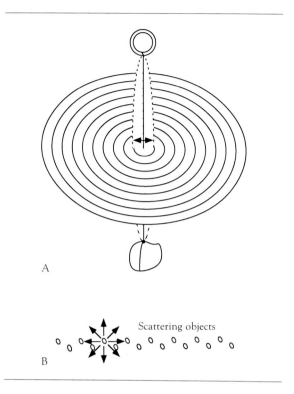

FIGURE 4-8. Scattering phenomenon. (A) The vibrating string would cause circular ripples in the surface of the water, similar to the reflections from a small scatterer. (B) In three dimensions, the vibrations would cause spherical waves, radiating out in all directions from the reflector.

When a large portion of the energy in the sound beam is absorbed or reflected, less is available for transmission to more distant interfaces along the line of travel. This sometimes creates a shadowing effect so that the more distant signals are extremely weak or undetectable. This is evident in hearts that contain large amounts of calcification, such as elderly patients with calcification of the mitral annulus or aortic valve. It is also seen in patients with prosthetic valves or Swan-Ganz catheters, and after injection of some of the newer, highly concentrated contrast microbubbles. The quantity of absorption varies among patients and even from one area to another in a single patient, so equipment settings require continuous adjustment to achieve meaningful results.

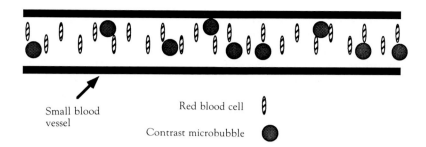

FIGURE 4-9. Artificial reflectors. With a quickly vibrating device called a sonicator, gas in liquids, such as iodinated radiographic dyes, 5% human albumin, and others, can be broken up into very small bubbles similar in size to red blood cells. The strong reflections from these bubbles can be used to examine blood flow patterns within the capillary bed of the myocardium.

## Signal Reception

Echoes that return to the transducer contain a tremendous amount of information, in some ways more than we know what to do with. The application that is most familiar, that is the creation of anatomic images of the heart, uses one portion of the available data. The equipment is calibrated to measure echo return time and calculate distance from the transducer face to the anatomic structure producing the echo (Fig. 4-10). This distance is calculated using the following formula:

$$\text{distance to reflector} = \frac{\text{round trip time(sec)} \times \text{velocity(cm/sec)}}{2}$$

The velocity of sound in the soft tissues of the body falls into a fairly small range, generally 1480 to 1640 m per second at normal body temperature. Therefore an average velocity of 1540 m per second is used in most imaging systems in this formula.[19] The ability of current electronics to accurately measure very short intervals has allowed the creation of the M-mode technique, which introduced echocardiography to the world of clinical cardiology. M-mode has been shown to be very accurate in distance measurements within the heart and is sensitive enough that it can record the rapid position changes of intracardiac structures. Newer beam-steering capability allows display of large cross sections of the anatomy. Derivation of dis-

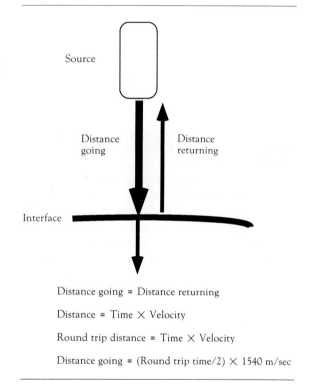

Distance going = Distance returning

Distance = Time × Velocity

Round trip distance = Time × Velocity

Distance going = (Round trip time/2) × 1540 m/sec

FIGURE 4-10. Reflector location. An echocardiography machine measures the time each echo takes to return, calculates distance travelled, and divides it in half to find the distance between the transducer and reflector. This information is combined with the position and angle of the transducer to locate the reflector.

tance data from the time to echo return is the portion of the returning signal that has been used for the longest time and is best understood and accepted by the medical community.

Another type of information is the frequency of the returning signal. Johann Christian Doppler theorized in the mid-nineteenth century that a regularly repeating waveform (i.e., a constant frequency) would be perceived as a different frequency if its source were moving relative to the observer or receiver.[39] Therefore, the detected frequency tells us a great deal about the motion of reflectors, such as groups of red blood cells. Acceptance of information derived from this aspect of the signal has caused an explosion of interest in the application of echocardiography to patients with valve disease, congenital disorders, and coronary artery disease during the mid-1980s.[16]

Strength or power of the returning ultrasonic impulse is widely used, although the exact meaning of this data is somewhat debatable. By interpreting strength relative to that of other signals in the same image or same patient, some useful conclusions can often be reached. More attention will be given to this issue in the discussion of signal amplification. Generally speaking, returned power is an indicator of the reflector's acoustic impedance mismatch and its size.

Much data arrive at the transducer crystal that are not used by current clinical ultrasound units. Information about selective frequency absorption is contained in a received signal. The phase of the echo and a great deal of angle information are ignored by our systems. Phased-array systems have the potential to detect and use a great deal of angle information, but very few have been equipped to do more than basic focusing of the return signals. Attempts to use more information, such as the previously mentioned O-mode prototype, are confounded by the problem of displaying and recording more information. The operator has trouble interpreting the deluge of data, as at a noisy party, when a person must filter out the voice of one person rather than listening to 50 people at once. The rest of the conversations are ignored, as are many incoming ultrasound signals.

The portions of the returning echoes that are accepted create extremely weak electronic signals and need to be amplified. In addition, reflections from

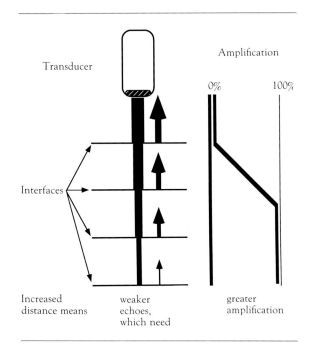

FIGURE 4-11. Signal amplification. Echoes from more distant reflectors are weaker than those from identical closer reflectors. In order to display the reflections on the left in a uniform way, those originating from distant interfaces require the greatest amplification (maximum 100%). The time gain compensation function accomplishes this goal.

an interface that is farther from the transducer than an identical interface will be weaker. Since the amount of energy reaching the second surface is already weaker and reflectance is a percentage of the incoming sound beam, the reflected signal will be proportionately weaker. More of the deeper reflector's return pulse will also have been absorbed, since it has passed through more material. The objective of a sonographic imaging system is to display an image of reflective characteristics of the body's interfaces, no matter where these interfaces are located in the body. It must, therefore, compensate for differences due to location or distance from the transducer (Fig. 4-11). Imagers provide controls that allow the operator to increase the strength of such weak echoes (overall gain or output) and to selectively compensate for the later-returning echoes (*Time Gain Compensation* {TGC} or depth compensation).

Knob
controls

TGC
display

Slide
potentiometers

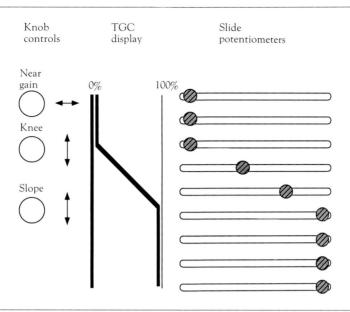

FIGURE 4-12. TGC control panel. The shape of the TGC curve, which represents the timing or depth of amplification changes, can be modified by a series of controls. The controls on the left of the diagram may be knobs on some units or computer software controls on others. Near Gain controls the percentage of amplification of the flat portion of the curve (at the top). The Knee controls the distance at which the angled or increasing portion of the curve begins without changing its angle. The Slope control changes the steepness of the angled portion of the curve. Different manufacturers use different terms to describe these controls. Controls on the right of the diagram are levers that slide left and right within grooves on the control panel. Each one controls a particular point on the TGC curve. As the top control is moved toward the right, amplification of structures at the top of the picture would increase toward 100%. An infinite variety of TGC curves can be created, many of which would introduce ambiguities or obscure valid information.

The time gain compensation provides increased amplification for echoes that originate from more distant structures.[8] This is often displayed as a curve which represents the level at which the amplifier is operating at each distance from the transducer. It shows low power near the crystal (usually the top of the screen), gradually increasing gain as depth increases (moving down on the screen), and then peak amplification in the more distant field, usually beginning about 8 to 12 cm from the body surface. The exact labelling and configuration of these controls varies from manufacturer to manufacturer, but they should be present in some form on all imaging instruments. It is important to understand how they operate—in general and specifically on each machine. Proper application of this knowledge prevents incorrect display of the patient's anatomy, either by overlooking or obscuring what is present. Some machines use knobs to control portions of the TGC curve, some use slide potentiometers to control specific depths in the image, and still others use software controls (Fig. 4-12). This is one of the most important functions to examine closely when inspecting a new unit. No matter how well a sonographer understands the theory of the TGC, he or she will still need to work with the controls to appreciate their effects.

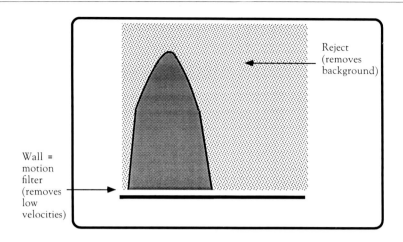

FIGURE 4-13. Filters. Reject, or amplitude filtering, removes weak signals such as background noise, helping to clarify the borders of a real signal. If the control is turned too high or if real signals are weak, real reflections can also be removed. Wall-motion (low-frequency or high-pass) filters remove signals from slow-moving reflectors. Compared to the flow velocity of red blood cells, the cardiac walls and valves are slow moving, but they return relatively powerful reflections, which can obscure important but weak signals from the blood cells. Proper use of this control is critical to good quality Doppler examinations.

## FILTERS

Returning signals quickly become contaminated by electronic noise within the ultrasound unit itself. Therefore, both real and contaminating "noise" needs to be removed from the signal before it is presented in its final display. Signal features that are often filtered are amplitude (using a reject control), direction (by a manufacturer-programmed receive focus), and frequency (via an operator-controlled wall motion or high-pass filter).

*Amplitude Filtering.* Reject filtering is a way of removing the weak electronic noise from the display (Fig. 4-13). When the reject level is set, all signals with powers below that level are removed from the image. Background "snow" that appears to be random can be eliminated this way, making real signals look sharper and easier to see. It is important to note that increasing amplifier gain tends to increase the strength of both the real and the noisy signals, negating the effect of the reject filter.

*Direction Filtering.* Phased- and annular-array systems are capable of removing signals that do not

arrive from the desired angles. A flat wavefront approaching the crystals from other than a 90-degree angle reaches the nearer crystals slightly before it reaches the more distant crystals. The timing of the arrival is characteristic of the incident angle. The delay line of the processor can be programmed to accept only signals that come from the expected direction. With parallel processing technology applied to phased array, multiple delay lines can be used to accept signals from more than one angle at a time, so more of the available information is used instead of being discarded.[30]

*Frequency Filtering.* Doppler ultrasound is used to study blood flow velocity. When the heart is diseased blood flow velocity tends to be high, but relatively slow-moving heart walls, which are much stronger ultrasound reflectors than red blood cells, are also encountered by the beam. It is the high-velocity signals that provide most of the clinically useful data, and this is much easier to display well if the stronger signals are removed. This is done by filtering out the low velocities which give low Doppler frequency shifts by using a high-pass

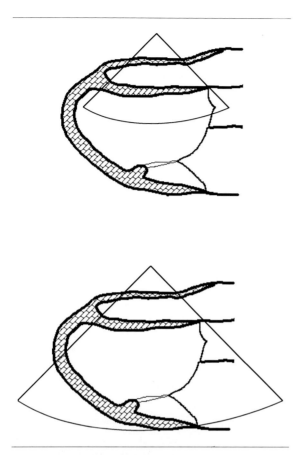

FIGURE 4-14. Depth control. (*Top*) Low depth settings will display only the portions of the heart seen within the sector arc shown above. This is all that would be seen with an 8- to 9-cm setting in most hearts, making it difficult to orient oneself to the displayed anatomy. (*Bottom*) A more appropriate depth setting (usually at least 15 cm) would include the recognizable motion of the mitral valve, shortening the search time. Greater depth settings would increase the odds of including the mitral valve in images of pathologically dilated hearts.

(often called wall motion) filter (see Fig. 4-13). There are usually at least three operator-selected settings for these filters. While the reject filter removes low power signals, the wall motion filter removes low frequency signals.

The display of any echocardiographic information concerning anatomic images or Doppler flow information is subject to a great deal of electronic manipulation. Another important operator control is that for the *scale* or *magnification* of the display. There is a tendency for students of the tech-

niques to want to enlarge, magnify, or—worst of all—use preset machine values of scale, even when they are having difficulty locating a structure. Typical imagers allow display of a range of tissue depths from 5 cm (designed for examining neonates) to about 24 cm. Typical Doppler units allow adjustments of up to ±6.0 m per second on the continuous-mode display. It is important to condense the image or Doppler display sufficiently so that all relevant data is displayed. If the maximum displayed image depth is 10 cm and the patient's mitral valve is 12 cm from the transducer, no usable data is obtained (Fig. 4-14). Good *minimum* settings for beginning an examination are: M-mode and two-dimensional, 15 cm; continuous-wave Doppler, ±3 m per second. It is unlikely that increasing the displayed depth to the maximum allowed by the scanner (minifying the image or Doppler display) would cause unnecessary confusion. When moving structures are imaged but are difficult to understand anatomically, greater depth settings often are helpful. All systems display some form of dots or dashes on the screen which represent a calibration factor (that is, they represent a centimeter of tissue depth or a velocity calibration). These data serve as visual reminders of the current magnification setting.

## Information Batching

Much of the function of an echocardiograph involves the grouping of numerical information into batches that can be displayed graphically in a way that the eye and the brain can easily comprehend. In a sense, the amount of information available is decreased to make it easier to interpret. As an example, say that we have information values 1 through 50, which will be assigned to 10 shades of gray. Numbers 6 to 10 are all seen as one shade. We can no longer tell the difference between value 7 and value 9. As long as there is no need to know this difference, that is fine. It is exactly what is done in 2-D gray-scale echocardiographic images. Shades of gray are used to represent the power of the signal returning from a location, white being a very strong signal and dark gray being a very weak one. Digital scanners offer a variety of ways of assigning these shades to the range of powers being shown, many of which are nonlinear. The precise selection of display parameters (often labelled preprocessing) is usually dictated by operator preference rather than any scientific rule. Systems are capable of offering large numbers of gray shades in their displays; however the eye is usually unable to detect and use more than 8 shades in a real image. More shades might be useful in some of the video-densitometry analysis that is done on off-line computer systems.[31,32]

Imaging systems also batch distance information. Careful examination of a magnified image shows that it is made up of small rectangles (pixels), each of which is assigned a shade of gray. There could be multiple signals originating from within the tissue volume represented by that pixel, but all are assigned one shade. The size of the pixel represents the limit of the resolution (ability to display detail) of the display system. Other factors also limit resolution of the ultrasound system, and the display components usually are not the limiting factor.

Batching of directional information may occur in some systems. Although the beam is not straight and narrow along its axis, the signals are processed as if they were. Also, in the case of a mechanical transducer that is constantly moving, the crystal is in a slightly different position while receiving than it was while sending; its position during the receive cycle is even slightly different when it receives near echoes than when it receives distant echoes.

Similar groupings occur in all types of Doppler velocity data displays.[2,27] In a graphic velocity versus time display, the velocities are grouped and displayed as rectangles on a graph. Each rectangle represents a small range of velocities over a small unit of time. The gray shade assigned to that block again represents the power of the signal returning at that velocity range (Figs. 4-15, 4-16). Similarly, in the color Doppler display, a small anatomic region on the two-dimensional image is examined for Doppler shift and is coded in a color and a brightness, depending on its direction and its velocity.

Integrated backscatter is a method of analyzing the returning ultrasound signal before it has been processed for the imaging display to determine the specific characteristics of a particular tissue.[22,25] The processor looks at the powers of different frequencies within the band emitted by the transducer being used and compares this to test values obtained from a known flat, ideal reflector. These values are then combined to give an integrated value

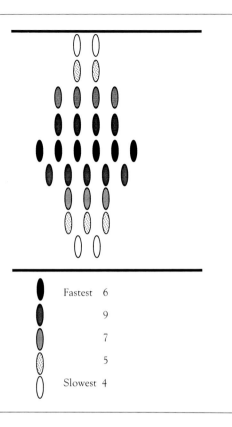

FIGURE 4-15. Red blood cell velocity. This diagram is an example of the velocity distribution of blood cells moving within a normal vessel. The fastest-moving cells (black) tend to be in the center, as the cells along the edges are slowed by friction from the vessel walls. The majority of cells tend to move at medium speeds (gray shades).

for the scatterers within the sample area. Specular reflectors are intentionally excluded, so that the value obtained depends only on information about non-angle-dependent reflectors. If this were not done, small changes in transducer position or angle would affect these measurements and make them undependable. These values have the capacity to differentiate between tissue types and to detect changes in the condition of the sample tissue. In normal myocardium, integrated backscatter values change with the cardiac cycle (high values near end-diastole, lower values near end-systole). Ischemia causes a higher total backscatter and loss of these cyclic changes, and collagen-infarcted tissue

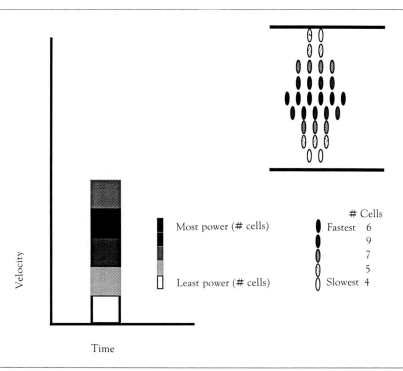

FIGURE 4-16. Spectral analysis. A spectral analysis display consists of an ongoing series of vertical time lines. The graph demonstrates how the spectral display would show velocity distribution during one short interval. The shades of gray represent the strength of the reflections, which is related to the number of cells moving at a particular velocity. Since larger numbers of cells are moving at the medium velocities, the middle-velocity blocks are assigned darker shadings.

has values that fall into a totally different range. These findings have been shown in experimental models and are being investigated in human subjects. Efforts are being made to display this type of data in clinically usable scanners. It is hoped that this capability will help us to obtain more information about tissue structure, physiologic state, and postoperative success or rejection.

The material wanted for display is compiled and digitized into a memory referred to as a digital scan converter.[9] This allows the information that has been accumulated as a plot on some form of an *x-y* graph to be stored and read out in another form, such as on video or a raster scan.

For instance, a single 2-D image is created by plotting the location of the transducer (the top of the screen), the angle of the beam (one line along the image), and a series of dots representing the dis-

tances of the reflectors from the transducer (Fig. 4-17). Each display point can be thought of as a point on an *x-y* axis. A full sweep of the ultrasound beam through its arc creates one picture. Such a picture could be displayed on an oscilloscope, but devices like television screens and videotape recorders do not accept information in this format. They require an image that consists of a series of horizontal lines covering the whole screen. This is discussed further below.

Because the ultrasound data is available in a numerical form in the digital scan converter, the display can be manipulated further in many systems through controls that are usually referred to as *postprocessing*. This means that algorithms (mathematical procedures) that change the gray scale assignments even further can be applied as the numbers are read out of the internal electronic memory

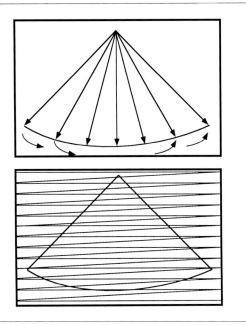

FIGURE 4-17. Scan conversion. *(Top)* An image is created by drawing a series of coordinates in the memory (DSC). As the echoes are received, a point is plotted along the known sending direction (vertical line). As the next pulse is sent, the line is moved along the arc and the received signals are plotted again. When a full sweep through the sector arc has been completed, the creation of the next image begins. *(Bottom)* An image is read from the memory (DSC) to the display screen and recording devices in this preset routine television format. The reading beam sweeps horizontally, reading the degree of brightness at each point along the line. It then moves quickly back to the beginning point and down one line, repeating this cycle until it reaches the bottom of the screen. The image has now been converted from the form in which it was created (a series of dots that can be randomly placed in a coordinate system) to one displayed in a standard television format.

without changing what is in the memory. This data is kept in the memory for only a very short time, so it has been of very little advantage in clinical echocardiography. It has the potential for looking at one image at multiple settings, but in practice very little decision-making is based on the appearance of an individual frame when a continuously moving structure is under examination.

## Display Screens

Current echocardiography systems use either a black-and-white or a color television monitor for their display. They are similar to a home television but don't have a channel selector. They cannot receive their own television signals and require an input from an external source.

The black-and-white monitor has the same basic structure as an oscilloscope (Fig. 4-18). It has a screen that is clear but is coated on the inside with a phosphorescent material that glows in any places where it is struck by a high-energy electron beam. The beam is created by an electron gun at the rear of the television. The gun creates a cloud of electrons, which are accelerated toward the screen by an anode (positive terminal) placed near it. The electron beam is steered through a raster pattern, consisting of 525 horizontal lines, sweeping horizontally across the screen, moving down one line and sweeping again. That is the current American television standard, although higher-resolution systems are currently being introduced for general use. To create this pattern automatically, a set of electromagnets placed around the circumference of the tube near the electron gun can be activated to attract or repel the electron beam, to "write" a pattern on the screen. As the beam position is steered, the incoming video signal modifies the force with which the electron beam strikes the screen, thereby creating dots of varying brightness. It does this by varying the voltage or potential difference between the electron gun and the anode near the screen, with greater voltage causing a brighter glow in that area of the phosphor. In order to create a coordinated raster pattern, a reference signal included in the video signal tells the television monitor when to begin a sweep.

It is interesting to consider what is different about black-and-white signals and color signals. It has long been obvious that a color video signal can be viewed on a black-and-white television. All the information that is needed is there, but there must be something additional that encodes the color data. That extra reference signal is a color burst, which is followed by phase shifts of the brightness voltages (Fig. 4-19). The triggering of the color display is caused by the phase of the video signal that controls the brightness (see above). How out of phase this is compared to a reference signal deter-

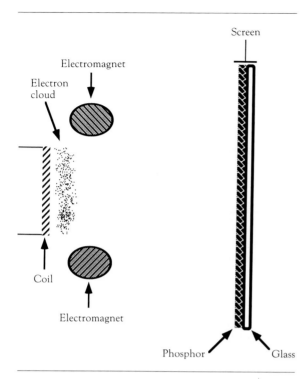

FIGURE 4-18. Television monitor. On the right side of the diagram is the screen: a sheet of glass coated with a phosphor, which glows when struck by high-energy electrons. On the left is a small coil that will produce a free cloud of electrons when heated by a small electrical current. These electrons gain a high level of energy because of acceleration toward an anode (not shown here) near the screen. The great voltage differential between the electron source and the anode (a positively-charged plate) creates high acceleration. Electromagnets focus the electrons into a narrow beam as they travel toward the screen.

mines the color assignment. The color burst follows the signal that triggers the horizontal sweep. This phase shift information is then used to trigger relative brightnesses of three color electron guns, which create combinations of red, green, and blue glowing phosphors on the screen. The balance or addition and subtraction qualities of these colors allows generation of other needed colors, although current color Doppler units use mostly red, blue, and green in their displays. It is interesting to note that brightness information of the colors is still

seen on a black-and-white screen and only the actual color assignment is lost.

## Mode Selection

Echocardiographic examinations are generally begun using *2-D imaging*.[5,15] It allows quick location of available ultrasound windows and a survey of the position and condition of anatomic structures. In a 2-D display, the top of the screen represents the location of the transducer. The image is shaped like a pie wedge, and distance down from the peak represents distance from the transducer. The triangle consists of many lines of information originating from the peak. Along each line a received reflection is displayed as a white dot whose brightness increases with reflection power. (In cardiac ultrasound, the video background is black.)

The features of individual units vary considerably, but some general restrictions and trade-offs are worth understanding. A major limit to the amount of information that can be received in a given amount of time is the velocity of ultrasound in soft tissue (average 1540 m per second). The human eye is usually unable to distinguish more than 25 separate pictures or frames per second, so a series of images displayed at a rate of 25 to 30 frames per second will appear to show continuous motion. To look at the effects of this limit let us say that the scanning process must be repeated every $\frac{1}{25}$ second. At the assumed velocity this would allow information from one line of sight to be obtained from up to 61.6 m away, much farther than the areas of interest in the human body, but many lines of information are needed to compose a cross-sectional picture. Up to a point, the more lines of data, the greater the detail in the image. There is a limit to the detail that the monitor can portray so that it becomes saturated with detail at some level. To continue with the example, if the image had 140 lines of data in its cross-sectional arc, each could be up to 0.44 meters (44 cm) long if the machine transmitted once and then listened for the whole $\frac{1}{25}$ second. Because the machine must interrupt the listen phase to send a pulse for each line, it cannot listen for that long and it can only display somewhat shorter lines. Some time is also lost in the electronic switching and processing. Slightly higher frame rates also decrease the depth of visu-

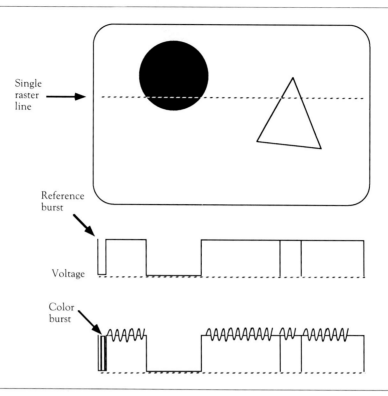

FIGURE 4-19. Creation of a television image. *(Top)* A television screen with an image. The voltage signal that modifies the high screen voltage to create one line of information *(dotted horizontal line)* is shown in the middle panel. *(Middle)* The reference burst signals the screen to begin a new line. High voltages produce a white read-out on the screen; low voltages cause the screen to go black. The shades of gray represent lower voltages. *(Bottom)* This diagram shows the addition of color information. A color burst sets the reference phase for the color display. The phase of the waveform in each voltage or brightness signal determines the color assignment of that signal. In order to display this information, the monitor needs additional color phosphors and electron sources. Colors usually displayed are a combination of red, green, and blue.

alization significantly. So a machine that attempts to display more than 20 to 22 cm of anatomic depth usually needs to switch to a frame rate of less than 20 frames per second. Parallel processing computer techniques allow these limits to be overcome to some degree by using multiple analyzers to accept multiple information lines from a single ultrasound burst, however this has been applied in very few commercial scanners. In fact, so much information can be accepted with some versions that the limiting factors become the screen's ability to display and the videotape system's ability to record

the volume of data. Computer spatial averaging of data can allow less lines of information to be acquired without having the image look incomplete, however this can be at least theoretically inaccurate in a fast-moving organ like the heart.

At 25 to 30 frames per second the machine needs at least 33 to 40 msec to compile enough information to compose one complete picture. This picture cannot truly represent the heart because the structures at the left of the screen are not in that position at the same time as those at the right of the screen. For most clinical applications, this does not seem to make much difference, but the much higher temporal resolution of M mode may still offer some significant advantages, especially when applied to the color Doppler mode.

Since a large number of pictures are being presented to the eye at a very rapid rate, it is sometimes difficult to make full use of the timing of the data and to make some reproducible measurements of structures of interest. Most 2-D echocardiographs have the capability of automatically freezing the image at an operator-selected time in the cardiac cycle as indicated on the simultaneous electrocardiogram (ECG) monitor. Often called ECG gating, this may be done in a split-screen format (i.e., one side of the screen shows the normal continuous image while the other side demonstrates the selected freeze-frames being updated with each cardiac cycle. This sequence can either be videotaped with the desired frozen image selected for analysis, or the proper images can be analyzed if the freeze button is activated before the next updated image replaces the desired one.

The sonographer should remember that, because the ultrasound beam possesses thickness, so does the cross-sectional plane. The anatomy seen in one 2-D image does not necessarily all fall within one plane. It is sometimes helpful to note that the display consists of ultrasound reflections from within the heart rather than a true visual image of cardiac anatomy and motion. Reports of "mistakes" often show that the referring physician misunderstands the information about the reflectance and transmission characteristics of the heart. We must avoid that trap ourselves and communicate such information accurately.

*M-mode* examination of the heart was the first clinically accepted form of echocardiography and is still performed routinely.[15] Most 2-D scanners are capable of producing the examination without changing transducers. M-mode scans can be recorded either on videotape, a video printer, or on a separate, expensive strip-chart recorder.

The M in M-mode stands for motion: it was the first mode that allowed tracking of the motion of particular interfaces.[8] The original units for making cross-sectional images, the static B scanners, required hand-moved single-crystal transducers that took 2 to 3 seconds to compile a single image. They were not useful for demonstrating rapidly moving cardiac structures as several cardiac cycles occur in this period. M-mode samples along the one direction of a single crystal at rates of 700 to 1000 times per second and automatically sweeps the display across a viewing screen. To interpret the display, one assumes that the transducer is at the top of the screen and that the distance downward represents distance from the crystal. The most recent line of information may be presented in one of two forms on the screen: For *sweeping* (Fig. 4-20) an invisible vertical baseline sweeps from left to right. Its position at any given moment represents the most current data. Therefore, the newest positions of structures may be along any vertical line on the screen, depending on the time in the sweep cycle. For *scrolling* (Fig. 4-20) the most recent data always appears at the right side of the display while the older data is constantly shifted toward the left side. The newest structure positions are always at the right of the display.

M-mode–only machines used the sweeping presentation with either a continuously fading (persistence) screen or an erase-at-end-of-sweep function. Digital units offered the capacity to present scrolling data, as it is being read constantly from the digital scan converter for display on the television monitor. The monitor can rearrange the screen's data with each raster scan, in either sweeping or scrolling form, with equal ease.

A dot is placed from top-to-bottom along the invisible baseline of the M-mode display at the distances where reflectors are detected. As the reflectors move and the sweep or scroll occurs, the dots go up and down to create wavy lines, which represent the motion patterns of the interfaces (Fig. 4-21). A rapidly rising line represents an interface moving quickly toward the transducer. A fairly horizontal line represents a surface whose distance from the transducer is relatively stable. All motion representation of the heart assumes that the transducer is stationary. Any motion perpendicular to the ultrasound beam goes unrecorded.

Because the sampling rate of the M-mode instrument is very fast, positional changes that occur in very short intervals (several milliseconds) can be well-demonstrated. Motions such as the fine fluttering of the anterior mitral leaflet seen in aortic insufficiency are demonstrated well by M-mode but are too fast to be seen on a slow 2-D scan. This can

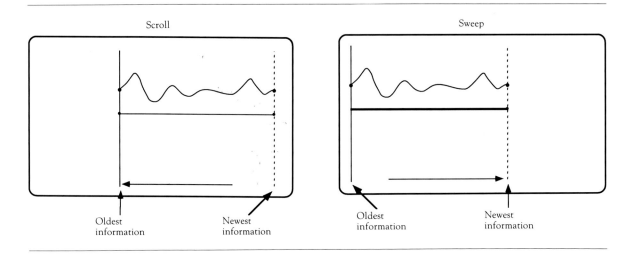

Figure 4-20. Motion-mode (M-mode) displays. Some echocardiography machines offer the ability to switch between scrolling and sweeping types of M-mode display. Neither has any diagnostic advantage over the other, but both presentations should be understood. In the scrolling format, new M-mode information appears on the right side of the screen. As more information appears it is moved toward the left, where old data disappears. In a sweeping presentation the line where the new M-mode information appears and moves from the left side of the screen toward the right. The old information remains still. New data overwrites the old data as the sweep begins again.

be very useful for timing intracardiac events, and it is unlikely that this degree of time resolution will ever be obtained with cross-sectional imaging systems.

The larger view of relative anatomy in cross sections is a powerful tool. Because of the restricted view that M-mode offers, its usefulness in making reproducible analyses and measurements depends on standardization of images produced. In other words, a position is used from which several interfaces are seen simultaneously. Usually this can be done only from a very limited area, requiring that repeat measurements be made from the same position.

*Doppler echocardiography* left the realm of research technique and entered the world of clinical application in the United States in 1982–1983. This was when Dr. Hatle's approach to the combined continuous- and pulsed-mode examination was understood and applied. She developed her approach after she was stimulated by Dr. Holen's ap-

plication of fluid dynamics principles, which allowed noninvasive prediction of hemodynamic measurements performed during cardiac catheterization. Doppler instruments use a different approach to analyzing reflected ultrasound. Instead of looking only at arrival time and power, these units also determine the returning frequency of the sound waves. The Doppler principle states that if a source of a waveform is moving relative to an observer (or a receiver) the perceived frequency and wavelength will be different from the transmitted frequency or wavelength. The formula for this relationship is as follows:

$$F_D = \frac{2F_O V \cos A}{C}$$

where $F_D$ = the observed frequency change from a moving reflector

$F_O$ = the transmitted frequency from the transducer

$V$ = the velocity of the reflector

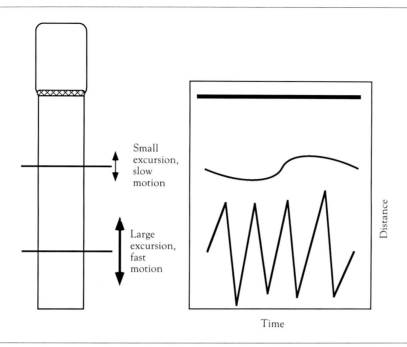

FIGURE 4-21. M-mode display of distance between the transducer and interfaces changes. On the left is the transducer, whose beam encounters two interfaces with similar reflective characteristics but different motion patterns. Any surface with a larger excursion will create an M-mode graph with a greater change between its top and bottom points. If a reflector moves faster, the slope of the line will be steeper.

A = the angle between the ultrasound beam and the direction of motion of the reflector
C = the velocity of sound in blood (1560 m/sec).[17]

Since $2F_O$ and C are constants, the observed frequency change measured by the machine depends on the velocity of the reflector (Fig. 4-22) and the angle between the ultrasound beam and the direction of reflector motion. That is,

$$F_D \sim V$$

By rearranging the first formula, the velocity of reflectors such as groups of red blood cells can be determined by solving:

$$V = \frac{F_D C}{2F_O \cos A}$$

The instrument can read out this velocity if the operator can align the beam so that it is parallel to the flow of blood. Since angle A becomes 0 or 180 degrees and cosine A is 1, this alignment makes the velocity directly proportional to the frequency shift. Such alignment is not always easy to sustain, as flow direction is not precisely predictable in a normal heart and is highly unpredictable in an abnormal heart. The trick is to utilize the sound signal that is presented along with pulsed and continuous-wave Doppler signals. A sound is created by feeding the $F_D$ value to a sound system. Doppler shift frequency values fall within the human audible range and can be easily converted into a sound signal. As the operator approaches a parallel alignment, the detected frequency shift—and therefore the pitch (frequency) of the audio signal—also rise. With practice and careful attention, the angle can usually be brought to under 20 degrees, which would cause an estimate error of under 6% in the velocity reading. Some machines have an angle

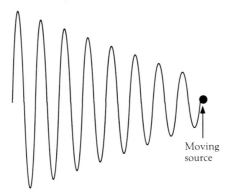

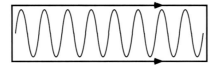

Source

Frequency sent = Velocity/Wavelength

Frequency received by the observer is altered by the
  velocity of the source.
Velocity is constant in the medium.
Wavelength is compressed when moving toward and vice versa.
Frequency is higher if toward and vice versa.

FIGURE 4-22. Doppler effect. When a sound source is moving, the waves in front of it are compressed (creating shorter wavelengths, higher frequency) whereas those in back of it are stretched (longer wavelengths, lower frequency). Waves spreading out to the sides are altered, depending on their angle; those going straight out to the side (perpendicular to the motion) are not stretched or compressed at all. As a result, if the motion of the reflectors is directly across the ultrasound beam, no Doppler frequency shift is detected. If the motion is directly toward or away from the transducer, the full value of the frequency shift is detected.

correction control that allows the operator to enter the angle A by using a cursor superimposed on the 2-D image. This is not usable in echocardiography because flow angles often are not predictably related to the walls of the surrounding structure. In fact, the studies that correlate Doppler with invasive hemodynamic data show no improvement and sometimes a poorer correlation when angle correction is attempted. This option should not be used in cardiac applications.

Continuous and pulsed-mode Doppler data are presented as a spectral analysis display. Each signal is decoded into its component frequencies. These exist, because in any volume of moving blood, not all the blood moves at the same velocity. To take an example in vitro, when blood moves through a tube the blood near the walls rubs against the walls and moves more slowly than the fluid in the middle of the tube. The relatively wide beam is likely to detect multiple velocities simultaneously. These frequencies are translated into velocities and arranged along a vertical line with distance from the zero line corresponding to the magnitude of the velocity. The more power registered at each velocity (theoretically representing the number of red cells moving at that velocity), the darker the gray shade

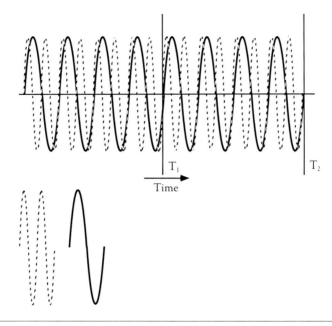

FIGURE 4-23. Aliasing or frequency ambiguity. The dotted waveform has twice the frequency of the solid waveform in this diagram. Imagine sampling a waveform at two times, $T_1$ and $T_2$. Both waveforms would appear at the same point in their cycle and it would be impossible to tell which frequency was being observed. If the sampling frequency is increased so that there are more sample points between the left side of the line and $T_1$, eventually enough samples will be produced to recognize the differences between the frequencies. In pulsed-mode Doppler, it is always assumed (sometimes incorrectly) that the lower frequency is correct. Increasing pulse repetition frequency increases the sampling rate and allows correct definition of higher-frequency Doppler shifts.

assigned to that velocity. As one moves to the right along the recording, the displayed velocities occur more recently in time.

Why do we use both continuous- and pulsed-mode Doppler? As with most choices in ultrasound, each option has advantages and limitations. Pulsed-mode scanning operates in a form similar to the imaging systems. By sending out a pulse of sound, it is possible to tell how far away a reflector lies by measuring the time it takes for the signal to return. This enables the sonographer to localize the origin of the signal and to sort out the signals that are near each other. The signal's frequency shift can then be analyzed to determine its velocity. In order to reconstruct the frequency information, multiple samples are needed. Each sample provides

only a single point along the waveform, and many points are used to define the overall signal. A series of waveforms possessing progressively higher frequencies can be constructed that will fit these sample points. Because the machine always selects the *lowest* frequency that fits the sample points, each pulsed system is limited in how high the frequency shift (or velocity) can be before it begins to misinterpret the velocity. Once the detected velocity exceeds this limit (the Nyquist limit, $N$), *aliasing,* or frequency ambiguity, occurs (Fig. 4-23).

The appearance of frequency ambiguity on a pulsed-mode recording is quite characteristic, but it may be somewhat difficult to understand, initially.[3,4,17] If a reflector whose velocity exceeds the $N$ of the system is moving toward the transducer the signal will rise above the baseline until it reaches $+N$. It will then appear at $-N$ and will continue to rise above $-N$ toward the zero line. It therefore appears as if there are velocities both toward and away from the receiver (above and below the baseline) at the same time. The precise value of $N$ on any system depends on the sampling rate or pulse-repetition frequency (PRF). If the PRF is increased, higher velocities can be reached before $N$ and frequency ambiguity are reached. When the PRF rises, a second pulse may be sent before all the relevant echoes from the first pulse have been received. This means that the machine may not know which pulse caused the reflection from an interface or the total travel time of that echo. Therefore *range ambiguity* (difficulty in determining the depth of the reflector) may occur.

Although this describes the appearance and control of frequency ambiguity (aliasing), the reason for the limitation may be better explained by using a different example of a pulsed sampling system. Imagine watching a solitary ice skater on a rink moving steadily forward around the rink at a rate of one trip every 4 seconds (It's a small rink!). If you look at him only once every second, you would see him advance one quarter of the way each second and would correctly judge that he went forward one round trip every 4 seconds (Fig. 4-24). Both speed and direction are correctly assessed. With the skater doing the same thing, now imagine that you look at him briefly half as often, or once every 2 seconds. Each viewing would show him halfway around, and you would have no way of knowing which way he was going (forward or backward), but you would correctly assess the speed as one round trip every two viewings (4 seconds). This is the beginning of the ambiguity. Now decrease your sampling rate to once every 3 seconds. On the second viewing, he would appear to have gone backward one quarter revolution from the position at the first viewing. The third viewing would show that he went backward a total of two quarters. He would appear to go around backward one time every four viewings (12 seconds). Both the direction and the speed are incorrect. This is true of the velocity registration on a pulsed Doppler system.

When the Nyquist limit is exceeded to $+N+x$, it is displayed as $-N+x$. The same is true in the

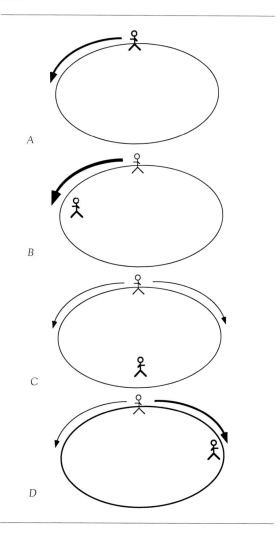

FIGURE 4-24. Aliasing. (*A*) The skater in this diagram moves counterclockwise at one revolution every 4 seconds. (*B*) An observer who looks at the action once every second correctly perceives that the skater moves counterclockwise one quarter revolution every second. (*C*) An observer who looks once every 2 seconds perceives that the skater moves one half revolution every 2 seconds but is unable to determine the skater's direction, clockwise or counterclockwise. It is at this point that ambiguity begins. (*D*) An observer who looks once every 3 seconds perceives that the skater moves clockwise one quarter revolution in 3 seconds. The observed velocity appears much slower than the true velocity and the direction is incorrect (*bold arrows* represent perceived direction of motion).

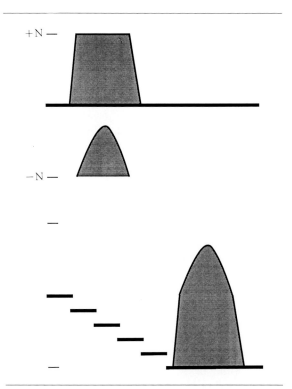

FIGURE 4-25. Baseline shifting. *(Top)* This shows velocity toward the transducer which exceeds the Nyquist limit (N). *(Bottom)* The baseline has been moved by the operator to the bottom of the scale. Any signals originally shown below the baseline have been placed electronically at the top of the display. All signals are now displayed above the baseline, regardless of their true direction. The baseline could also be shifted to the top of the display, all signals being displayed below the baseline. This maneuver allows measurement of velocities up to $+2N$ or down to $-2N$ in pulsed mode, but it introduces direction ambiguity.

other direction (away from the transducer). When the velocity is $-N-x$, the unit calls it $+N-x$. It always puts the velocity ($V$) between the positive and negative limits:

$$-N<V<+N$$

and does not display anything outside these limits. Most machines have controls that enable you to shift the baseline so that you can increase the capability to measure velocity in one direction by sacrificing the other direction (Fig. 4-25). That is, measurement can be made in either of these ranges:

$$-2N<V<0 \quad \text{or} \quad 0<V<+2N,$$

but you are always restricted to a range equal to $2N$. Some manufacturers introduced equipment with high PRF capabilities; that is, they intentionally use a PRF that introduces range ambiguity (and introduce sample volumes at multiple depths within the heart) to overcome some of the frequency ambiguity, using a single crystal transducer. Such designs have been shown to be less effective than continuous wave and to have very little clinical advantage.[35]

This serves as an introduction to the major advantage of continuous-mode Doppler. Since one of the two continuous-wave transducer crystals is constantly sending, it would be the equivalent of pulsed mode with an infinitely high PRF. There would be no Nyquist limit, so it is capable of measuring velocities as high as is required. Extremely high velocities ($>5.5$ to $6.0$ m/sec) can occur in pathologies such as aortic stenosis and mitral regurgitation, and these can be demonstrated and measured accurately with continuous-mode Doppler. However, since the PRF is infinitely high, there is total range ambiguity. In other words, there is nothing that defines the distance to the reflector. Sometimes the velocity pattern itself tells the experienced examiner the origin of the signal. Using the velocity pattern to determine the location of the flow requires a great deal of practice and experience. Dr. Hatle's original work also made use of phonocardiographic recordings to help define the origins of the velocity patterns. Another advantage of continuous wave is its convenience as a searching mode. When pointing a continuous-wave beam in one direction, all signals that exist in that direction are usually detected. In order to search the same amount of area with a pulsed wave, the operator would have to aim in that direction and slowly adjust the range control so that you have sampled along the entire length of the beam.

So the answer to Why do we use both continuous-wave and pulsed-mode Doppler? is that with the former we can measure the velocity of blood flow and with the latter locate and map the extent of particular velocity patterns. Each of these pieces of information has its uses, as will be described in the pathology sections of this text. However, the significance of blood flow velocity measurements should be discussed. In 1976, Dr. Holen showed both theoretically and in practice that pressure gradient (the force that drives blood through a narrow opening) is proportional to the square of the velocity at which the blood moves. He proposed that pressure gradients (which are commonly measured across stenotic heart valves during cardiac catheterization) could be predicted by noninvasive Doppler measurements using Holen's modification of Bernoulli's equation which says:

$$P = 4V^2$$

Highlighting this formula is a subtle hint that it is extremely powerful for providing critical clinical information. It has been validated many times; the best correlations appear in simultaneous catheter-Doppler comparisons. There are some circumstances in which it may not apply perfectly, not all of which are well-understood, but it has made echocardiography a *quantitative* tool for the evaluation of valvular and other types of heart disease. One should think carefully about what is being done when this formula is used:

The ultrasound *frequency shift* is being *measured*.
The *velocity of blood* flow is being *calculated*.
The *instantaneous pressure gradient* is being *estimated*.

In some circumstances, derived information may be less meaningful or reliable than measured data. Also, the gradients measured during cardiac catheterization are not always instantaneous gradients and may appear to show differences from Doppler results in some circumstances. It is hoped that clinicians will be comfortable enough with the concepts behind Doppler application to resist being overwhelmed by the mathematical-sounding discussions that arise in presentations of Doppler methods. It is important to keep in mind that Doppler equipment presents data about blood speed, direction, and location, and that each presentation mode has inherent advantges and shortcomings, including the dramatic advance of color-flow Doppler.

*Color-flow Doppler* concepts have been applied to M-mode scanning but did not gain acceptance until the technology for 2-D application was developed.[23,24] Anything that flashes bright blues, reds, greens, and yellows during a sonographic examination tends to attract and excite, but it is important to look at the precise meaning of the display to use it well. Current color-flow units include both 2-D and M-mode displays, and a sonographer will recognize early on that the M-mode display is extremely useful for timing the rapidly changing color patterns. Correct timing of velocity patterns has prevented many incorrect conclusions.

Color-flow technology allows display of velocity data in a cross-sectional format that can be superimposed on a 2-D anatomic image. A standard gray-scale 2-D image is seen, but instead of black spaces representing the homogeneous blood pool there are color signals that represent the motion of the red blood cells. Each colored dot represents motion in a small area of the blood pool. By convention motion toward the transducer is coded red and motion away from the transducer is coded blue. This should not be confused with the colors of arterial and venous blood. They only indicate direction relative to the transducer. Not all signals are easily interpreted by the system as moving either toward or away from the transducer. In the diseased heart, blood flow sometimes is very disturbed or changes rapidly. A machine that is attempting to detect a pattern of velocities in the small area of a pixel will conclude that the velocity has a great deal of *variance*. This typically occurs in areas where there are eddies, or swirls of blood that change direction often. To represent this, the coder adds green to the dominant direction color, red or blue, to create another color, either yellow or blue-green. This is *not* the same effect seen with *aliasing* of a flow signal, in which a fairly smooth signal is represented by an incorrect color. For instance, when a stenotic mitral valve is viewed from the apex, the diastolic inflow signal often appears to be red at the edges and blue in the middle. This must be aliasing in the color mode, since blood in the center of the inflow could not be moving in the reverse direction.

The color image is composed by creating range gates or sample volumes along each pulse direction (250 to 500 such gates are available in some units)

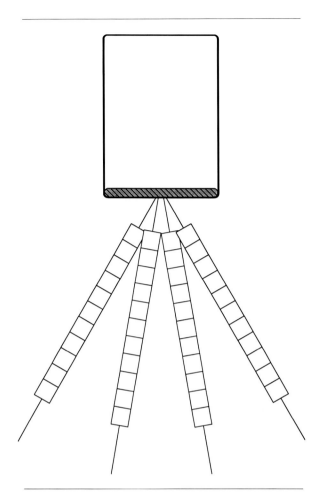

FIGURE 4-26. Color Doppler samples. A color Doppler image is composed of many samples perceived along each line of ultrasound investigation. The pixels that represent each sample are very small and actually represent the motion over a relatively large area. Experiments in vitro on flow through a tube suspended in a water tank have demonstrated that the color Doppler signal is wider than the tube itself. The lateral resolution of the color system, however, is still limited by the width of the ultrasound beam.

from a cardiac structure is displayed in the grayscale image, the color information is eliminated in those pixels. This means that the gain of the imaging part of the unit will have a reverse effect on the color-flow display; when more pixels have image displayed in them (whether real signals or just noise), fewer pixels have color in them. The instruments determine flow direction and velocity through somewhat different techniques, including autocorrelation, instantaneous frequency estimation, and combinations of the above.

The methods appear to have similar requirements and restrictions. They require sampling in each area of color assignment several times (eight is a typical average) to be able to compare signals and determine changes that represent frequency shifts. This means that a great deal of time is spent sampling along each line of information. The total number of lines acquired is usually very small, so the sector arc is narrower than when the system is not displaying color-flow information. The Nyquist limit is also usually low. With typical settings used in adult echocardiography and a 2.5-MHz transducer, it is not unusual for aliasing to occur at velocities greater than about 0.75 m per second.

It is also useful to recognize that the output of the color unit's velocity estimator represents the mean velocity within the sample volume. A reasonable guess is that within a small volume the mean and the maximum velocity are similar, so in these cases the color display can be viewed as presenting data about the maximum values present; however, since the lateral resolution is still equal to the width of the ultrasound beam, the size of the blood volume being evaluated is much greater than the size of the pixels on the color display. Recognizing the true meaning of the display is important when trying to make quantitative velocity or volume assessments from the color image.

This discussion of mode presentations available to the echocardiographer shows the tools available for the performance of a composite comprehensive cardiac examination. Each mode offers to examiner and interpreter a particular type of information:

2-D: Cross-sectional anatomic display of the entire heart
M-mode: Definition of rapid motions and standardized dimension measurements

that will each be coded to represent velocities in that region (Fig. 4-26). Since it is desirable to encode only reflections representing blood cells, reflections from larger moving structures like valves and walls are sorted out by devices such as moving target indicators. In other words, when a reflection

Continuous-wave Doppler: Searching the heart and measuring high velocities

Pulsed Doppler: Localization of signals and measurement of low-velocity signals

Color 2-D: Rapid survey of an entire cross section of velocity patterns, identification of disturbed flow areas, demonstration of eccentric flow patterns (particularly useful in congenital heart disease)

Color M-mode: Timing of rapidly changing patterns seen on the color 2-D image and recording of signals of brief duration

While all examinations not performed during life-threatening emergencies should be used to make a general survey of the heart in search of unexpected abnormalities that may affect patient therapy, it is not cost- or time-effective to do everything on every patient. Special procedures such as contrast echocardiograms may also be appropriate sometimes, but not always. Therefore, careful selection of modes and approaches should be used to optimize relevant results.

## Recording of Echocardiographic Data and Images

Several types of recording devices can be used in echocardiography instruments. The most universally accepted units are videotape recorders based on the VHS system of recording. Some units have offered other formats for video recording, but all manufacturers have switched to VHS. Industrial quality instruments are used that can tolerate a great deal of stop, play, and rewind activity, as well as long periods in the pause mode between recordings. Many systems are also able to search for some particular location on the videotape and stop automatically.

Videotape decks require that the echocardiograph have a video output signal, which all machines except the extremely small battery-powered units (sometimes called ultrasound stethoscopes) provide. Audio outputs are also provided for Doppler units and are sometimes recorded in stereo (one channel records flow toward and the other flow away from the transducer). This medium is good quality for two-dimensional and color Doppler, as the recording resolution of the tape system is often at least as good as the quality of the image itself, but they are not capable of recording the full resolution capability of M-mode or continuous-wave and pulsed-wave Doppler. New products incorporating super-VHS and high-definition television (HDTV) may improve videotape recordings.

*Strip-chart recorders* made M-mode recordings practical and were widely used.[18] There were two major types, which had some desirable characteristics: (1) They were able to reproduce the image with very high resolution, even at very expanded recording scales. (2) They could produce continuous recording of cardiac events over long periods of time utilizing a long roll of paper. (3) They required no additional equipment such as film processors. The early strip charts used a pink paper that was sensitive to light and developed its latent image when exposed to ultraviolet light (flourescent or sunlight). The image consisted of shades of pink and purple. Units built after 1979 use paper that produces a black image on a white background. It is necessary to heat the paper to develop the image. Images on pink paper tended to fade after about 5 years; those on white paper should last indefinitely, as long as they are protected from excessive heat.

A strip chart receives a direct (not scan-converted) analog signal, which is fed to a fiberoptic cathode ray tube (FOCRT). Instead of a viewing screen opposite the electron gun of this tube, there is a narrow band of fiberoptic material, which collects the light from the phosphors and concentrates it into a fine, intense line. This bright light exposes the paper as a motor drive moves it past the FOCRT.

The paper used in these units is expensive and bulky to file. To economize, some users record only brief frozen images of the M-mode or Doppler recordings. Because the images are frozen, they are already in video format and resolution is much poorer than that of unprocessed recordings made with continuous strip-chart recording. The value of these records is that one does not need a videotape system to review them later. Because strip-chart recorders usually cost over $12,000, they add a great deal of expense to the system.

A reasonable alternative to the strip chart is the *video page printer*. Such units are much less expensive and add some attractive features to the recording capability. They accept a video format image (already processed through the scan converter) and print a high-resolution copy for a few pennies per page. The cost of the printer depends on the size and quality of print desired, but all black-and-white models cost less than 10% of what a strip-chart recorder costs. They can print images of any mode that is displayed on the television screen, so M-mode, continuous-wave, and pulsed-wave Doppler, and frames of 2-D studies can all be reproduced. Because they have their own memory, some of the printers even permit recording a picture without freezing the image. This is advantageous because the picture taking does not slow down the examination. Color printers are also available at a higher price.

Another recording modality that was used with early M-mode technology and that has resurfaced on color-flow units is *Polaroid photography*. While Polaroid also gives good resolution reproduction with little equipment, it is very expensive for black-and-white recordings. It is very convenient for color, since film is readily available, but it is still an expensive way to record.

ARTIFACTS AND RESOLUTION

The dictionary defines an artifact as "a product ... of artificial character due to extraneous ... agency."[38] To apply this concept to echocardiographic imaging, we propose the following definition of artifacts: *signals that are displayed in such a way that they do not accurately represent the anatomic or flow characteristics of the subject.* Many types of artifacts are possible, and when viewing sonographic information it may be difficult to be sure which type of artifact is present. *Frequency shift artifacts* in Doppler have been discussed at length in the Mode Selection section. *Location* and *power amplitude* artifacts will now be discussed.

Location of a reflector may be improperly displayed along the path of the ultrasound transmission (axially) or from side to side (laterally). An echo may not be visible if it originates directly behind another echo when the distance between reflectors is less than the axial resolution of the system (i.e., if the reflectors are too close). *Axial resolution* (ability to identify separate reflectors) improves with higher transducer frequency and lower gain setting (Fig. 4-27). Transducer frequencies of

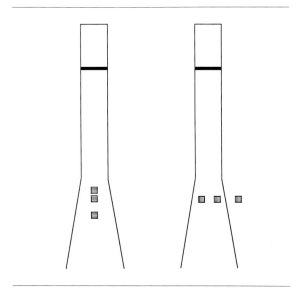

FIGURE 4-27. Axial and lateral resolution. *(Left)* Reflectors that lie behind one another tend to blend into one signal if they are closer together than half the length of the ultrasound pulse. The shorter the pulse, the greater the ability of the system to sense the separation of two surfaces. This ability is called axial resolution. *(Right)* Reflectors that lie next to each other will not appear as separate objects if they are both seen within the beam at the same time. The narrower the beam, therefore, the greater the chance that the system will be able to differentiate between the reflectors (i.e., the greater its lateral resolution capability). Since the length of an ultrasound pulse is much smaller than the width of the beam, axial resolution is usually better than lateral resolution.

approximately 3.5 MHz provide the best balance of optimal resolution and penetration for adult imaging.

The machine determines the axial location of a reflector according to the time of echo return and the assumed speed of ultrasound travel. In some circumstances, such as the presence of artificial materials, this speed may be incorrect. This is commonly seen in patients with ball-and-cage–type prosthetic valves. The speed within the ball is often much slower than in the average soft tissue, causing the echo from the far surface of the ball to appear farther away than it really is.

Some echoes may bounce off multiple surfaces or back and forth between two highly reflective surfaces before returning to the transducer. They appear on the display at a depth where no real interface exists. Many mechanisms can produce an incorrect display in the axial dimension, but they are usually recognizable because they do not make anatomic and physiologic sense.[18]

The *lateral resolution* of a system (ability to distinguish signals from reflectors that are side by side when viewed from the transducer) is determined by the effective width of the ultrasound beam (Fig. 4-27). Influencing factors are the crystal width, frequency, distance from the transducer, focusing, and receiver gain. Because crystal width also influences the length of the narrow near field, a narrower crystal does not improve lateral resolution in all circumstances. When creating the 2-D image, the processor takes information from a fairly wide beam (usually 5 to 10 mm) and displays all returned signals along one fairly thin line (Fig. 4-28). One reflector may appear in multiple lines of the image as the interface is within the beam when they are recorded. A single strong reflector, such as a wire, will be imaged as a line across a section of the display. The length of the line is equal to the width of the ultrasound beam. Reflectors that are next to each other at a distance less than the beam width blend together into one line. Also, a strong reflector at the edge of a fluid-filled chamber appears to extend into a chamber. (Because of this, pacemaker wires sometimes appear to cross the interventricular septum.)

In addition to the central ultrasound beam, most transducers, especially phased-array transducers, also produce side lobes, or extra skirts of ultrasound energy, around the central beam.[8] When echoes from interfaces within these lobes are very strong, they are also displayed and greatly degrade the lateral resolution of the system. When discussing cross-sectional image lateral resolution, one must realize that it is difficult to separate reflectors next to each other both within the plane of the section and perpendicular to that plane. In other words, the "slice" of the heart that is looked at also has thickness. Since annular-array transducers have the potential to reduce the thickness of the slice and to improve resolution within the slice, their resolution is the best currently available. In all systems, lateral resolution is less reliable than axial resolution.

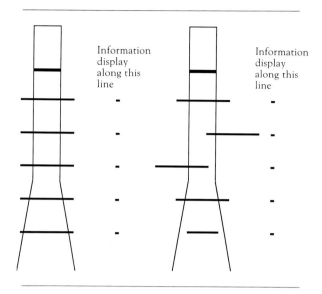

FIGURE 4-28. Lateral resolution artifacts. The width of the ultrasound beam in three-dimensional space is much greater than the width of one image line on the display screen. Both of the relationships shown in the diagram above would give the same display in that one information line. In fact, on a 2-D image, each reflector would appear longer than it actually is because it would continue to be displayed as long as it lay within the beam. The width of the reflector would be overestimated by approximately the width of the beam.

*Power artifacts* are created because the amplitude of the signal displayed is out of proportion to the acoustic impedance mismatch of the interface. That is, if the same reflector were in another location, the strength of its echo would be either greater or less (Fig. 4-29). For instance, some structures (like calcified aortic valves) greatly decrease the amount of energy transmitted to the structures behind them (like the left atrial wall). They cast a shadow, and interfaces within the shadow appear weaker than one might expect. In contrast, large fluid-filled areas (like pericardial effusions) tend to transmit more ultrasonic energy than average soft tissue, so that reflectors behind the fluid appear much brighter than expected. These characteristics can be very useful in differentiating tissue types. Structures or masses that are solid usually do not have bright reflections behind them. Since some solid structures are relatively homogeneous and do

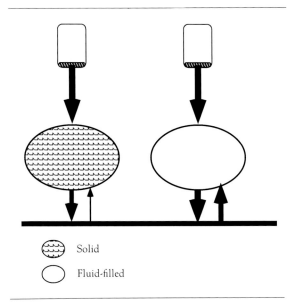

Solid

Fluid-filled

FIGURE 4-29. Power artifacts. The strength of a reflection from an interface is partially determined by the amount of energy that reaches the interface. In the diagram, the echo from the part of the interface that is behind a fluid-filled structure *(right)* is much stronger than the signal that had to pass through a solid structure with internal reflectors *(left)*. While TGC gives greater amplification to more distant structures, it does not account for differences along different image lines. Identical interfaces may have different appearances depending on the structures that lie in front of them.

not have internal echoes, the lack of enhancement of distant areas may be the only indication that they are not fluid filled.[18]

## Computers in Echocardiography

Computers are incorporated into almost every echocardiograph now marketed and also appear in increasing numbers as separate items in laboratories. Their applications fit into three major categories: measurement and calculation, image manipulation, and data storage. All cardiac ultrasound scanners with digital scan converters now contain some form of *measurement and calculation* package. These usually contain a linear measurement that measures distance, time, slope, and velocity depending on the active scan mode. Some may also

perform automatic conversions, such as calculating the gradient that corresponds to the measured velocity through $P = 4V^2$. Measurements may also be taken on multiple cycles, and some units have the capacity to average the values obtained. Also included is the capacity to trace an outline in order to calculate an area (on an image) or an integral (on a velocity recording). These numbers can then be used in formulas for estimating other values such as left ventricular volumes, aortic valve area, and mean gradients.[1] Although some units have offered automated tracing ability, it should be recognized that the data is either entered or approved at the judgment of a human operator and is not infallible. Data from poor quality examinations is not improved through computer measurement. Most units allow measurements to be performed on frozen images during the patient examination, without calibrating the machine. Since this is time-consuming, many prefer to make the measurements later from the videotaped image. Some machines are coded to tell them the scale settings of recorded images, but if calibration is needed, it must be done carefully to achieve accurate measurements. Separate computers have the ability to do these same measurements with a great deal more flexibility. They also serve as off-line review centers for physicians who are not present during the examinations, but this use alone does not justify the cost of these systems. Some of the following tasks can now be performed by computers installed within scanning equipment, but most analysis beyond quick review is more effectively performed off-line.

A great deal of *image manipulation* can be performed by redigitizing the analog data recorded on the videotape. One of the popular operations performed on the digitized image is the storage of a "cine loop" in the computer's video memory. This allows continuous replay of a selected set of video frames for an indefinite period. Since many echocardiographic recordings vary in image quality during the taping (owing to respiration, movement, arrhythmias), this allows concentration on the information in a single well-demonstrated cardiac cycle as well as the ability to store the selected cycle in computer memory or diskettes. Images made under different conditions (e.g., before and after stress, before and after infarction) can be presented side by side for comparison or to look at multiple views simultaneously by splitting the screen in half or in quadrants. Creation of the cine loop (often referred to as frame grabbing) can also be performed on-line without degrading the image by recording it on videotape. Since video images are usually presented in a 512 × 480 pixel presentation, storage of the image at full resolution takes a great deal of memory (245,760 bytes). To reduce the computer space problem, some units store at lower resolution or use compression algorithms to store repetitive information (such as the black background) in less memory. Computers may also be used to decode and compare the brightness of signals in particular areas. In images, this is called the videodensity, and measurements of it are called videodensitometry.[21,41] This, for example, can be measured in images before and after contrast injections to try to quantify the amount of contrast that has reached the area of interest. The relationship between videodensity and contrast flow is difficult to define because of the variation in processing that occurs in ultrasound units and even in one unit at different operator-controlled settings. Some attempts at calibration and standardization have been made, but they are not easily performed with equipment available in the average clinical laboratory. In color-flow maps, the brightness represents the velocity information in the reflected ultrasound. These velocities can also be decoded with computers. Some computer algorithms attempt to unwrap aliased velocity representations, but the problems involved in this process are still being solved.

Postprocessing and subtraction of images can be achieved with off-line computers, but no clinical application of such capabilities has yet been shown (though some interesting psychedelic effects have been produced). Color coding of image amplitude data is being investigated as a way of enhancing visual analysis of tissue characteristics.

*Data storage* of measurements obtained allows the generation of reports from the computer. Well-designed ones offer advantages in professional appearance, clarity and highlighting of important data, selection of pretyped phrases, artificial-intelligence stringing of phrases, easy correction, instantaneous production and future retrieval, and data basing.

Production of a good-looking, informative, instantaneous, and accessible report makes the computer a powerful tool. The ability to create a data base is useful in all laboratories for billing, budgeting, and planning, and for research and quality control. For financial analysis, a computer can save a great deal of time and revenue. For research and quality control, it is desirable to be able to retrieve information about patients with particular diseases. The computer can compile a list of reports containing specific diagnoses or phrases and can cross-reference this list against another data base containing results of other diagnostic tests, surgery, pathology, or clinical outcome. To foresee such needs and questions that will arise in the future requires a well-planned, flexible data base.

It is important for users to be aware of the functions programmed into commercially available computer systems, for instance, what formulas are being used by a particular instrument to calculate left ventricular volume and function. When multiple views are entered or multiple cycles of one view, how is the data being integrated? One unit does not average images whose results have been stored in memory with newly entered images. It also does not reconstruct a three-dimensional plot from multiple views in all appropriate situations. It does suggest that it has solved formulas from a particular method when it has not been given enough data to do so. Some careful testing protocols using these capabilities can be designed to reveal these functions.

## Bioeffects of Ultrasonography

A great deal of effort has been put into investigating the possible effects and hazards of applied ultrasound, but few results are conclusive. By learning about the mechanisms that are thought to play a part in these effects—thermal, cavitation, and mechanical stress—we will see the difficulties encountered in investigating them *in vivo*. Much of the energy that is lost from the ultrasound beam is converted to heat.[26] Some consider a temperature change of 1°C acceptable as this is within the range that body temperature may vary during a normal day and as it is does not persist very long.

Cavitation may occur in some situations when small bubbles exist in the body. These situations are rare with the exception of decompression or intentional injection of bubbles for contrast echocardiograms. In stable cavitation, the bubbles resonate and create stress on the surrounding materials. In transient (or collapsing) cavitation, the gas collapses and causes high energy but very localized energy release, which may generate free radicals (charged particles that may interact with biologic molecules such as DNA and disrupt their structure and function). There is currently no reproducible evidence that these events occur in the clinical setting.

It has taken a long time to achieve standardization in exposure measurements. Spatial location of the area of measurement changes the value as the ultrasound beam is not uniform in its cross-sectional distribution. Temporal peak values are quite different from temporal average values. Also, some equipment operates in continuous modes and other in pulsed modes.[36] The duty factor, or ratio between time on and time off, must be considered. Commonly referred measurements of intensity tend to be $I_{(spatial\ peak\ temporal\ average)}$ and $I_{(spatial\ peak\ pulse\ average)}$ when measured in a water tank. Some units have controls that alter the output, and it is suggested that attempts be made to limit patient exposure without sacrificing diagnostic accuracy. Operators should be aware that Doppler units often have significantly higher energy output than imagers and that fetal Doppler studies should be controlled as much as possible. Standards for acceptable exposure and output have been set arbitrarily, without much scientific basis. Organizations such as the American Institute of Ultrasound in Medicine, National Electrical Manufacturers Association, Center for Devices and Radiologic Health of the Food and Drug Administration, American Society of Echocardiography, National Council of Radiation Protection and Measurements, and the National Institutes of Health all have expressed opinions on regulation of ultrasound outputs. Machines with potential outputs above the arbitrary limits set for fetal use have been labelled "not for fetal use," in ways that may be visible—and sometimes upsetting—to patients.

There is still much work to be done to reach a rational balance between patient benefit and patient risk. It is encouraging to note that after more than two decades of clinical use, no documentation of ultrasonic damage to a living human has been shown.[34] It is also interesting to note that the mechanisms of extracorporeal shock-wave lithotripsy, which produces energy capable of breaking up renal calculi, are not even understood. In the end, the total level of exposure a patient receives during an echocardiogram depends on the knowledge and skill of the examiner.

## Acknowledgments

The author would like to offer special thanks to Larry Waldroup, who first taught me to think creatively about ultrasound principles and equipment; Dennis Schubert, who used both his engineering and his interpersonal skills to translate many of the developments of the last decade into understandable terms; and Richard Meltzer, who encourages his employees to grow and undertake projects like this one.

## References

1. Amico AF, Lichtenberg GS, Reisner SA, et al. Assessment of left ventricular ejection fraction by two-dimensional echocardiography: Are computers necessary? Am Heart J. 1989; 118:1259–1265.

2. Angelsen BAJ. A theoretical study of the scattering of ultrasound from blood. IEEE Trans Biomed Eng. 1980; 27:61–67.

3. Berger M. Doppler echocardiography in heart disease. New York: Marcel Dekker; 1987.

4. Bom K, deBog J, Rijsterborgh H. On the aliasing problem in pulsed Doppler cardiac studies. J Clin Ultrasound. 1984; 12:559–567.

5. Bom N, Lancee CT, Honkoup J, et al. Ultrasonic viewer for cross-sectional analyses of moving cardiac structures. Biomed Eng. 1971; 6:500.

6. Bom N, Lancee CT, Ligtvoet CM. Improvement of lateral resolution in ultrasonic systems. Acta Med Scand. {Suppl} 1979; 627:41–47.

7. Eggleton RC. Interim AIUM standard nomenclature. Reflections. 1978; 4:275.

8. Feigenbaum H. Echocardiography. 4th ed. Philadelphia: Lea & Febiger; 1986.

9. Goldberg PR. Principles of two-dimensional real-time echocardiography. Acta Med Scand. {Suppl} 1979; 627:7–24.

10. Goldman DE, Jeuter TF. Tabular data of the velocity and absorption of high-frequency sound in mammalian tissues. J Acoust Soc Am. 1956; 28:35.

11. Goss SA, Frizzell LA, Dunn F. Ultrasonic absorption

and attenuation in mammalian tissues. Ultrasound Med Biol. 1979; 5:181–186.

12. Gramiak R, Holen J. CW and pulsed Doppler echocardiography utilizing a stand-alone system. Ultrasound Med Biol. 1984; 10(2):215–224.

13. Gramiak R, Shah PM. Echocardiography of the aortic root. Invest Radiol. 1968; 3:356–366.

14. Gramiak R, Shah PM, Kramer DH. Ultrasound cardiography: Contrast studies in anatomy and function. Radiology. 1969; 92:939–948.

15. Harrigan P, Lee R. Principles of Interpretation in Echocardiography. New York: John Wiley; 1985.

16. Hatle L. Introduction to Doppler echocardiography. Acta Paediatr Scand. {Suppl} 1986; 329:7–9.

17. Hatle L, Angelsen B. Doppler Ultrasound in Cardiology: Physical Principles and Clinical Applications. 2d ed. Philadelphia: Lea & Febiger; 1985:32.

18. Kremkau FW. Diagnostic Ultrasound: Principles, Instrumentation and Exercises. Orlando, FL: Grune & Stratton; 1984.

19. McDicken WN. Diagnostic Ultrasonics: Principles and Use of Instruments. 2d ed. New York: John Wiley; 1981.

20. Melton HE, Thurstone FL. Annular-array design and logarithmic processing for ultrasonic imaging. Ultrasound Med Biol. 1978; 4:1.

21. Meltzer RS, Roelandt J, Bastiaans OL, et al. Videodensitometric processing of contrast two-dimensional echocardiographic data. Ultrasound Med Biol. 1982; 8:509–514.

22. Miller JG, Perez JE, Mottley JG, et al. Myocardial tissue characterization: An approach based on quantitative backscatter and attenuation. Proc IEEE Ultrason Symp. 1983; 83:782.

23. Miyatake K, Okamoto M, Kinoshita N, et al. Clinical application of a new type of real time, two-dimensional Doppler flow imaging system. Am J Cardiol. 1984; 54:857–869.

24. Omoto R, Yokote Y, Takamoto S, et al. The development of real-time, two-dimensional Doppler echocardiography and its clinical significance in acquired valvular disease. Jpn Heart J. 1984; 25:325–340.

25. Perez JE, Miller JG, Barzilai B, et al. Progress in quantitative ultrasonic characterization of myocardium: From the laboratory to the bedside. J Am Soc Echocardiogr. 1988; 1:294–305.

26. Porder JB, Porder KN, Meltzer RS. Ultrasound bioeffects. Echocardiography. 1987; 4(2):89–99.

27. Rabiner LR, Gold B. Theory and Application of Digital Signal Processing. Englewood Cliffs, NJ: Prentice-Hall; 1975.

28. Schluter M, et al. Transesophageal cross-sectional echocardiography with phased-array transducer system: Technique and initial clinical results. Br Heart J. 1982; 48:67.

29. Seward JB, Khandheria BK, Oh JK, et al. Transesophageal echocardiography: Technique, anatomic correlations, implementation, and clinical applications. Mayo Clin Proc. 1988; 63:649–679.

30. Shattuck DP, Weinshenker MD, Smith SW, et al. Explososcan: A parallel processing technique for high-speed ultrasound imaging with linear phased arrays. J Acoust Soc Am. 1984; 75:1273–1282.

31. Sinclair RBL, Oldershaw PJ, Gibson DG. Computing in echocardiography. Prog Cardiovasc Dis. 1983; 25:456.

32. Skorton DJ, McNary FC, Shah PM. Digital image processing of two-dimensional echocardiograms: Identification of the endocardium. Am J Cardiol. 1981; 48:479.

33. Snyder JE, Disslo J, VonRamm OT. Real-time orthogonal-mode scanning of the heart: I. System design. J Am Coll Cardiol. 1986; 7:1279–1285.

34. Stewart WJ, Galvin KA, Gillam LD, et al. Comparison of high pulse-repetition frequency and continuous-wave Doppler echocardiography in the assessment of high flow velocity in patients with valvular stenosis and regurgitation. J Am Coll Cardiol. 1985; 6:565–571.

35. Stewart HD, Stewart HF, Moore RM, et al. Compilation of reported biological effects data and ultrasound exposure levels. J Clin Ultrasound. 1985; 13:167.

36. Taylor KJW. Current status of toxicity investigation. J Clin Ultrasound. 1974; 2:149.

37. VonRamm OT, Thurstone FL. Cardiac imaging using a phased-array ultrasound system. Circulation. 1976; 53:258.

38. Webster's New Collegiate Dictionary. Springfield, MA: G. & C. Merriam Company; 1977.

39. Weld PW. Early history of echocardiography. J Cardiovasc Ultrasonography. 1986; 5(2):169–175.

40. Wells PNT. Absorption and dispersion of ultrasound in biological tissue. Ultrasound Med Biol. 1975; 1:369.

41. Xie F, Meltzer RS. Ejection fraction determination by contrast echocardiography: An in vitro study. J Ultrasound Med. 1988; 7:581–587.

# CHAPTER 5

# M-Mode Echocardiography

SUE A. GEORGE, MARVEEN CRAIG

Echocardiography is the study of the position and movement of cardiac acoustic interfaces by means of reflected ultrasound. The images obtained provide both anatomic and functional information about the heart's circulatory performance. In the more than 25 years since the concept was first introduced by Edler, echocardiography has proved to be one of the most valuable tools for studying cardiovascular disorders.

## Operating Modes

Because the heart beats constantly, the technique for examining it sonographically is different from that for observing more quiescent organs. Originally, in order to visualize the motion of the heart, two basic formats were devised for recording echocardiographic data: A-mode (amplitude modulation) and B-mode (brightness modulation). Both formats displayed echoes along a baseline representing the beam axis. The essential difference between the two formats lies in the method of depicting echo amplitude. The A-mode format displays individual echoes as spikes or deflections along a vertical baseline or beam axis, whereas B-mode echocardiography transmits the amplitude of echoes to the electron gun of a cathode ray tube (CRT) in the form of bright dots, or points of light. The distance between the points along the vertical or horizontal axis represents the depth of the encountered echo-producing structures. The bright-

ness of the points indicates the sonodensity of their reflectors (Fig. 5-1).[3,4,7]

The first modification of B-mode technology was the introduction of M-mode, or time-motion, display. Utilizing a slow-sweep or x-axis generator, it was possible to sweep sequential B-mode lines across the face of the CRT. With an appropriate amount of persistence in the phosphor of the CRT, the B-mode lines left a trail of echoes as they moved. The high resolution, rapid sampling rate, and convenient graphic format of M-mode echocardiography were ideal for imaging localized areas of the heart and analyzing time-related events. As a result, M-mode became the primary echocardiographic method until the advent of the two-dimensional (2-D) format (see Fig. 5-1).[3,7]

M-mode echocardiography provides information concerning structural motion and depth only. Its usefulness is limited because it fails to convey the true lateral distances between structures and to accurately reflect off-axis motion and depth.[3,7] M-mode technique produces a continuous readout of reflected sound in a graphic one-dimensional rather than a pictorial 2-D display.

Two-dimensional systems have expanded the visualization and appreciation of the heart by permitting viewing of selected structures in two dimensions. Additionally, through its expanded field of view and real-time capabilities it is possible to view not only the structure of interest but its relationship to surrounding structures.

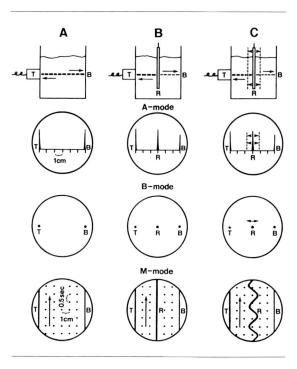

FIGURE 5-1. Diagrams illustrating the principles of acoustic imaging using pulsed, reflected ultrasound. T, transducer; B, beaker; R, rod. (From Feigenbaum H, Zaky A. Use of diagnostic ultrasound in clinical cardiology. Indiana Med 1966; 59:140. By permission of the Indiana State Medical Association.)

Today, M-mode echocardiography is often used in conjunction with 2-D echocardiography. One of the early difficulties encountered with M-mode prior to the availability of 2-D techniques was the fact that the M-mode studies were performed blindly, as it was not possible to determine the angle at which the beam was striking structures within the chest wall. By using both techniques, both cardiac structures and their motions can be imaged and analyzed. The use of dual techniques also affords the opportunity to visually check the angle of incidence and achieve correct angulation for structure investigation with the M-mode beam at a known anatomic site (Fig. 5-2).

Because 2-D echocardiography precisely demonstrates anatomic structures the extent and use of M-mode formats has declined. Many still use M-mode for taking measurements and for gathering or correlating other data, because M-mode pro-

vides far better time resolution and allows analysis of the temporal relationships of intracardiac events.

## Technique

M-mode is an exacting technique, in spite of the fact that 2-D echocardiography has alleviated some of the difficulties of ensuring that the sound beam is perpendicular to the structures of interest. Now, by simply placing a cursor on the 2-D display so that it passes through the desired structures and then switching to M-mode format, the examiner can be assured that the angle of beam incidence to the target is always 90 degrees. Thus, the most serious pitfall of M-mode echocardiography has essentially been eliminated.

Perpendicularity of the acoustic beam to the structures of interest is a critical factor in all echocardiography techniques; without it, images of structures can be distorted and data derived from them, erroneous. For example, if the left ventricle (LV) is imaged improperly, not only will its dimensions be altered but an abnormal septal wall and abnormal motion will be displayed as well. For these reasons, it is important to use the 2-D image as a guide for placing the M-mode cursor.

It is critical for sonographers to be familiar with normal echo patterns before attempting to deal with the abnormal patterns caused by disease. As with all diagnostic tests, it is also very important to obtain a brief history of the patient's problem before beginning any study.

A routine M-mode study of the heart includes identification and recording of the following structures: mitral valve, aortic valve, left atrium, interventricular septum (IVS), left ventricle, posterior wall of the left ventricle, right ventricle, tricuspid valve, pulmonic valve, and a sweep from the left ventricle to the aorta. The echo characteristics of these various structures are depicted in detail in this chapter. Appropriate measurements must also be taken. (Techniques for measurement are described in Chapter 7.)

It becomes necessary to angulate or change transducer positions in small to moderate increments in order to record all structures of interest. Standard beam directions and transducer placements are demonstrated in Fig. 5-3. These basic approaches may not produce very satisfactory images of the tri-

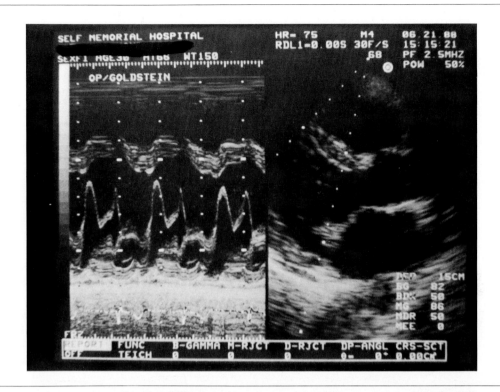

FIGURE 5-2. Split-screen display of an M-mode scan *(left)* and a correlating 2-D image *(right)*. Note M-mode scan plane indicated by cursor.

cuspid and pulmonic valves; detailed instructions for imaging them are presented in Chapters 9 and 10.

To obtain diagnostic quality echocardiograms, attention must be given to the patient's position and breathing during the study. Routine echocardiograms may be recorded with the patient lying supine and breathing normally, but if the sonographer has difficulty obtaining satisfactory scans it may be helpful to examine the patient in the left lateral decubitus (LLD) position and to instruct the patient to suspend breathing at full inspiration.

## M-Mode Protocols

### MITRAL VALVE

This cardiac structure is one of the easiest to recognize. The mitral valve is a strong reflector of sound and exhibits the greatest amplitude of all of the valves. Another identifying feature of the mitral valve is its double or biphasic kick. Conse-

quently, the mitral valve serves as a constant reference point in M-mode examination of the heart (Fig. 5-4).[4,6]

With the transducer placed perpendicular to the chest wall in the third, fourth, or fifth intercostal space (ICS) and along the left sternal border, the search for the mitral valve begins (Fig. 5-5). It is sometimes necessary, if 2-D assistance is not available, to employ slight medial or lateral angulation of the transducer toward the sternum to visualize this valve.

The anterior mitral valve leaflet (AML) usually lies at a depth of 6 to 9 cm from the chest wall (average 7 cm; see Fig. 5-5). With the transducer positioned slightly inferior and lateral, it should be possible to see the valve move 2 to 3 cm toward the anterior wall during systole and then move downward, registering two peaks during diastole. The deflection points in the echo trace of the AML are depicted in Fig. 5-6 as A through F.

The valve opens to a peak at point A by atrial

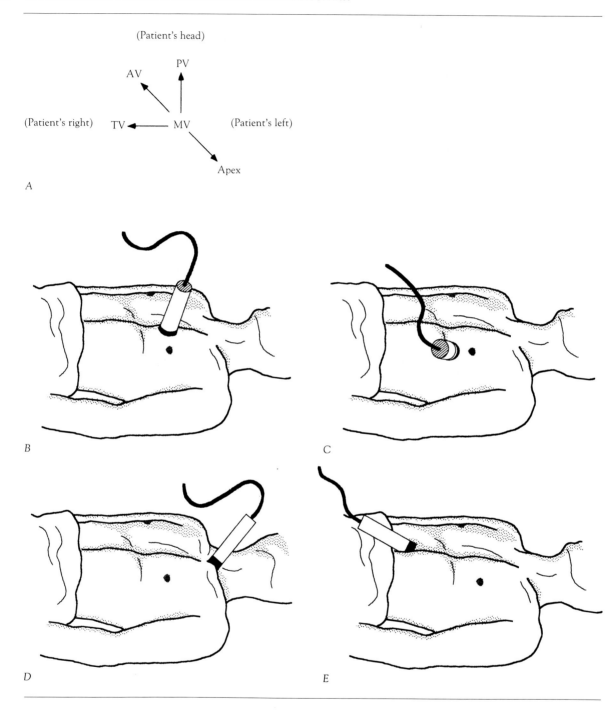

FIGURE 5-3. (A) Structural atlas indicating proper transducer placements for imaging the mitral valve (MV), aortic valve (AV); tricuspid valve (TV); and pulmonic valve (PV). (B) Transducer placement along the left sternal border. (C) Apical transducer placement. (D) Suprasternal transducer placement. (E) Subcostal or subxyphoid transducer placement.

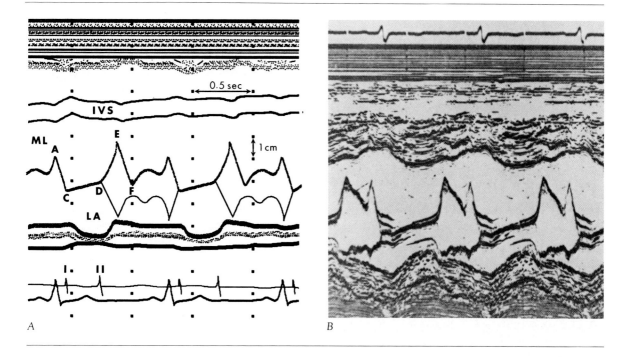

FIGURE 5-4. (A) Schematic representation of an M-mode scan of the mitral valve. (IVS, interventricular septum; ML, mitral leaflet; LA, left atrium; A-F, labeling of mitral leaflet openings and closings.) (B) M-mode scan of the mitral valve.

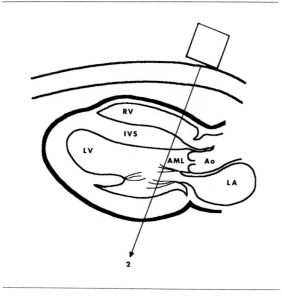

FIGURE 5-5. Schematic representation of ultrasound beam direction during mitral valve scanning. (RV, right ventricle; IVS, interventricular septum; LV, left ventricle; Ao, aorta; LA, left atrium; AML, anterior mitral leaflet.)

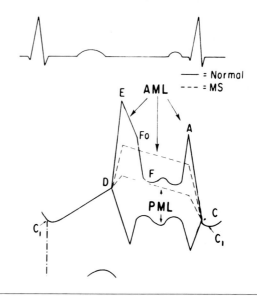

FIGURE 5-6. Labeling of the anterior and posterior mitral valve leaflets as they would appear using M-mode technique.

contraction and begins to close after atrial relaxation. Following ventricular contraction, it closes completely at point C. The valve opens again rapidly after the second heart sound and reaches a peak at point E. Then, the leaflet moves posteriorly, reaching a semiclosed position at point F. The motion pattern observed during this maneuver has been compared to hands clapping.[4]

Behind the AML, in the vicinity of the mitral ring, the left atrial wall is recorded across the left atrial cavity. By directing the transducer inferolaterally from this point it is possible to record the chordae, papillary muscles, left ventricle, and apex of the heart. The mitral ring (or annulus) forms the superior border of the valve, whereas the multiple chordae tendineae attach the anterior and posterior leaflets to the papillary muscle of the left ventricular wall.[1,3,4,7]

### Aortic Valve and Left Atrium

The base of the aorta as it leaves the left ventricle is called the aortic root. It contains three cusps to regulate the flow of blood to the body.[4,6] To properly record the aortic root, semilunar cusps, and left atrial cavity it is necessary to return to the original reference point (the mitral valve) and to direct the transducer superomedially, or toward the patient's right shoulder (Fig. 5-7). In this way it is possible to visualize the AML blending with the posterior aortic wall echoes. The aortic cusps will appear within the two parallel echoes generated by the aortic root.

The area behind the posterior aortic wall represents the left atrial cavity, which can be recognized by its immobile wall.

Although it is easy to record the aortic valve during diastole, in systole recording of echoes from the cusp is made more difficult as they occur less frequently and may appear less defined.[4] It is important to remember that echoes from the aortic root should be parallel and should move upward and anteriorly in systole and downward in diastole. The cusps form a box shape and usually separate approximately 2 cm (16 to 20 mm) during ejection. The anterior echo generally originates from the right coronary cusp and the posterior echo from the noncoronary cusp. The echo appearing in the center of the box represents movement of the left coronary cusp (Fig. 5-8). If difficulty is encountered in imaging cusp movement, it may be helpful to

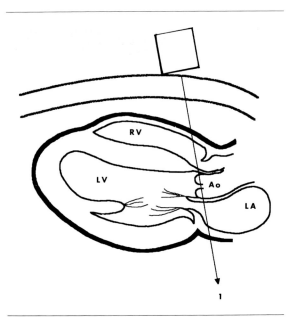

FIGURE 5-7. Schematic representation of ultrasound beam direction during scans of the aortic cusps. (RV, right ventricle; LV, left ventricle; Ao, aorta; LA, left atrium.)

direct the transducer medially, laterally, downward, or upward in small increments. Likewise, if there is any difficulty recording the noncoronary cusp, it is helpful to move the transducer slightly posterolateral and to ask the patient to hold a breath. Other useful maneuvers might be to try other intercostal spaces or to roll the patient onto the left side during the study.[4]

### Left Atrium

The left atrium is located posterior to the aortic root. Measurement of this structure should be made during end-systole. The points to be measured are from the leading edge of the posterior aortic wall to the leading edge of the left atrial wall.

### Left Ventricle, Interventricular Septum, and Posterior Left Ventricular Wall

The transducer should be positioned in the fourth intercostal space at the left sternal border, with the beam directed caudad and slightly to the left (lateral to the mitral valve). As the beam is directed toward the left ventricle, it will cross over the right

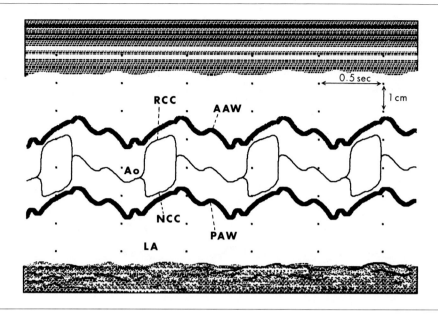

FIGURE 5-8. Schematic representation of an M-mode scan of the aortic valve. (Ao, aorta; RCC, right coronary cusp; NCC, non-coronary cusp; AAW, anterior aortic wall; PAW, posterior aortic wall; LA, left atrium.)

ventricle, the IVS, the left ventricular cavity, and the posterior wall of the left ventricle (Fig. 5-9).[4,5]

The right and left sides of the IVS will be represented as two linear echoes. The thickness of the IVS is represented by the distance between these two lines (Fig. 5-10). In normal patients, this structure lies approximately 4.5 cm from the chest wall and moves posteriorly during systole and anteriorly during diastole. The space behind the IVS represents the left ventricular cavity. In the middle of this cavity, thin echoes, representing the chordae tendineae, are seen during systole, particularly with lowered gain settings.

On the M-mode tracing the posterior wall of the left ventricle is actually made up of echoes emanating from the endocardium and the epicardium. It is important to measure the diameter of the left ventricular cavity at end-diastole and end-systole. The left ventricular wall (LVW) moves anteriorly during systole and posteriorly during diastole. In order to delineate the three layers of the LVW, it may be necessary to reduce the gain settings of the ultrasound system. The strongest moving echoes reflected back to the transducer represent the pericardial echo.[4]

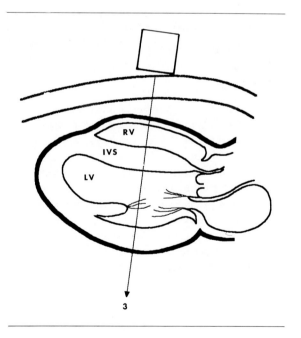

FIGURE 5-9. Schematic representation of ultrasonic beam direction during left ventricle scanning. (RV, right ventricle; IVS, interventricular septum; LV, left ventricle.)

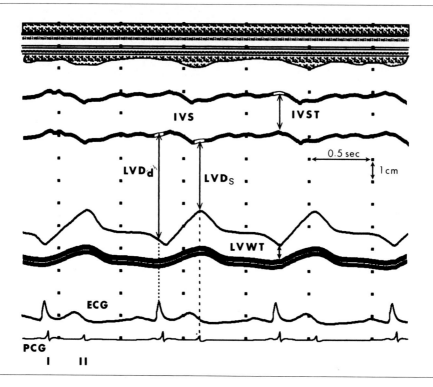

Figure 5-10. Schematic representation of an M-mode scan of the left ventricle. (IVS, interventricular septum; IVST, arrows indicate thickness of the IVS; LVD$_d$, left ventricular dimension at end-diastole; LVD$_s$, left ventricular dimension at end-systole; LVWT, thickness of the left ventricular wall (*arrows*); ECG, electrocardiogram; PCG, phonocardiogram.)

An interesting feature of the left heart is that the IVS and LVW contract during systole and relax during diastole. In the normal heart, the IVS and LVW move toward one another. Paradoxical septal motion indicates that the IVS is moving opposite the left ventricle in systole.

The LVW is composed of endocardium, epicurdium, and pericardium. The endocardium displays a characteristic "notch" that is not evident on the adjacent chordae tendinae (Fig. 5-9)[4] and produces the greatest amplitude of motion in the LV wall vicinity.

### Right Ventricle

As the most anterior chamber of the heart, the right ventricle's anterior wall may be difficult to recognize without lowering the near gain setting of the ultrasound unit. With proper settings, the an-

terior wall of the right ventricle can be recognized as the first *moving* echo, directly beneath the immboile chest wall echoes. Patient position can affect measurement of the right ventricle (see Chapter 7).[7]

### Tricuspid Valve

The tricuspid valve is more difficult to image because it is usually overshadowed by the sternal border. Through the same window that produced the aortic root image the transducer should be angled inferiorly and slightly medial, pointed toward the patient's right foot (Fig. 5-11). Another option is to return to the mitral valve position and angle medially toward it. It is usually the whiplike initial opening of the anterior valve that is recorded in systole and early diastole (Fig. 5-12).[4]

Occasionally, the tricuspid valve is difficult to

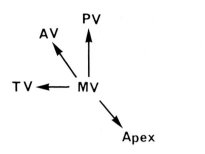

FIGURE 5-11. Interrelationship of cardiac valves and apex of left ventricle. (MV, mitral valve; PV, pulmonary valve; AV, aortic valve; TV, tricuspid valve.)

distinguish from the pulmonic valve. Several facts are helpful in such situations. The tricuspid valve is always inferior and medial to the aortic root, whereas the pulmonic valve is situated more superiorly and laterally. Tricuspid valve motion moves anteriorly during atrial contraction; pulmonic valve motion drops posteriorly.

## PULMONIC VALVE

The pulmonic valve is a semilunar three-cusp valve. Only the left (posterior) cusp can be adequately imaged on M-mode echocardiography, but with 2-D technique, two, and often all three, cusps can be seen. It is best to start imaging at the aortic root, angling superolaterally, toward the patient's left shoulder (the anterior aortic root forms the posterior boundary of the area containing the pulmonic valve). Because the posterior cusp motion of the pulmonic valve is very fleeting, it may be helpful to watch for its parallel motion on an A-mode screen. The M-mode appearance of the pulmonic

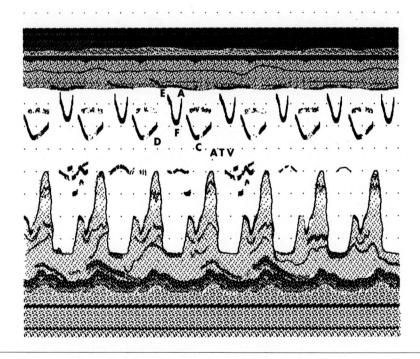

FIGURE 5-12. Schematic representation of an M-mode scan of the tricuspid valve. (ATV, anterior tricuspid valve leaflet; A–C, valve openings and closings.)

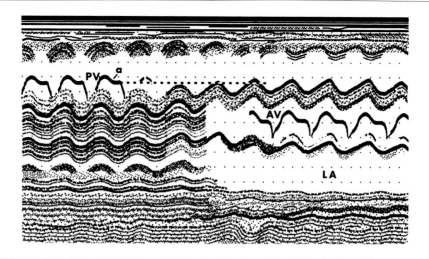

FIGURE 5-13. Schematic representation of an M-mode scan of the pulmonic valve. Note relationship to the aortic valve. (PV, pulmonic valve; AV, aortic valve; LA, left atrium.)

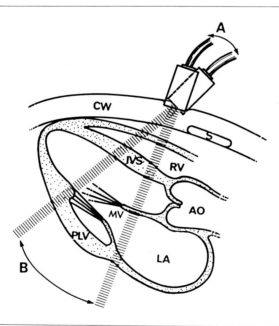

FIGURE 5-14. Schematic representation of the transducer angulations required to perform a sweep from the left ventricle to the aorta. (CW, chest wall; IVS, interventricular septum; RV, right ventricle; S, sternum; AO, aorta; LA, left atrium; PLV, posterior left ventricular wall.) (From Feigenbaum H. Clinical applications of echocardiography. Prog Cardiovasc Dis. 1972; 14:531. By permission of W.B. Saunders Company.)

valve is reminiscent of the aortic cusp. When correctly imaged, the left posterior valve cusp lies posteriorly within the right ventricular outflow space. For patients who are difficult to examine, a change to supine position is sometimes helpful (Fig. 5-13).[4] Moving down to the next intercostal space can also be helpful.

### M-MODE CARDIAC SWEEP

A sweeping scanning motion from the left ventricle to the aortic root is valuable in demonstrating the anatomic continuity of the intracardiac struc-tures (Figs. 5-14 to 5-16). Starting at the apex of the heart with the standard left ventricle view and sweeping up toward the base of the heart, the papillary muscle and chordae tendinae can be seen, changing to the anterior mitral leaflet.

### Conclusion

M-mode echocardiography was used initially as a qualitative technique. With advances in technology it became more widely used in quantitative ways. Although there will be continued reliance in

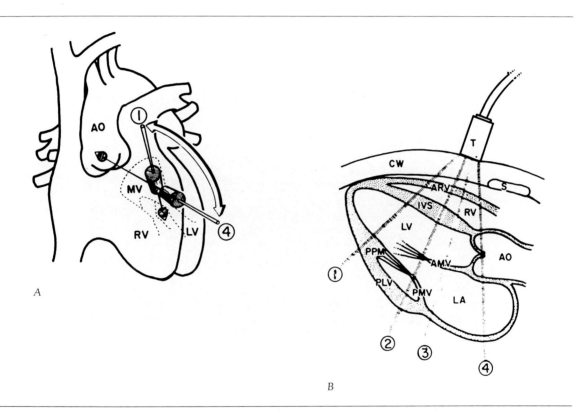

FIGURE 5-15. M-mode scan of sweep from left ventricle to aorta. (A) Angulation of transducer from mitral position to aortic position; (B) structures transected as transducer is angled from mitral valve area to aorta. (AO, aorta; MV, mitral valve; RV, right ventricle; LV, left ventricle; CW, chest wall; T, transducer; ARV, anterior right ventricular wall; PPM, posterior papillary muscle; PLV, posterior left ventricular wall; AMV, anterior mitral valve; PMV, posterior mitral valve; LA, left atrium; S, sternum; IVS, interventricular septum.) (From Feigenbaum H. Clinical applications of echocardiography. Prog Cardiovasc Dis. 1972; 14:531. By permission of W.B. Saunders Company)

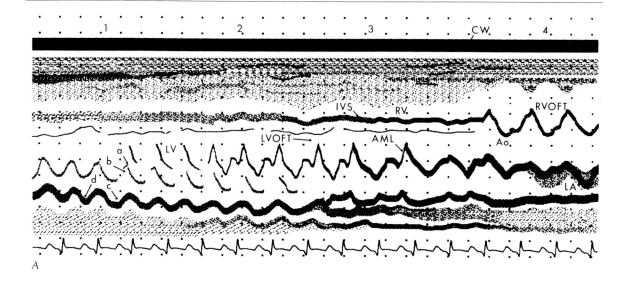

*A*

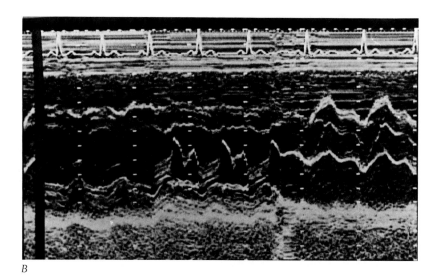

*B*

FIGURE 5-16. Schematic representation of an M-mode scan of the sweep from the left ventricle to the aorta. (IVS, interventricular septum; RV, right ventricle; RVOFT, right ventricular outflow tract; LV, left ventricle; LVOFT, left ventricular outflow tract; AML, anterior mitral leaflet; Ao, aorta; LA, left atrium; a, chordae tendineae; b, endocardium; c, epicardium; d, pericardium.)

measuring and evaluating the heart with 2-D echocardiography, M-mode techniques are assured a place in the diagnostic workup of the patient because the two techniques complement each other. Two-dimensional echocardiography affords better analysis of shape, but it suffers from a limited sampling rate (15 to 60 samples per second of the cardiac structures). M-mode, in contrast, offers a higher sampling rate (500 to 1000 samples per second), yielding continuous and greater accuracy.[3]

Historically, the greatest experience has been with M-mode displays. With the advent of 2-D echocardiography and cardiac Doppler techniques, echocardiographers are faced with the obligation to employ whatever techniques will provide the answers to clinical questions.

## References

1. Chang S. M-Mode Echocardiographic Technique and Pattern Recognition. Philadelphia: Lea & Febiger; 1982.
2. Chang S, Feigenbaum H, Dillon R. Condensed M-mode echo scan of the symmetrical left ventricle. CHART. 1975; 00:68–93.
3. Feigenbaum H. Echocardiography. 3d ed. Philadelphia: Lea & Febiger; 1981.
4. Hagen-Ansert S. Textbook of Diagnostic Ultrasonography. 2d ed. St. Louis: CV Mosby; 1983.
5. Omoto R, Kobayashi M (eds). Atlas of Essential Ultrasound Imaging. Tokyo: Igaku-Shoin; 1981.
6. Salcedo E. Atlas of Echocardiography. Philadelphia: WB Saunders; 1978.
7. Weyman AE. Cross-Sectional Echocardiography. Philadelphia: Lea & Febiger; 1981.

CHAPTER **6**

# Two-Dimensional and Doppler Echocardiography

PAMELA HARRIGAN

Over the past 20 years ultrasound technology has evolved and expanded considerably. As a result, the echocardiographic examination now consists of a series of subprocedures designed to take advantage of technical developments in M-mode and two-dimensional (2-D)-echocardiography and in spectral Doppler and color-flow mapping. Examiners are required to integrate many varieties of anatomic and physiologic data in order to appropriately demonstrate normal and pathologic conditions.

At one time M-mode was the only ultrasound modality available to examine the heart. Although the examination was technically straightforward, it was diagnostically quite limited. Because it involved only a single beam of ultrasound swept manually through cardiac structures, the examiner was required to mentally reconstruct three-dimensional anatomy by analyzing the strip chart recordings. Physiologic information was gathered inferentially, by relating the M-mode patterns to certain physiologic events, such as diastolic fluttering of the mitral valve in aortic regurgitation, decreased diastolic closure rate of the anterior mitral leaflet in decreased left ventricular diastolic compliance, and decreased excursion of the mitral and aortic valves in low-flow states. As only one-dimensional images were available, this technique was clearly limited in its ability to image cardiac anatomy, a particular disadvantage in conditions in which

morphology is markedly abnormal such as congenital heart disease.

Because 2-D echocardiography allows examination of tomographic slices of cardiac anatomy and is a clearly superior method of defining spatial relationships, it has dramatically enhanced the diagnostic usefulness of echocardiography. The structural information provided by 2-D echocardiography is complemented by Doppler spectral analysis and color-flow mapping, which permits a dynamic assessment of the direction and velocity of blood flow. The latter techniques allow assessment of the hemodynamic state by estimates of intracardiac pressures and gradients.

Modern echocardiography involves applying all these imaging modalities. The operator is required to have a thorough understanding of the techniques and information being generated. Also, as the examination is often tailored to specific issues or abnormalities detected along the way, the examiner is required to make interpretive decisions as the study is being performed. All this requires a familiarity with normal findings and knowledge of cardiac pathophysiology. In this sense, echocardiography differs from most medical technical procedures. Although this makes performance of a good echocardiographic examination technically demanding, it also makes it very rewarding, because a great variety of pathophysiologic information can be gathered from this noninvasive technique.

## Examination Technique: An Integrative Approach

The sequence and manner in which imaging is performed and Doppler information is acquired and recorded varies considerably from institution to institution. Generally, an integrative approach is preferable to a fractionated one because it allows the examiner to better use the acquired information to tailor and specialize the examination to the observed abnormalities. Examinations can fall short, diagnostically, if the operator regards the study as merely a series of views or Doppler samplings without considering the significance of the physiologic information that is obtained and how it fits into the clinical problem that is being addressed. In order to establish consistency, views can be obtained in a specific order from each patient. After a view is visualized in detail for the purpose of recording *anatomic* information, the Doppler examination is performed in the same view to add *physiologic* information. When that view has been assessed completely, the examination proceeds to the next view and the procedure is repeated. In this way, echocardiographic data is correlated in an efficient manner and an understanding of the relationship between anatomy and physiology is achieved.

### EQUIPMENT AND PATIENT PREPARATION

The importance of proper equipment maintenance cannot be overstated. Any change in equipment performance or in the quality of displayed images should be noted, and regular preventive maintenance by the manufacturer is essential. This helps prevent gradual deterioration of study quality due to technical factors and helps avoid significant down time due to equipment failure.

Ideally, the operator can choose from a variety of transducers of different frequencies and focal depths, in order to maximize the amount of information obtained from each patient. Generally, the 2-D study is best carried out with the highest-frequency transducer that allows imaging in the patient under study and the Doppler examination with a lower-frequency transducer. In most adult studies, a 2.5- or 3.5-MHz transducer is adequate for both purposes. In pediatric studies, a 5-MHz transducer gives better image quality and is often adequate for Doppler analysis, although occasion-ally a 3.5- or 2.5-MHz transducer may be necessary to optimize Doppler data.

After the transducer has been selected, consideration must be given to how to position the patient so as to optimize the position of the heart within the chest and the availability of acoustic windows. A small proportion of adult patients can be scanned best in the supine position, but with the majority of adults optimal visualization of cardiac structures is obtained with the patient rotated into the left lateral decubitus position. Elevating the head sometimes is helpful. The patient's left arm should be tucked upward under the head so that it does not interfere with positioning of the transducer. The patient's right arm lies along the right side. Because optimal patient positioning increases the probability of producing a high-quality study, it should be exploited to its fullest by positioning each patient as necessary to enhance the findings of the study.

Patient respiration has multiple effects on cardiac parameters imaged by echocardiography, and in some patients the orientation of the heart and lungs in the chest is such that images of the heart can be obtained only at certain points in the respiratory cycle. It may be necessary to have the patient suspend respiration at certain points during the cycle so that images can be obtained. In addition, the physiologic effects of respiration on blood flow and chamber size can be used to diagnostic advantage in certain conditions. Generally, image quality in the parasternal and apical views improves with deflation of the lungs. In the subcostal position, deep, sustained inspiration displaces the heart downward and often brings it into a more optimal position for viewing.

### TRANSDUCER MANIPULATION

In most echocardiography systems, the plane of the 2-D sector scan is indicated by a marker located on the transducer that corresponds to that aspect of the sector plane that is displayed on the right side of the image.

Three aspects of transducer orientation are important to achieving optimal 2-D images: (1) *positioning*, to locate the best imaging sites; (2) *angulation*, to image structures of interest; and (3) *rotation*, to fine-tune the image. Each of these maneuvers must be adjusted constantly by the examiner throughout the procedure, and will be subsequently discussed for each 2-D view.

After acoustic gel has been applied liberally to the left sternal area and the transducer face, the transducer is placed along the left parasternum. It is important to map the entire left parasternum as completely as possible as the examination begins, in order to locate the best imaging sites. One approach is to begin with the transducer along the left sternal edge, below the clavicle. The transducer should be moved laterally, toward the shoulder, then down an intercostal space and back toward the sternum, then down another intercostal space and back toward the axilla. This pattern is repeated from the level of the clavicle to the lower sternal edge, so that the operator can assess imaging sites from the entire left parasternum. In this way, the operator is assured of exploring all potentially useful imaging sites, can concentrate on areas that produce optimal images, and avoids spending too much time attempting to manipulate a view that is not adequate.

Even if a reasonably good picture is obtained on the initial attempt, the examiner should not be reluctant to experiment with variations in transducer alignment. This willingness to explore multiple combinations of transducer adjustments significantly increases the number of successful examinations. It is by modifying the standard views that the examiner's repertoire expands and maximum clinical benefit is obtained. Individual variations in heart size and position, window availability, and distortion of anatomy by disease make firm rules of examination impossible and demand flexibility on the part of the examiner.

## Parasternal Long-Axis Views

### LEFT SIDE OF THE HEART

In most cases, the parasternal long-axis view of the left side of the heart is optimized when the transducer is in the third, fourth, or fifth intercostal space along the left sternal border. The acoustic beam is perpendicular to the chest wall. With the reference marker oriented toward the right shoulder, the scan plane is oriented along a plane running from the right shoulder to the left hip. This produces an image that incorporates the left ventricular outflow tract and aorta on the right side of

the sector display, the mitral valve near the center of the image, and the ventricular structures inferior to the mitral valve along the left side of the sector. This long-axis view of the left side of the heart allows observation of both the inflow tract and the outflow tract of the left ventricle. Figure 6-1 illustrates the anatomy imaged in this view.

In the ideal cross-sectional image of the parasternal long-axis view of the left side of the heart, the transducer is positioned so that the interventricular septum is the same distance from the transducer as the anterior aortic root. In this way both are roughly perpendicular to the sound beam, as is the posterior wall of the heart. M-mode tracings should be taken from this scan plane. If this optimal acoustic window is not accessible in a given patient (or as an adjunct to the standard view), the transducer can be positioned in a lower intercostal space. In this case, the apical half of the interventricular septum is closer to the transducer (closer to the top of the sector on the image), and the aortic root appears to be deeper in the image (Fig. 6-2). This view often permits optimal visualization of the left ventricular structures, but it is not appropriate for some short-axis views.

Once the optimal parasternal long-axis view of the left side of the heart is obtained, varying transducer angulation and rotation permits the examiner to image other aspects of cardiac anatomy. For example, mediolateral angulation and slight rotation of the scan plane in the image permits the examiner to (1) visualize the pulmonary venous entry into the left atrium, (2) optimize opening excursion of the mitral and aortic valves, and (3) visualize the left ventricular papillary muscles and chordal structures. Superior and inferior angulation of the scan plane in this image permits (1) recording of a larger extent of the ascending aorta, (2) improved visualization of the left atrial cavity, and (3) visualization of the apical half of the left ventricle.

Figure 6-3 illustrates the movement of the cardiac structures throughout the cardiac cycle in a normal patient as viewed from the parasternal long-axis perspective. At the onset of diastole (frame A), the mitral valve opens wide to permit rapid filling, and the left ventricle relaxes to accept the incoming blood. The aortic valve is closed. In middiastole (frame B), the mitral leaflets float toward each other as early filling slows. Having filled

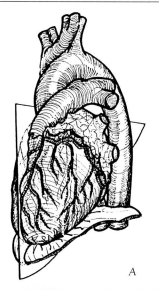

FIGURE 6-1. (A) Schema of scan plane through the heart in the parasternal long-axis view of the left side of the heart (B). In this standard view, the transducer is positioned so that the acoustic beam is perpendicular to the ventricular septum (VS) and left ventricular posterior wall (PW). Note that the anterior wall of the aortic root (ao) is the same distance from the transducer (represented by the top of the sector triangle) as the ventricular septum. The small arrow points to the coronary sinus; the large arrow to the descending thoracic aorta (LA, left atrium; LV, left ventricle; RV, right ventricle; MV, mitral valve). (Harrigan P, Lee R. Principles of Interpretation in Echocardiography. New York: John Wiley & Sons; 1985.)

A

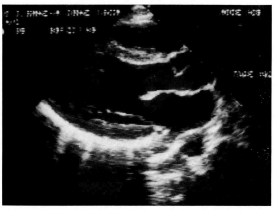

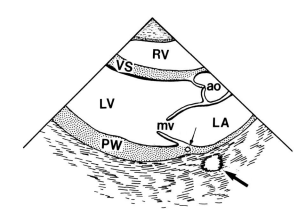

B

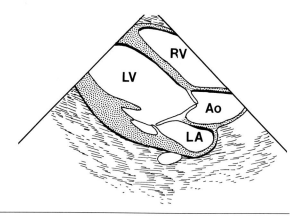

FIGURE 6-2. Parasternal long-axis view from a relatively low transducer position. Note that the acoustic beam is no longer perpendicular to the major intracardiac structures, but more of the left ventricular cavity is available for imaging (Ao, aorta; LA, left atrium; LV, left ventricle; RV, right ventricle).

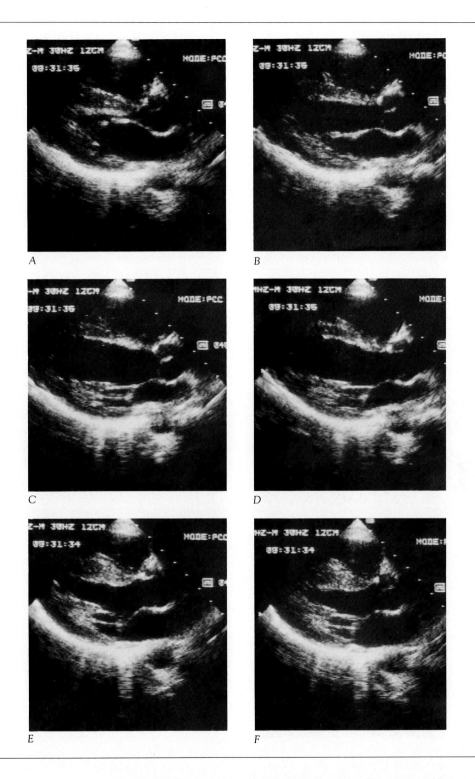

FIGURE 6-3. The sequence of cardiac motion from the parasternal long-axis orientation. (A) Early and (B) mid-diastole. (C) Isovolumic contraction phase of systole. (D) Early and (E) end ejection phases of systole. (F) Isovolumic relaxation.

with blood, the left ventricle expands. The left atrial dimension is reduced somewhat, because it is now emptying. After atrial systole and slight reopening of the mitral valve (frame C), ventricular systole ensues and the mitral leaflets close. This frame represents the period of isovolumic contraction, when the left ventricle has not yet generated enough pressure to open the aortic cusps. When left ventricular pressure exceeds that in the aorta (frame D), the aortic cusps open and ejection commences. During systole, the left ventricular myocardium thickens, decreasing the internal dimension of that chamber. Note that (from frames C to E) the mitral annulus, particularly the posterior portion, is drawn inferiorly and slightly anteriorly. Left atrial filling has resulted in expansion of that chamber. At end-systole, when the myocardium is thickest and the left ventricular dimension is smallest, ejection slackens and the aortic valve closes. During isovolumic relaxation (frame E), left ventricular pressure falls below that in the left atrium, coincident with rapid, early filling of the left ventricle (as seen in frame A). Figure 6-4 illus-

trates some measurements commonly taken on images made through the parasternal long-axis view.[2]

### COLOR-FLOW IMAGING AND DOPPLER SPECTRAL ANALYSIS

Doppler assessment of flow velocities across the mitral and aortic valves is not optimized in this view, as the direction of these flows is almost perpendicular to the sound beam. However, a qualitative impression can be obtained that is useful in detecting normal and abnormal flow patterns (Fig. 6-5). Abnormal turbulent flow resulting from either mitral or aortic regurgitation can be observed in this view. In the case of mitral regurgitation, abnormal flow is observed behind the mitral leaflets into the left atrium in systole. With aortic regurgitation, the abnormal flow occurs in diastole and is located in the left ventricular outflow tract.

Other flows that can be appreciated in this view with slight alterations of the scan plane include normal pulmonary venous inflow to the left atrium, shunt flow due to ventricular septal defects, turbulent left ventricular inflow due to mitral stenosis, and abnormal inflow and regurgitant patterns secondary to valve prostheses.

It is important to note that the 2-D image may be significantly altered when the color map is optimized. When utilizing Doppler the examiner must focus only on the flow information rather than on the quality of the 2-D image.

In performing Doppler spectral analysis it is often helpful to use the color-flow image as a guide

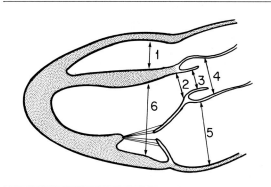

FIGURE 6-4. Cross-sectional measurements obtained from the pasternal long axis view.

| | | |
|---|---|---|
| 1. | right ventricular internal dimension in diastole | 25 to 38 mm |
| 2. | aortic annulus | 16 to 26 mm |
| 3. | aorta at level of sinuses of Valsalva | 24 to 39 mm |
| 4. | aorta at level of sinotubular junction | 21 to 34 mm |
| 5. | left atrial anteroposterior dimension (end-systole) | 25 to 38 mm |
| 6. | left ventricular internal dimension at end-diastole and end-systole | 37 to 53 mm  23 to 36 mm |

FIGURE 6-5. (See color insert for parts C and D.) (A) ▶ Parasternal long-axis view during systole, with the Doppler sample volume positioned behind the mitral leaflets to examine for mitral regurgitation. (B) In this diastolic image this Doppler sample volume was positioned in the left ventricular outflow tract to assess for aortic regurgitation. Color-flow map in diastole (C) and systole (D) from the parasternal long-axis perspective. Although the direction of flow relative to the acoustic beam is not optimal for qualitative assessments, qualitative judgments regarding the characteristics of flow can be made. Note the absence of turbulent flow behind the mitral valve in systole in this normal patient (Ao, aorta; LA, left atrium; MV, mitral valve).

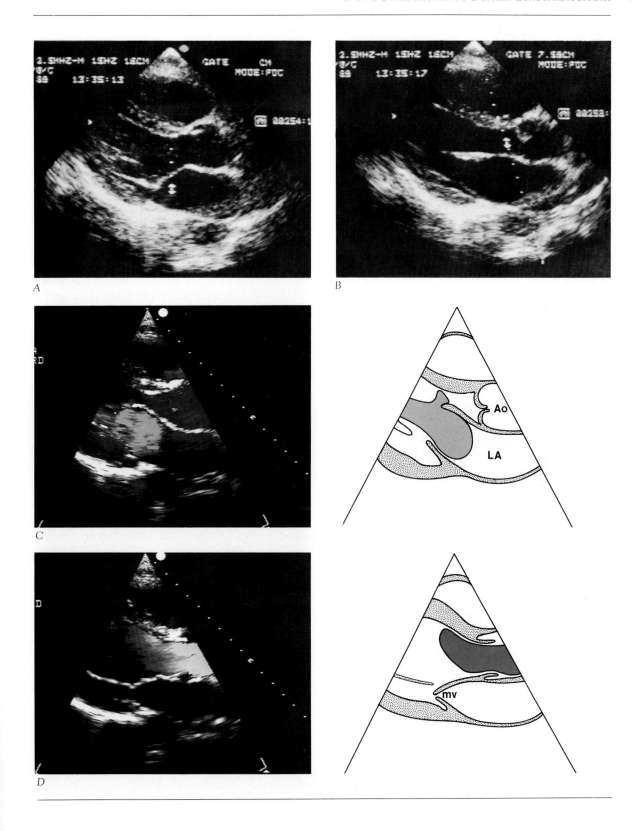

*A*

*B*

*C*

*D*

Ao

LA

mv

for sample volume placement. To sample for the turbulence of mitral regurgitation, the sample volume is placed immediately behind the coaptation point of the mitral leaflets in the left atrium. *It is important to listen carefully to the audio component of the Doppler signal and to use the sounds as a guide while moving the sample volume in the area of interest.* Care must be taken to sample as thoroughly as possible behind the valve to rule out abnormal flow. In certain valve lesions, the regurgitant jet may have an unusual direction or may change its direction with time. Careful sampling is required to avoid missing these jets.

The same technique is used for the aortic valve. The sample volume is positioned just below the coaptation point of the cusps in the left ventricular outflow tract and is moved by the operator into different positions below the valve in order to capture possible abnormal flow. Once regurgitation of either the mitral or aortic valve is found, the sample volume should be moved farther and farther from the valve to document the depth and width of the area of turbulence.

Whenever possible, is it useful to combine color-flow mapping and Doppler spectral tracings. The color map can be used first to document the presence of a particular flow and to obtain information on its direction and magnitude. Spectral tracings then permit observation of the velocity distribution within the flow of interest. If a particular flow has a sufficiently high peak velocity to produce aliasing on the pulsed Doppler spectral tracing, the peak velocity can only be quantitated with a continuous-wave Doppler approach. Either an image-guided transducer or one that has a dedicated continuous-wave probe can be used. The continuous-wave Doppler examination usually is not useful in the standard parasternal long-axis view of the left side of the heart, since most flow is perpendicular to the Doppler beam. An exception is the flow associated with ventricular septal defect, which, in many cases, travels axial to the transducer; in such cases velocities can be documented accurately. Table 6-1 illustrates the velocities detected by Doppler in normal adult hearts.

## THE RIGHT VENTRICULAR INFLOW TRACT

Because the anatomy of the normal right ventricle makes it impossible to visualize the inflow tract and

TABLE 6-1. Normal Doppler velocities in normal adults

| STRUCTURE | AVERAGE VELOCITY (RANGE) (M/SEC) |
| --- | --- |
| Mitral valve | 0.90 (0.6–1.3) |
| Tricuspid valve | 0.50 (0.3–0.7) |
| Pulmonary valve | 0.75 (0.6–0.9) |
| Aortic valve | 1.35 (1.0–1.7) |

(From Hatle L, Angelsen B. Doppler Ultrasound in Cardiology. 2nd ed. Philadelphia: Lea & Febiger, 1985.)

the outflow tract in the same scan plane, each area of the right ventricle must be visualized separately. The long-axis view of the right ventricular inflow tract is obtained by slight clockwise rotation and inferomedial angulation from the parasternal long-axis view of the left side of the heart. In order to omit any left heart structures from the image, this angulation may have to be quite acute. Occasionally, this view is optimized by moving to a window slightly inferior and lateral to the window that provided optimal images of the left side of the heart. This orientation permits visualization of the right atrium, tricuspid valve apparatus, and inflow portion of the right ventricle. Often, the mouth of the inferior vena cava is also seen. This is an excellent view for assessing the morphology of the tricuspid valve (Fig. 6-6).

The color-flow image reveals diastolic flow across the tricuspid valve toward the transducer encoded in shades of red (Fig. 6-7). If there is any degree of tricuspid regurgitation, the retrograde turbulent flow can be seen as shades of blue, yellow, and green behind the tricuspid leaflets. Often, caval flow is documented; it can be red if the velocity is relatively low, or a mosaic pattern if velocity is high. Other abnormal flow patterns that can be observed in this view include that of atrial septal defect, which appears as turbulence within the right atrium, and that of ventricular septal defect, which appears as turbulence within the right ventricle. Tricuspid stenosis and prostheses can also be examined with Doppler imaging from this view.

Spectral analysis is done in a similar fashion to the examination of the mitral valve. The sample volume is placed first immediately behind the valve, to document any possible trace of regurgitation. The sample volume is then moved carefully

FIGURE 6-6. (A) Schema of the scan plane through the heart in the parasternal long-axis view of the right ventricular inflow tract (B). In this systolic image the entrance of the inferior vena cava (ivc) is seen entering the right atrium (RA). (C) Diastole (atl, anterior tricuspid leaflet; ptl, posterior tricuspid leaflet; RV, right ventricle). (Harrigan P, Lee R. Principles of Interpretation in Echocardiography. New York: John Wiley & Sons; 1985.)

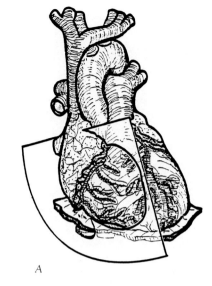

A

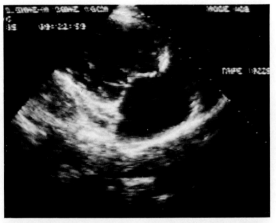

B

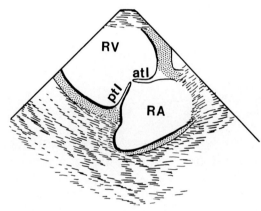

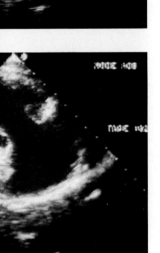

C

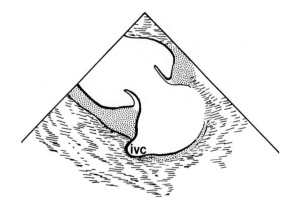

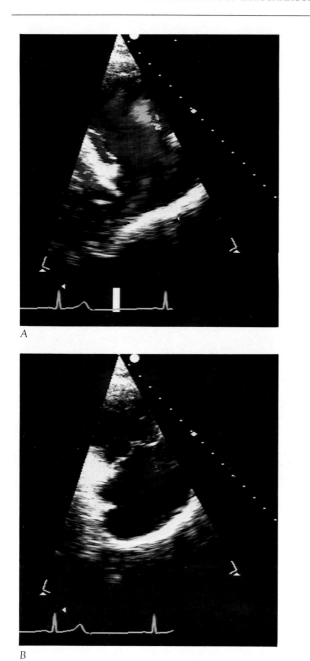

A

B

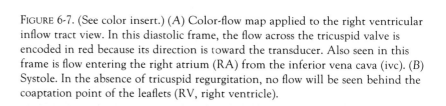

FIGURE 6-7. (See color insert.) (A) Color-flow map applied to the right ventricular inflow tract view. In this diastolic frame, the flow across the tricuspid valve is encoded in red because its direction is toward the transducer. Also seen in this frame is flow entering the right atrium (RA) from the inferior vena cava (ivc). (B) Systole. In the absence of tricuspid regurgitation, no flow will be seen behind the coaptation point of the leaflets (RV, right ventricle).

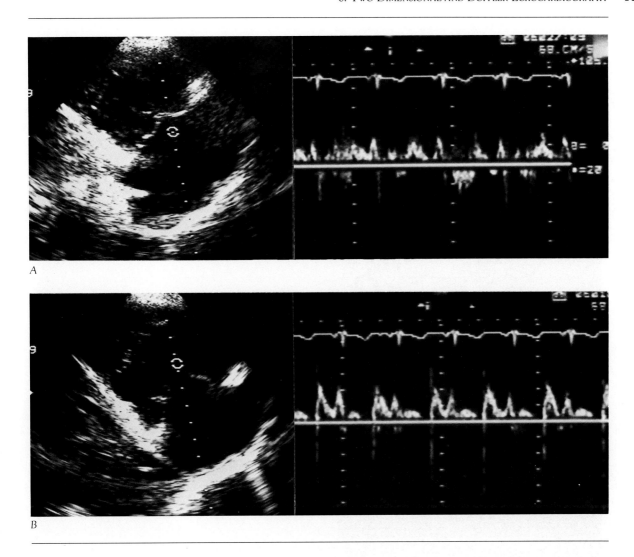

FIGURE 6-8. Pulsed-wave Doppler spectral tracings of tricuspid valve flow. (A) Sample volume in right atrium behind the coaptation of the leaflets reveals the prevalvular velocities and tricuspid regurgitation, if present. (B) Sample volume positioned at peak opening of the leaflets to record the peak velocity across the valve. See Table 6-1 for normal values.

and methodically within the chamber behind the valve to assess the size of any abnormal regurgitant jet. Timing the flow in the right atrium helps differentiate tricuspid regurgitation, caval inflow, and atrial septal defect. The sample volume is then positioned on the forward flow side of the tricuspid valve in the right ventricle in order to demonstrate the peak velocity and optimal flow profile of tri-

cuspid diastolic flow. Once again, the sample volume must be placed in a variety of positions to ensure complete inspection. Figure 6-8 demonstrates the tricuspid valve flow profile of a normal heart. With this scan plane orientation, flow across the tricuspid valve is toward the transducer in diastole. Therefore, the spectral tracing demonstrates positive displacement above the baseline. The rapid

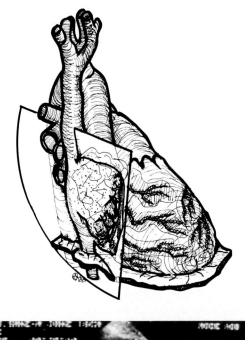

FIGURE 6-9. (A) Schema of the scan plane through the heart in (B) the parasternal long-axis view of the right ventricular outflow tract (rvot). In this diastolic frame, the pulmonary valve (PV) and main pulmonary artery (MPA) are recorded. (C) Systole.

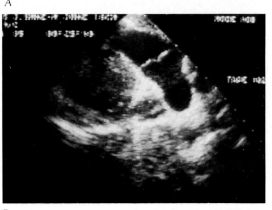

*A*

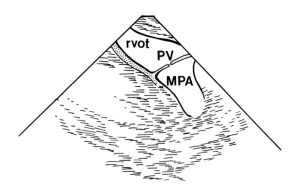

*B*

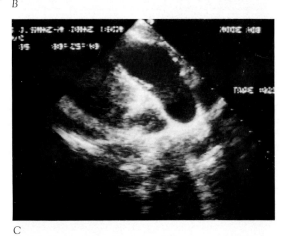

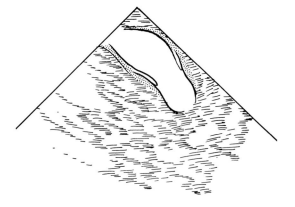

*C*

filling phase of diastole, as well as the additional inflow coincident with atrial contraction, produces two velocity peaks of blood flow. The exact pattern varies according to heart rate, flow volume, the relative compliances of the atria and ventricles as well as other factors.

THE RIGHT VENTRICULAR OUTFLOW TRACT

The long-axis view of the right ventricular outflow tract has two components: the proximal right ventricular outflow tract and pulmonary valve and the distal right ventricular outflow tract (pulmonary artery bifurcation). Images of the proximal right ventricular outflow tract can be obtained by slight clockwise rotation and superolateral angulation of the transducer from the position for a parasternal long-axis view of the aorta. The view can sometimes be improved by positioning the transducer at an intercostal space higher than that which optimized viewing of the left side of the heart. Variations of this view can be made by locating the transducer within inferior intercostal spaces and maintaining the original angulation and plane position. Visualization of the right ventricular infundibulum, pulmonary valve, and main pulmonary artery can be obtained (Fig. 6-9). Often two of the pulmonary valve cusps are seen, making this a very useful view for assessing pulmonary valve structure and function. Pulmonary valve morphology, infundibular stenosis, and pulmonary artery dilatation or hypoplasia are examples of anatomic information revealed in this view.

In this plane, the color-flow image reveals the systolic flow in the pulmonary artery, encoded in shades of blue. If any degree of pulmonary insufficiency is present, a turbulent jet encoded in shades of red, yellow, and green is observed in diastole (Fig. 6-10). Careful maneuvering of the scan plane may be necessary to document the small jets, which are quite common in normal subjects. Spectral tracings can be recorded by placing the sample volume immediately behind the pulmonary valve in the right ventricular outflow tract and carefully mapping to document the presence or absence of pulmonary regurgitation. Peak forward velocities are then obtained by placing the sample volume on the forward flow side of the pulmonary valve in the main pulmonary artery (Fig. 6-11). With the sample volume positioned at the level of the pulmo-

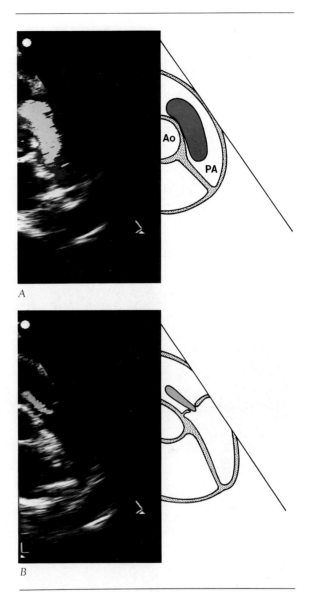

FIGURE 6-10. (See color insert.) Color-flow map applied to the right ventricular outflow tract view. (A) Systolic view reveals flow across the pulmonary valve into the pulmonary artery (PA), which is encoded in shades of blue, because of its direction away from the transducer. (B) Diastolic frame demonstrates pulmonary regurgitation that is commonly seen in normal patients (Ao, aorta).

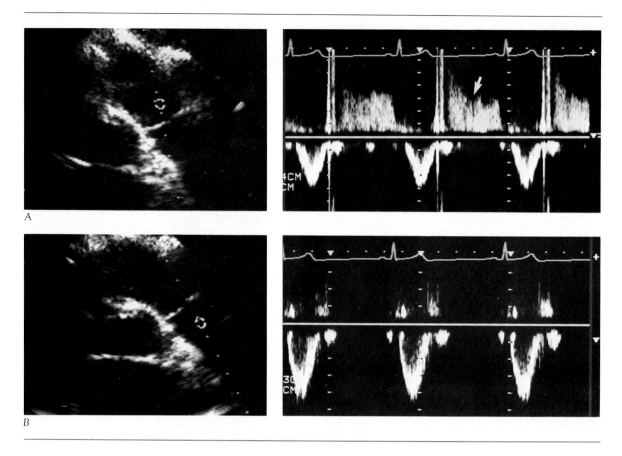

FIGURE 6-11. Pulsed-wave Doppler spectral tracings of pulmonary valve flow. *(A)* Sample volume placed in the right ventricular outflow tract behind the coaptation point of the leaflets to record the prevalvular velocities and any pulmonary regurgitation that may be present *(arrow).* *(B)* Sample volume is placed within the pulmonary artery just distal to the tips of the valve leaflets to record the peak velocity.

nary valve from the parasternal perspective, flow is away from the transducer in systole. Negative displacement of the spectrum is recorded in systole. Again, it is important to select a variety of positions from which to visualize this flow in order to find the optimal signal. The physiologic information obtained in this view includes pulmonary regurgitation, high-velocity flow across a stenotic pulmonary valve, shunt flow across a supracristal ventricular septal defect, and flow disturbance in the main pulmonary artery from pulmonary stenosis or persistent patent ductus arteriosus.

With further clockwise rotation and more marked superior angulation from the proximal right ventricular outflow tract view the beam can be oriented to pass through the long axis of the more distal aspects of the pulmonary artery. The pulmonary valve sometimes is not recorded optimally in this view, but the relative size of the aorta and pulmonary artery can be studied, as well as the anatomy of the right and left pulmonary arteries as they bifurcate from the main pulmonary artery. Occasionally persistent patent ductus arteriosus can be identified as it joins the proximal left pulmonary artery. This view is especially helpful when using color flow mapping and spectral Doppler to

FIGURE 6-12. (A) Schema of the scan plane through the heart in the parasternal long-axis view of the distal main pulmonary artery (MPA). The bifurcation to the right pulmonary artery (rpa) and left pulmonary artery (lpa) can be recorded. The relationship of the pulmonary artery and its branches with the ascending aorta (aao) and descending aorta (dao) can be appreciated. (Harrigan P, Lee R. Principles of Interpretation in Echocardiography. New York: John Wiley & Sons; 1985.)

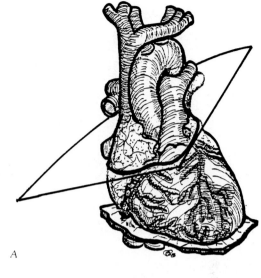

A

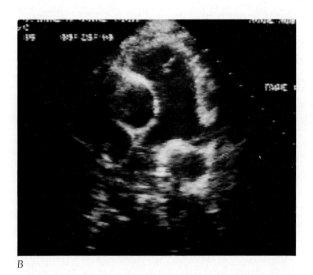

B

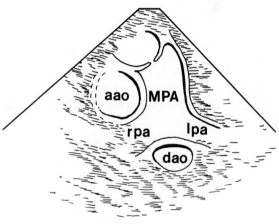

assess the presence of ductal flow. Note that in this view, the short axis of the descending thoracic aorta is visualized between the two pulmonary branches (Fig. 6-12).

## Parasternal Short-Axis Views

As the scan plane has been gradually rotated clockwise to record the distal pulmonary artery, it has now essentially come around into a short-axis orientation relative to the aorta and ventricles. Therefore, the operator can now continue the study with examination of the short-axis views. The parasternal short-axis views are perpendicular to the left ventricular long axis. The transducer position is often identical to the one that was established for optimal parasternal long-axis visualization, and transducer angulation may be similar or identical to that used for long-axis imaging.

Rotation is the parameter of transducer alignment that requires the greatest change in the transition from parasternal long-axis to short-axis scanning. As we have seen, the direction of rotation is clockwise from the long-axis orientation. This ori-

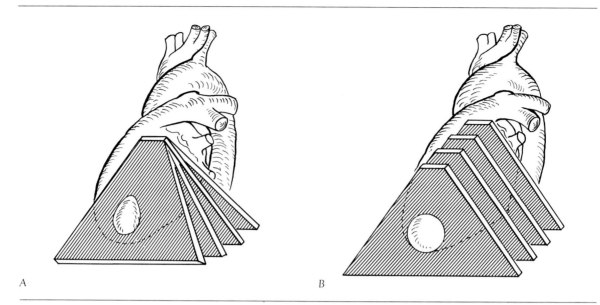

A                                          B

FIGURE 6-13. Schematic drawing illustrating the two methods of short-axis imaging of the heart. (A) Tilting permits appreciation of the anatomic continuity of structures but may result in oblique cuts. (B) "Bread-loafing" assures a perpendicular relationship between the acoustic beam and the structures of interest. Illustrated here is the left ventricle; however, this technique is applicable to the structures at the base of the heart as well.

entation causes the sector aspect that had previously been superior and medial (visualizing the aorta) to be rotated to the patient's left. The plane marker on the transducer will now be directed generally toward the patient's left shoulder.

The operator should employ two maneuvers in order to scan through the short axis of the heart: (1) the transducer in a fixed *position* can change the *angle* to pass the beam through different areas and (2) incrementally move the transducer to different levels of tissue in order to "bread loaf" the area of interest. Both maneuvers are important. The first may optimize appreciation of the anatomic continuity of intracardiac structures; the second ensures that the sound beam is perpendicular to the structures under study, an ideal orientation for imaging spatial resolution (Fig. 6-13).

### PROXIMAL CORONARY ARTERIES

As the scan plane, which has previously been angled superiorly toward the pulmonary artery bifurcation, is angled inferiorly toward the aortic valve,

it may pass through the proximal right and left coronary arteries (Fig. 6-14). Sometimes only the ostia are visualized; in other cases, several centimeters of these vessels can be seen. Often slight clockwise rotation of the scan plane improves visualization. This view is important for assessing for anomalous origins of the right or left coronary arteries, coronary artery dilatation secondary to aortic regurgitation or to such entities as Kawasaki's disease, and coronary artery fistula.

### THE AORTA AND BASAL STRUCTURES

As the scan plane is angled slightly inferiorly, or if the transducer is moved to a slightly inferior position, the short axis of the aortic valve is seen. In many cases, continuous visualization of the full extent of aortic valve motion requires that the transducer be placed in a more inferolateral position in order to look upward into the left ventricular outflow tract at the valve. If this maneuver is employed, it is important to return the transducer to its original position when examining inferior left-

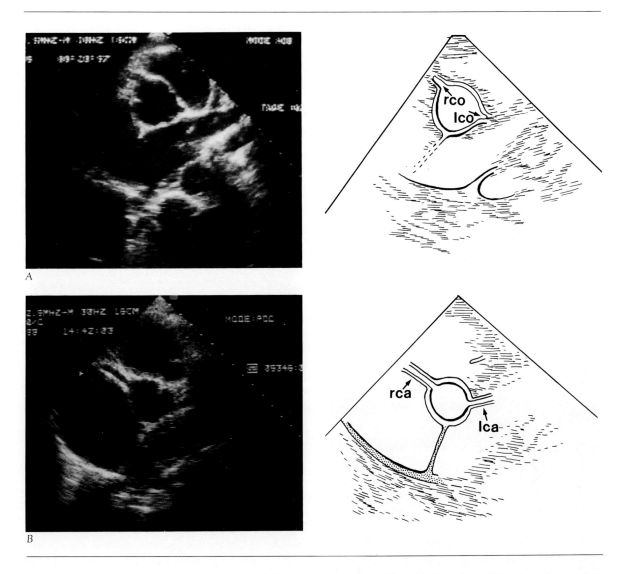

FIGURE 6-14. (A) Parasternal short-axis view of the aorta revealing the right and left coronary artery ostia (rco, lco). (B) Occasionally longer segments of the right and left coronary arteries are recorded (rca, lca).

sided heart structures (mitral valve and left ventricle).

The short axis of the aortic root can be seen as a circular structure within which the aortic cusps are visualized. In diastole, the closed cusps form a Y shape. In systole, the orifice is roughly triangular. In normal to high-output states, a more rounded appearance may be noted; in low-output states, a smaller, more defined triangular shape may be present. Figure 6-15 illustrates this view, with the associated surrounding anatomy. The left atrium is noted posterior to the aorta, often with good visualization of the left atrial appendage. The interatrial septum can be seen separating the two atria, while portions of the tricuspid valve can be seen between the right atrium and right ventricular outflow tract. The pulmonary valve is seen at the root of the main pulmonary artery.

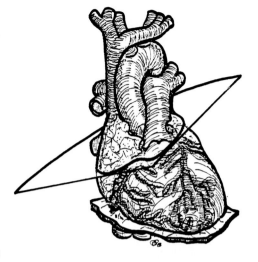

A

Figure 6-15. (A) Schema of the scan plane through the heart in the parasternal short-axis view of the aortic root, aortic valve, and surrounding structures (B). (C) In systole, the aortic orifice is visualized and the pulmonary cusp has moved out of the sound beam. The left atrial appendage (laa) is often visualized as the scan plane is moved inferiorly from the level of the sinotubular junction to the aortic valve level (RA, right atrium; ias, interatrial septum; LA, left atrium; rvot, right ventricular outflow tract; pv, pulmonary valve; r, right coronary cusp; n, noncoronary cusp; l, left coronary cusp). (Harrigan P, Lee R. Principles of Interpretation in Echocardiography. New York: John Wiley & Sons; 1985.)

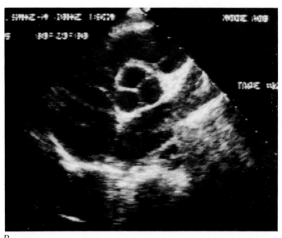

B

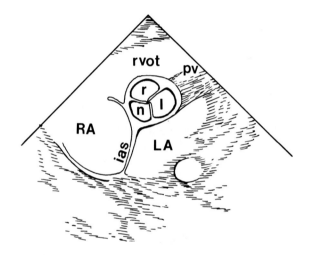

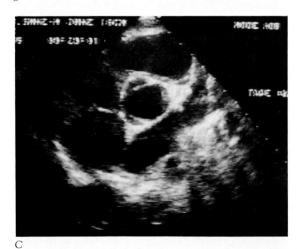

C

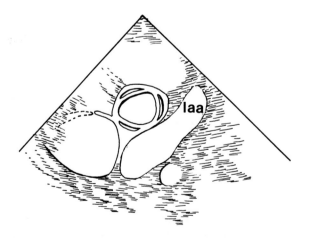

Abnormalities of the aortic valve morphology can be well appreciated in this view, as all the cusps are imaged. The presence of thickening, calcification, fusion of commissures, bicuspid valve with or without a raphe, inappropriate closure secondary to dilatation of the proximal aorta, aortic sinus dilatation, and aortic sinus of Valsalva aneurysm can be assessed. Left atrial masses, such as thrombi in the chamber or appendage or tumors with or without attachments to the left atrial walls, can be observed. Atrial septal defects are often recorded in this view.

There are several instances when color-flow mapping in this view may be useful. The location of aortic regurgitant orifices can be recorded. This is particularly important when assessing the presence or absence of valvular versus paravalvular leak of a prosthetic valve in the aortic position. Spectral tracings can be obtained by placing the sample volume in positions all around the sewing ring and within the central portion of the prosthesis. This view can be used to assess shunt flow across an atrial septal defect of the primum or secundum type. As previously mentioned, with slight inferior angulation of the scan plane toward the basal portion of the left ventricular outflow tract, the flow disturbance associated with shunt across a perimembranous or supracristal ventricular septal defect can be appreciated.

### THE MITRAL VALVE

The short axis of the mitral valve and the basal segments of the left ventricle are examined by positioning the sector plane posteriorly, perpendicular to the mitral valve. Figure 6-16 illustrates the motion of the mitral valve at various points in the cardiac cycle.

An important consideration must be addressed at this point. Short-axis imaging is much more subject than long-axis imaging to distortion by misalignment of the scan plane. Careful adjustment of the rotation aspect of transducer manipulation is critical in short-axis imaging. There are visual clues, however, that the operator can use to optimize the short-axis recordings and avoid error. Regarding the mitral valve, it is important that both the medial and lateral commissures be visualized, with the separation of the anterior and posterior leaflets from these two points completely visualized

throughout the cardiac cycle. If the scan plane has been underrotated to the short axis of the mitral valve, the lateral commissure may be seen to open up and will not be visualized completely. If the scan plane is overrotated beyond the short axis of the mitral valve, the medial commissure may show the same appearance (Fig. 6-17).

The parasternal short-axis view is important to appreciate diffuse or focal thickening of the mitral valve leaflets and to assess the mitral valve orifice size in normal hearts and in disease states such as mitral stenosis. The morphologic abnormalities of the leaflets and chordal structures in cleft mitral valve, mitral valve prolapse, and hypertrophic obstructive cardiomyopathy can be demonstrated.

Color-flow mapping can be useful to assess the area occupied by a jet due to aortic insufficiency and to appreciate in a plane orthogonal to the long axis the spatial distribution of mitral regurgitation. It may also help to outline the mitral orifice in patients with mitral stenosis. Shunt flow across ventricular septal defects located at this level of ventricular septum can also be demonstrated. Pulsed-wave and continuous-wave Doppler equipment permit observation of the duration and velocity of these shunt flows.

### THE LEVEL OF THE LEFT VENTRICULAR PAPILLARY MUSCLES

With slight inferolateral angulation or positioning of the scan plane from the mitral valve, the midventricular region is visualized. The posteromedial and anterolateral papillary muscles can be seen. Figure 6-18 consists of diastolic and systolic parasternal short-axis images. In this example, systolic motion of the myocardium is normal in all regions of the left ventricle. This view is useful for assessing papillary muscle morphology and hypertrophy. Myocardial hypertrophy can also be detected and sometimes shows regional variability in conditions such as hypertrophic cardiomyopathy. The principal role of this view, as well as the other short-axis views of the left ventricle, is to assess regional wall motion. Patients with coronary artery disease and certain cardiomyopathies may develop either diffuse or segmental changes in myocardial performance which can be effectively documented by echocardiography. Additionally, the thinning and scarring characteristics seen with fibrotic myocar-

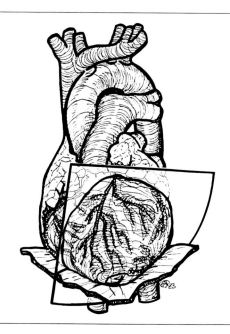

FIGURE 6-16. (A) Schema of the scan plane through the heart in the parasternal short-axis view of the mitral valve. The anterior and posterior mitral leaflets (aml, pml) are seen in (B) early diastole, (C) atrial contraction, and (D) early systole. Note that both the medial and lateral hinge points are recorded (arrows), ensuring proper scan plane orientation through the mitral valve (RV, right ventricle). (Harrigan P, Lee R. Principles of Interpretation in Echocardiography. New York: John Wiley & Sons; 1985.)

A

dium can be noted along with any aneurysmal expansion of weakened heart muscle.

Another abnormality that can be demonstrated in this cross-sectional view is ventricular septal systolic or diastolic flattening seen in right ventricular pressure and volume overload states.

ANGULATION ARTIFACTS

A caveat regarding short-axis imaging must be discussed. It is important to find a scan plane that is truly parallel to the short axis, especially when evaluating segmental dysfunction. Both the shape of the ventricle and the amplitude of wall motion are altered by surprisingly small amounts of transducer misalignment. If the transducer is placed somewhat low, relative to the position of the heart in the chest, the sector plane passes obliquely through the left ventricle, producing a vertical oval shape or a keyhole appearance (Fig. 6-19). The lower the transducer is in relation to the heart, the more the shape of the left ventricular short axis view is distorted. In these cases, it is difficult to know precisely which level of the left ventricle is being visualized. In addition, assessment of wall motion is fraught with error.

Owing to factors such as patient body habitus or surgical dressings, it may not be always possible to image a successive series of parallel sectors of the left ventricle from base to apex. In such cases, it may be necessary to angulate the transducer from one scan plane to another in order to obtain short-axis images of the left ventricle. Alternatively, a low window may be the only available site for imaging, in which case wall motion must be interpreted with caution.

ROTATION ARTIFACTS

Improper rotation of the scan plane can also produce a misshapen left ventricle. In this situation, a somewhat horizontal oval shape is created as the left ventricle is imaged. As the transducer is rotated farther and farther from the ideal short axis, the image becomes more oval until eventually a full long-axis orientation is reached. One of the most common artifacts caused by slight overrotation of the scan plane in the short axis of the left ventricle is flattening of the ventricular septum. As one of the uses of the parasternal short-axis view of the left ventricle is to assess changes in ventricular septal configuration secondary to right ventricular pressure or volume overload, it is critical for the operator not to create this appearance in a patient who does not have this abnormality.

Figure 6-20 illustrates the pattern of ventricular

(Text continues on page 117.)

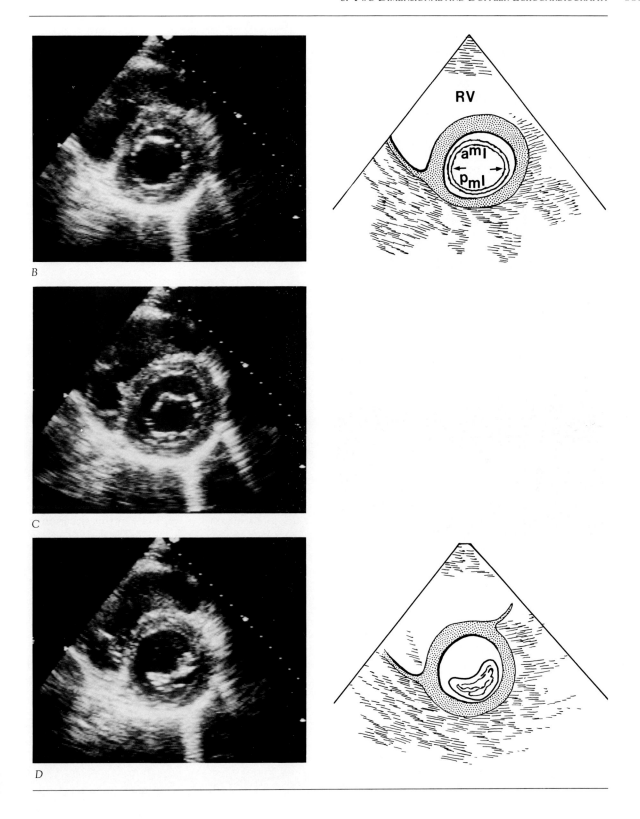

B

C

D

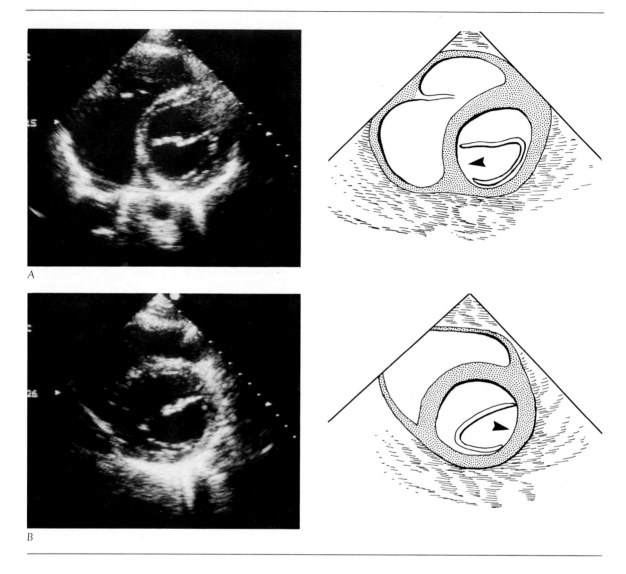

FIGURE 6-17. (A) Parasternal short-axis view of the mitral leaflets with the scan plane underrotated. Note that the medial hinge point is "open," indicating a full short-axis orientation has not been achieved (*arrow*). (B) Overrotation of the scan plane through the mitral valve illustrating the resultant open lateral commissure (*arrow*).

FIGURE 6-18. (A) Schema of the scan plane through the heart in the (B) parasternal short-axis view of the left ventricle (LV), taken at the level of the papillary muscles in diastole and systole (C). Note the normal thickening of the ventricular septum and free wall (al, anterolateral papillary muscle; pm, posteromedial papillary muscle; RV, right ventricle). (Harrigan P, Lee R. Principles of Interpretation in Echocardiography. New York: John Wiley & Sons; 1985.

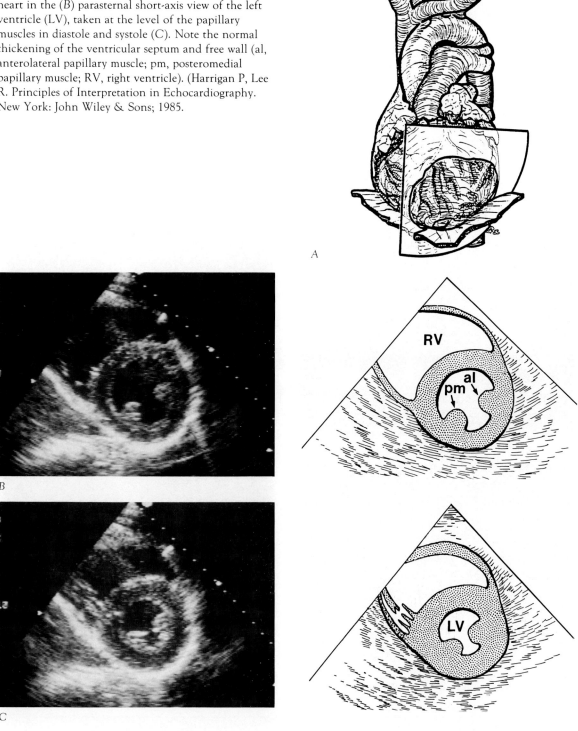

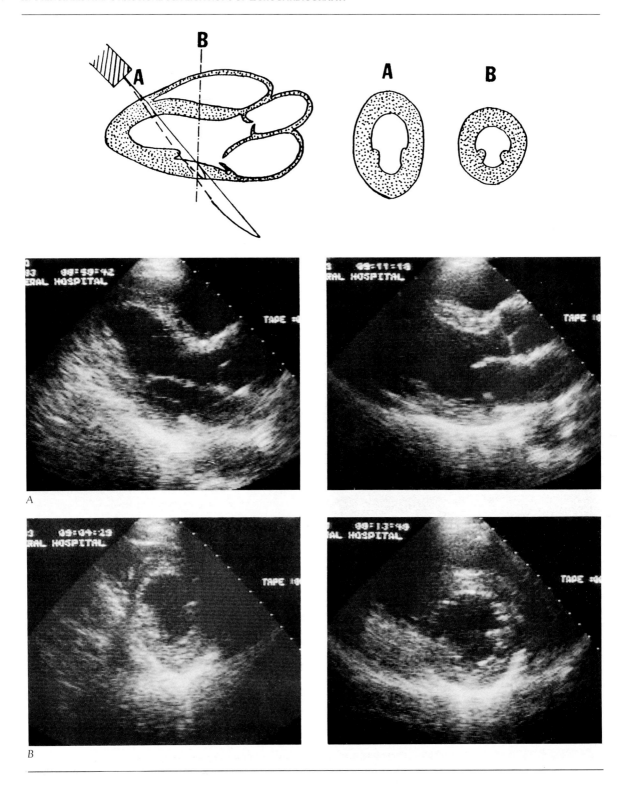

A

B

◀ FIGURE 6-19. (A) Parasternal long- and short-axis views obtained from a low transducer position relative to the position of the patient's heart within the chest. The apex of the heart occupies more of the near field, whereas the aorta appears deeper within the sector display. The distorted image of the left ventricular short axis is observed as a vertical oval, and assessment of wall function may be hindered. Also, an M-mode tracing obtained from this transducer position would produce erroneously increased internal dimensions and wall thickness. In contrast, optimal placement of the transducer, (B) will position the ventricular septum and anterior aortic wall at approximately equal distances from the transducer. The short-axis configuration of the left ventricle is more rounded, which would permit more accurate analysis of left ventricular performance. An M-mode tracing obtained from this transducer position would be through the true minor axis of the left ventricle and perpendicular to the ventricular septum and the posterior wall. (Harrigan P, Lee R. Principles of Interpretation in Echocardiography. New York: John Wiley & Sons; 1985.)

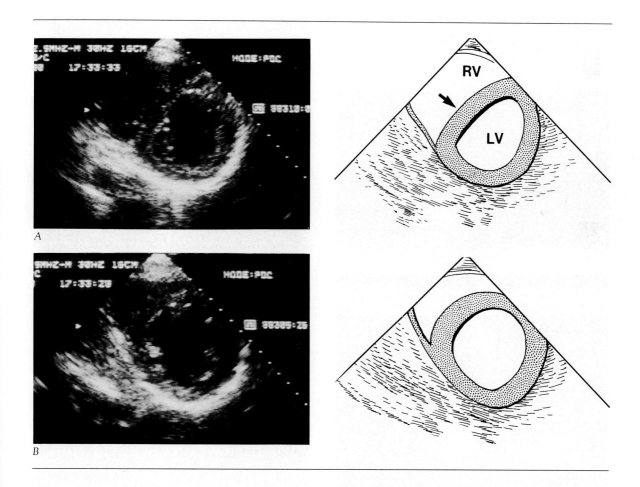

FIGURE 6-20. (A) Parasternal short-axis view of the left ventricle (LV) in which the sector plane has been overrotated, resulting in a perceived "flattening" of the interventricular septum (arrow). (B) Correct plane orientation demonstrates normal septal configuration (RV, right ventricle).

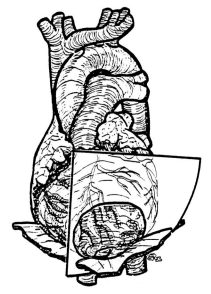

A

FIGURE 6-21. (A) Schema of the scan plane through the heart in the parasternal short-axis view of the left ventricle (lv) over the apex, inferior to the papillary muscles (B). This view is particularly important in patients with ischemic heart disease. (C) Long axis of the apical tip (rv, right ventricle). (Harrigan P, Lee R. Principles of Interpretation in Echocardiography. New York: John Wiley & Sons; 1985.)

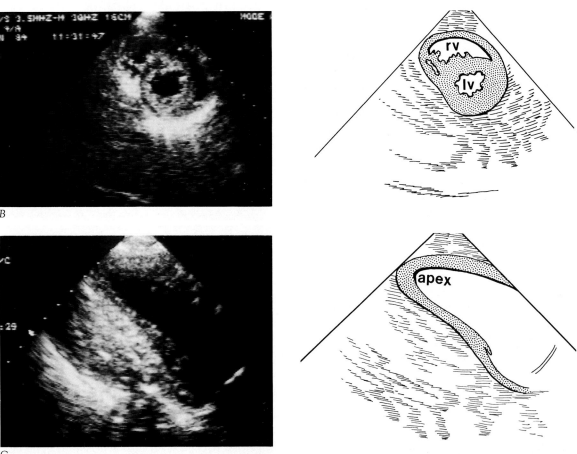

B

C

septal configuration with slight overrotation of the scan plane in the short-axis view. The examiner must recognize the potential for creating this pattern and must make every attempt to find a transducer position and rotation that results in a round appearance of the left ventricle. If this pattern cannot be found, a right ventricular overload pattern should be sought.

### The Apical Portion of the Left Ventricle

In Figure 6-21 the transducer has been positioned below the papillary muscle level and over the left ventricular apex in order to assess wall motion at this level. This view is critical because it often permits the best visualization of apical function.

It is also useful to rotate the transducer 90 degrees counterclockwise into a long-axis view of the apical tip. These views are especially important for assessment of ischemic heart disease.

## Apical Views

The apical views are vital in 2-D imaging, as very large cross-sectional areas of anatomy are visualized at once, providing an enormous amount of anatomic and physiologic data. Significant changes in transducer adjustment are required when proceeding from parasternal imaging to apical imaging.

### Four-Chamber View

The transducer should initially be placed in an extreme lateral position along the posterior axillary line. The plane marker should point roughly toward the patient's left posterior axilla. This ensures that the left side of the heart is displayed on the right of the sector display, as recommended by the American Society of Echocardiography.[2] The scan plane is directed toward the base of the heart (toward the patient's right shoulder) in order to fully record the atria. Then, in a fashion similar to the initial sweeping done at the beginning of the parasternal study, the transducer is moved medially as well as superiorly and inferiorly until all potential imaging sites have been explored. The operator can then exploit the areas that are most useful. Recording the apical myocardium can be problematic in the apical views, owing to its proximity to the transducer. Care should be taken to ensure that the transducer is positioned at the true apex. There

are indicators to assist the examiner. In most cases, the left ventricle tapers at the apex. If the apex appears very rounded, it is likely that the transducer is positioned near the anterior wall of the apex rather than at the apex itself. In addition, the examiner should be able to record the moderator band in the right ventricle.

In the standard apical four-chamber view, the interventricular and interatrial septa have a vertical orientation in the sector image. Because the interatrial septum is membranous at the level of the fossa ovalis, it is a relatively poor reflector of sound. In this transducer orientation, the beam is more or less parallel to it, and dropout of echo signal can occur, giving the false impression of a defect. Therefore, modification of the scan plane may be necessary to better define the exact anatomy of the interatrial septum. One such variation will be described later.

Once portions of all four chambers have been displayed, the scan plane can be carefully rotated, using the mitral and tricuspid valves as landmarks. The major left ventricular walls displayed will be the interventricular septum and the posterolateral wall. Because they are oriented parallel to the ultrasound beam, the endocardium may occasionally be less than optimally visualized. Again, scan plane modification can provide better images of these areas, as will be illustrated later.

Identification of the right and left sides of the heart can be accomplished in several ways in order to ensure proper scan orientation. Demonstration of the moderator band identifies the right ventricle. The septal tricuspid valve leaflets insert into the septum more apically than the anterior mitral valve leaflet. This also aids in identifying the ventricles. The pulmonary veins can be seen to enter the left atrium, and by scanning the plane along the floor of the heart, the coronary sinus is visualized entering the right atrium. In the absence of complex congenital heart disease, these landmarks can be used to identify the cardiac anatomy to ensure proper plane orientation.

Figure 6-22 illustrates the apical four-chamber view during various phases of the cardiac cycle: onset of systole, immediately after closure of the atrioventricular valves (Fig. 6-22A); systole, when the atrioventricular annuli descend inferiorly and the atria dilate (Fig. 6-22B); onset of diastole, as the

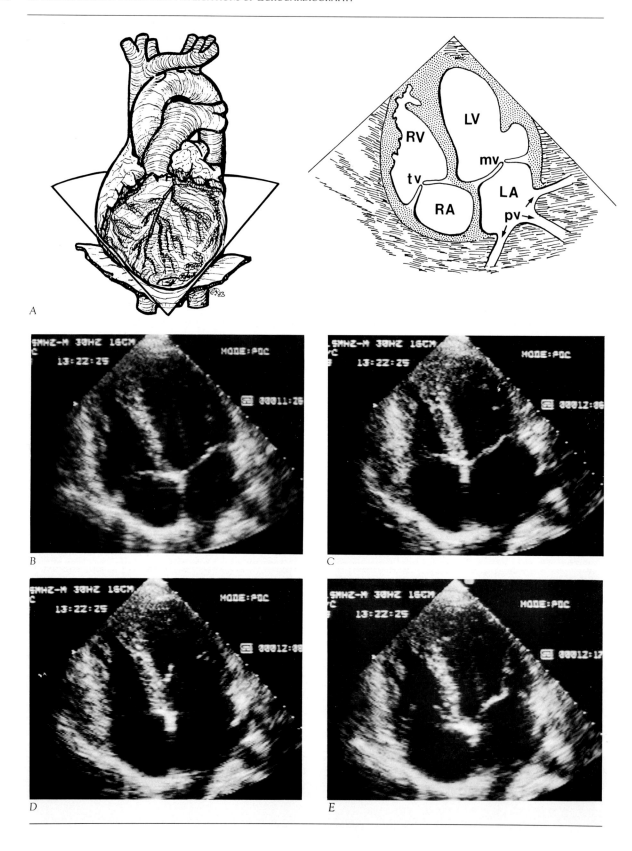

atrioventricular valves open wide for early rapid filling of the ventricles, the atrial blood enters the ventricles, and the atrioventricular annuli ascend as the ventricles dilate (Fig. 6-22C); and atrial contraction, when the leaflets reopen, although to a lesser extent than in the early filling phase (Fig. 6-22D). Often, more detailed visualization of the right side of the heart can be obtained by placing the transducer slightly to the left side of the apex and angling sharply medially (Fig. 6-23).

Another useful variation of the four-chamber view is obtained by placing the transducer on the right ventricular side of the apex and angling the scan plane laterally. As mentioned earlier, this permits more optimal visualization of the apex, lateral wall, and septa. Mitral valve morphology, as well as subvalvular structures, chordae, and papillary muscles, are visualized more clearly. Defects in the ventricular and atrial septa are more likely to be optimized. In addition to these imaging advantages, the quality of color-flow mapping and Doppler spectral tracings is sometimes improved with this transducer orientation (Fig. 6-24).

### The Left and Right Ventricular Outflow Tracts

With slight superior angulation from the standard apical four-chamber view the sector plane is moved anteriorly and the outflow tracts can be visualized (Fig. 6-25). From the standard apical four-chamber view, the beam is tilted up to scan through the left ventricular outflow tract, the aortic valve, and a portion of the ascending aorta. This view is also known as the apical five-chamber view. Often, the atrioventricular valves are less well-defined in this view. With further anterior angulation, the more

superior aspects of the ascending aorta may be seen. Scanning further, the more anteriorly positioned right ventricular outflow tract can occasionally be viewed.[3] The relationship between the great arteries, the pulmonary valve, and occasionally the pulmonary artery bifurcation can be recorded.

Imaged optimally the apical views can yield a significant amount of the diagnostic information obtained in an echocardiographic study. Assessment of biventricular internal dimensions, wall thickness, and function can be made. Atrioventricular valve morphology and function, the integrity of the septa, and the state of the atria can be observed, as can fixed or dynamic left ventricular outflow tract obstruction, disease of the aorta, intracardiac masses, and pericardial disease.

*Color-Flow Mapping and Doppler Examination of the Apical Views* A sizable portion of cardiac anatomy is examined in the apical views, so it follows that a significant amount of flow information can be obtained from this scanning orientation. The apical placement of the transducer is such that the majority of intracardiac flow is nearly parallel to the sound beam, which is ideal for Doppler assessments. Because of the wide range of flow information, it is helpful to approach the apical Doppler examination in a systematic manner that affords an understanding of the hemodynamics involved.

*The Left Side of the Heart.* After the apical four-chamber view is optimized, the color-flow map can be applied to the image. Once the Doppler spectrum or color map has been employed, the examiner must focus on *this* information in order to optimize the Doppler exam and must not rely on the

---

◀ FIGURE 6-22. (A) Schema of the scan plane through the heart in the standard apical four-chamber view. Images represent early (B) and end-systole (C) and early (D) and end-diastole (E). Note the inferior insertion of the septal tricuspid leaflet into the ventricular septum relative to the anterior leaflet. Also note the more heavily trabeculated right ventricle. Significant changes in chamber size can be observed as the atrioventricular annuli descend in systole and ascend in diastole (LA, left atrium; LV, left ventricle; tv, tricuspid valve; mv, mitral valve; pv, pulmonary veins; RA, right atrium; RV, right ventricle). (Harrigan P, Lee R. Principles of Interpretation in Echocardiography. New York: John Wiley & Sons; 1985.)

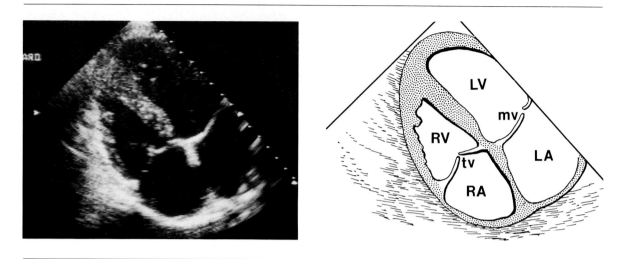

FIGURE 6-23. Apical four-chamber view with sharp medial angulation to optimize visualization of the right ventricle (RV). (LA, left atrium; LV, left ventricle; MV, mitral valve; RA, right atrium; tv, tricuspid valve.)

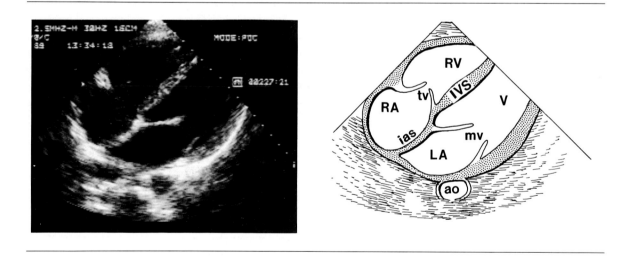

FIGURE 6-24. Four-chamber view of the heart obtained by placing the transducer on the right ventricular side of the apex and angling the sound beam laterally. This view is a very useful adjunct to the standard four-chamber view (LA, left atrium; LV, left ventricle; ias, interatrial septum; IVS, interventricular septum; RA, right atrium; RV, right ventricle; ao, aorta; mv, mitral valve; tv, tricuspid valve.

appearance of the view. *Often the Doppler data are of highest quality in a scan plane that is not optimal for tissue imaging definition.* The examiner should focus on the area immediately behind the mitral valve in the left atrium to locate any possible systolic turbulent flow from mitral regurgitation. The scan plane should be carefully scanned anteriorly and posteriorly, medially and laterally within the left atrium, to document the full extent of the mitral regurgitant jet, if present.

During diastole, the operator can follow the flow across the mitral valve into the left ventricle (encoded in shades of red), along the lateral half of the chamber, around the apex toward the medial aspect of the chamber, along the left ventricular outflow tract (encoded in shades of blue), and across the aortic valve. Each aspect of these flow patterns can be optimized by moving the scan plane within the color map. It is important to understand the normal pattern of flow within the left ventricular inflow and outflow tracts, because abnormal flows may occur concurrently or may be superimposed and, therefore, need to be recognized and differentiated.

Figure 6-26 illustrates schematically the pattern of normal flow that is seen in this view. It can be shown that the Doppler examination allows the examiner to follow this flow systematically from the mitral valve, through the inflow tract, into the left ventricle (where flow is toward the transducer in diastole), and then to the outflow tract, to the subaortic area, and across the valve into the aorta (where flow is away from the transducer in systole). The Doppler spectral traces illustrate typical flow in a normal heart at various points along the left ventricular inflow and outflow tracts: (1) behind the coaptation point of the mitral valve at annular level (prevalvular acceleration), and farther into the left atrium if mitral regurgitation necessitates, (2) point of peak mitral valve inflow profile, (3) midventricular region (will begin to record some outflow tract velocities), (4) left ventricular outflow tract (mitral valve flow becomes less prominent), (5) subaortic area (prevalvular flow), and (6) aortic valve, for peak transvalvular aortic flow velocities.

After flow in the left side of the heart has been assessed, the color-flow map and spectral tracings of tricuspid valve flow can be examined. Although these velocities have already been recorded from the parasternal right ventricular inflow view, it is important to corroborate findings in as many views as possible.

### Apical Two-Chamber View

To obtain the apical two-chamber view, the scan plane is rotated counterclockwise from that of the standard apical four-chamber view. As the transducer is rotated, the right side of the heart gradually disappears from the image until only the two left heart chambers are seen. This is a very important view of the left ventricle, since it permits visualization of the entire length of the anterior and inferior walls (Fig. 6-27). Color-flow mapping and Doppler spectral tracings are helpful, as it is important to document abnormal flow from multiple scan planes in order to appreciate the three-dimensional size of the disturbed flow.

Slight lateral angulation and fine tuning with rotation of the scan plane often reveals a large extent of the descending thoracic aorta (Fig. 6-28). This view is extremely important for assessing disease of the aorta.

### Apical Long-Axis View

Continued counterclockwise rotation from the position for the apical two-chamber view brings the scan plane through the aorta, and the apical long-axis view is obtained. The structures seen are similar to those seen from the parasternal location, although the apex now occupies the tip of the sector triangle and the basal structures are distal within the field of view (Fig. 6-29). This is an excellent view for assessment with color-flow mapping, because flows are parallel to the beam and both inflow and outflow tracts are visualized simultaneously in this plane.

(Text continues on page 129.)

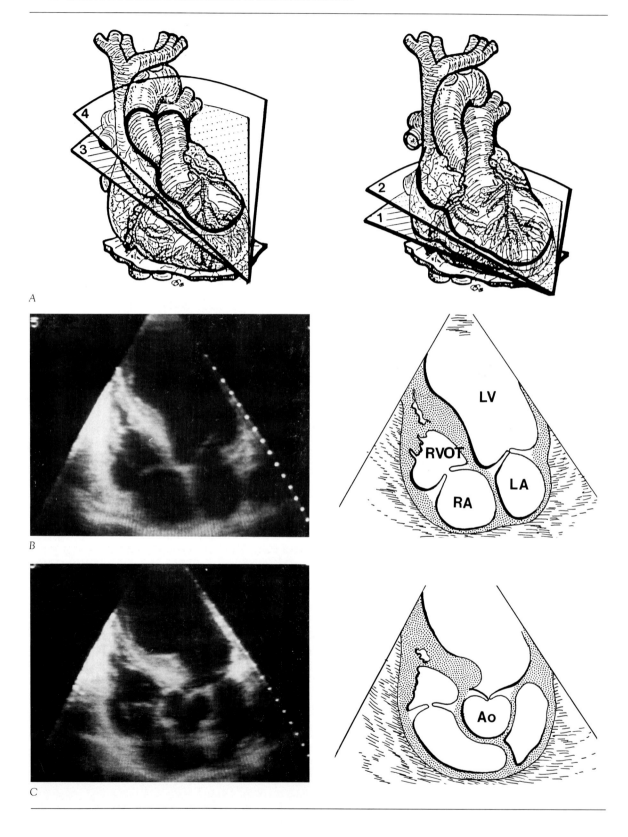

A

B

C

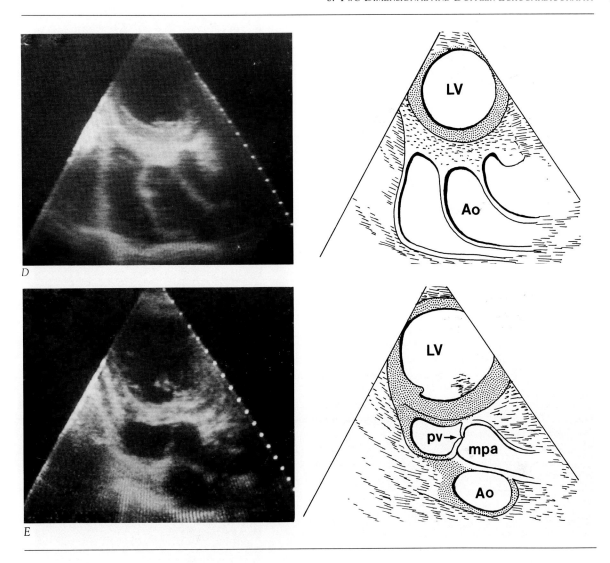

FIGURE 6-25. (A) Schema of the scan plane through the left and right ventricular outflow tracts from the apex. (B) Standard apical four-chamber view (plane position 1). (C) With slight anterior angulation, the sector plane passes through the proximal aorta (Ao) and reveals the subaortic area (plane position 2). (D) With further anterior angulation, the more distal segment of the ascending aorta may be seen (plane position 3). Further anterior angulation may occasionally permit visualization of the main pulmonary artery (mpa) as it courses leftward (E, plane position 4). The pulmonary valve (pv) cusps may also be recorded (LA, left atrium; LV, left ventricle; RA, right atrium; RVOT, right ventricular outflow tract). (Harrigan P, Lee R. Principles of Interpretation in Echocardiography. New York: John Wiley & Sons; 1985.)

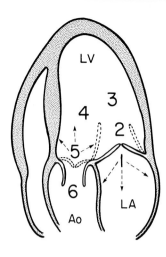

A

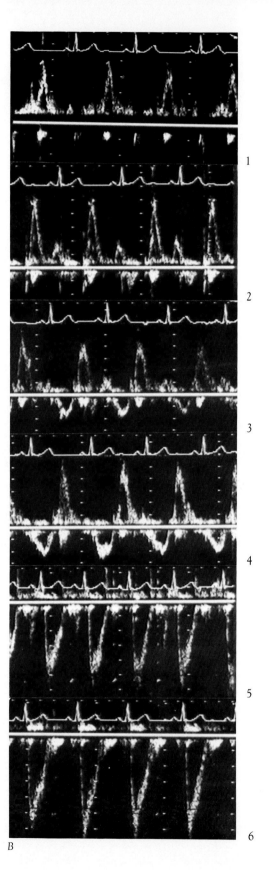

B

FIGURE 6-26. (See color insert for parts C, D, and E.) (A) Schematic drawing illustrates the positions of the sample volume across the left ventricular (LV) inflow and outflow tracts. (B) Pulsed-wave Doppler spectral tracings taken at each of these points. As the sample volume is brought across the mitral valve, the filling flows predominate. As the sample volume is positioned into the left ventricle and then toward the outflow tract, mitral valve flow diminishes on the spectral tracing and LV outflow tract flow predominates as the sample volume is moved across the aortic valve. The arrows behind the mitral valve and below the aortic valve indicate that the sample volume should be moved carefully in all directions to assess for possible mitral or aortic regurgitation. Color-flow map applied to the apical "five-chamber" view in diastole (C) and systole (D). Flow across the mitral valve into the left ventricle is toward the transducer in this orientation and, therefore, is encoded in red. Flow across the left ventricular outflow tract into the aorta (Ao) is moving away from the transducer and is encoded in blue. (E) Pulmonary venous inflow, encoded in red, is seen entering the left atrium (LA).

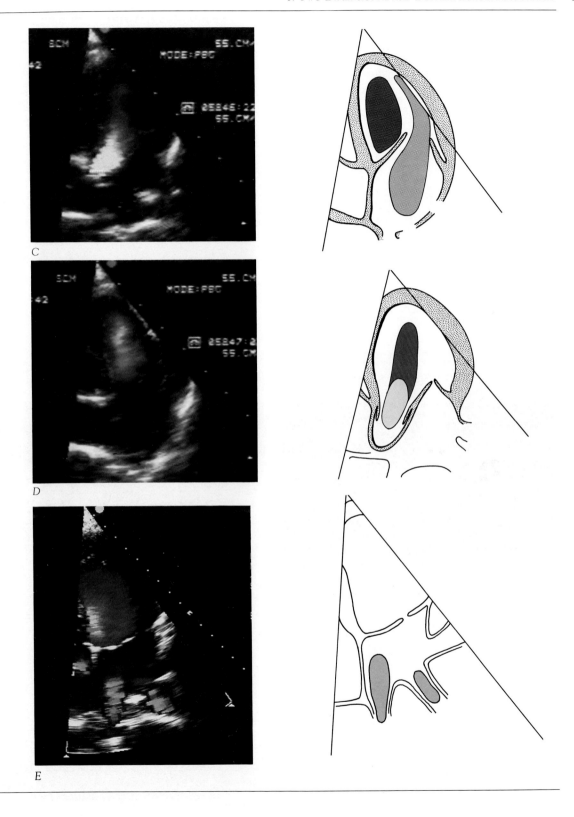

C

D

E

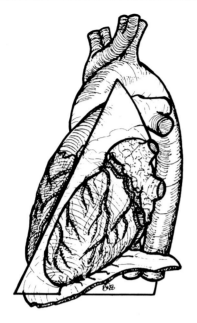

A

FIGURE 6-27. (A) Schema of the scan plane through the heart in the apical two-chamber view (B). The sector plane has been rotated counterclockwise from the standard apical four-chamber view and no longer passes through right-sided structures (aw, anterior wall; iw, inferior wall; LA, left atrium; LV, left ventricle; mv, mitral valve).

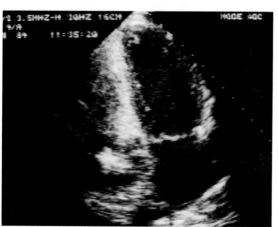

B

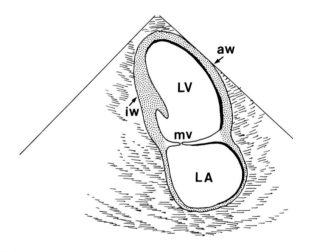

FIGURE 6-28. (A) Schematic drawing illustrating the scan plane for the (B) long-axis view of the descending thoracic aorta (DTA) imaged from the apex (lv, left ventricle).

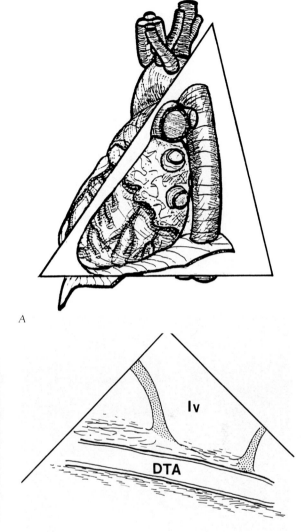

A

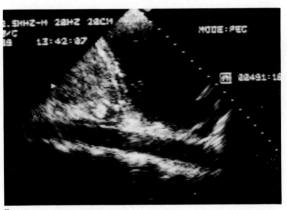

B

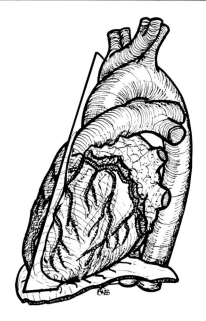

*A*

FIGURE 6-29. (A) Schema of the scan plane through the heart in the apical long-axis view of the left heart (B). The left ventricular (LV) apex occupies the near field, while the aorta (AO), owing to its increased distance from the transducer, occupies the far field (ao, descending thoracic aorta; LA, left atrium; mv, mitral valve). (Harrigan P, Lee R. Principles of Interpretation in Echocardiography. New York: John Wiley & Sons; 1985.)

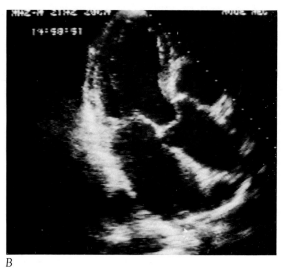

*B*

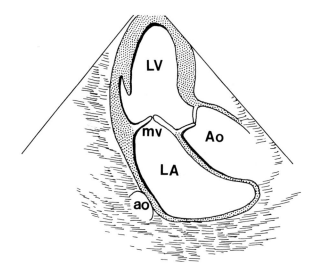

(Text continues from page 121.)
## Subcostal Views
Use of the subcostal views significantly increases the percentage of patients from whom clinically useful information can be derived by echocardiography. High-quality diagnostic images can be obtained, and are most appreciated when technical limitations with the parasternal or apical approach preclude the gathering of optimal images.

Patient positioning can assist greatly in obtaining these images. The patient should be supine, with the knees elevated and the feet on the bed, to relax the abdominal muscles. Lowering of the head to raise the rib cage can facilitate access to the subcostal region. Deep, sustained inspiration usually improves image quality, as the heart is forced inferiorly toward the transducer as the lungs inflate and the diaphragm moves downward.

Images may be obtained at or below the level of the subxyphoid process, and from beneath the left and right sides of the rib cage. Occasionally, depending on the heart position, images can sometimes be recorded by placing the transducer farther down on the abdomen, above the umbilicus, and directing the beam toward the heart. It is important to fully exploit all possible imaging sites. The transducer should be held in an overhand approach, in order to keep the hand from being an obstruction and to allow the index finger to keep firm pressure on top of the transducer. The examiner should begin the subcostal examination gently, so that the patient will tolerate the gradually increasing pressure that may be necessary to optimize the images. Any sudden pressure applied to the patient's abdomen in a hasty attempt to obtain views may produce reflexive tightening of the abdominal muscles, which impedes the examination.

## Four-Chamber View
The plane marker on the transducer should point approximately toward the patient's left hip. In this way, the apex of the heart will be positioned at the right of the sector display and the base of the heart will be at the left of the image. Because the transducer has been positioned on the abdomen, liver tissue will occupy the near field of the image (Fig. 6-30). Segments of all four chambers are seen separated inferosuperiorly by the atrioventricular valves and laterally by the ventricular and atrial septa. Because the septa are nearly perpendicular to

the sound beam in this view which is optimal for ultrasound imaging, the presence of septal defects can often be observed; however, these structures are in the far field, where spatial imaging resolution can be suboptimal. This view is also useful when assessing the distribution of pericardial fluid, and geometry-distorting abnormalities such as apical aneurysm.

Technical note: The central aspect of the scan plane can be angled toward the apex to bring that segment into the center of the sector image or scanned more medially to bring the atria into the center of the sector display.

### LONG-AXIS VIEW OF THE LEFT AND RIGHT VENTRICULAR OUTFLOW TRACTS
The left ventricular outflow tract can be visualized by slight anterior angulation from the four-chamber view. Further anterior angulation may result in images of the ascending aorta and the superior vena cava. The latter will occupy a position to the right of the aorta and extending into the right atrium (Fig. 6-31).

If the scan plane is moved farther anteriorly beneath the rib cage, the right ventricular outflow tract, including the infundibulum, pulmonary valve, and main pulmonary artery, may be seen (Fig. 6-32).

### LONG-AXIS VIEW OF THE INFERIOR VENA CAVA
With slight counterclockwise rotation and more medial angulation, the inferior vena cava can be seen entering the right atrium. The Eustachian valve, located at the mouth of the inferior vena cava, is often seen in this scan plane. Visualization of the hepatic vasculature, which can be helpful in assessing right heart function, is also possible (Fig. 6-33).

Color-flow mapping and pulsed Doppler can be useful in these views, particularly when assessing the presence of shunt flow. Also, the extent of tricuspid regurgitation into the right atrium or reflux into the inferior vena cava and hepatic veins can be recorded; however, the clinical utility of Doppler and color-flow mapping studies can sometimes be limited by the fact that the subcostal transducer position requires that outgoing sound pulses and incoming echoes traverse liver tissue, which is highly echo attenuating.

(Text continues on page 134.)

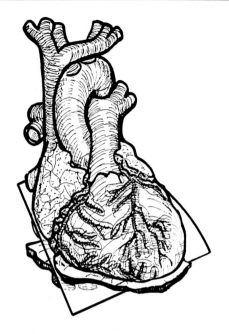

A

Figure 6-30. (A) Schema of the scan plane through the heart in the subcostal long-axis view at the level of the atrioventricular valves (B). The interventricular and interatrial septa (IVS; IAS) are often well-visualized owing to their perpendicular relationship to the acoustic beam (LA, left atrium; LV, left ventricle; RA, right atrium; RV, right ventricle; tv, tricuspid valve; mv, mitral valve; pv, pulmonary valve). (Harrigan P, Lee R. Principles of Interpretation in Echocardiography. New York: John Wiley & Sons; 1985.)

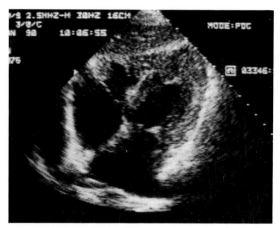

B

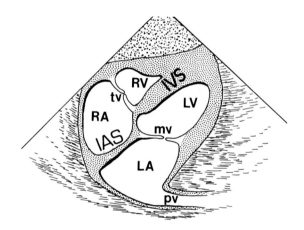

FIGURE 6-31. (A) Schema of the scan plane through the heart in the subcostal long-axis view of the left ventricular outflow tract (plane position 1). (B) By tilting the scan plane anteriorly from the subcostal four-chamber view, the aortic valve and aorta (Ao) can be recorded. Note the superior vena cava (svc) entering the right atrium (RA) (RV, right ventricle; LV, left ventricle). (Harrigan P, Lee R. Principles of Interpretation in Echocardiography. New York: John Wiley & Sons; 1985.)

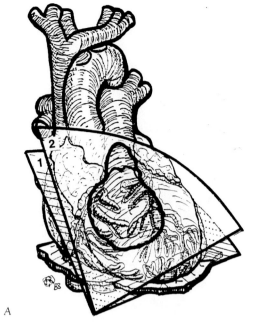

A

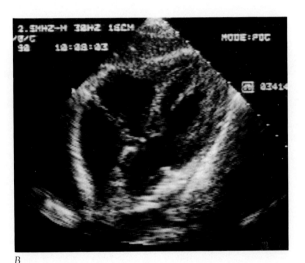

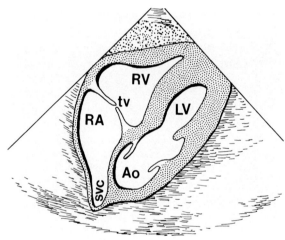

B

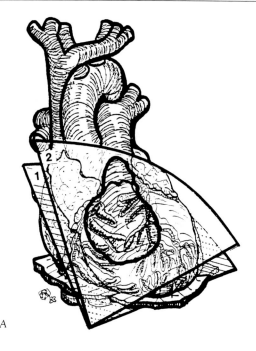

FIGURE 6-32. (A) Plane position 2. (B) Further anterior angulation beyond the scan plane in Fig. 6-31 will pass the sector plane through the right ventricular outflow tract (rvot), including the infundibulum, pulmonary valve (pv), and a portion of the main pulmonary artery (mpa).

A

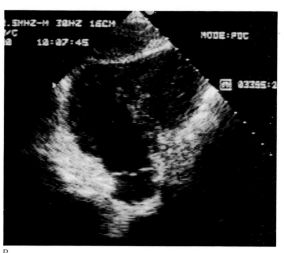

B

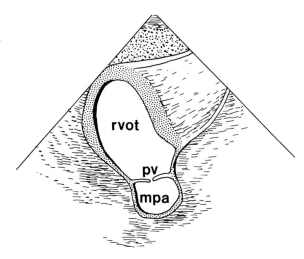

FIGURE 6-33. (A) Schema of the scan plane through the heart in the (B) subcostal long-axis view of the inferior vena cava (ivc) entering the right atrium (RA). Some hepatic veins (hv) can also be visualized (ev, eustachian valve; svc, superior vena cava). (Harrigan P, Lee R. Principles of Interpretation in Echocardiography. New York: John Wiley & Sons; 1985.)

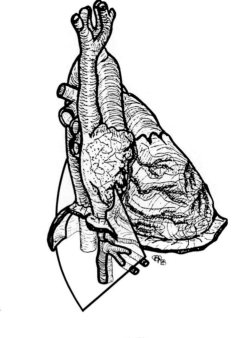

A

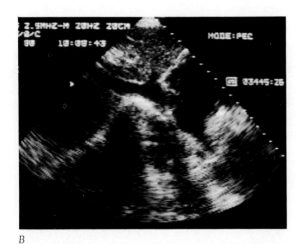

B

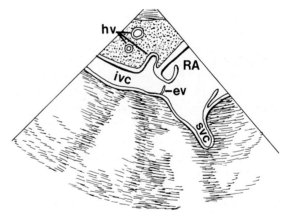

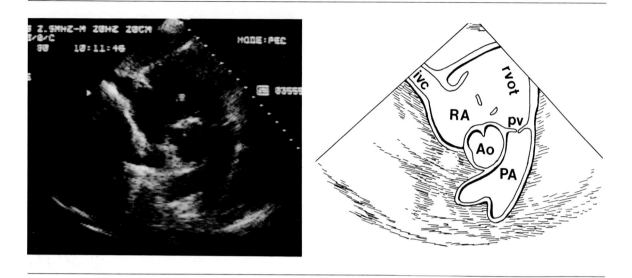

FIGURE 6-34. Subcostal short-axis view at the base of the heart. The aortic root (Ao) and valve are seen in short axis with the right ventricular outflow tract (rvot) and pulmonary artery (PA) coursing away from the transducer (ivc, inferior vena cava; RA, right atrium; pv, pulmonary valve).

(Text continues from page 129.)

SHORT-AXIS VIEWS

Short-axis views of the heart can also be recorded from this perspective. Variations on these views are often used in the assessment of congenital heart disease in children. Many of the same images are of use in the adult patient, as well, since additional regions of anatomy are seen, revealing the spatial relationships of structures.

*Base of the Heart.* As the scan plane is brought back toward the heart from the long axis of the inferior vena cava it moves into position to record the short axis of the cardiac structures. Figure 6-34 reveals the subcostal short-axis view at the level of the outflow tracts. This view reveals similar anatomy to that seen in the parasternal short-axis views with the image rotated somewhat clockwise. Therefore, the same diagnostic assessments can be made in both views.

*Level of the Mitral Valve and Left Ventricle.* With gradual angulation of the scan plane toward the left ventricle, the mitral valve orifice (Fig. 6-35) and short axis of the left ventricle (Fig. 6-36) at all levels can be recorded. If the images are satisfactory, assessment of left ventricular function is possible in these views, particularly if the parasternal short axis approach was suboptimal. M-mode tracings can be taken in these views when proper scan orientation is possible.

THE ABDOMINAL AORTA

Another useful view from this transducer orientation is of the abdominal aorta. Assessment of this segment of the aorta is important in any patient with disease of the thoracic aorta. It is also useful to determine Doppler flow characteristics in such entities as coarctation of the aorta and severe aortic regurgitation.

The transducer can be placed on the abdomen, just below the xyphoid process. The scan plane is directed posteriorly to transect the body in a sagittal plane. The plane marker points to the patient's left. The inferior vena cava should be seen in short axis to the patient's right (left on image) and the aorta is seen in short axis to the patient's left (right side of image). Differentiation of these vessels is made by their pulsatile characteristics.

FIGURE 6-35. (A) Schema of the scan plane through the heart in the subcostal short-axis view at the level of the mitral valve (mv). Note the clockwise orientation of the image compared to the parasternal short-axis view (RV, right ventricle). (Harrigan P, Lee R. Principles of Interpretation in Echocardiography. New York: John Wiley & Sons; 1985.)

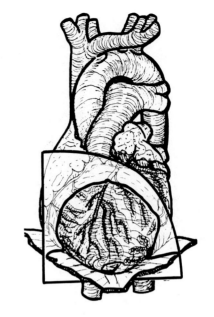

A

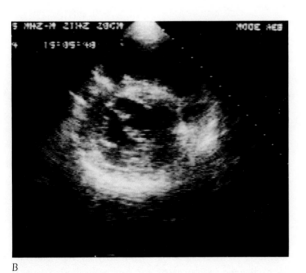

B

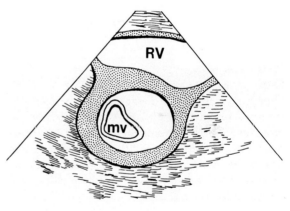

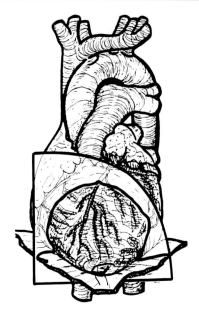

A

FIGURE 6-36. Subcostal short-axis view at the level of the papillary muscles (LV, left ventricle; RV, right ventricle).

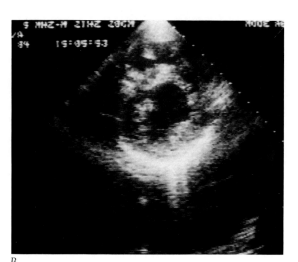

B

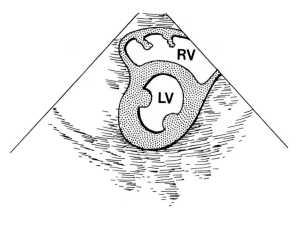

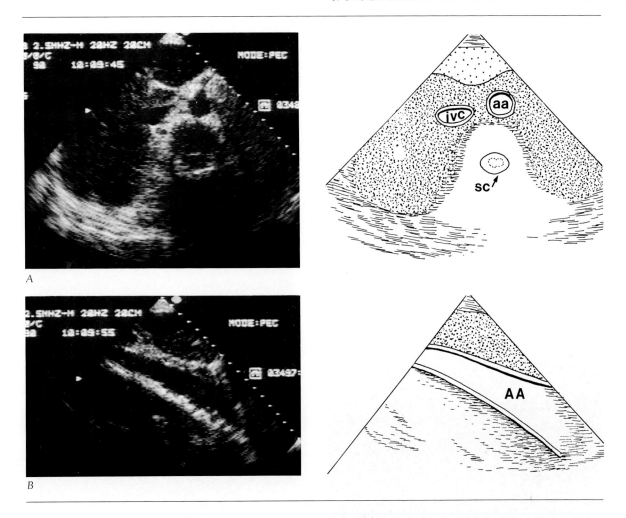

FIGURE 6-37. (A) Transverse plane through the abdomen below the xyphoid process. The inferior vena cava (ivc) and abdominal aorta (aa) can be differentiated by their pulsatile qualities. (B) With rotation of the scan plane, the long axis of these vessels can be imaged, here the abdominal aorta (AA) (sc, spinal cord).

The inferior vena cava exhibits respiratory expansion and contraction; the aorta expands with each systole.

To visualize the long axis of the aorta, the scan plane is rotated 90 degrees counterclockwise, in such a way that the superior portion of the aorta is to the right of the image and the inferior portion is to the left. The transducer can be moved along the surface of the body to record as much of the length of the aorta as possible (Fig. 6-37).

## Suprasternal Views

### Long-Axis View of the Aorta

The suprasternal notch provides an examination site that often permits visualization of the arteries and veins located at the base of the heart. The transducer is placed in the notch, angled inferiorly and posteriorly, with the plane marker aimed toward the left jaw. The ascending aorta is displayed to the left of the image and the descending thoracic aorta to the right (Fig. 6-38). The arterial branches,

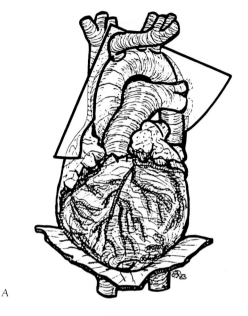

A

FIGURE 6-38. (A) Schema of the scan plane through the heart in the (B) suprasternal notch long-axis view of the aorta and transverse arch (ta). The right pulmonary artery is seen in short axis *(arrow)*, with the left atrium (la) positioned posteriorly (aa, ascending aorta; da, descending thoracic aorta). (Harrigan P, Lee R. Principles of Interpretation in Echocardiography. New York: John Wiley & Sons; 1985.)

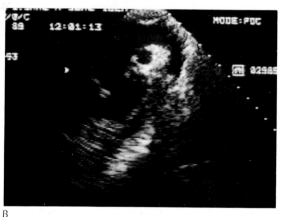

B

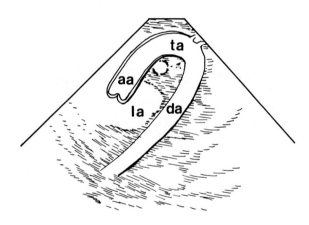

the innominate artery, left common carotid artery, and the left subclavian artery can be recorded with superolateral angulation of the scan plane (Fig. 6-39). The right pulmonary artery is seen in its short axis, with the left atrium located posteriorly.

These views are useful when assessing regional or diffuse dilatation of the aorta, aneurysm formation, aortic dissection, or coarctation. Color-flow mapping permits characterization of turbulent or high-velocity flow in the aorta, which can result from such entities as aortic stenosis and coarctation. Color-flow mapping may also be useful in determining the true versus the false lumen in the presence of aortic dissection. Diastolic reversal of flow may be seen in the descending thoracic aorta in patients with severe aortic insufficiency. Figure 6-40 illustrates the color-flow map from this scan plane. Pulsed Doppler examination is done by placing the sample volume in the ascending aorta to record the positively directed spectral tracing; it is then

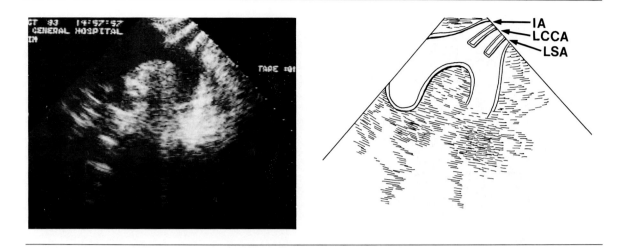

FIGURE 6-39. Superolateral angulation from the previous scan plane often permits better visualization of the arch vessels (IA, innominate artery; LCCA, left common carotid artery; LSA, left subclavian artery).

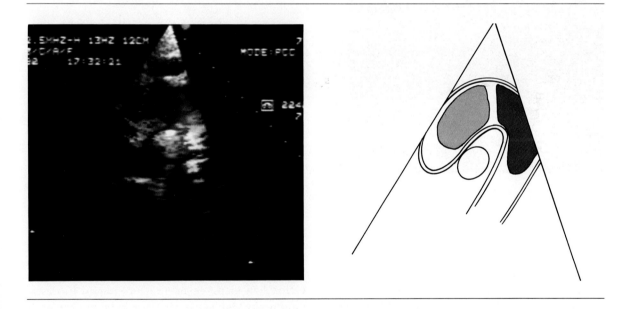

FIGURE 6-40. (See color insert.) Color-flow map applied to image of the transverse arch. The ascending aortic flow is encoded in red as it flows toward the transducer and descending aortic flow is encoded in blue as it flows away from the transducer.

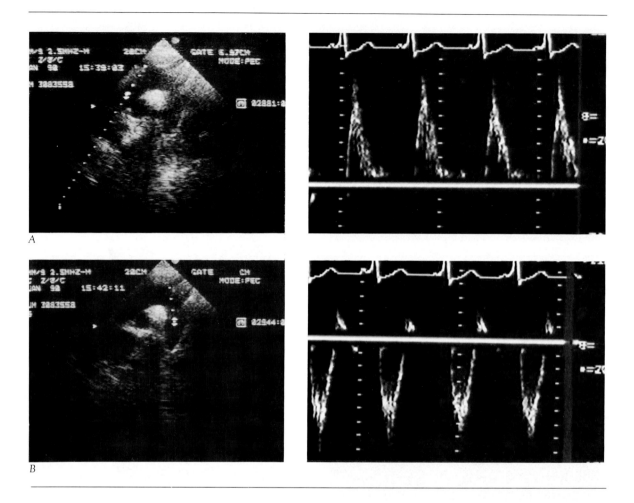

FIGURE 6-41. (A) Pulsed-wave Doppler spectral tracing from the ascending thoracic aorta obtained from the suprasternal notch imaging site. The displayed signal is above the baseline, reflecting flow toward the transducer. (B) Descending thoracic aortic flow is displayed below the baseline, since it travels away from the transducer.

moved to the descending thoracic aorta to record the negatively directed spectral tracing (Fig. 6-41). In any case where aliasing occurs on the pulsed Doppler examination, continuous-wave Doppler should be employed, using either a stand-alone continuous-wave probe or an image-guided continuous-wave transducer to fully display these high-velocity jets.

LONG-AXIS VIEW OF THE RIGHT PULMONARY ARTERY With a clockwise rotation of 90 degrees from the long axis of the thoracic aorta, the sector plane will pass through the long axis of the right pulmonary artery and the short axis of the transverse aortic arch. Often, the convergence of the innominate veins into the superior vena cava can be recorded. Also of importance is the ability to record the entry of the right and left pulmonary veins into the left atrium (Fig. 6-42).

FIGURE 6-42. (A) Schema of the scan plane through the heart in the (B) suprasternal notch short-axis view of the transverse arch (ta). The right pulmonary artery (rpa) is now seen in short axis. The left and right brachiocephalic (innominate) veins (lbcv, rbcv) can be seen entering the superior vena cava (svc), which courses inferiorly. The four pulmonary veins are often visualized entering the left atrium (la). (11 pv, left lower pulmonary vein; lupv, left upper pulmonary vein; rlpv, right lower pulmonary vein; rupv, right upper pulmonary vein.) (Harrigan P, Lee R. Principles of Interpretation in Echocardiography. New York: John Wiley & Sons; 1985.)

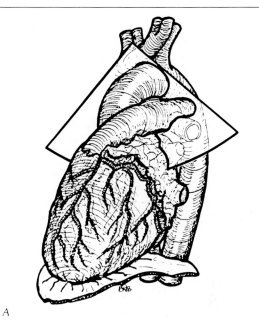

A

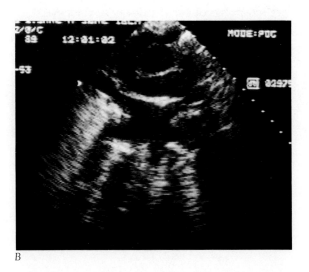

B

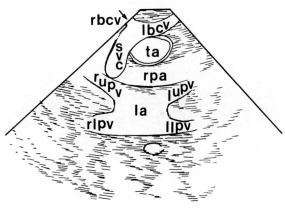

## Right Parasternal Views

It had long been assumed that using the chest wall to the right of the sternum as an imaging site was of little assistance in producing diagnostic images of the heart. However, if this examination site is used routinely high-quality diagnostic images can be recorded in a surprising number of patients. For this reason it is helpful to routinely attempt echocardiographic imaging from this examination site, as it is difficult to predict on the basis of standard imaging what will be recorded in these views. Routine use of this examination site will also maintain examination skills for those instances when such views are critical to diagnosis.

Any number of possible images of the heart may be available. In a certain percentage of patients in whom the standard left parasternal views are inadequate, significantly better right parasternal images can be obtained, including the parasternal long-axis and short-axis views. These were described as performed from the left parasternum; on the right side the position of the plane marker of the transducer is the same, the transducer being positioned at multiple imaging sites. Color-flow mapping and Doppler spectral tracings can be obtained where appropriate.

### ADDITIONAL IMAGING VIEWS FROM THE RIGHT PARASTERNUM

*The Thoracic Aorta.* Images of the ascending aorta can often be obtained by placing the transducer below the clavicle in the first or second interspace, usually at the right sternal edge. In some patients this view is optimized by moving the transducer more laterally, sometimes to the anterior axillary margin. The plane marker points cephalad and slightly left. Directing the scan plane toward the aortic valve usually reveals the full length of the ascending aorta (Fig. 6-43). This scan plane is also critically important when the peak velocity across the aortic valve must be obtained in patients with aortic stenosis. By directing the Doppler beam toward the aortic valve, this view often reveals the best recordings of aortic valve peak velocities.

Bringing the transducer down one or two interspaces may permit visualization of the entire tho-

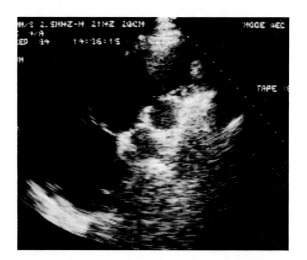
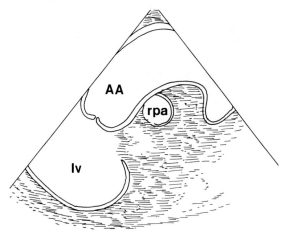

FIGURE 6-43. Right parasternal view of the ascending aorta (AA). This view is usually obtained from a high intercostal space in order to image directly down the ascending aorta and is a helpful way to determine optimal sites for Doppler sampling across a stenotic valve (lv, left ventricle; rpa, right pulmonary artery). (Harrigan P, Lee R. Principles of Interpretation in Echocardiography. New York: John Wiley & Sons; 1985.)

Figure 6-44. (A) Schema of the scan plane through the heart in the right parasternal view of the thoracic aorta (B). The short axis of the right pulmonary artery (rpa) is usually seen. This view is helpful in assessing diseases of the aorta (AA, ascending aorta; DTA, descending thoracic aorta). (Harrigan P, Lee R. Principles of Interpretation in Echocardiography. New York: John Wiley & Sons; 1985.)

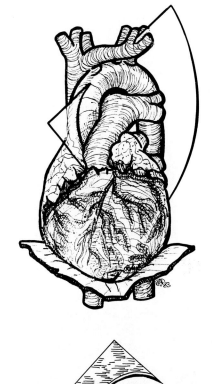

A

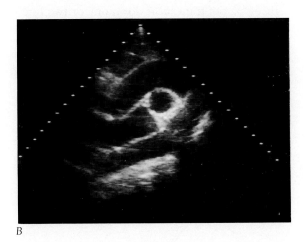

B

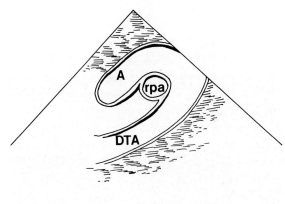

racic aorta, a view that is especially important for assessing a patient with disease of the aorta (Fig. 6-44).

*Superior Vena Cava.* The superior vena cava is located to the right of the ascending aorta and can be recorded by tilting the scan plane laterally, or to the right, from a view that demonstrates the ascending aorta. Usually the transducer is positioned in the second, third, or fourth intercostal space with the plane marker pointing cephalad in order to display the long axis of the superior vena cava. Occasionally the inferior vena cava can also be recorded simultaneously, with both cavae entering the right atrium. The right pulmonary artery and right pulmonary veins are also visualized behind the right atrium (Fig. 6-45). Color-flow mapping in this view reveals the superior vena caval flow encoded in blue and the inferior vena caval flow encoded in red (Fig. 6-46).

FIGURE 6-45. (A) Schema of the scan plane through the heart in the (B) right parasternal view of the superior vena cava (SVC) and inferior vena cava (IVC) draining into the right atrium (RA). The right pulmonary artery (rpa) and right pulmonary veins (pv) are demonstrated in this patient. (Harrigan P, Lee R. Principles of Interpretation in Echocardiography. New York: John Wiley & Sons; 1985.)

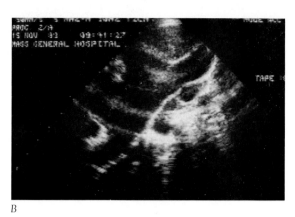

*B*

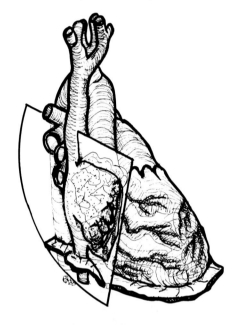

*A*

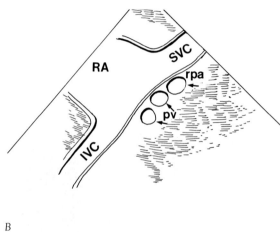

*B*

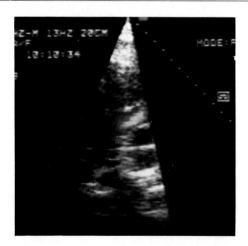

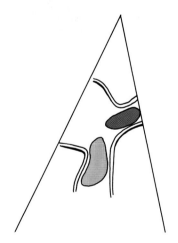

FIGURE 6-46. (See color insert.) Color-flow map applied to the image of the venae cavae illustrated in the previous figure. The superior vena caval flow, moving away from the transducer, is encoded in blue. The inferior vena caval flow, moving toward the transducer, is encoded in red.

FIGURE 6-47. (A) Schema of the scan plane through the heart in the (B) right parasternal short-axis view of the superior vena cava (svc), aorta (ao), and pulmonary artery (pa). The right atrium (RA) is noted posteriorly. (Harrigan P, Lee R. Principles of Interpretation in Echocardiography. New York: John Wiley & Sons; 1985.)

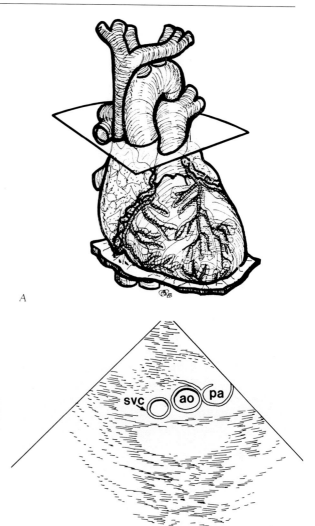

A

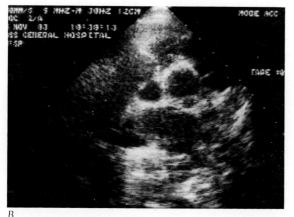

B

With a 90-degree clockwise rotation from this scan plane, a short-axis view of the superior vena cava, aorta, and pulmonary artery may be recorded (Fig. 6-47).

*Right and Left Atria.* The two atria and the interatrial septum can often be recorded by positioning the transducer along the right parasternum, usually in the second, third, or fourth intercostal space, and directing the sector plane medially. The plane marker should point inferomedially, toward the ventricular apex. This view often permits an im-

proved view of the interatrial septum, which is especially useful when examining a patient for defects in this area. (Fig. 6-48A.) In some patients, a four-chamber view can be obtained by placing the transducer in a lower interspace along the right parasternum and pointing the plane marker toward the ventricular apex (Fig. 6-48B).

Color-flow mapping and spectral Doppler tracings can be done in this view to assess possible shunt flow. Where available, the right parasternal approach is superior for evaluating patients with atrial septal defects because it has the advantages

FIGURE 6-48. (A) Schema of the scan plane through the heart in the (B) right parasternal view of the two atria. This view often permits an improved image of the interatrial septum and can be used for flow analysis with spectral Doppler and color-flow mapping. (C) Right parasternal four-chamber view in a patient with biatrial enlargement (ias, interatrial septum; IVS, interventricular septum; LA, left atrium; LV, left ventricle; mv, mitral valve; RA, right atrium; RV, right ventricle; tv, tricuspid valve). (Harrigan P, Lee R. Principles of Interpretation in Echocardiography. New York: John Wiley & Sons; 1985.)

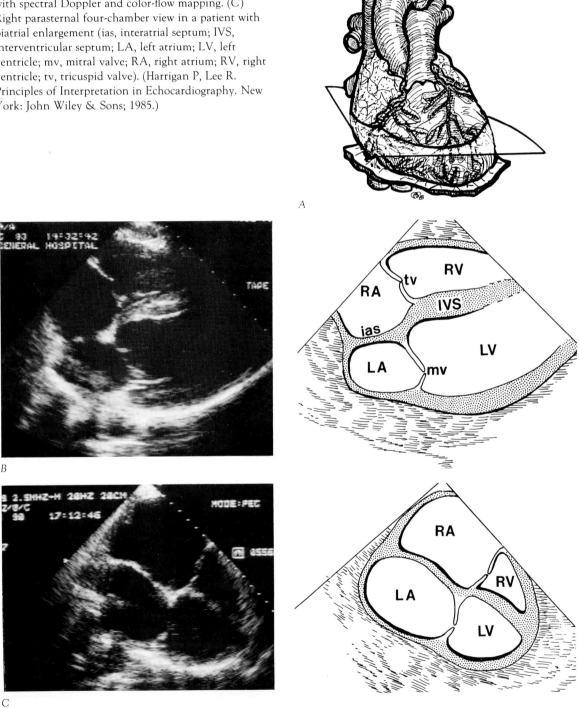

FIGURE 6-49. (A) Schema of the scan plane through the heart in the (B) right parasternal long-axis view of the right ventricular inflow tract (atl, anterior tricuspid leaflet; ptl, posterior tricuspid leaflet; RA, right atrium; RV, right ventricle). (Harrigan P, Lee R. Principles of Interpretation in Echocardiography. New York: John Wiley & Sons; 1985.)

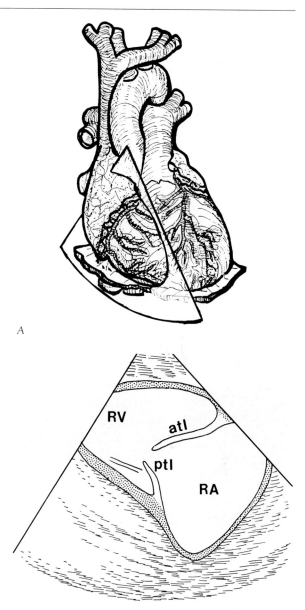

A

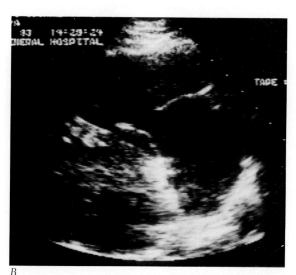

B

of confining the area of interest within the transducer focal zone and of imaging structures in a plane perpendicular to the acoustic beam.

*Right Ventricular Inflow Tract.* The right ventricular inflow tract can be recorded by positioning the transducer in the third or fourth interspace, directing the plane marker toward the patient's right shoulder, and angling the beam posteriorly (Fig. 6-49). The tricuspid valve orifice can be observed by rotating the scan plane 90 degrees clockwise (Fig. 6-50). This orientation also permits improved appreciation of the configuration of the right ventricle as the sternum is not an obstacle in this view.

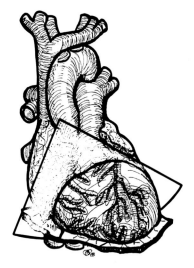

A

FIGURE 6-50. (A) Schematic drawing illustrating the scan plane of the (B) right parasternal short-axis view, which often permits visualization of the tricuspid orifice (tvo) (LV, left ventricle; RV, right ventricle).

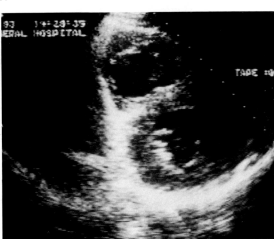

B

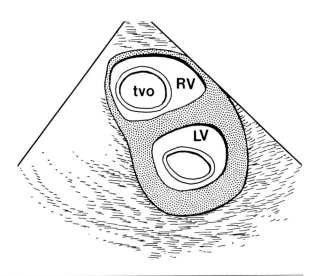

## Summary

The previous discussion has described the standard as well as some nonstandard images of the heart. Color-flow mapping and spectral Doppler technique have been suggested as integrated functions in the examination process. It is important to establish consistency in examination protocol in order to ensure a thorough examination of every patient. It is equally important not to feel confined by these standard views and to be creative, in order to use echocardiography to its fullest.

## Acknowledgments

The author is very grateful to colleague and friend, Anthony J. Sanfilippo, M.D., Hotel Dieu Hospital, Kingston, Ontario, for editorial input; and to Nancy Kriebel and Bernie Reisen for artwork.

## References

1. Harrigan P. Echocardiographic examination of the ventricular outflow tracts and great vessels: Use of the cardiac apex as an examination site to record the RVOT. Med Ultrasound. 1984; 8:137–144.
2. Henry WL, et al. Report of the American Society of Echocardiography Committee on Nomenclature and Standards in Two-Dimensional Imaging. Circulation. 1980; 62:212.
3. Weyman AE. Cross-Sectional Echocardiography. Philadelphia: Lea & Febiger; 1982.

# CHAPTER 7

# Essentials of Echocardiographic Measurements

SALLY MOOS

**M**easurements are an important part of the echocardiographic examination as chamber size, wall thickness, Doppler velocities, and other quantitative parameters of a patient's heart are compared to normal established values or monitored in serial studies. These values, which can be obtained relatively quickly, repeatedly, and noninvasively, have been well accepted by the medical community as a useful part of the examination, but, because echocardiographic results are operator dependent, measurements can be accurate or invalid. It is the sonographer's responsibility to understand how the various measurements are made and to acquire adequate images to ensure that the results are valid. This chapter is an overview of some of the most popular measurement techniques and calculations available for two-dimensional (2-D), M-mode, and Doppler echocardiographic examinations. The methods covered should be varied enough to allow the echocardiographer to apply these concepts readily to other calculations not covered in this text.

## Considerations

Controversy persists over whether 2-D or M-mode technique should be used to measure chamber and artery size and wall thickness and whether measurements should be made from a hard copy of the M-mode or 2-D image or on line, off the monitor. As long as the position is standardized and compared to normal values obtained in a similar plane, whichever method is the least time consuming is recommended. After establishing a standardized position where the cursor line transects the interfaces perpendicularly, one can usually measure from the 2-D image. If the acoustic window is limited and the plane is not optimal, the examiner should make no exact measurements but should give only a subjective impression of grossly normal or abnormal chamber size and wall thickness. When an image in the correct plane is available, the measurements from 2-D and M-mode images will be approximately the same. Data that does not display the specific interfaces should be considered technically poor for measurement. Specific guidelines available from the American Society of Echocardiography (ASE) for 2-D and M-mode measurements are reviewed in detail below. These serve as a reliable standard for measuring technically adequate data. The Penn convention for M-mode measurements is another alternative. Whichever method is used, the sonographer must be sure to consult corresponding normal value tables.[10,13,46]

Many measurements and calculations are available for Doppler data: pressure gradients, cardiac output, and left ventricular diastolic function, among others. The list is extensive and will continue to increase as new and better parameters for interpretations are developed. Application of certain measurements and calculations is reliable only if specific criteria are met; these have been listed for the individual calculations in this text. It is important to remember that measurements are operator dependent and small errors can produce grossly different results when entered into various calculations. Common sense as well as the following guidelines should be applied to each measurement.

### Guidelines for Making Echocardiographic Measurements

The reference for end-diastolic measurements is the Q wave on the electrocardiogram or the maximum left ventricle (LV) dimension, the thinnest walls, or deepest aortic position from the transducer. The reference for LV end-systolic measurements is at (1) the peak inward motion of the ventricular septum (VS), if motion is normal, or (2) the peak inward motion of the LV posterior wall (PW), if VS motion is abnormal, or at (3) the maximum left atrial (LA) dimension. Mitral valve (MV) closure imaged by M mode or cessation of flow across the MV imaged by Doppler also serve as references for end-diastole, whereas aortic valve closure or the cessation of aortic flow indicates end-systole.[46]

Data should be measured only when interfaces (such as the endocardium or the right side of VS or the Doppler spectral peak velocity) are clearly available. In other words, the examiner must not guess where the structure or point to be measured is.

Many measurements become impossible to take or, if they can be taken, are invalid when the heart rate (HR) is greater than 100 beats per minute (tachycardia). If the HR is rapid, measurements should be deferred until it drops below 100 beats per minute. Measurements should not be taken after a premature ventricular contraction (PVC). If the patient's echocardiogram rhythm is bigeminy the measurements become invalid. If a patient is experiencing atrial fibrillation, measurements are taken during a cardiac cycle of fairly normal HR (60 to 100 beats per minute) or a series of at least three to five measurements is averaged.

For Doppler calculations involving velocity, the examiner should always measure the highest velocity that is recorded. Guiding the spectral Doppler (continuous-wave, pulsed, or high pulse repetition frequency) with color-flow mapping Doppler can facilitate positioning parallel to flow. The spectral waveform should be complete throughout the phase of the cardiac cycle (systole or diastole) of interest. Maximum flow is displayed while minimizing artifact by optimal equipment control adjustment. Any timing measurements are more precise if the recording speed is 100 mm per second. This allows 1 mm on a ruler to equal 1 mm per second on the strip-chart recording. In addition, Doppler spectral amplitude measurements are more precise when the scale is set so that the maximum vertical display is used.

The sonographer must know the calibration on the system in use. The depth markers (distance) occur each 1 cm or 10 mm but may be subdivided into 5- or 2-mm increments. The amplitude divisions (velocity) occur 0.2, 0.25, 0.5, or 1 m (or 20, 25, 50, 100 cm). Horizontal divisions (time) may occur each 0.04, 0.2, 0.5, or 1 second.

In this chapter, values for measurements and calculations are displayed in brackets. If abnormal, they are preceded by Ab., and if for children, by P. Otherwise the numbers reflect *approximate* adult normal values. It is most beneficial if individual laboratories establish normal values that accurately reflect their specific patient population; these can be arranged by age and body size for more accuracy.

## Left and Right Ventricles

### Measuring Dimensions from Two-Dimensional or M-Mode Images

The examiner should establish a standardized position from the 2-D echocardiogram.[13] On the parasternal long axis, the VS should be fairly horizontal, not vertical. From the short axis, the LV should appear circular, not oblong.

The cursor line should be perpendicular to both the VS and LVPW and should, therefore, cross the VS and LVPW at approximately the same level within the LV. From the short-axis plane the cursor must be in the middle of the circle. For the left and right ventricles (RV) the cut should be between the free edge of the MV leaflets and the tips of the papillary muscle.

According to the standards established by the ASE[46] (Fig. 7-1) and guidelines described above, the examiner obtains a recording of the LV and RV at end-diastole (Dd) and measures the following

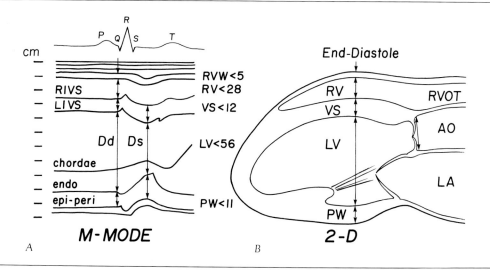

FIGURE 7-1. (A) On an M-mode tracing, chamber size and wall thickness are measured from leading edge to leading edge of the tissue interfaces which are compared to the cm calibration markers using calipers. Upper normal values are listed. (B) From a standard plane, similar dimensions can be obtained from the 2-D data at end-diastole and end-systole. (RIVS, right interventricular septum; LIVS, left interventricular septum; endo, endocardium; epiperi, epipericardium; RVW, right ventricular wall; RV, right ventricle; VS, ventricular septum; LV, left ventricle; PW, posterior wall; RVOT, right ventricular outflow tract; Ao, aorta; LA, left atrium.)

structures to calculate chamber size and wall thickness and at end-systole (Ds) for LV function:

*LV Size.* Leading edge of left side of VS to leading edge of endocardium {Dd, <5.6 cm}.

*RV Size.* Leading edge of RV endocardium to leading edge of right side of VS {Dd, <2.8 cm}.

*VS Thickness.* Leading edge of right side to leading edge of left side. Be sure to exclude tricuspid apparatus, which may lie along the right VS {Dd, < 1.2 cm}.

*LVPW Thickness.* Leading edge of endocardium to leading edge of epicardium {Dd, <1.1 cm}.

*RVW Thickness.* Leading edge of epicardium-pericardium to endocardial interface {Dd, <0.5 cm}. This may be defined more clearly from the subcos-

tal view. The RVW must not be measured at the level of the papillary muscle.

*Asymmetric Septal Hypertrophy (ASH).* Calculate the ratio of VS to LVPW, {Ab, ≥1.5}.

SYSTOLIC FUNCTION
*Percentage of Fractional Shortening (FS).* {(LVDd − LVDs)/(LVDd)} × 100 {>30%}.[20,42]

*Velocity of Circumferential Fiber Shortening (VCF) Circumference per Second.* (LVDd − LVDs)/(LVDd × LVET) or FS/LVET [≥1.1][43]

*Volumes and Ejection Fraction.* Echocardiography underestimates volume calculations compared to other methods of volume calculations, but this error is cancelled out in the ejection fraction calculation.[13] Serial follow-up changes are not affected in individual patients. The most accurate method of calculating volume is the geometric Simpson (apical four- and two-chamber views) and Bullet (apical four-chamber and parasternal short-axis views) biplanar formulas, which require planimetry. This is best obtained with a computer program available on many echocardiography systems and on all off-line analysis systems.[11,19,48]

When no segmental wall motion abnormality is present a single-plane (apical four-chamber or apical two-chamber) method provides fairly reliable ejection fraction results.[61] A simplified point-to-point method can be used when the image of the endocardial surface is incomplete, either with a single short-axis cut if no wall motion abnormality is present (method A) or with a triple short-axis cut if segmental wall motion abnormalities are present (method B).[1] This method can be applied without computer assistance by using hard copy recordings. Finally, volume and ejection fraction calculations can be obtained from M-mode data, subject to the following conditions: (1) the remaining myocardium is contracting similarly, and (2) the LV is ellipsoid.

*Two-dimensional (point-to-point) echocardiographic approach.* Apical four-chamber or two-chamber views are obtained at end-diastole (largest LV volume) and end-systole (smallest LV volume). For method A the sonographer should measure the length (*l*) from the base of the MV to the apex and the internal diameter (*d*) midposition at end-diastole (ED) and end-systole (ES). For method B the sonographer should measure the length (*l*) from the base of the MV to the apex and three equidistant diameters—1 cm above the base of the MV ($d_1$), midcavity ($d_2$), and at an equal distance toward the apex ($d_3$) at ED and ES (Fig. 7-2).

Calculate the following:

$A = \pi r^2$

where $\pi = 3.14$, $r = d/2$

$A = 3.14 \times (d/2)^2$

*Diastolic volume (EDV) or systolic volume (ESV):*
$$5/6 \, (A \times L) \text{ ml/min.}^{68}$$
*Ejection fraction (EF), method A:*
$$[(\text{ED}d)^2 \times \text{ED}l] - [(\text{ES}d)^2 \times \text{ES}l]/(\text{ED}d)^2 \times \text{ED}l \times 100 \, [>50\%].^1$$
*Ejection fraction (EF), method B:*
$$(\text{EF}_1 + \text{EF}_2 + \text{EF}_3)/3, \, [\text{Ab.} < 50\%].^1$$

*M-mode approach.* An M-mode image of LV is

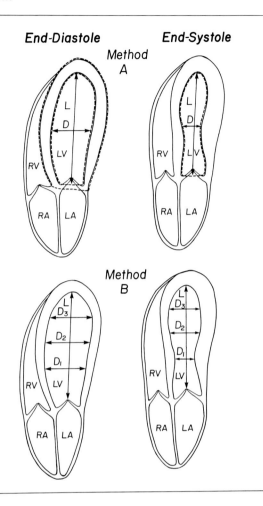

Figure 7-2. For a simplified point-to-point LV ejection fraction calculation from apical views at end-diastole and end-systole, measure the internal length (L) and diameter (D) on a frozen image or hard copy recording for method A. For method B also measure diameters ($D_1$ and $D_3$) at points equidistant from $D_2$. Using the modified Bullet formula available on many echocardiographic system calculation packages, trace the endocardial border and measure the length (L) at end-diastole and end-systole (*top*). Deriving LV mass from a single-plane method requires calculating the volume from the endocardial area and length and the epicardial area and length (*top left*). (RV, right ventricle; LV, left ventricle; RA, right atrium; LA, left atrium.) (Modified from Baron AO, Rogal GJ, Nanda NC. by two-dimensional echocardiography: A new method. J Am Coll Cardiol. 1983; 1:1471–1473. Reprinted with permission from the American College of Cardiology.)

obtained following guidelines for dimensions above. LVDd and LVDs are measured from

*End-diastolic volume (EDV)*
$$= \{7.0/(2.4 + LVDd) \times (LVDd)\} \text{ ml/m}^2,$$
$$\{\text{about 70 ml/min}^2\}.[3]$$

*End-systolic volume (ESV)*
$$= \{7.0/(2.4 + LVDs) \times (LVDs)\}^3 \text{ ml/m}^2,$$
$$\{\text{about 25 ml/min}^2\}.[13,59]$$

From volumes measured on either 2-D or M-mode images the following values are calculated:

*Stroke volume (SV):* EDV − ESV {about 45 ml/min}.

*Ejective fraction (EF):*
$$\{(EDV − ESV)/EDV\} \times 100, \{>50\%\}.[6,13,29]$$

*Note: For the most accurate results, use a biplanar computer program for ejection fraction calculations.*

RV ejection fractions (EFs) have proved to be accurate, particularly when they are calculated with a biplanar formula (RV four-chamber and subcostal views or RV two-chamber and RV parasternal long-axis views).[40] The guidelines for LVEF, above, apply.

*Cardiac Output.* Cardiac output (CO) must not be estimated across stenotic or regurgitant valves or in patients with complex arrhythmias.

*Two-dimensional approach.* The guidelines under Volumes and Ejection Fractions, above, are applied to obtain stroke volume (SV) from a 2-D image,[15] which is usually underestimated with this method. Measure the RR interval on the electrocardiogram to determine the HR.

$$HR = 60/R − R, \{60 \text{ to } 100 \text{ beats/min}\}.$$

$$CO = (SV/1000) \times HR, \{\text{about 5 l/min}\}.$$

*Doppler approach.* The guidelines under Considerations, above, apply (Figs. 7-3, 7-4). Values needed to calculate CO are the flow velocity integral (FVI), cross-sectional area (CSA), and HR.[21,28]

FVI and CSA can be obtained from Doppler recordings parallel to flow and 2-D- or M-mode-based diameters of the aorta, LV outflow tract, pulmonary artery, RV outflow tract, across mitral or tricuspid valves. In adults the most accurate CO is obtained from the LV outflow tract (LVOT) or aorta.

The Doppler spectral tracing should show

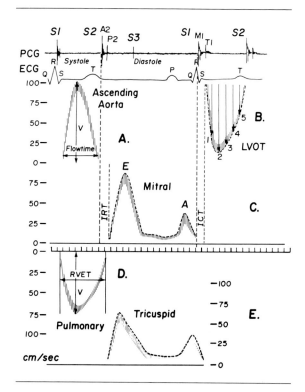

FIGURE 7-3. Timing of the Doppler systolic and diastolic duration in normal persons are represented in this schematic drawing. (A) LV flow time and volocity (V) can be measured for the flow velocity integral calculation. (B) Velocities 1 to 5 can be measured at regular intervals and averaged to obtain the mean velocity. (B,C,E) For the most accurate calculation of mean velocity, use a planimetry method and trace around the outer border of the spectral tracing. (D) Right ventricular ejection time (RVET) and velocity (V) measurements are displayed. (PCG, phonocardiogram; S1, first heart sound; A2, aortic closure of the second heart sound; P2, pulmonic closure of the second heart sound; S2, second heart sound; ECG, electrocardiogram; LVOT, left ventricular outflow tract; IRT, isovolumetric relaxation time; ICT, isovolumetric contraction time.)

clearly the onset and end of flow, a narrow bandwidth, and consistent peak velocity from beat to beat. Measurements described below for calculating velocity (V) should be made from the baseline to the peak of the flow and expressed in centimeters. For the most accurate results three or more complexes should be averaged.

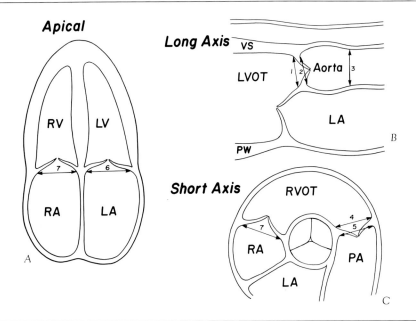

FIGURE 7-4. Various positions are available for measuring cardiac outputs. An accurate diameter measurement is crucial for calculating cardiac output. Internal dimensions should be taken from well-defined tissue interfaces, as noted from positions 1 (left ventricular outflow tract, LVOT), 2 (aortic root), 3 (ascending aorta above the level of the sinus of Valsalva), 4 (right ventricular outflow tract, RVOT), 5 (pulmonary artery, PA), 6 (mitral annulus), 7 (tricuspid annulus) and as described on pages 154–155. (VS, ventricular septum; PW, posterior wall; LA, left atrium; RV, right ventricle; LV, left ventricle; RA, right atrium.)

For the CSA calculation the internal diameter of the outflow tract, artery, or valve annulus is measured on the clearest view. Precision is imperative, as a 0.1- or 0.2-cm error can be magnified by the formula. It may not be possible to use the same view from which the Doppler tracing was obtained, but the same area or level should be used.

The HR is determined by measuring the RR interval on the electrocardiogram. To calculate FVI, planimetry is used to determine mean velocity by computer or by measuring velocities at regular intervals (e.g., 2 mm) from beginning to end of the spectral tracing that are averaged and multiplied by the time of the spectral waveform (see Fig. 7-3B). For aortic or pulmonic FVI, a simplified formula shown in Figure 7-3A can be applied:

$$FVI = (Peak\ V \times Flow\ time)/2$$

This underestimates the true value but is useful for serial measurements in individual patients. The following formula produces a more accurate calculation:

$$1.14\ [(Peak\ V \times Flow\ time)/2] + 0.30$$

$$CSA\ cm^2 = \pi r^2 \qquad \pi = 3.14 \qquad r = d/2$$

$$\text{or} \qquad 3.14 \times (D/2)^2$$

FVI and CSA calculations can be made from the areas listed below.

*Calculations for flow velocity integral and cross sectional areas (see also Fig. 7-4).*

Obtain the LVOT velocity using PW Doppler and diameter from the 2-D or M-mode measurement just proximal to the aortic valve.

Obtain the aorta velocity by CW or PW Doppler and internal diameter at aortic annulus or 2 to 3 cm distal to aortic valve and above aortic sinuses.

Obtain the RVOT velocity by PW Doppler and internal diameter just proximal to the pulmonic valve.

Obtain the PA velocity by CW or PW and PA diameter.

Obtain the MV velocity by CW or PW and MV annulus diameter (and minimum/maximum leaflet separation by M-mode).

Obtain the TV velocity by CW or PW and TV annulus diameter.

*Stroke volume* = FVI × CSA {about 45 ml/m$^2$}

*HR* = 60/R − R sec {60 to 100 beats/min}

*CO* = (SV/1000) × HR {about 5 L/min}

CO can be calculated more precisely across the mitral valve by obtaining an M-mode image of the mitral valve and measuring the maximum ($S_M$) and minimum ($S_m$) separation between the anterior and posterior leaflets[14]:

CO = FVI × CSA × ($S_m$/$S_M$) × HR

In normal persons aortic or mitral (systemic) CO is equal to pulmonic or tricuspid (pulmonary) CO.[12,18]

For follow-up of patients undergoing therapy or following an exercise program, it may be useful to evaluate the percentage of change of the aortic FVI. This also avoids the inherent errors associated with estimates of CSA. Aortic FVI is measured at baseline ($FVI_1$) and on follow-up ($FVI_2$).

*Aortic FVI (% change)* = ($FVI_1$ − $FVI_2$)/$FVI_1$

[if FVI % change is >20%, then SV change is >20%.][12,18]

*Other Doppler Parameters.* *Peak ejection velocity* is determined by measuring baseline to peak velocity (*V*, Fig. 7-5B) and is expressed in meters per second.[12,18] *Acceleration time (AT)/deceleration time (DT)* (a way of serially following LV function) is determined by measuring the time from onset of systolic flow to peak velocity (*V*) and dividing it by the measured time from peak velocity (*V*) to cessation of flow (Fig. 7-5B).[12,18] In patients with aortic stenosis the peak velocity (*V*) across aortic valve in systole is measured simultaneously with brachial systolic blood pressure (BP).

*LV systolic pressure* =
$$4V^2 + \text{(systolic BP)}, \{<150 \text{ mm Hg}\}.[21]$$

*Systolic Time Intervals (STIs).*

*Left side of the heart.* M-MODE APPROACH. An M-mode image of the *aortic valve* is obtained using the parasternal or apical approach, showing clearly the exact points of complete *opening* (separation of anterior and posterior leaflets) and *closing* (coaptation of anterior and posterior leaflets). A2 (aortic valve closing sound) recorded from a phonocardiogram tracing can be substituted for aortic valve closure by echo (Fig. 7-5A).

DOPPLER APPROACH. A clean spectral trace of *aortic flow velocity* is obtained from the suprasternal, apical, or right parasternal view using a low filter that shows clearly the *initial rise* and *return to baseline* (see Fig. 7-5B).

M-MODE AND DOPPLER. The electrocardiogram must show clearly the onset of the *Q wave*. (Lead II—left arm, left leg, and right leg usually displays it well.) A phonocardiogram recording that displays clearly the onset of the first heart sound (S1, mitral valve closure) and the second heart sound (S2, aortic valve closure, A2), is optional (see Fig. 7-5). The parameters are measured for three to five cardiac cycles and are recorded at 100 mm/sec and are averaged. All are expressed in millimeters per second.

The *electromechanical interval (EMI)* is measured from Q-wave to aortic valve closure (A2). *Isovolumetric contraction time* is measured from mitral valve closure (S1) to onset of aortic valve opening, or systolic flow {<0.05 m/sec}. *LVET* is measured from aortic valve opening to closure (A2), or onset of end of systolic flow {280 to 320 m/sec}. The *preejection period (PEP)* is the difference between EMI and LVET, or the period from Q wave to aortic valve opening, or the time from Q wave to onset of systolic flow. The normal range of the PEP-LVET ratio is 0.27 to 0.43.[64]

*Right side of the heart.* The pulmonic valve (PV) or pulmonary artery (PA) Doppler tracing is used for measuring right-sided systolic time intervals following the method for the left side of the heart, above.

*Wall Motion Score.* Echocardiographic evaluation of wall motion abnormalities requires establishing

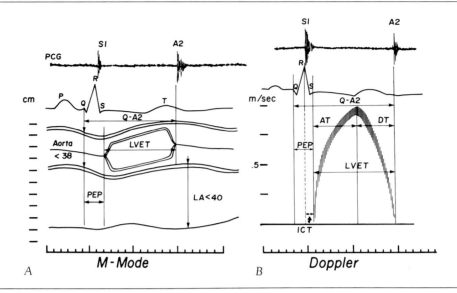

FIGURE 7-5. (A) For systolic time interval calculations from an M-mode tracing, measure the LVET and Q to aortic valve closure on any echocardiogram or phonocardiogram (A2). The dimensions from leading edge to leading edge of the aorta at end-diastole and the LA at end-systole are normally less than 38 and 40 mm, respectively. (B) The Doppler calculation of systolic time intervals requires a low filter to allow accurate identification of the initiation and cessation of flow. Acceleration time (AT) and deceleration time (DT) calculations also require a well-defined peak velocity. Isovolumetric contraction time (ICT) can be measured from the start of the mitral closure sound (S1) to the initiation of the Doppler systolic flow. (PCG, phonocardiogram; PEP, preejection period.)

identifiable segments of the LV walls and describing the wall motions. The ASE has specific recommendations for the wall segment division.

A simplified 14-segment model (Fig. 7-6) has been used to evaluate the LV wall motion score (WMS).[39] To analyze wall motion using the WMS index, both endocardial motion and myocardial thickening must be visualized. The WMS is derived by numerically rating wall motion in each segment visualized (see Fig. 7-6): 0, hyperkinetic; 1, normal; 2, hypokinetic; 3, akinetic; 4, dyskinetic; 5, aneurysm. The WMS index is the average of these scores {1.0}.[39]

### DIASTOLIC FUNCTION
*Doppler Approach.* The Doppler spectrum of the LV inflow is imaged just distal to the annulus, near the MV leaflet tip at end expiration. The peak rapid filling point (E) and peak atrial contraction

point (A) must be clearly visible. The Doppler guidelines listed in Considerations and Figure 7-7 provide more detail on where to measure.[9,32,37,52,58] The sonographer must be aware that age, presence of mitral regurgitation, diastolic BP, and position of the pulsed Doppler sample volume are major considerations when analyzing diastolic Doppler flow data.

*Velocities. E velocity,* in meters or centimeters per second, is measured from the baseline to peak rapid filling point, {about 0.8 m/sec}. A *velocity* is measured from baseline to peak A point, {about 0.5 m/sec}. The ratio of E to A should be >1.0 and that of A to E, <1.0 in normal subjects.[16,54] *Acceleration half-time* is the elapsed time from peak E to 50% of E velocity on the upslope, {62 ± 18 m/sec}.[17] *Deceleration half-time* is the elapsed time from peak E to 50% of E velocity on the downslope, {73 ± 24 m/sec}.[17] *One-half filling fraction* is the FVI during

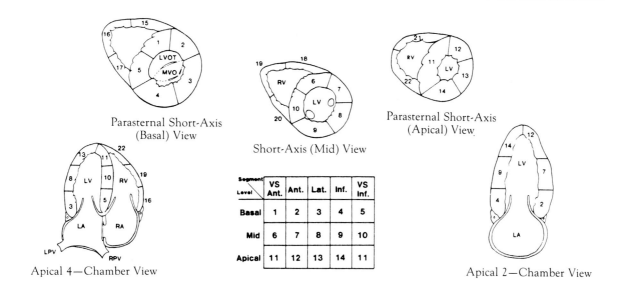

| Segment<br>Level | VS<br>Ant. | Ant. | Lat. | Inf. | VS<br>Inf. |
|---|---|---|---|---|---|
| Basal | 1 | 2 | 3 | 4 | 5 |
| Mid | 6 | 7 | 8 | 9 | 10 |
| Apical | 11 | 12 | 13 | 14 | 11 |

Parasternal Short-Axis (Basal) View

Short-Axis (Mid) View

Parasternal Short-Axis (Apical) View

Apical 4—Chamber View

Apical 2—Chamber View

FIGURE 7-6. Segmental motion of the LV walls at the basal, middle, and apical levels can be divided into 14 segments. The number for each wall segment is identified on the tomographic views and on the center graph. Enter the number for the wall motion (0, hyperkinetic; 1, normal; 2, hypokinetic; 3, akinetic; 4, dyskinetic; 5, aneurysm) in each section of the center graph for each wall segment visualized. Add these together and divide by the number of segments visualized. (LVOT, left ventricular outflow tract; MVO, mitral valve orifice; RV, right ventricle; LV, left ventricle; RA, right atrium; LA, left atrium; RPV, right pulmonary vein; LPV, left pulmonary vein; Ao, aorta; VS Ant, ventricular septum anterior wall; Ant, anterior wall; Lat, lateral wall; Inf, inferior wall; VS Inf, ventricular septum inferior wall.) (From Nishimura RA, Tajik AJ, Shah C, et al. Role of two-dimensional echocardiography in the prediction of in-hospital complications after myocardial infarction. J Am Coll Cardiol. 1984; 4:1080–1087.)

the first half of diastole divided by the total FVI, {>0.55}. *One-third filling fraction* is the FVI during the first third of diastole divided by the total FVI [$p$ .58 ± 8].[66] *Isovolumetric relaxation time* is the time from A2 (aortic valve closure on a phonocardiogram) to the beginning of the Doppler diastolic waveform, {<0.05 sec}.

*Other Doppler parameters.* Many other diastolic function measurements and calculations, including indexes of peak and mean filling rates, areas, and area fractions, may be useful. The measurements and calculations described above can be applied to assessment of RV diastolic function but normal values are presently unavailable.

*Left ventricular end-diastolic pressure (LVEDP).* With continuous-wave Doppler technique, a recording is obtained of the aortic regurgitation (AR) flow throughout diastole displaying clearly the peak velocity at end-diastole. The maximum AR velocity ($V$) is measured at the end of diastole (from baseline to peak; Fig. 7-13A). The diastolic blood pressure is determined with a brachial cuff.

$$LVEDP = \text{Diastolic BP} - 4V^2, \{<12 \text{ mm Hg}\}.[53]$$

LEFT VENTRICULAR WALL MASS
*Two-Dimensional Approach.* The guidelines for obtaining EDV or ESV, above, apply; a planimetry

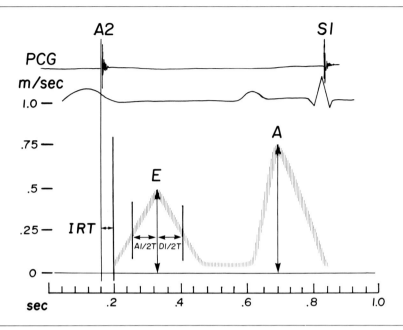

Figure 7-7. For analysis of diastolic left ventricular filling, measure the peak velocity from the baseline to the peak velocity of the E and A waves. Isovolumetric relaxation time (IRT) is measured from the beginning of the aortic closure (A2) on the phonocardiogram (PCG) to the initial diastolic flow. The time from the initial flow to 50% of the peak E is the acceleration one-half-time (A ½ T) and from E to 50% of the downslope is the deceleration one-half-time (D ½ T). (S1, first heart sound.)

method such as Simpson's or Bullet's is preferred. The EDV$_{endo}$ and EDV$_{epi}$ are determined by measurement of the endocardial and epicardial border, respectively. A single-plane formula is used if wall thickness is symmetric. A biplanar formula is used if it is asymmetric. The epicardial measurement must include the entire thickness of the septal and apical walls (see Fig. 7-2).

For the single-plane method, the formula for *LV wall mass*[5], in grams, is: 1.04 × (EDV$_{epi}$ − EDV$_{endo}$).

*M-Mode Approach.* The guidelines on pages 149–150 for obtaining diastolic LV chamber (LVDd) and wall thickness measurements apply (see Fig. 7-1). The formula for *LV wall mass*[10], in grams, is: 1.04 {(LVDd + LVPWd + VSd)$^3$ − (LVDd)$^3$}. *Body surface area (BSA)*, in square meters, is determined by plugging the patient's height and weight into a nomogram for BSA or by calculating as follows:

1/99.093 [(height in inches)$^{0.725}$ + (weight in lbs)$^{0.425}$],

or 0.007184 [(height in cm)$^{0.725}$ + (weight in kg)$^{0.425}$]

The formula for *LV wall mass index*, in grams per square meter, is: LV wall mass/BSA [<100 g/m$^2$].

## Mitral and Tricuspid Valves

### Prolapse

No standardized, widely accepted measurements are available for this controversial syndrome because the echocardiographic and clinical findings are so varied. Attempts to establish reliable criteria based on M-mode or 2-D echocardiograms of the mitral or tricuspid valve have been unsuccessful.

### Stenosis

The Doppler computer calculation package supplied with ultrasound equipment provides a quick and accurate means for calculating peak and mean velocities and gradients and measuring pressure half-time and valve areas. If such software is not available a hard copy should be made at the fast recording speed (100 mm/sec). A Doppler complex should be chosen for measurements that clearly exhibits the maximum peak velocity and defines the spectral velocities throughout the flow phase. To obtain the mean gradient, peak gradients should be calculated at regular intervals (e.g., every 2 mm) for the duration of the diastolic flow and averaged. (See guidelines in Considerations, above, and review Figure 7-8A for more details.[21,24,45])

*Peak Velocity (V), in m or cm*, is measured from the baseline to the peak of the flow excursion during initial diastole. *Peak gradient, in mm Hg, is $4V^2$* {mild 4 to 10; moderate 11 to 20; severe >20}. *Mean gradient, in mm Hg*, is the average of several peak gradients ($4V^2$) calculated at regular intervals (about every 2 mm) over the flow duration.

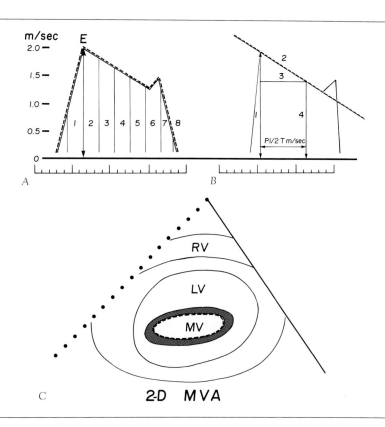

Figure 7-8. (A) In AV valve stenosis or prosthetic replacement, obtain peak velocity by measuring from the baseline to E. Use the equipment planimetry method to trace around the outer spectral envelope for the mean gradient or average the peak gradients obtained at equidistant points (1 to 8). (B) Calculation of mitral valve area by the pressure one-half-time method can be made from a hard copy recording by following steps 1–8 on page 160. (C) Using the calculation package on the echocardiographic equipment, trace the inner border of the mitral valve orifice to obtain the mitral valve area (MVA) on the 2-D tracing. (RV, right ventricle; LV, left ventricle; MV, mitral valve.)

*Pressure Half-Time and Valve Area.* The examiner should choose a complex that exhibits a clear peak and a straight downslope during the first third of diastole. It need not be the same complex used to calculate gradients. Calculations of pressure half-time and mitral valve area are described below and in Figure 7-8B.[25,33,34] {P half-time <60 m/sec is normal. MVA <1.0 cm² represents severe stenosis}.

*Calculation of pressure half-time and mitral valve area*

1. A vertical line is drawn from the point of peak velocity to baseline (line 1).
2. Line 1 is measured and the value divided by 1.4 ($\sqrt{2}$). This value (point) is marked on line 1.
3. A straight line (line 2) is drawn from line 1 through the diastolic downslope, following the initial slope of the velocity profile.
4. A horizontal line (line 3) is drawn from the peak velocity (V/1.4 point on line 1) to line 2.
5. A vertical line (line 4) is drawn from the intersection of lines 2 and 3 to the baseline.
6. The time between the intersection of line 1 and line 4 on the baseline (line 5) is measured. This value is the pressure half-time.
7. Lines 1 to 3 to 4 must lie at right angles to each other.
8. The mitral *valve area*, in square centimeters, is equal to 220 divided by the pressure half-time.

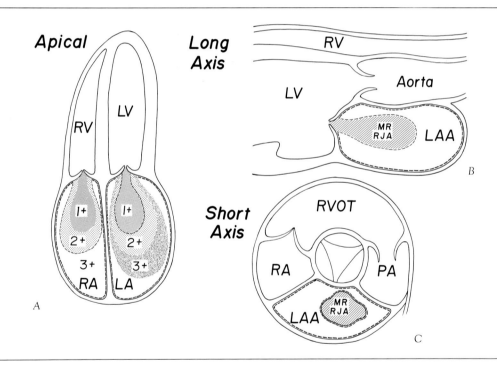

FIGURE 7-9. (A) For mitral regurgitation (MR) measure the area of the regurgitation jet (RJ) and compare to the measured left atrial area (LAA). A ratio of RJA to LAA less than 20% denotes mild disease (grade 1/3), whereas a value over 40% denotes severe disease (grade 3/3). (B) It is necessary to evaluate multiple planes to obtain the maximum jet area. (C) To establish the symmetry of the three-dimensional jet, it is useful to evaluate two orthogonal planes such as the parasternal long axis and short axis. (RV, right ventricle; LV, left ventricle; RA, right atrium; LA, left atrium; RVOT, right ventricular outflow tract; PA, pulmonary artery.)

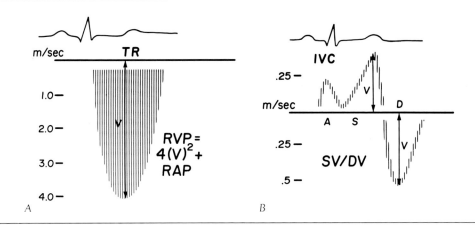

FIGURE 7-10. (A) Calculation of the right ventricular pressure (RVP) requires obtaining a peak velocity (V) of the tricuspid regurgitation (TR) flow. A constant of 10 mm Hg can be used for the right atrial pressure (RAP). (B) From an inferior vena cava (IVC) or vertical hepatic vein Doppler recording, measure the systolic (S) and diastolic (D) flow from the baseline to the peak velocity. The ratio of SV/DV should normally be less than 1.0.

*Calculation of Valve Area from a Two-Dimensional Tracing.* From a 2-D short-axis view, an image is obtained that shows the maximum orifice area at the tips of the valve leaflets. This may require scanning from the annulus to the chordae. The *valve area, in* $cm^2$, is determined by careful planimetry of the inner border of the orifice (Fig. 7-8C).[27,35]

REGURGITATION

*Regurgitant Fraction.* The regurgitant fraction should be calculated only when the regurgitant lesion is isolated. From the Doppler spectral trace, stroke volume (SV) across the atrioventricular valve (mitral or tricuspid) and semilunar valve (aortic or pulmonic) is determined using the method described under Cardiac Output, above. The following calculation is appropriate for mitral or tricuspid valve regurgitant fraction (RF): RF in % is (Mitral SV − Aortic SV)/Mitral SV.[21,57]

*Regurgitation Quantitation from Color Doppler Images.* The severity of regurgitation can be quantitated from color Doppler images. Because of limitations in this technique, results are not always accurate. The maximum jet area is recorded from a well-de-fined image of the atrial cavity. In some patients optimal visualization is afforded by an apical four- or two-chamber view; in others, by a parasternal long- or short-axis view. The entire jet area (RJA) and the atrial area (AA) are measured by planimetry. Results may be improved by averaging the RJA from views in two orthogonal planes (Fig. 7-9). The formula for *MR*, in percent, is RJA/AA; {grade 1/3, <20%; grade 2/3, 20 to 40%; grade 3/3, >40%}.[26] The same method can be applied to calculate tricuspid valve regurgitation (TR), but values for grading regurgitation on the right side are not as well established.

*RV Systolic Pressure and Pulmonary Artery Systolic Pressure Quantitation from Tricuspid Regurgitation.* From a spectral tracing of TR, the maximum (peak) velocity of regurgitation is measured. Right atrial (RA) pressure is estimated from the jugular venous pulse or the RA line, or the constant 10 mm Hg is used (see Fig. 7-10A). The formula for *RV systolic pressure, in mm Hg*, is $4 V^2 + 10$, or $4 V^2 + (JVP + 5)/1.3$.[4,8,69] If there is no right-sided valvular or sub-valvular obstruction *RV systolic pressure* is equal to *pulmonary artery pressure* {about 25 mm Hg}.

## Aortic and Pulmonic Valves

### STENOSIS

*Gradients.* The guidelines in Considerations and in Stenosis, above, apply, as does Figure 7-11D.[3,7,22,23,55] The *velocity* (*V*) is measured from the baseline to the peak systolic excursion of flow. The formula for the *peak gradient, in mm Hg,* is $4V^2$ or $4(V_1^2 - (V_2^2))$, {mild about 5 to 35, moderate 35 to 65, severe > 65}. The *mean gradient* is the average of several peak gradients ($4V^2$) calculated at regular intervals (about every 2 mm) over the flow duration.

*Aortic Valve Area (AVA).* From a parasternal long-axis view, the diameter (*D*) of the LV outflow (LVOT) is measured just distal to the aortic valve. From the apical four-chamber view, the peak LVOT velocity (*V*) is obtained by pulsed-wave Doppler technique just distal to the aortic valve. Care must be taken to avoid sampling in the flow of the stenosis jet. The peak velocity is measured by continuous-wave Doppler scanning across the aortic valve (aortic peak velocity; see Fig. 7-11).[45,51,55,60,67]

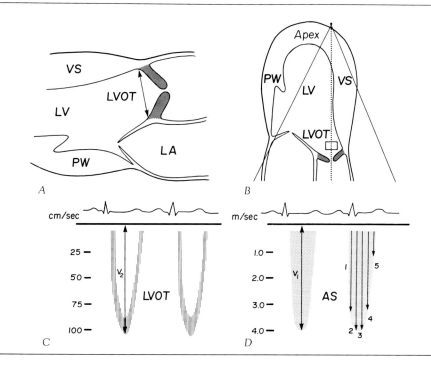

FIGURE 7-11. (A) In the calculation of aortic valve area, the left ventricular outflow tract (LVOT) diameter is measured just proximal to the thickened aortic valve on the parasternal long-axis view. (B) The LVOT velocity is obtained by pulsed-wave Doppler technique from the apical view just proximal to the aortic valve. The spectral flow should be laminar. (C) Measure the LVOT velocity ($V_2$) from the baseline to the peak flow. (D) To obtain the peak gradient ($4V^2$) and the final measurement to solve for aortic valve area, measure the velocity ($V_1$) from baseline to peak flow. The mean gradient can be obtained from hard copy by averaging peak gradients at equidistant points 1 to 5. (VS, ventricular septum; LV, left ventricle; PW, posterior wall; LA, left atrium; AS, aortic stenosis.)

Calculate the following:

Area $(A) = \pi r^2$,

or $3.14 \times (d/2)^2$

$AVA$, in $cm^2$, =

(LVOT $V$ × LVOT $A$)/Aortic peak velocity.

## REGURGITATION

*Regurgitant Fraction.* The regurgitant fraction must be calculated only when the regurgitant lesion is isolated. From the Doppler spectral tracing, stroke volume (SV) across the semilunar valves is determined using the method described in Cardiac Output, above. The formula for aortic regurgitant fraction (RF)[30], in percent, is:

(Aortic SV − Pulmonary SV)/Aortic SV or
          (Aortic SV − Mitral SV)/Aortic SV.

*Quantitation of Regurgitation from Color Doppler Images.* The severity of regurgitation can be roughly quantitated from color Doppler images. As with mitral regurgitation, limitations in this technique provide results that are not always accurate. The jet is recorded at its largest (height and width) as seen at its origin from the valve in a well-defined LVOT, which usually is displayed best in parasternal long- and short-axis views or in a low parasternal long-axis view but occasionally may be seen better from an apical or right parasternal approach. The height of the RJ is measured as it initially enters the LVOT, before fanning out. LVOT diameter is measured at the same level (Fig. 7-12). The percentage of *AR* is calculated by dividing the height of the jet by the diameter of the LVOT[41]: {grade 1/4, <25%; grade 2/4, 25 to 45%: grade 3/4, 46 to 63%; grade 4/4, >64%}. This method also can be applied to pulmonic regurgitation, but a grading system has not been established.

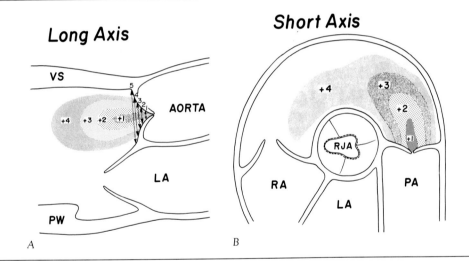

FIGURE 7-12. (A) For the quantitation of aortic regurgitation (AR) severity, measure the regurgitation jet (RJ) size and LVOT dimension (5) from a parasternal long-axis view. Four gradings (1 to 4) of severity can be differentiated. (B) Evaluate the aortic regurgitation jet area (RJA) from the parasternal short axis just proximal to the aortic valve as well to better define the symmetry of the lesion. Severe pulmonic regurgitation (PR) (grade 4/4) will extend to the tricuspid leaflets, whereas mild PR (grade 1/4) usually extends less than 1.0 cm from the pulmonic valve. (RV, right ventricle; LV, left ventricle; LA, left atrium; VS, ventricular spetum; PW, posterior wall; RA, right atrium; MPA, main pulmonary artery; LPA, left pulmonary artery.)

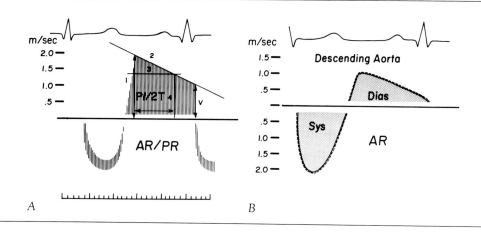

FIGURE 7-13. (A) For the steps to obtain the pressure one-half-time (P ½ T) calculation for the severity of aortic regurgitation (AR) see steps 1 to 7 on page 160. The velocity (V) is measured from baseline to peak flow at end-diastole for the calculation of the left ventricular end-diastolic pressure in AR and the pulmonary artery diastolic pressure in pulmonic regurgitation (PR). (B) The presence of significant AR can be determined by the appearance of diastolic backflow in the descending aorta from the suprasternal view. The ratio of the systolic (Sys) forward flow to the diastolic (Dias) regurgitant flow can be calculated by planimetry around the outer envelope of the flows.

*Severity of Aortic Regurgitation.*
*Pressure half-time or slope.* An image with a clearly defined peak and deceleration (downslope) of the AR jet is obtained by pulsed- or continuous-wave Doppler technique. A clear downslope may be recorded in only about 50% of patients with AR. The sonographer should follow steps 1 to 7 on page 160 and Figure 7-13A. A *pressure half-time* greater than 250 m/sec represents severe regurgitation.

*Backflow in the aorta.* This measurement requires a clearly defined pulsed-wave Doppler image of the descending aorta from the suprasternal view that shows clearly the entire cardiac cycle in systole and diastole. The area of the systolic flow is measured below the baseline and the area of the diastolic flow, above the baseline (see Fig. 7-13B). The *regurgitant fraction at the descending aorta* is the area measured during diastole divided by the area measured during systole and is expressed as a percentage.

To enhance the validity of this ratio, the aorta should be measured at the maximum ($d_{max}$) and minimum diameter ($d_{min}$) on an M-mode tracing.

The *diastolic diameter* ($d_d$) is the average of the two values, and the *systolic diameter* ($d_s$) is the maximum diameter. The formula for the *ratio* is:

(diastolic area/systolic area) $\times$ ($d_d^2/d_s^2$) $\times$ 100.

A value greater than 70% represents severe AR.[30] Backflow seen only at the beginning of diastole is a normal recoil phenomenon and does not indicate aortic regurgitation.

*Pulmonary Artery Diastolic Pressure.* A clearly defined pulsed-wave Doppler recording of the pulmonic regurgitation (PR) flow from a parasternal or subcostal view is needed (see guidelines on page 150). Maximum velocity (V) is measured at the end of diastole (see Fig. 7-13A). RA pressure is determined from the jugular venous pulse or the RA line. The formula for *pulmonary artery diastolic pressure*[36], in *mm Hg*, is:

$4V^2$ + RA pressure.

## Prosthetic Valves

All prosthetic valves develop some degree of stenosis, and the gradient formulas for calculating native stenosis can be applied in this situation. Many prostheses also have inherent regurgitation; again the methods already described for quantitating regurgitation apply. Because of the prosthesis artifact, imaging the regurgitation in front of or to the side of (rather than behind) the prosthesis improves results. If gradients are to be calculated the beam must be aligned parallel to the flow to obtain the maximum velocity.[44,65] No accurate Doppler calculations for determining valve area in prosthetic valves have been established.

### MITRAL AND TRICUSPID VALVE PROSTHESES

*Peak and Mean Gradients.* Guidelines for these calculations are described on pages 159 and 160; see also Figure 7-8A. The *peak gradient, in mm Hg,* is $4V^2$. For the *mean gradient, in mm Hg,* peak gradients are calculated at regular intervals (e.g., every 2 mm) for the duration of the diastolic flow and these values are averaged. The area of the *prosthetic valve, in square centimeters,* is 220 divided by the pressure half-time.

*Regurgitation.* The guidelines described on pages 150 and 161 and Figure 7-9 apply. The *regurgitation grading (RJA/AA)* is calculated as the grading for mitral regurgitation is.

### AORTIC AND PULMONIC VALVE PROSTHESES

*Peak and Mean Gradients.* Guidelines are described on pages 162 and 163 and in Figures 7-3B and 7-11. *Peak gradient, in mm Hg,* is $4V^2$. If the LVOT velocity is more than 1.0 m/sec, then, for *peak gradient, in mm Hg,* $4V_1^2 - V_2^2$. For mean gradient, in mm Hg, peak gradients are calculated at regular intervals (e.g., every 2 mm) for the duration of systolic flow and these values are averaged.

*Regurgitation.* Guidelines are described on pages 163 and 164 and in Figures 7-12 and 7-13A, B. The *regurgitation grading* of RJ height divided by LVOT diameter, *pressure half-time divided by slope (in meters per second),* and *aortic backflow ratio (diastolic area/ systolic area)* are calculated as is aortic regurgitation.

## The Atria

### DIMENSIONS

According to the standards established by the ASE (see Fig. 7-5A) and the guidelines described on page 150, a recording is obtained of the left atrium and aorta.[46] A standardized position is obtained from the 2-D image, either a parasternal long-axis or short-axis view that displays a circular aorta where the cursor line crosses perpendicular to the aorta. The cursor must be in the middle of the circle, not to either side. The cut should be made at the level of the aortic valve.

The *LA dimension* is measured in centimeters from the leading edge of the posterior aortic wall to the leading edge of the LA wall at the maximum dimension (at end-systole). A normal value is 4.0 cm or less. The RA can be subjectively compared with the LA from apical four-chamber, parasternal short-axis, or subcostal views. The RA should be about the same size as a normal left atrium.

*Ratio of Dimensions of Left Atrium and Aorta.* To better determine LA enlargement, the LA dimension can be compared to the size of the aortic root. The method of measuring the aorta is described on page 166. This *ratio* is normally less than 1.2 in adults and less than 1.1 in children.[13]

*Left Atrial Systolic Pressure.* To calculate the LA systolic pressure, measure the maximum mitral regurgitation velocity ($V$) and the brachial (arm) systolic blood pressure (BP). It is assumed that the LV systolic pressure is equal to the brachial arm pressure in the absence of aortic stenosis.

*LA systolic pressure, in mm Hg,* is the systolic BP minus $4V^2$ [mean 8 mm Hg].[21]

## The Left and Right Ventricular Outflow Tracts

### DIMENSIONS

Guidelines for these calculations are described on page 154. A perpendicular plane is established (parasternal long or short axis) to the LVOT or RVOT, if possible. The narrowest diameter is measured during systole; for example, from the left side of the VS to the anterior leaflet of the MV or just below the aortic valve in the LVOT (see Fig. 7-4)

{1.6 to 2.6 cm; in hypertrophic cardiomyopathy may be <1.0}.

### Subvalvular Obstruction

*Peak and Mean Gradients.* High–pulse repetition frequency (extended range) or continuous-wave Doppler is used to image the point of maximum velocity ($V_1$) across the obstruction. With pulsed Doppler mode the velocity ($V_2$) proximal to the obstruction is imaged and measured. Guidelines for these measurements are on page 150 (see Fig. 7-11B, C).[21,22] The formula for the *peak gradient, in mm Hg,* is $4(V_1^2 - V_2^2)$. The *mean gradient* is the average of five peak instantaneous gradients measured at regular intervals (e.g., every 2 mm).

## The Aorta and Pulmonary Artery

### Dimensions

According to the guidelines on pages 149 and 150 the left atrium and the aorta are imaged (see Fig. 7-5A).[13] The *aortic dimension* is measured from the leading edge of the anterior wall of the aorta to the leading edge of the posterior wall of the aorta at end-diastole {<3.8 cm}. The *pulmonary artery size* can be compared subjectively to the aorta from the parasternal long- or short-axis view. The artery should be about the same size as a normal aorta.

### Pulmonary Hypertension

Calculation of pulmonary artery pressure from tricuspid and pulmonic regurgitation, and ventricular septal defect are described on pages 161, 164, and 166. With pulsed Doppler, a recording is made of the pulmonary artery flow which clearly displays the systolic onset, the maximum flow during systole, and the end of systolic flow (see Fig. 7-3D). The *acceleration time* is the interval from onset of ejection to peak velocity, measured in millimeters per second. The *ratio* is the quotient of acceleration time divided by RV ejection time {40 to 50%} or of the acceleration time divided by the preejection period {<110%}.[21]

## Other Measurements

### The Inferior and Superior Vena Cava

By 2-D or M-mode tracing, the IVC is examined from subcostal or right parasternal views and the SVC from the suprasternal or right parasternal view, and the internal dimension is measured. It should be less than 1.0 cm.

On pulsed-wave Doppler tracing, the IVC flow is recorded, clearly displaying the systolic and diastolic velocities. The peak retrograde (above the baseline) systolic and diastolic velocities are measured from baseline to peak (see Fig. 7-10B).

The *ratio* of systolic to diastolic velocity should be less than 1.0. A value greater than 1.0 indicates significant TR.

### Ventricular Septal Defect

*Pulmonary Artery Pressure.* In the absence of LVOT and RVOT obstruction, the maximal VSD velocity from a left to right shunt is obtained by measuring the velocity ($V$) from baseline to peak. The brachial systolic BP is also measured. The formula for pulmonary artery pressure, in mm Hg, is systolic BP $- 4V^2$.[38,49]

*QP-QS Ratio.* Following the guidelines on pages 153–155 the pulmonic and systemic COs are measured. With a moderate-sized to large VSD, pulmonic CO or mitral CO is used for the right side (QP) and aortic CO for the left side (QS). The *QP-QS ratio* is the ratio of pulmonic CO to systemic CO.[2,62,70]

### Atrial Septal Defect

Following the guidelines on pages 153–155 the pulmonic and systemic CO are obtained. With a moderate-sized to large ASD, pulmonic CO is used for the QP and aortic or mitral for the QS. The *QP-QS ratio* is the ratio of pulmonic CO to systemic CO.[2,31,47,63]

### Patent Ductus Arteriosus

*Timing and Systolic PAP.* In the presence of pulmonary hypertension, a complete recording is obtained of the ductal flow from a high parasternal view. The beam should be parallel and in the jet throughout the cycle. The duration of diastole (the time from the end of systolic flow away from the baseline to the next systolic flow) is measured on the spectral waveform and the duration of the diastolic ductal flow is measured above the baseline. The ratio is diastolic duration divided by PDA diastolic flow.

In the absence of pulmonary hypertension, the maximum ductal flow is measured with high–PRF or extended-range Doppler or continuous-wave Doppler, displaying clearly the end-systolic velocity ($V$), which is usually around 4.0 m/sec. The brachial systolic BP is measured. The *systolic PAP, in mm Hg,* is the systolic BP minus $4V^2$.

*QP-QS Ratio.* Pulmonic and systemic COs are measured according to the guidelines on pages 153–155. RV outflow CO is used for the QS (systemic venous return) and the mitral CO for the QP (pulmonary venous return). QP/QS Ratio is the ratio of pulmonic CO to the systemic CO.[2]

### COARCTATION OF THE AORTA, CONDUITS, AND BANDS

With a continuous-wave spectral Doppler tracing, the peak velocity from the obstruction, conduit, or band ($V_1$) is measured. With pulsed-wave Doppler instrumentation, the velocity proximal to the obstruction, conduit, or band ($V_2$) is measured. Guidelines are provided on pages 150 and 162 (see Fig. 7-11D).[56] The *peak gradient, in mm Hg,* is $4(V_1^2 - V_2^2)$. The *mean gradient* is the average of several peak gradients ($4V^2$) calculated at regular intervals (e.g., 2 mm) over the flow duration.

## Acknowledgments

The author would like to acknowledge the valuable assistance of Dr. Kanwal Kapur and Dr. Rajendra Mehta in the preparation of this chapter.

## References

1. Baron AO, Rogal GJ, Nanda NC. Ejection fraction determination without planimetry by two-dimensional echocardiography: A new method. J Am Coll Cardiol. 1983; 1:1471–1473.
2. Barron SJ, Sahn DJ, Valdes-Cruz LM, et al. Clinical utility of two-dimensional echocardiography techniques for estimation of pulmonary to systemic blood flow ratios in children with left to right shunting atrial septal defect, ventricular septal defect and patent ductus arteriosus. J Am Coll Cardiol. 1984; 54:857.
3. Berger M, Berdoff RL, Gallersteen PE, et al. Evaluation of aortic stenosis by continuous-wave Doppler ultrasound. J Am Coll Cardiol. 1984; 3:150.
4. Berger M, Haimowitz A, Vantosh A, et al. Quantitative assessment of pulmonary hypertension in patients with tricuspid regurgitation using continuous-wave Doppler ultrasound. J Am Coll Cardiol. 1985; 6:359.
5. Byrd BF III, Wahi D, Wang YS, et al. Left ventricular mass and volume/mass ratio determined two-dimensional echo in normal adults. J Am Coll Cardiol. 1985; 6:1021.
6. Carr KW, Engler RL, Forsythe JF, et al. Measurement of left ventricular ejection fraction by mechanical cross-sectional echocardiography. Circulation. 1979; 60:320.
7. Currie PJ, Seward JB, Reeder JS, et al. Continuous wave Doppler echocardiographic assessment of severity of calcific aortic stenosis: A simultaneous Doppler-catheterization correlative study in 100 adult patients. Circulation. 1985; 71:1162.
8. Currie PJ, Seward JB, Chan K, et al. Continuous-wave Doppler determination of right ventricular pressure: Simultaneous Doppler catheterization study in 127 patients. J Am Coll Cardiol. 1976; 6:75.
9. Danford DA, Huhta JC, Murphy DJ Jr. Doppler echocardiographic approach to ventricular distolic function. Echocardiography. 1986; 3:181.
10. Devereux RB, Reichek N. Echocardiographic determination of left ventricular mass in men: Anatomic validation of the method. Circulation. 1977; 55:613.
11. Eaton JW, Maughan WL, Shoukas AD, et al. Accurate volume determination in isolated ejecting canine left ventricle by two-dimensional echocardiography. Circulation. 1979; 60:320.
12. Elkayam U, Gardin J, Berkley R, et al. Doppler flow velocity measurements in assessment of hemodynamic response to vasodilator in patients with heart failure. Circulation. 1982; 67:377.
13. Feigenbaum H. Echocardiography. 4th ed. Philadelphia: Lea & Febiger; 1986.
14. Fisher DC, Sahn, DJ, Friedman MJ, et al. The mitral valve orifice method for noninvasive two-dimensional echo Doppler determinations of cardiac output. Circulation. 1983; 67:872.
15. Folland ED, Parisi AF, Moynihan PF, et al. Assessment of left ventricular ejection fraction and volumes by real-time two-dimensional echocardiography. Circulation. 1979; 60:760.
16. Friedman BJ, Drinkovic N, Miles H, et al. Assessment of left ventricular diastolic function: Comparison of Doppler echocardiography and gated blood pool scintigraphy. J Am Coll Cardiol. 1986; 8:1348.
17. Fujii J, Yazaki Y, Sawada H, et al. Noninvasive assessment of left ventricular and right ventricular filling in myocardial infarction with two-dimensional

Doppler echocardiographic method. J Am Coll Cardiol. 1985; 5:1155.

18. Gardin JM, Iseri LT, Elkayam U, et al. Evaluation of dilated cardiomyopathy by pulsed Doppler echocardiography. Am Heart J. 1983; 106:1057.

19. Gordon EP, Schnittger I, Fitzgerald PJ, et al. Reproducibility of left ventricular volume by two-dimensional echocardiography. J Am Coll Cardiol. 1983; 2:506.

20. Gutgsell HP, Paquet M, Duff DF, et al. Evaluation of left ventricular size and function by echocardiography results in normal children. Circulation. 1977; 56:457.

21. Hatle L, Angelsen B. Doppler Ultrasound in Cardiology. Philadelphia: Lea & Febiger; 1985.

22. Hatle L. Non-invasive assessment and differentiation of left ventricular outflow obstruction with Doppler ultrasound. Circulation. 1981; 64:380.

23. Hatle L, Angelsen BA, Tromsdol A. Noninvasive assessment of aortic stenosis by Doppler ultrasound. Br Heart J. 1980; 43:284.

24. Hatle L, Angelsen B. Doppler Ultrasound in Cardiology: Physical Principles and Clinical Applications. Philadelphia: Lea & Febiger; 1982.

25. Hatle L, Angelsen B, Tromsdol A. Noninvasive assessment of atrioventricular pressure half-time by Doppler ultrasound. Circulation. 1979; 60:1096.

26. Helmcke F, Nanda NC, Hsiung MC, et al. Color Doppler assessment of mitral regurgitation with orthogonal planes. Circulation. 1987; 75:175.

27. Henry WL, Griffith JM, Michaelis LL, et al. Measurement of mitral orifice area in patients with mitral valve disease by real-time two-dimensional echocardiography. Circulation. 1975; 51:827.

28. Huntsman LL, Stewart DK, Barnes SR, et al. Noninvasive Doppler determination of cardiac output in man. Circulation. 1983; 67:593.

29. Kan G, Visser CA, Lie KI, et al. Left ventricular volumes and ejection fraction by single plane two-dimensional apex echocardiography. Eur Heart J. 1981; 2:339.

30. Kitabatake A, Ito H, Inoue M, et al. A new approach to noninvasive evaluation of aortic regurgitant fraction by two-dimensional Doppler echocardiography. Circulation. 1985; 72:523.

31. Kitabatake A, Inoue M, Asao M, et al. Noninvasive evaluation of ratio of pulmonary to systemic flow in atrial septal defect by duplex Doppler echocardiography. Circulation. 1984; 69:73.

32. Kitabatake A, Inoue M, Asao M, et al. Transmitral blood flow reflecting diastolic behavior of the left ventricular in health and in disease: A study of pulsed Doppler technique. Jpn Circ. 1982; 46:92.

33. Libanoff A, Rodbard S. Atrioventricular pressure half-time, measure of mitral valve orifice area. Circulation. 1968; 38:144.

34. Libanoff A, Robard S. Evaluation of severity of mitral stenosis and regurgitation. Circulation. 1966; 33:218.

35. Martin RP, Rakawski H, Kleman JH, et al. Reliability of reproducibility of two dimensional echocardiographic measurements of stenotic mitral valve orifice area. Am J Cardiol. 1979; 43:560.

36. Masuyama T, Kadama K, Kitabatake A, et al. Continuous wave Doppler echocardiographic detection of pulmonary regurgitation and its application to invasive estimation of pulmonary artery pressure. Circulation. 1986; 74:484.

37. Miyatake K, Okamoto M, Kinashiba N, et al. Augmentation of atrial contribution to left ventricular inflow with aging as assessed by intracardiac Doppler flowmetry. Am J Cardiol. 1984; 53:586.

38. Murphy DJ Jr, Ludomirsky A, Huhta JC. Continuous wave Doppler in children with ventricular septal defect: Noninvasive estimation of intraventricular pressure gradient. Am J Cardiol. 1986; 57:428.

39. Nishimura RA, Tajik AJ, Shah C, et al. Role of two-dimensional echocardiography in the prediction of in-hospital complications after myocardial infarction. J Am Coll Cardiol. 1984; 4:1080.

40. Panidis S, Ren J, Kotler M, et al. Two-dimensional echocardiographic estimate of right ventricular ejection fraction in patients with coronary artery disease. J Am Coll Cardiol. 1983; 5:911.

41. Perry GJ, Helmcke F, Nanda NC, et al. Evaluation of aortic incompetence by Doppler color flow mapping. J Am Coll Cardiol. 1987; 9:952.

42. Quinones MA, Pickering E, Alexander JG. Percentage of shortening of echocardiographic left ventricular dimensions: Its use in determining ejection fraction and stroke volume. Chest. 1978; 74:59.

43. Quinones MA, Gaasch WH, Alexander JG. Influence of acute changes in preload, afterload, contractile state and heart rate on ejection and isovolumetric indices of myocardial contractility in man. Circulation. 1976; 53:293.

44. Reisnor S, Meltzer R. Normal values of prosthetic valve Doppler echocardiographic parameters: A review. J Am Soc Echocardiogr. 1988; 3:201.

45. Requarth JA, Goldberg SJ, Vasko ST, et al. In vitro verification of Doppler prediction of transvalve pressure gradient and orifice area in stenosis. Am J Cardiol. 1984; 53:1369.

46. Sahn DJ, DeMaria A, Kisslo J, Weyman A. Recommendations regarding quantitations in M-mode echocardiography: Results of a survey and echocardiographic measurements. Circulation. 1978; 58:1072.

47. Sanders SP, Yeager S, Williams RG. Measurements of systemic and pulmonary blood flow and QP/QS ratio using Doppler and two-dimensional echocardiography. Am J Cardiol. 1983; 51:952.

48. Schiller NB, Acquatella H, Ports TA, et al. Left ventricular volume from paired bi-planed two-dimensional echocardiography. Circulation. 1979; 60:547.

49. Silbert BR, Brunson AC, Schiff R, et al. Determination of right ventricular pressure in presence of ventricular septal defect using continuous wave Doppler ultrasound. J Am Coll Cardiol. 1986; 8:379.

50. Silverman NH, Lewis AB, Heymann MA, et al. Echocardiographic assessment of ductus arteriosus in premature infants. Circulation. 1974; 50:821.

51. Skjaepe T, Hergrenaes L, Hatle L. Noninvasive estimation of valve area in patients with aortic stenosis by Doppler ultrasound and two-dimensional echocardiography. Circulation. 1985; 72:810.

52. Snider AR, Gidding SS, Raechini AP, et al. Doppler evaluation of left ventricular diastolic filling in children with systemic hypertension. Am J Cardiol. 1985; 56:921.

53. Snider AR. Prediction of intracardiac pressures and assessment of ventricular functions with Doppler echocardiography. Echocardiography. 1987; 8:305.

54. Spirito B, Maron BJ, Bonaw RO. Noninvasive assessment of left ventricular diastolic functions: Comparative analysis of Doppler echocardiography and radionuclide angiographic techniques. J Am Coll Cardiol. 1986; 7:518.

55. Stamin RB, Martin RP. Quantitation of pressure gradients across stenotic valves by Doppler ultrasound. J Am Coll Cardiol. 1983; 2:707.

56. Stevensen JG, Kawabori I. Noninvasive determination of pressure gradients in children. J Am Coll Cardiol. 1984; 179–192.

57. Stewart WJ, Palacios I, Tiang L, et al. Doppler measurements of regurgitation fraction in patients with mitral regurgitation: A new technique (abstr). Circulation. 1983; 68(suppl 3):111.

58. Takenaka K, Dabestani A, Gardin J, et al. Left ventricular filling in hypertrophic cardiomyopathy: A pulsed Doppler study. J Am Coll Cardiol. 1986; 7:1263.

59. Teichholz LE, Kreulen T, Herman MV, et al. Problems in echocardiographic volume determinations: Echocardiographic-angiographic correlations in the presence or absence of asynergy. Am J Cardiol. 1976; 37:7.

60. Teirstein P, Yeager M, Yack PG, et al. Doppler echocardiographic measurement of aortic valve area in aortic stenosis: Noninvasive application of Gorlin's formula. J Am Coll Cardiol. 1986; 8:1059.

61. Tortolado FA, Quinones MA, Fenandes GC, et al. Quantification of life ventricular volume from two-dimensional echocardiography: Simplified and accurate approach. Circulation. 1983; 67:579–584.

62. Valdes-Cruz LM, Horowitz S, Mesel E, et al. Pulsed Doppler echocardiographic method for calculation of pulmonary and systemic flow: Accuracy in a canine model with ventricular septal defect. Circulation. 1983; 68:597.

63. Valdes-Cruz LM, Horowitz S, Mesel E, et al. A pulsed Doppler echocardiographic method for calculating pulmonary and systemic blood flow in atrial level shunts: Validation studies in animals and initial human experience. Circulation. 1984; 69:80.

64. Weissler AM, Lewis RP, Leighton RF: The systolic time intervals as a measurement of left ventricular performance in man. In: Yu PN, Goodwin JF, eds. Progress in Cardiology. Philadelphia: Lea & Febiger; 1972; 1.

65. Williams G, Labovitz A. Doppler hemodynamic evaluation of prosthetic (Starr Edwards and Bjork-Shiley) and bioprosthetic (Hancock and Carpentier-Edwards) cardiac valves. Am J Cardiol. 1985; 56:325.

66. Wind BE, Snider AR, Buda AG, et al. Pulsed Doppler assessment of left ventricular diastolic filling in patients with coronary artery disease before and immediately after coronary angioplasty. Am J Cardiol. 1987; 59:1041.

67. Worth DC, Stewart WJ, Black PC, et al. A new matter to calculate aortic valve area without left heart catheterization. Circulation. 1984; 70:978.

68. Wyatt HL, Mierbaum S, Heng MK, et al. Cross-sectional echocardiography: III. Analysis of mathematical models for quantifying volume of symmetric and asymmetric left ventricle. Am Heart J. 1980; 100:821.

69. Yock P, Popp R. Noninvasive measurement of right ventricular systolic pressure by Doppler ultrasound in patients with tricuspid regurgitation. Circulation. 1984; 70:657.

70. Yokai K, Kambe T, Ichiniya S, et al. Pulsed Doppler echocardiographic evaluation of shunt flow in ventricular septal defect. Jpn Heart J. 1983; 24:175.

# CHAPTER 8

# Laboratory Development and Professional Interactions

Barbara Sternlight

## Managing an Ultrasound Laboratory

A sonographer in charge of an echocardiography laboratory is confronted with certain questions. Whether there is an established department or the sonographer must build a laboratory from scratch, the suggestions in this chapter are designed to provide a framework for this project.

### ADMINISTRATIVE FLOW CHART

A thorough understanding on the supervisor's part of the departmental personnel flow chart is essential. Knowing the players makes the job easier: questions, suggestions, and material will be directed to the proper persons the first time around, and knowing who has final authority on various issues saves everyone from wasting effort and time.

### BUDGET

The budget constraints of the laboratory or department are extremely important: What funds are available for each necessary item? Can funds be borrowed from one expense category to add to another? (For example, if funds allotted for travel are not used in a given period, can they be applied to the purchase of reference books for the library?) How are disbursements made? Are there any limitations?

### LABORATORY DESIGN

A needs analysis is a prerequisite to designing a diagnostic ultrasound laboratory or restructuring (or even understanding) an existing one. The following questions must be asked:

1. What kind of clinical work will be done?
   a. What specific examinations will be performed?
   b. Will collected data be used for medical management? Research? Teaching?
2. What type of patients will be examined?
   a. What is their age?
   b. What is their body *habitus*?
   c. What pathology typically is seen?
   d. What is the daily study volume?
3. What kind of equipment will be needed?
   a. What is the necessary complement of equipment and accessories?
   b. Does the laboratory already possess it?
   c. Can it be purchased? If so, what is the budget and who requests, evaluates, and authorizes purchases (Table 8-1).
4. Who are the laboratory personnel?
   a. Technical staff
      i. How many?
      ii. What are their roles?
      iii. To whom do they report?
      iv. How is work performance measured and evaluated?

171

b. Physicians
  i. How many?
  ii. What are their roles (readers or interpreters, teachers, scanners)?
  iii. What are the expectations of each (e.g., Dr. Jones likes page prints; Dr. Smith prefers strip-charts; Dr. Brown likes images with high contrast; Dr. Vega prefers softer gray scale)?
c. Administrators
  i. How many?
  ii. What are their job definitions and expectations?
d. Clerical Staff
  i. How many?
  ii. What are their roles?
  iii. To whom do they report?
5. What supplies are needed in the laboratory?
  a. What general clerical and clinical supplies are needed?
  b. What specific supplies are needed for the equipment and procedures (see Fig. 8-1)?
  c. What personal supplies are needed?

### POLICIES AND PROCEDURES MANUAL

All of the items already presented should be incorporated into a manual of policies and procedures (P&P), which must be explicit and concise. All employees in the echocardiography laboratory should receive a copy of the manual at the time of hire and should sign a form acknowledging that they have read it and understand the contents.

The P&P manual will become a reference for all personnel, new and old. In the following section, sample pages of a P&P manual are presented for review. None of the categories is absolutely exhaustive. Every laboratory is different and has special requirements. The samples provide a foundation upon which to build guidelines specific to individual laboratories, and they can be adapted to specific needs.

*Personnel Issues.* An orientation program for new employees is extremely important. Even when a medical facility has an introductory program, it is advantageous to create a procedure specific to the echocardiography department. When employees clearly understand the organization of a department and its expectations, performance appraisal

TABLE 8-1. Inventory checklist

*Personal*
  Lab coats, uniforms, spare shoes (In a pediatric laboratory, a complete change of clothes may be a good idea.)
  Calipers
  Calculator
  Textbooks, reference charts
*Clinical*
  Gel
  Strip-chart paper and film
  Videotapes
  Electrodes
  Syringes
  Saline
  Contrast material
  Gloves, masks
  Tissues
  Alcohol swabs
  Paper towels
  4 × 4 gauze pads
  Linen
  Pillows
  Wedges (for patient positioning)
  Drugs (e.g., chloral hydrate for pediatric sedation)
  Cleaning supplies (disinfectant, sponges)
  Trash bags

and evaluation are much easier for all concerned. When policies are published and followed, departments run more smoothly and efficiently.

Other important personnel issues to be addressed in the P&P manual include job descriptions, salary ranges, overtime provisions and absence rules, vacation and sick time standards, dress code, termination procedure, pregnancy policy (exposure to patient infection; duration of maternity leave), and CME expectations and travel opportunities.

A current file of ultrasound courses and meetings (local and national) is useful to everyone in the department. It is important to allow time for staff to attend conferences whenever possible. Employees who are challenged stay clinically interested and informed. Interdisciplinary conferences in the hospital are an excellent vehicle for echocardiographers' growth: putting together parts of the diagnostic puzzle keeps the mind sharp. Staying current with the latest ultrasound imaging technologies helps echocardiographers run an efficient and reliable clinical laboratory. Also, technicians

VENDOR
Location _____
Phone number _____
Sales representative _____

SIZE AND WEIGHT OF EQUIPMENT
Dimensions
Height _____ Weight _____
Depth _____ Width _____
Portability of system _____

PRICES
Cost of system and accessories _____
Cost of paper/film _____
Cost of Polaroid film _____
Cost of color print paper _____
Cost of videotape _____

WARRANTY
Cost _____
Breakdown _____
Terms _____
_____

SERVICE
Process _____
_____
Turnaround time _____
Location of service support _____
Service representative _____
Phone number _____

COMMENTS
Ease of use (ergonomics and portability) _____

Flexibility of software _____
_____

Image (2-D and M-mode)
  Presentation _____
  _____
  Flexibility _____
  _____

Doppler
  Display _____
  _____
  Sensitivity _____
  _____
  Flexibility _____
  _____
  Ease of use _____

Other important features
  Measurement package _____
  _____
  On-line?___ Yes ___ No ___
  Comprehensive package?___ Yes ___ No ___
  Computer hookup?___ Yes ___ No ___
  Auto-annotation?___ Yes ___ No ___
  Body marks?___ Yes ___ No ___
  User programmability _____
  _____
  System upgradability _____
  _____
  Delivery date _____

EDUCATION
Applications provided _____
_____
Training programs _____
_____
_____

FIGURE 8-1. Equipment evaluation form.

who keep up with technology and new techniques are more apt to enjoy their work. Courses that offer CME credits are particularly important for those who have licenses to maintain and an identified career path. Time off and travel and education funds enhance employees' job satisfaction.

*Laboratory Maintenance.* The basics of laboratory upkeep are supplies, laboratory cleaning, and equipment maintenance. It is vital that an accurate inventory be created and that it be updated at regular intervals (Table 8-2). A comprehensive checklist of laboratory supplies is important, particularly when more than one person is responsible for checking inventory and placing orders. Cleaning procedures must be described in specific detail.

Equipment is expensive and preventive maintenance pays off. Service representatives can help develop a troubleshooting guide for the imaging equipment if the equipment manual does not con-

TABLE 8-2. Inventory ordering information

Supplies (List all items in separate columns, separating general stock vs. items for specific equipment)
Amount at stocking time
Purchasing procedures
Vendors, phone numbers, addresses
Prices
Turnaround time
Date ordered
Date received
Contact persons
*Equipment and supplies requisition procedure*
What forms must be submitted?
Who authorizes and signs purchase requests?

Patient's name _____
Address _____
Phone number _____
Referring physician _____
Diagnosis _____
Type of examination _____
Date and time of examination _____
Dates of any previous studies _____

FIGURE 8-2. Patient scheduling form.

tain one. If the guide is consulted carefully before a call for help is made, the relationship with service people is enhanced. A laboratory's credibility is very important. Too many customers call for service unnecessarily, when they could correct a problem themselves. Service persons' names and numbers should be filed, and a log of service problems and repairs should be kept.

*Emergency Procedures.* Everyone in the laboratory should know what to do and whom to call in an emergency. *All* numbers should be posted prominently. The location of emergency equipment in the laboratory should also be posted.

*Sterilization Protocol.* Employees should follow the hospital's established protocol to protect themselves and their patients. Equipment vendors can provide guidelines for protecting imaging equipment. Other questions should be referred to an imaging society such as the Society of Diagnostic Medical Sonographers (SDMS), which publishes protocols. Cleaning the laboratory and equipment daily helps to prevent problems.

*Patient Scheduling Form.* A schedule (Fig. 8-2) kept carefully up to date, eliminates problems of examination overbooking. A conveniently located and visible schedule is also helpful to physicians and ancillary personnel on site, who will understand the laboratory's time constraints when referring patients for appointments.

*Patient Scheduling Procedure.* In order to develop a patient scheduling procedure, the following information should be gathered and analyzed:

How many patients are to be scheduled each day?
When are exceptions made (e.g., emergencies)?
Who is responsible for scheduling?
What are the criteria for ordering scans (acceptable diagnoses, patient mobility, etc.)?
How long does each type of study take?
How long is the interval between patients?
What equipment is used for each study?
What patient preparation is involved in each study, and how is this information conveyed to the patient?
When is a patient consent form used? What is the procedure?
What is the procedure for bedside studies?
What is the procedure for "dismissing" a patient? Are scans reviewed first by a physician?
Is an exit interview conducted with the patient? How is an inpatient returned to his/her room? What is the billing policy?
Who is responsible for reading, measuring, and sending reports? When, where, and with whom will this take place?
What measurement standards are used? (Samples of all report forms and normal measurement values should be a part of the P&P manual.)
Are measurements done during the exam or off-line?
To whom are the patient's reports sent?
What items are filed or stored and in what form (e.g., videotapes, hard copy, patient reports)?

*Log Book Format.* A log book (Fig. 8-3) is an excellent reference for all laboratory personnel who need to retrieve information about patients who have undergone echocardiography. This log is an effective organizational tool, and one of the most important items in any laboratory.

Patient's name _____

Date of examination _____

Dates of previous studies _____

Diagnosis _____

Referring physician _____

Reading or interpreting physician _____

Videotape number, counter number _____

Technologist's initials _____

Figure 8-3. Log book format.

*Scanning Protocol.* This section of the P&P manual must be very explicit and include all procedures carried out in the laboratory—everything from the patient's position, to the probe's orientation, to views that must always be recorded.

Forms, Files, and Reference Materials for an Echocardiography Laboratory

Samples of each item should be included in the P&P manual.

Administrative flow chart
Budget
Laboratory design
Equipment evaluation form (Fig. 8-1)
Service log book
Vendor list and brochures and files of operating manuals
Addresses and phone numbers
  Physicians in the hospital
  Other important numbers: labs, nursing stations, emergency personnel
  Referring physicians
  Vendors (all)
  Societies
    Local professional societies are also an excellent vehicle for learning about new developments in the field of diagnostic imaging. If none exists in the area, the sonographers in the laboratory may consider starting a group of their own. Equipment representatives might help a laboratory network with other interested persons in their area.
  Local colleagues
Inventory of supplies and order requisition forms
Library cardex file

Textbooks (include the laboratory's purchasing protocol)
Journals
Articles
Teaching file
  Strip-charts
  Videotapes
  Films
  Polaroid photographs
  Slides
  Handouts and manuals
  Journal articles
Schedule book
Patient log book
Report forms
Insurance and billing forms
Patient consent forms
Filing system
  Tapes
  Hard copy
  Reports
  Patient card file

Useful Items for the Echocardiography Laboratory

| For Adults | For Children |
|---|---|
| Patient education brochures | Toys (pre-echo, too) |
| | Puppets, stuffed animals |
| Patient eduction tapes | Musical toys |
| Designs on the ceiling | Hanging things (kites, pinwheels, mobiles) |
| | Entertainment videos |
| | Designs on the ceiling |

## Interacting with Medical Staff and Patients

Once an echocardiography laboratory is set up and operating, the staff will find themselves interacting with other medical staff and, of course, with patients. The key to managing or working in a smoothly functioning laboratory is to keep daily procedures consistent. One must follow protocols religiously and educate the medical personnel who refer patients to the laboratory about the way the department is organized. Occasional deviation is a way to demonstrate flexibility, but it is important to adhere to an established protocol. If the familiar structure is modified too frequently, laboratory personnel will lose control.

INTERACTING WITH PHYSICIANS

Interacting with physicians can be an interesting challenge for sonographers. Like other professionals, physicians exhibit a variety of personality characteristics and possess different degrees of echocardiography experience and expertise. There will be some whose presence is always a joy, whose love of teaching, guiding, and sharing make the day pleasurable. There will also be some difficult ones.

*The Physician Who Orders the Wrong Examination.* Inappropriate requisitions or referrals for echocardiography usually result from inexperience with the modality. The service can *educate* referring physicians. It can publish a standard list of examinations, define them, and list the indications for ordering them and explain what patient preparation is necessary. Education of referring physicians illustrates for them what examination limitations might exist in a laboratory setting, ensuring appropriate examination requests. If it is practical, physicians should be invited to observe occasionally to see what kinds of patients are difficult to scan and what various studies typically look like. Physicians who understand the limitations of the laboratory environment make more reasonable requests. An additional effort to educate support staff in the facility is also worthwhile. Nurses and ward clerks who appreciate scanning time, patient preparation, transport needs, and examination indications are usually more sensitive and cooperative.

*The Physician or Nurse Who Hovers.* There will always be persons who position themselves a few inches behind the sonographer's shoulder and stay there. The sonographer should try to be calm, stay in control, and maintain a sense of humor. Such hoverers may actually contribute excellent suggestions about the study. Others may truly appreciate what they can learn watching a scan in progress. At all times, the sonographer must maintain a professional, polite attitude toward *any* medical personnel in the laboratory.

Depending on the size of the institution, sonographers may be asked to interact with or teach referring physicians, fellows, residents, interns, sonography students, or visitors. Following the fixed protocol is important at all times, making as few exceptions as possible. Consistency makes newcomers feel more secure.

INTERACTING WITH PATIENTS

*The Difficult Patient.* Patients can be uncooperative because they are frightened or physically uncomfortable or because they don't understand what is happening to them. The short time it takes to put a patient at ease saves time and patient-related problems during the examination. Some suggestions for dealing with a difficult patient follow:

*Educate* the patient. Carefully explain the examination to be performed. Emphasize the noninvasive nature of the medium and be sure to inform the patient about everything that will happen (e.g., body position changes, injections, expected duration of the procedure). An informed person is less apt to be frightened. *This is particularly important when dealing with children!*

Families of patients (particularly children) are as entitled to information as patients. If they are told as much as possible about what is going on with their relative, they will not only be less anxious but can frequently help to calm the patient.

Printed brochures and posters on the wall are excellent adjuncts to the few minutes of explanation at the start of a study. Some laboratories have videotapes that can be viewed before an examination that provide explanations of Ultrasound as a diagnostic tool. Equipment vendors and medical education film distributors are sources of such materials.

Creative *distractions* in the lab may help a patient relax during an examination. Soft music, entertaining videotapes, pleasant pictures on the wall (although lighting is a problem in a completely darkened room), and mobiles hanging from the ceiling can keep a patient's mind off temporary discomfort.

It is a good practice to *play* with young children in the laboratory. If the examiner takes a few minutes to make friends with them at the start of an examination, they are more apt to cooperate. A child needs a little time to adjust to the laboratory environment and to establish trust before the study begins. Toys often help to make a child feel at home. Some laboratories routinely sedate young patients; others do so only if absolutely necessary. Pacifiers and bottles can be offered when possible, and a mother may be encouraged to breast feed if it helps.

In dealing with anxious and uncooperative patients of any age a sonographer's *attitude* is of the utmost importance. Calm and professionalism are in order at all times. If a sonographer's affect is calm, friendly, and straightforward, patients are less apt to be edgy. A patient's modesty and privacy should always be respected. Patients should be carefully draped, particularly if additional personnel or students are present during an exam. Reflecting on one's own feelings about undergoing echocardiography may be helpful. It is important to be aware of a patient's psychological and physical needs.

A sonographer discussing examination findings with patients should answer questions generally without making comments that resemble diagnoses. That is the domain of the physician who interprets the study.

## Setting Up a Mobile Ultrasound Service
### MOBILE SERVICE

The process of planning and setting up a mobile ultrasonography laboratory is quite similar to that of establishing a hospital-based laboratory. Special attention to detail is called for, because the sonographer and equipment must be absolutely self-sufficient, regardless of their location.

First, a company must be formed and a charter developed. A checklist of items that need to be addressed next follows:

*Equipment.* Item 3 regarding equipment under Laboratory Design, above, should be consulted. Special care must be taken to choose equipment that is truly portable. Think ahead about moving equipment on and off vans and in and out of hospitals. Try to avoid systems that are too heavy, too large, or too cumbersome to be easily maneuvered. Carefully evaluate a manufacturer's service record and service availability in out-of-the-way locations. If peripheral equipment is used, a cart may be necessary to transport it from van to bedside.

*Vans.* Vans may need special adaptations, such as bubble tops, to accommodate monitors and ancillary equipment. They should also be equipped with a lift gate (which must not be built until *after* the dimensions of the equipment are established!). Sheet metal is often used to reinforce van floors, and special brackets or straps must be installed to secure the equipment during transport.

Vans must have a cabinet of some sort to store supplies like gel, electrodes, and film. Each van should contain a log book for gasoline purchases and maintenance records. Company credit cards may be issued to sonographers to avoid confusing reimbursement calculations.

*Insurance.* Insurance is critically important in a mobile environment. The following types of insurance are necessary in addition to that of the account hospitals:

Workman's Compensation. The cost depends on the number of employees covered.

Malpractice Insurance and General Liability. Cost is generally based on a percentage of the mobile service's income. It is advisable to state in contract with each subscribing hospital that this kind of insurance is carried by the service.

Automobile Insurance. The cost depends on the deductible amounts chosen.

Health Insurance. Different insurance carriers may be chosen for each item listed above. An insurance broker might be selected who can shop around for the best policies to suit the service's needs.

*Marketing and Sales.* Marketing and sales often require separate management personnel. Both go hand in hand with education. In a community whose hospitals do not have in-house laboratories referring physicians may need extensive education regarding indications for diagnostic ultrasonography, clinical findings, and even pathophysiology. Often, potential hospital accounts may contract with a mobile service only if they receive educational materials and programs as part of the service.

Brochures designed for patient education/scheduling purposes are excellent marketing tools to develop. In addition, established mobile services may assist an account hospital in planning and hosting an "open house" for community physicians and potential patients. Such an affair gives the hospital greater visibility and helps advertise its state-of-the-art diagnostic capabilities. Public relations is a term that should be as familiar to a mobile service as echocardiography.

*Education.* Education, beyond that used for marketing, should extend to the account hospitals' support staff (nurses, ward clerks), so that they understand who and what the mobile service is and what examination protocols and patient preparation involve. Such education may spare the mobile sonographer from driving long distances to perform inappropriate studies.

Mobile staff training is very important as well. Continuing education keeps "mobile sonographers" current with accepted scanning techniques. The key here is quality control. Their loyalty will also be maintained if they are provided assistance in accruing CME credits to qualify for certification or license renewal. Offering opportunities for education may help to compensate for the lack of interaction with medical personnel and teachers inherent in working in the field, moving from site to site.

*Hiring.* Hiring should be approached very thoughtfully. Mobile sonographers must be extremely experienced and particularly independent. Typically they have no one to consult on questions in the field, so their clinical and administrative judgment must be excellent.

*Personnel Issues.* Overtime, vacation, and other considerations are critical in a mobile environment where back-up personnel are less accessible. Other personnel issues are essentially the same as those of an in-house laboratory.

*Billing.* Billing also demands careful consideration. Many mobile services prefer to bill hospital or clinic facilities on a fee-for-service basis rather than take on the insurance reimbursement and collection problems that accompany direct billing. Account invoices must be designed that show the type of study, its cost, and extra charges for items such as special procedures and emergency call-back.

*Readers (Quality Control).* If the account hospitals do not have physicians experienced in interpreting ultrasound examination results, it will be necessary to contract with outside physicians on a fee-per-reading basis. Results of an examination should not be left in a hospital where no one is qualified

to generate an *accurate* diagnostic report that can be submitted to the referring physician.

*Logistics.* Logistics is the toughest assignment. Certain elements of a mobile service must function smoothly. A capable and careful logistics coordinator must log hospital calls for scheduling and chart sonographer assignments. A phone system is needed that is designed to handle incoming calls from field sonographers and accounts on some lines and reserves other lines for marketing and other business. A reliable answering service is also important. Pagers are a necessity for all sonographers on staff.

P&P manuals must be prepared for *all* account sites, and every van should carry a copy. Clear protocols should be included for sterilization procedures, particularly as equipment is moved not only from patient to patient but from institution to institution. (Some institutions will require a special Biomedical Engineering Department check of your equipment.)

## Summary

In this chapter general guidelines are presented for the development and organization of an echocardiography laboratory. Each laboratory has unique requirements and must be structured accordingly. The key to success is first to evaluate input from all of the significant participants in the laboratory's operation and second to be explicit about all operational issues.

The manager of an echocardiography laboratory has an important responsibility to see that the laboratory operates smoothly. Good managers deserve to be proud of the effort put into this operation. An organized laboratory earns the respect of hospital personnel and sets an example for other divisions. A successful manager can be proud of his or her accomplishments and can share that pride with everyone in the department.

The most important priority at all times is patient care. None of the other necessities of laboratory operation should ever interfere with a patient's well-being!

# PART THREE

# Acquired Heart Disease

# The Mitral and Tricuspid Valves

Sue A. George

## The Mitral Valve

Historically the mitral valve has been a structure of principal echocardiographic interest because of its high reflectivity, its characteristic motion pattern (Fig. 9-1), and its location directly beneath the parasternal echocardiographic window. All of these factors facilitate its location and recording. Because of its central position in the heart, the mitral valve has always been a valuable sonographic landmark by which important surrounding structures are located. Because it is frequently involved in a variety of disorders that affect structure and function, it continues to have great clinical interest and importance.[3,4,7,13]

### ANATOMY

Anatomically, the mitral valve is a complex structure composed of the mitral leaflet tissue, chordae tendinae, papillary muscles, left ventricular myocardium (subjacent to the papillary muscles), and fibromuscular mitral annulus (Fig. 9-2A).

The mitral leaflets actually represent a continuous veil of fibrous tissue whose base is attached around the entire circumference of the mitral valve orifice to the fibromuscular ring, the mitral annulus. The free edge of this veil contains several indentations. Two of these, the anterolateral and posteromedial commissures, divide the mitral valve into an anterior and a posterior leaflet. The anterior leaflet is relatively long and semicircular or triangular. Although the posterior leaflet is shorter,

its attachment to the annulus is more extensive. The distal third of both leaflets is roughened and opaque, whereas, the proximal two thirds is smooth and clear. The roughened area receives the insertion of the chordae tendineae on the ventricular surface. A ridge at the superior margin of the roughened area marks the line of coaptation of these two (anterior and posterior) leaflets.[3–5,11,13]

Using two-dimensional (2-D) echocardiography, the mitral valve can be imaged from many views, including the parasternal long axis (Fig. 9-2B, C) the parasternal short axis (Fig. 9-3), and the apical views (two, three, four, and five chambers; Fig. 9-2B, C). Subcostal views may also be used (Fig. 9-4). The best view for high-frequency interrogation is the parasternal long-axis view, in which both leaflets can be seen. It is here that mitral valve prolapse can best be noted, as can ruptured chordae, flail mitral valve leaflet, and systolic anterior motion (SAM). The distinctive "bent-knee" motion of mitral stenosis is best identified here (Fig. 9-5). Parasternal short-axis views demonstrate the "fish-mouth" motion of the mitral valve. Orifice size is best seen in this view and lends itself to planimetry to determine size in conditions such as mitral stenosis. The apical view is usually used to gather additional information and to verify findings obtained from other planes.

Mitral valve motion is influenced by many factors, including: (1) the relative pressures within the left ventricle and left atrium, (2) the velocity and

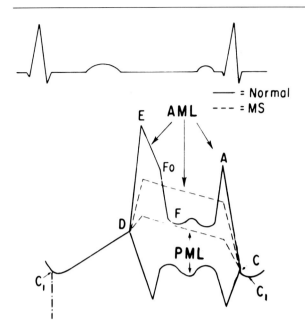

FIGURE 9-1. Schematic drawing of the mitral valve as seen in M-mode echocardiography.

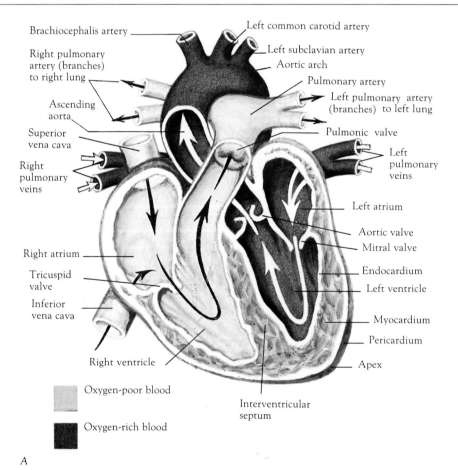

*A*

FIGURE 9-2 (*Continued*)

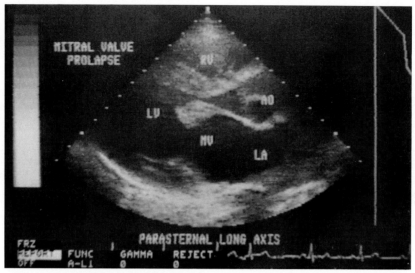

B

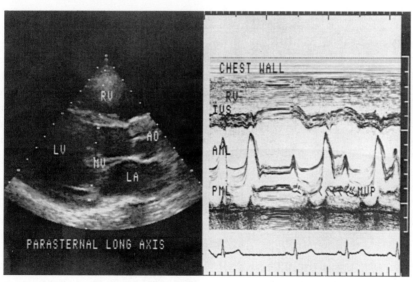

C

FIGURE 9-2. (*A*) (See color insert.) Anatomy of the heart. (*B*) Two-dimensional echocardiographic view of the mitral valve. (RV, right ventricle; LV, left ventricle; MV, mitral valve; LA, left atrium; AO, aorta.) (*C*) Left sternal border, long-axis view of the mitral on 2-D echocardiogram. (*A* From Memmler RL, Wood DL. Structure and Function of the Human Body. 4th ed. Philadelphia: J.B. Lippincott, 1987; 135.)

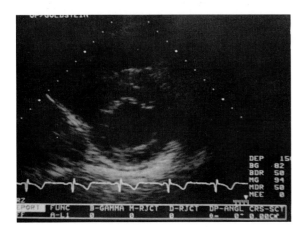

Figure 9-3. Left sternal border, short-axis view of the mitral valve.

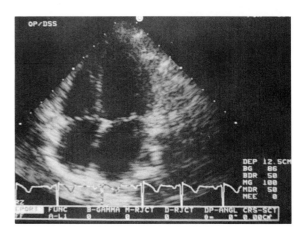

Figure 9-4. Four-chamber apical view of the mitral valve.

volume of blood flow through its orifice, (3) the motion of the leaflets in reference to their annular attachment, (4) the left ventricle diastolic compliance, and (5) the systolic performance of the left ventricle.

### PATHOLOGIC LESIONS

*Mitral Valve Stenosis.* Rheumatic mitral stenosis is the leading cause of obstruction to left ventricular inflow, but not all persons with rheumatic fever develop mitral stenosis. Estimated at 40 to 50%, the prevalence of mitral stenosis is decreasing every year, owing to antibiotic therapy and the decreasing prevalence of rheumatic fever.[3,13] Stenosis of the mitral valve is an acquired form of chronic valvular heart disease characterized by diffuse thickening of the mitral leaflets, fusion of the commissures, and shortening and fusion of the chordae tendineae. These characteristics combine to decrease the size of the mitral valve orifice, thereby reducing blood flow into the left ventricle.[3,7,11,13,14]

Mitral stenosis produces the following echocardiographic patterns: (1) increased echogenicity in the thickened and deformed leaflets, (2) abnormal diastolic leaflet motion, and (3) reduction of the mitral valve orifice. In patients with mitral stenosis, the anterior and posterior mitral leaflets are thickened and diastolic bowing or doming can be noted

(on two-dimensional studies) with varying degrees of restriction to the orifice and top leaflet excursion. The reduction in orifice size is the hallmark of mitral stenosis. Increased echo production from the deformed mitral leaflets can be observed in almost every instance of rheumatic mitral stenosis; calcification is noted in varying degrees.

Calcification of the rheumatic mitral valve begins at the tips of the leaflets and spreads upward toward the annulus. The pattern is in contrast to mitral annulus calcification, which is distinctly different. Abnormal mitral leaflet motion may be evident throughout diastole or only during the initial phase. This finding is best recorded in the parasternal long-axis view (Fig. 9-5). Changes in the anterior mitral valve leaflet are the most evident and are characterized by (1) restricted excursion of the leaflet tips, (2) diastolic doming of the anterior leaflet into the left ventricular outflow tract (bent-knee motion), and (3) lessening in the initial diastolic closing motion of the anterior mitral valve leaflet (E-F slope). Upon opening of the mitral valve in diastole the motion of the anterior leaflet is quickly halted, owing to fusion of the commissures. This tethering of the leaflets appears to tie them down, reducing their excursion. In contrast, the body of the leaflet continues anteriorly, and it is this continuation of motion by the body of the

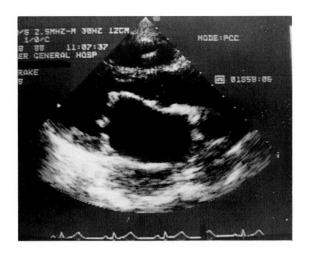

FIGURE 9-5. Parasternal long-axis view of the mitral valve demonstrates mitral stenosis. Note the "bent-knee" motion of the anterior mitral valve leaflet.

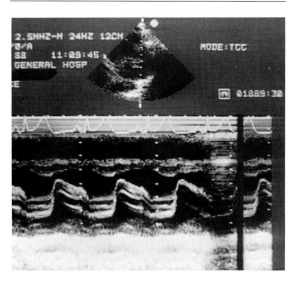

FIGURE 9-6. M-mode tracing demonstrates mitral stenosis. Note the concordant motion of the posterior mitral valve leaflet.

leaflet that produces the bent-knee action that is so indicative of mitral stenosis. The posterior mitral valve leaflet is pulled anteriorly due to the fusion and the velocity of blood flow. This anterior motion of the posterior leaflet during diastole, called concordant motion, is seen in the more severe forms of mitral stenosis (Fig. 9-6).

It should be noted that although diastolic doming is a relatively specific characteristic of mitral stenosis, there are at least three situations in which apparent doming of the valve may occur in the absence of stenosis. The most common of these are the redundant, floppy valves seen in mitral valve prolapse and mass lesions or vegetations involving the free edge of the anterior mitral valve leaflet.

The reduction in mitral valve orifice size is the hallmark of mitral stenosis and severity is assessed by the degree of reduction. The mitral valve orifice is best seen in the parasternal short-axis view, where the orifice can be planimetered (Fig. 9-7).

Doppler echocardiography and color-flow mapping can enhance the diagnosis and correlate well with 2-D and M-mode studies (Fig. 9-8). Pressure half times correlate well with catheter laboratory data.[3,13] Increased blood flow velocity across the mi-

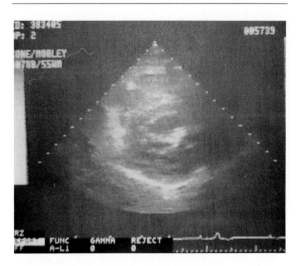

FIGURE 9-7. The mitral valve orifice is best demonstrated in the parasternal short-axis view, as seen here.

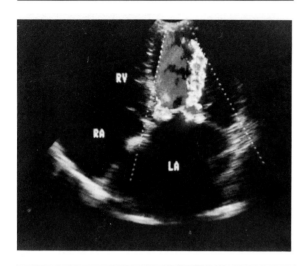

FIGURE 9-8. (See color insert.) Doppler color-flow map demonstrates mitral stenosis. Note the flow jet showing increased velocity and turbulence.

tral valve is frequently noted in patients with mitral valve stenosis. When prolapse is associated with mitral stenosis, it almost invariably involves the anterior leaflet and is associated with extreme leaflet pliability and prominent diastolic doming.

The clinical manifestations of mitral stenosis include dyspnea with orthopnea and occasional attacks of frank pulmonary edema, which may be precipitated by a variety of systemic stresses that increase blood flow across the stenotic valve. Additional symptoms may include hemoptysis, chest pain, and thromboembolism, and occasionally the patient presents with infective endocarditis. On physical examination the characteristic auscultatory findings include an opening snap, a presystolic murmur, and most characteristically, a diastolic, low-pitched, rumbling murmur that is well-localized between the point of maximum impulse and the midaxillary line, all of which are decreased during inspiration and increased during expiration. The electrocardiogram may demonstrate left atrial enlargement with frequent atrial fibrillation and left ventricular hypertrophy. Chest radiography demonstrates left atrial enlargement, and fluoroscopy may demonstrate calcification of the mitral valve.[5] In the United States, the incidence of mitral

stenosis has decreased so dramatically that it is now a relatively rare condition. Treatment is primarily surgical—commissurotomy and mitral valve replacement are the principal procedures. Alternatively, percutaneous balloon mitral valvuloplasty is performed in selected patients.

*Congenital Mitral Valve Stenosis.* Congenital mitral stenosis is a rare disorder of the mitral valve characterized by deformity of the valve apparatus that may include thickening, fibrosis, and nodularity of the leaflets. Fusion may occur, and sometimes commissures are absent. Abnormalities of the chordae are also noted, as are changes in the papillary muscles. The valve may appear to be thickened, funnel-shaped, or flat, with stiff and restricted leaflet motion. Diastolic excursion is usually reduced; on more pliable leaflets diastolic doming has been noted. Although diastolic vibration of the leaflets can be noted occasionally, the reason for this appearance is not clear.[1,3,5,7,13]

As in adult mitral stenosis, which is usually secondary to rheumatic disease, the clinical consequences are secondary to obstruction of left ventricular inflow. Generally, onset of clinical symptoms due to pulmonary venous obstruction occurs during infancy. Unless the obstruction is corrected surgically, patients usually die.

*Parachute mitral valve.* Parachute mitral valve is a congenital form of mitral stenosis characterized by a single large papillary muscle that originates from the floor of the left ventricle. The leaflets and chords appear normal. Usually, reflectivity is increased and leaflet motion is reduced. The characteristic feature of this disorder is the recording from the short axis of a single, large papillary muscle positioned posteriorly in the center of the left ventricle.[10]

As a subset of lesions causing anatomic obstruction to left ventricular inflow, the incidence, physical findings, prognosis, and treatment of parachute mitral valve are similar to those of other varieties of congenital mitral stenosis.

*Mitral Valve Regurgitation.* Mitral valve regurgitation can be associated with any abnormality in which the leaflets fail to close properly and allow backflow of blood into the left atrium. Thus, left atrial enlargement is noted. With Doppler echocar-

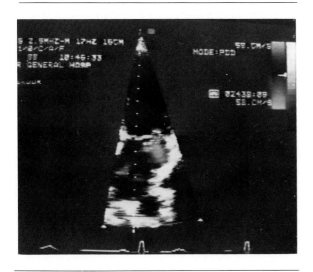

FIGURE 9-9. (See color insert.) Doppler color-flow map demonstrates mitral regurgitation.

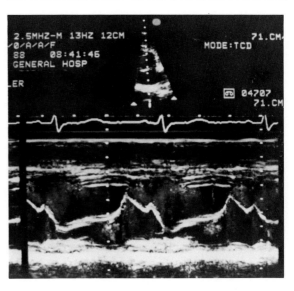

FIGURE 9-10. (See color insert.) Color M-mode image demonstrates mitral regurgitation.

diography one can reliably determine the amount of insufficiency (Figs. 9-9, 9-10).[3,5,7,13]

Chronic mitral regurgitation is distinguished from the acute form by its duration. Clinical findings are closely related to severity, time course, and association with other cardiac disease. The physical examination generally discloses a harsh systolic murmur throughout systole, primarily in the area of the cardiac apex and radiating through the axilla, with associated left ventricular hypertrophy and left atrial enlargement on electrocardiograms and echocardiograms. Chest radiographs show moderate enlargement of the entire cardiac silhouette and of the left atrium. Cardiac catheterization generally demonstrates elevated pressures in the right side of the heart with additional elevation in pulmonay capillary wedge pressure in the presence of v waves on the tracing. Ventricular cineangiography demonstrates various grades of regurgitation. The treatment and prognosis depend on a variety of factors ranging from normal life span without treatment for patients with chronic regurgitant lesions to a high mortality rate unless there is prompt surgical intervention in acute, severe cases of mitral regurgitation (flail leaflet).

*Mitral valve prolapse.* Mitral valve prolapse describes a heterogeneous group of anatomic and functional abnormalities of the mitral valve that are generally characterized by the displacement of all or any part of one or both mitral valve leaflets into the left atrium during ventricular systole (preferably mid- to late systole (Figs. 9-11, 9-12). From an anatomic standpoint, true prolapse relates only to the abnormal leaflet position and does not imply any underlying mechanism or clinical syndrome. The mitral valve itself (one or both leaflets) may be stretched, elongated, or redundant.

The cause of mitral valve prolapse is not known, but many theories have been proposed. Prolapse is suggested clinically on auscultation by the presence of a midsystolic click, and frequently a late systolic murmur. This association is not consistent, and other cardiac findings can be associated with a midsystolic click or a late systolic murmur.

It should be observed that a number of morphologic changes have been noted in mitral leaflets over the last several years. These include an increase in the size and length of the posterior leaflet relative to the anterior leaflet, thickening of both anterior and posterior leaflets (myxomatous degeneration, especially of the anterior leaflet), and in

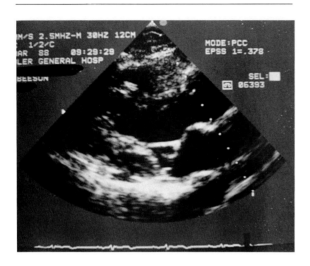

FIGURE 9-11. Parasternal long-axis 2-D scan demonstrates mitral valve prolapse.

some cases, marked leaflet redundancy and infolding. Prolapse is usually best seen in the left parasternal long-axis view (Fig. 9-13) and can sometimes be noted from the apical four-chamber view (Fig. 9-14).[3-5,7-9,11-14]

As in many causes of mitral regurgitation, a systolic murmur is classically associated with significant mitral valve prolapse, but in addition, a mid-systolic click is also heard in most patients. The overwhelming majority of patients have no symptoms and no significant sequela of mitral valve prolapse. Ordinarily the electrocardiogram is normal, as is the chest radiograph. Echocardiography is the primary diagnostic modality after auscultation. The heterogeneous nature of mitral valve prolaspe also encompasses more severe forms with significant regurgitation and its associated sequela. These require individualized medical and surgical management. An important preventive measure against mitral valve prolapse and other valvular lesions is antibiotic prophylaxis during dental and surgical procedures known to seed the bloodstream with bacteria that can cause infective endocarditis.

*Ruptured chordae tendineae.* The most common cause of acute, severe mitral valve insufficiency is

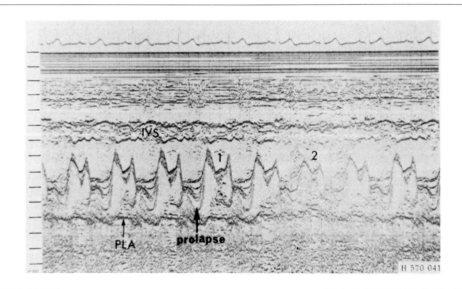

FIGURE 9-12. M-mode image demonstrates mitral valve prolapse. (IVS, interventricular septum; PLA, posterior left atrial wall)

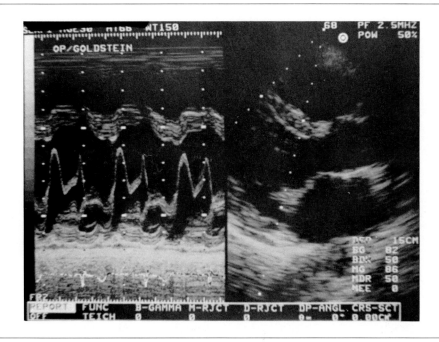

FIGURE 9-13. M-mode and 2-D echocardiograms show mitral valve prolapse.

ruptured chordae tendineae. Rupture of the chordae may occur in the absence of underlying disease or secondary to rheumatic heart disease, bacterial endocarditis, mitral valve prolapse, connective tissue disorders, myocardial infarction, idiopathic hypertrophic subaortic stenosis (IHSS), and trauma. Patients with spontaneous (primary) rupture most often have posterior leaflet involvement, whereas secondary chordae rupture usually is found to involve either the anterior or posterior leaflets.

The echocardiographic findings of chordae rupture vary. In some cases, a form of exaggerated mitral valve prolapse is noted; in more severe cases, the chordae themselves may be seen flying about wildly in the left ventricular cavity (Figs. 9-15 to 9-17).[3–5,7,11,13]

Regardless of the cause, ruptured chordae tendineae ultimately result in mitral regurgitation, the onset of which is often abrupt and acute. This generally requires surgical management, and the findings are related to the hemodynamics associated with the rupture.

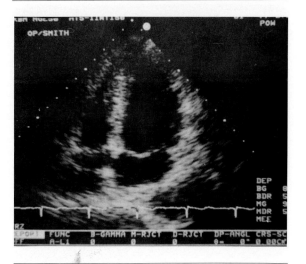

FIGURE 9-14. Mitral valve prolapse as seen from the four-chamber apical view.

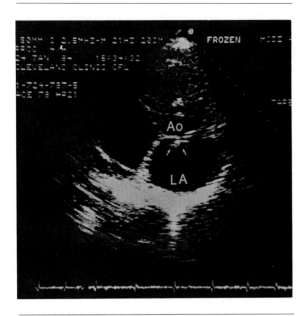

Figure 9-15. Echocardiographic findings of chordal rupture (short-axis, left parasternal view). (Ao, aorta; LA, left atrium.)

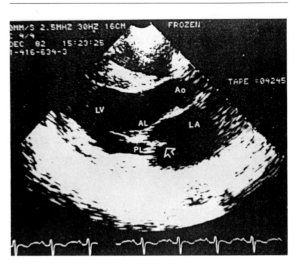

Figure 9-16. Two-dimensional echocardiographic finding of chordal rupture taken from the parasternal long-axis view. (Ao, aorta; LV, left ventricle; AL, anterior leaflet; LA, left atrium; PL, posterior leaflet.)

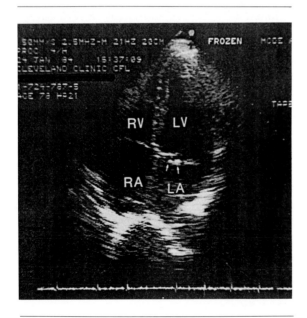

Figure 9-17. Two-dimensional four-chamber apical view of ruptured chord. (RV, right ventricle; LV, left ventricle; RA, right atrium; LA, left atrium.)

*Flail mitral valve leaflet.* Flail mitral leaflet, the most severe mitral leaflet motion disturbance, results from disruption of the supporting apparatus (chordae tendineae, papillary muscles). This condition is usually best seen in the left parasternal long-axis view (Fig. 9-18) and has also been seen from the apical four-chamber view (Fig. 9-19). Only a small portion of the mitral leaflet may flail. The characterized motion to be sought is the flipping motion of the affected leaflet, which has been compared to a sail flapping in the wind.[3,5,7,13,14]

Generally, flailing of a mitral valve leaflet is due to either papillary muscle rupture or rupture of multiple chordae tendineae. Again, it may result in acute mitral regurgitation and the associated clinical and prognostic findings and features may depend on the hemodynamic sequelae of such valve disruption. Surgical intervention may become necessary.

*Papillary muscle dysfunction.* Papillary muscles provide the foundation of support for the mitral leaflets during ventricular systole. Abnormal function of the muscles can produce improper closure of the leaflets, in which case mitral regurgitation can be

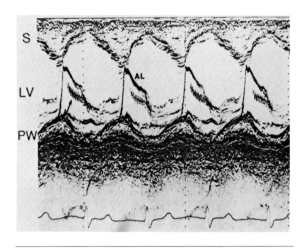

FIGURE 9-18. M-mode recording of flail mitral valve leaflet. (S, septum; LV, left ventricle; PW, posterior wall; AL, anterior mitral leaflet.)

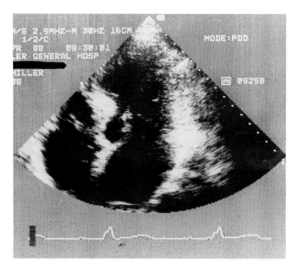

FIGURE 9-19. Apical four-chamber 2-D scan of flail mitral valve leaflet.

noted by Doppler echocardiography. This dysfunction is most commonly associated with ischemic heart disease; however, other causes have been noted, such as cardiomyopathy, left ventricular dilatation, trauma, and other endocardial and myocardial disorders. Dysfunction of the papillary muscle appears to be related to concomitant dysfunction of the myocardium at the papillary muscle base.[3,5,13]

As in the disorders discussed above, the severity of regurgitation determines the findings and treatment.

*Cleft Mitral Valve.* Clefts in the anterior mitral valve leaflet can occur as part of or in association with other defects, such as endocardial cushions or as an isolated lesion. The anterior leaflet may be entirely or partially cleft. Cleft valves are best visualized in the short axis configuration from the left sternal border (Figs. 9-20, 9-21). Mitral regurgitation is usually noted from these valve types.[3,13]

Clinically, the cleft mitral valve presents as mitral regurgitation in the presence of endocardial cushion defects. Management is dictated by the severity of the condition and often includes mitral valve repair or replacement. The clinical findings depend on the associated cardiac lesions.

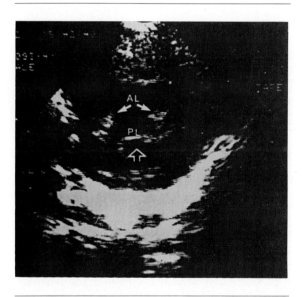

FIGURE 9-20. Short-axis, 2-D scan of cleft mitral valve. (AL, anterior leaflet; PL, posterior leaflet.)

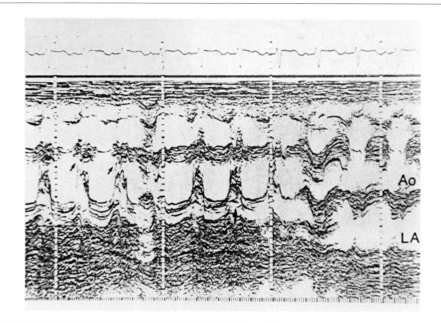

FIGURE 9-21. M-mode image demonstrates cleft mitral valve. (Ao, aorta; LA, left atrium.)

*Mitral Annulus Calcification.* Calcification of the mitral annulus is a degenerative disorder that usually occurs with advancing age and is characterized by calcium deposits on the mitral annulus area (Fig. 9-22) or the angular space adjacent to the posterior mitral leaflet. It sometimes encompasses the posterior mitral valve leaflet. Mitral regurgitation has been associated with mitral annulus calcification, as have conduction abnormalities, congestive heart failure, and when severe, obstruction of the left ventricular inflow. Two-dimensional echocardiography quickly identifies mitral annulus calcification (Fig. 9-23), demonstrating a dense, localized, highly reflective area at the base of the posterior mitral leaflet. The posterior mitral annulus is approximately five times more likely to become calcified than the anterior annulus.[2-5,7,11,13]

Generally, mitral annulus calcification produces no symptoms and has no effects demonstrable by examination or electrocardiography. Occasionally, mitral annular calcification is seen on a chest film or during fluoroscopy. If extremely severe, it may impair mitral valve function and it occasionally

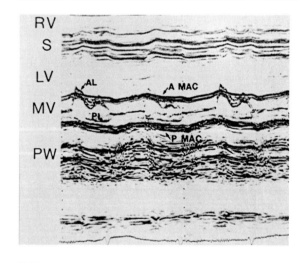

FIGURE 9-22. Mitral annulus calcification (anterior and posterior) as seen on M-mode echocardiography. (RV, right ventricle; S, septum; LV, left ventricle; MV, mitral valve; PW, posterior wall; AL, anterior mitral leaflet; PL, posterior mitral leaflet; MAC, mitral annulus calcification.)

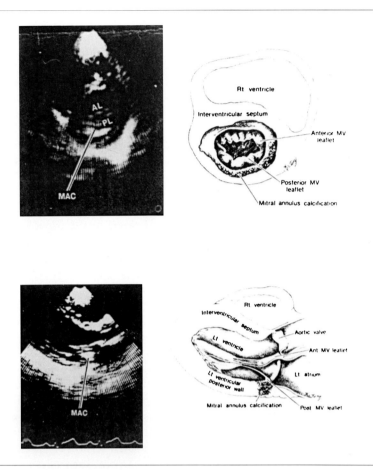

FIGURE 9-23. Two-dimensional echocardiographic view of mitral annulus calcification.

leads to mitral regurgitation with attendant sequelae. Surgical repair is complicated by the calcific annulus, which makes it difficult to sew a prosthetic ring in place or to repair the valve.

*Mitral Valve Vegetations.* Valvular vegetations are the result of bacterial endocarditis. These friable masses composed of clumps of bacteria, fungi, platelets, fibrin, white and red blood cells, and necrotic tissue are usually located in areas that were previously altered by rheumatic, congenital, or syphilitic cardiac lesions, but they also may be found on apparently normal valves. Vegetations can be eroded or weakened by valve leaflet motion and the entire structure or pieces of the vegetation

may break off and may dislodge, becoming a source of cardiac emboli. Treatment may produce healing or the areas may remain roughened and can calcify with time.[3,6,7,13]

Echocardiographically, vegetations appear as irregular masses of echoes attached to the valve leaflet (Fig. 9-24). They may look thickened, irregular, "smeared," or like cotton. Some patients show no changes on echocardiography, even in the presence of documented endocarditis, so it is quite helpful clinically to take blood specimens for culture as an adjunct to echocardiography. Echocardiography has enhanced evaluation of vegetative lesions on valves, but results are not diagnostic 100% of the time. Doppler echocardiography is extremely use-

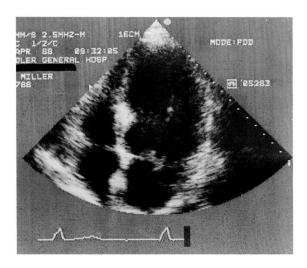

FIGURE 9-24. Mitral valve vegetations as seen on a four-chamber, apical view, 2-D scan.

ful for analyzing new regurgitant lesions resulting from infected cardiac structures.

Clinically, the history suggests an infectious process, either chronic or acute, depending on the type of organism and the route through which it is seeded into the bloodstream. Usually, the auscultatory findings are those of mitral insufficiency with a systolic murmur, although the electrocardiogram and chest radiograph may show little early on. Laboratory documentation of bacteremia in the appropriate clinical setting confirms the diagnosis, and echocardiography identifies the vegetations noninvasively. The incidences and prognosis are determined entirely by the type and severity of the infection; treatment ranges from several weeks of antibiotic therapy to surgical valve replacement with prolonged antibiotic management.

## Tricuspid Valve

Historically, the tricuspid valve has been one of the most difficult structures to record with M-mode echocardiography. The difficulty is related to its location immediately beneath the sternum and its plane of motion relative to the anterior chest wall. The improved visualization of the right side of the heart provided by 2-D echocardiography has facil-

itated recording and interrogation of the tricuspid valve.[2-4,12-14]

### ANATOMY

The tricuspid valve is a complex anatomic structure composed of leaflet tissue, chordae tendineae, papillary muscles, and the supporting annular ring and right ventricular myocardium (Fig. 9-25). Larger and more structurally complex than its mitral counterpart, the tricuspid valve has a larger and more irregular orifice. The tricuspid leaflets are actually a continuous veil of thin, fibrous tissue with a basal portion attached around the entire circumference of the tricuspid annulus. This fibrous tissue veil can be separated into three distinct leaflets by indentations along its free edge, though these areas of separation are less distinct than those of the mitral valve. There are three major tricuspid leaflets: anterior, septal, and posterior. The anterior leaflet is the largest, stretching from the infundibular region anteriorly to the inferolateral wall posteriorly. The septal leaflet stretches posteriorly along the interventricular septum from the infundibulum to the posterior ventricular border and attaches to the muscular and membranous areas of the septum. The insertion of the septal leaflet is characteristically inferior or apical, compared to the septal insertion of the anterior mitral valve leaflet. The posterior leaflet attaches along the posterior margin of the annulus, from the septum to the inferolateral wall. All of these relationships can be seen in short-axis views of the tricuspid valve.

Three papillary muscles support the tricuspid leaflets and lie beneath each of the three commissures. The anterior papillary muscle is largest and lies beneath the commissure between the anterior and posterior leaflets. It arises from the moderator band and from the "free" anterolateral wall of the right ventricle. The posterior papillary muscle lies inferior to the junction of the posterior and septal leaflets, whereas, a small septal papillary muscle originating from the septal border of the infundibulum tethers the anterior and septal leaflets high against the infundibular wall. Occasionally this papillary muscle is absent, in which case the chordae tendineae may arise from small tendinous connections in the infundibulum. Arising from each of these papillary muscles, the chordae tendineae attach to the free edges and the proximal ventric-

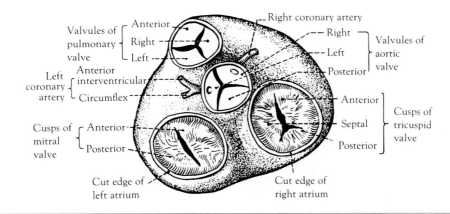

FIGURE 9-25. Anatomic view of the tricuspid and mitral valves. (From Hollinshead WH. Anatomy for Surgeons. The thorax, abdomen, and pelvis. 2nd ed: New York: Harper & Row; 1971; 2:129.)

ular surfaces of each of the leaflets supported by the papillary muscle.

Several unique morphologic features distinguish the tricuspid valve from its mitral counterpart: (1) three leaflets, (2) three distinct and separate papillary muscles, (3) the inferior or apical insertion point of the septal leaflet, and (4) the partial origin of the anterior papillary muscle on the moderator band. These features can be particularly valuable when ventricular structure is questionable. The tricuspid valve has always attracted much attention among clinicians, physiologists, surgeons, and pathologists, and much has been written on it.[2]

PATHOLOGY

The pathologic changes that affect the tricuspid valve can be congenital or acquired. The most common congenital malformation is Ebstein's anomaly. Other pathologic changes affecting this valve are infective endocarditis, stenosis, valve prolapse, and (rarely) ruptured chordae tendineae, among others.

The functional anatomy and pathology of the tricuspid valve can be readily assessed with 2–D echocardiography. All three leaflets can be visualized. Two of the best views for interrogating the tricuspid valve are that from the left sternal border, and the parasternal long-axis right ventricular inflow view, in which both anterior and posterior leaf-

let are easily identified. Other helpful views include the left sternal border short-axis view and the four-chamber view, in which the anterior and the septal leaflet are seen, and the subcostal, short-axis view, in which all three leaflets can be visualized.

*Ebstein's Anomaly.* Ebstein's anomaly is a congenital deformity characterized by downward displacement of a part of a malformed tricuspid valve into the right ventricular cavity. This feature of Ebstein's anomaly can be visualized best echocardiographically from the apical four-chamber view (Fig. 9-26). The anterior tricuspid leaflet characteristically is the largest and the one least affected in Ebstein's anomaly. The septal and posterior leaflets are more deformed, and the posterior leaflet may be rudimentary or absent. The right atrium is almost always dilated (Fig. 9-27), and atrial septal defect may be associated with this malformation.[3,4,6-9,11,12,14]

Many patients with Ebstein's anomaly present as adults in the third or fourth decade of life. The severity of symptoms correlates principally with the degree of severity of the associated anomaly. Most important is the predisposition toward arrhythmogenic foci, occasional paradoxical emboli, and brain abscesses. Auscultation demonstrates a systolic murmur characteristic of tricuspid insuffi-

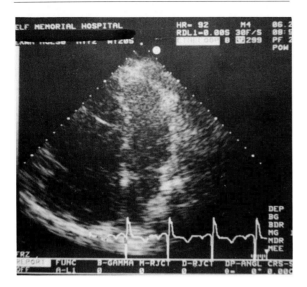

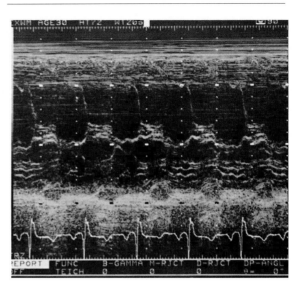

FIGURE 9-26. Ebstein's anomaly from the 2-D apical view.

FIGURE 9-27. Ebstein's anomaly recorded on M-mode echocardiography.

ciency and the electrocardiogram may show marked peaking of the P waves in as many as 10 to 25% of patients—and occasionally Wolf-Parkinson-White syndrome. Cardiac catheterization usually is not necessary and is not recommended unless absolutely indicated, because of the high incidence of arrhythmias during the procedure. Often patients can be managed medically, and occasionally, tricuspid valve annuloplasty or replacement is required.

*Tricuspid Vegetations.* Involvement of the tricuspid valve by endocarditis is relatively infrequent: the reported prevalence is 4% or less.[3–13] Tricuspid endocarditis is typically acute rather than subacute. *Staphylococcus aureus* is the most common infecting organism. Predisposing factors include intravenous drug abuse, alcohol abuse, skin infections, and infected venous catheters.

Echocardiographically, vegetations appear as irregular masses of echoes attached to the valve leaflet (Fig. 9-28). They may look thickened, irregular, "smeared," or like cotton (Fig. 9-29). There are patients in whom no apparent changes are noted echocardiographically in the presence of documented endocarditis. Blood culture is a quite helpful adjunct to echocardiography.

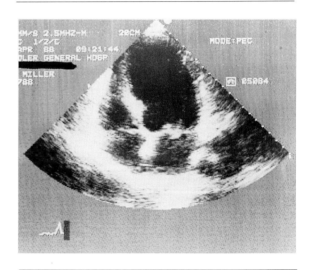

FIGURE 9-28. Tricuspid and mitral vegetations seen from the 2-D apical view.

Infective endocarditis is one of the most common causes of nonrheumatic tricuspid insufficiency. It often presents with fever, bacteremia, and a clinical picture consistent with endocarditis. The

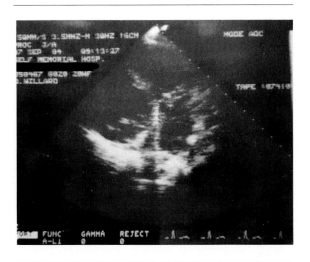

FIGURE 9-29. Two-dimensional scan of tricuspid vegetations (right ventricular inflow view).

clinical examination often discloses only slight systolic murmur of tricuspid insufficiency, but echocardiography confirms the presence of vegetations. Often, only standard antibiotic therapy is neces-

sary, and it is a rare case that requires surgical removal of the tricuspid valve tissue for management of the infection.

*Tricuspid Valve Prolapse.* Tricuspid valve prolapse can be identified as the anatomic displacement of one or more of the tricuspid leaflets, or part of those leaflets, into the right atrium during ventricular systole. Tricuspid prolapse appears to involve the septal and anterior leaflets primarily (Figs. 9-30, 9-31).[3,4,6,12,14] Like mitral valve prolapse, tricuspid valve prolapse involves incompetence of the tricuspid leaflets; in both instances the result is tricuspid insufficiency, with its clinical and systemic manifestations. The typical tricuspid regurgitant systolic murmur may also be associated, but in addition there may be a midsystolic click that varies with respiration, indicating that it is produced by a right-sided heart lesion. Therapy is rarely required, though surgical valvuloplasty sometimes is.

*Tricuspid Insufficiency.* Tricuspid insufficiency can be caused by any of a number of disorders.[14] Anything that causes the tricuspid valve to close incompletely can cause tricuspid insufficiency—among others valve prolapse, rheumatic heart disease, stenosis, bacterial endocarditis, carcinoid syndrome,

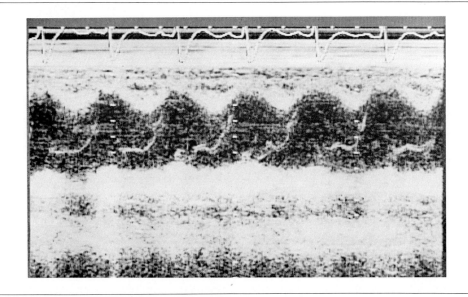

FIGURE 9-30. Tricuspid valve prolapse recorded on M-mode echocardiography.

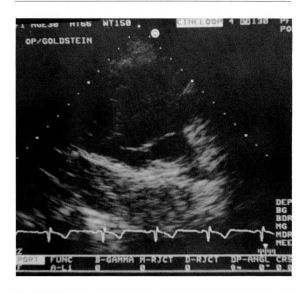

FIGURE 9-31. Tricuspid valve prolapse presented on 2-D echocardiography (left parasternal, right ventricular inflow view).

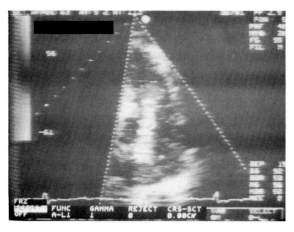

FIGURE 9-32. (See color insert.) Color-flow scan of tricuspid insufficiency.

trauma, and congenital disorders such as cusp differentiation or chordal malformation that prevents normal closure and Ebstein's anomaly. Tricuspid insufficiency has been found in normal persons and may or may not be a normal finding. Tei and associates measured the tricuspid annulus in normal patients and in patients with tricuspid insufficiency. Their findings demonstrated that the annular circumference was significantly larger in the patients with tricuspid insufficiency.[15] Color-flow mapping (Fig. 9-32) has made it much easier to assess the severity of tricuspid insufficiency.[2–4,6,10,12] In general, it is due to right ventricular enlargement with attendant stretching of the tricuspid valve annulus. Usually, the tricuspid valve itself is anatomically intact and the clinical findings are those of the causes of right ventricular enlargement with the murmur of tricuspid insufficiency. It is not uncommon to document some tricuspid insufficiency by Doppler studies in normal persons, but this does not necessarily reflect pathologic situations. Pacer wires are a known cause of tricuspid insufficiency as well. In tricuspid insufficiency secondary to diseased tricuspid valve tissue, the clinical findings and treatment vary with the underlying cause.

*Tricuspid Stenosis.* In the past, it was difficult to diagnose organic acquired tricuspid valve stenosis, but with the advent of 2-D echocardiography it has become quite easy. Rheumatic fever is the most common cause of acquired tricuspid valve stenosis. Rheumatic inflammation can produce scarring and fibrosis of the valve leaflets, resulting in fusion of the leaflet commissures and associated fibrosis and thickening of the chordae tendineae. This can limit leaflet mobility and reduce the size of the orifice. Tricuspid stenosis occurs less frequently than mitral stenosis, but when it does occur it is almost invariably associated with mitral stenosis. The tricuspid lesion is usually less severe than its mitral counterpart.[3,4,6,7,10,12,14]

Tricuspid stenosis is characterized echocardiographically by (1) increased echogenicity in the thickened deformed leaflets, (2) abnormal diastolic leaflet motion, and (3) reduced tricuspid valve orifice size (Fig. 9-33).

Another type of acquired tricuspid stenosis originates in the endomyocardium. Löeffler's endocarditis is characterized by deposition of fibrinous or fibroelastic material on the endocardial and valvular surfaces, which may lead to restriction of tricuspid leaflet motion and stenosis.[6–10] It has a somewhat different appearance than valves with rheumatic involvement and it is mentioned here only in passing.

Tricuspid stenosis is a very rare condition man-

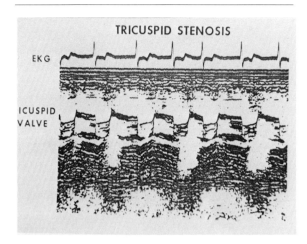

FIGURE 9-33. Tricuspid stenosis as seen on M-mode echocardiography.

ifested as an obstruction to right ventricular inflow with attendant reduction in cardiac output. Generally, the auscultatory findings suggest mitral stenosis and the finding suggestive of tricuspid stenosis—a very soft diastolic rumble at the lower left sternal edge that varies with inspiration—is difficult to discern. The electrocardiogram demonstrates marked right atrial enlargement, greater than expected for the degree of right ventricular hypertrophy. Usually, there is marked cardiomegaly secondary to enlargement of the right atrium. The primary therapy is surgical, and it is generally done in conjunction with repair of a coexisting mitral valve lesion.

## Conclusion

One of the principal uses of echocardiography is in examination of the cardiac valves. The attributes of M-mode technique, which permits excellent recordings of individual valve motion; the spatial orientation provided by 2-D echocardiography; and the imaging of blood flow through diseased valves with the techniques of Doppler echocardiography are the qualities that have made echocardiography the examination of choice in the evaluation of valve disease. Only by integrating the various echocardiographic techniques mentioned above can the most complete information be derived to aid in the management of patients with acquired valvular disease.

## Acknowledgment

Special thanks is given to Robert Rollings, M.D., for his clinical assistance and editing.

## References

1. Cope GD, Kisslo JA, Johnson ML, et al. A reassessment of echo in mitral stenosis. Circulation. 1975; 52:664–670.
2. D'Cruz IA, Panettia F, Cohen HC, et al. Submitral calcification or sclerosis in elderly patients. Am J Cardiol. 1979; 44:31–38.
3. Feigenbaum H. Echocardiography. 4th ed. Philadelphia: Lea & Febiger; 1986; 249–365.
4. Goss CM, ed. Gray's Anatomy: Anatomy of the Human Body. 29th ed. Philadelphia: Lea & Febiger; 1973; 455–473.
5. Harris A, Sutton GC, Tower M. Physiological and Clinical Aspects of Cardiac Auscultation. Philadelphia: Lippincott; 1979.
6. Martinez EC, Burch GE, Giles TD. Echocardiographic diagnosis of bacterial endocarditis. Am J Cardiol. 1974; 34:845–849.
7. Nasser FN, Guilliam E. Clinical Two-Dimensional Echocardiography. Chicago: Year Book Medical Publishers; 1983; 67–87; 106–117.
8. Popp RL, Brown OR, Silverman JF, et al. Echocardiographic abnormalities in mitral valve prolapse syndrome. Circulation. 1974; 49:428–433.
9. Sahn DJ, Allen HD, Goldberg SJ. MVP in children. Circulation. 1976; 53:651–657.
10. Shone JD, et al. The developmental complex of "parachute mitral valve," supraventricular ring of left atrium, subaortic stenosis and coarctation. Am J Cardiol. 1963; 11:714–725.
11. Tajik AJ, et al. Two-dimensional real-time ultrasonic imaging of the heart and great vessel. Mayo Clin Proc. 1978; 53:271–303.
12. Weyman AE. Clinical applications of cross-sectional echo. In: DeVlieger (ed.). A Handbook of Clinical Ultrasound. New York: John Wiley; 1978.
13. Weyman AE. Cross-Sectional Echocardiography. Philadelphia: Lea & Febiger; 1982; 137–192; 338–367.
14. Weyman AE, Wann LS, Rogers EW, Godley RN, et al. Five-year experience in correlating cross-sectional echo assessment of the mitral valve with hemodynamic valve area determination. Am J Cardiol 1979; 43:386.
15. Tei C, Shah PM, Ormiston JA, et al. Echocardiographic evaluation of tricuspid annulus size and function in normal and in tricuspid regurgitation. Am J Cardiol. 1981; 47:412.

# CHAPTER 10

# Acquired Aortic and Pulmonic Valvular Heart Disease

PAULA K. LOGAN

## Aortic Valve

The normal aortic valve has three leaflets. It allows blood to flow from the left ventricle into the aorta. The valve opens at the end of isovolumic contraction, when left ventricular pressure rises above aortic pressure, and closes when aortic pressure exceeds left ventricular pressure.

On M-mode echocardiography, the noncoronary and right coronary cusps are seen to open in a parallelogram fashion during systole and then close, occupying a position in the center of the aorta throughout diastole (Fig. 10-1). The cusps open to the extent of the aortic root walls and the cusps shudder during systole. It is important to remember that a valve affected by congenital aortic stenosis has the same motion by M-mode as a normal aortic valve.

With two-dimensional (2-D) echocardiography the aortic valve is studied in the parasternal long-axis view to visualize leaflet opening (Figs. 10-2, 10-3). The sinuses of Valsalva can be evaluated, as can a short segment of the ascending aorta. The parasternal short-axis view detects the number of cusps on the valve and areas of thickening (Figs. 10-4, 10-5). Other views can be used to assess the aortic valve, should the parasternal view be inadequate. Although apical five-chamber, apical long-axis, and subcostal views can provide information on valve thickening, they cannot demonstrate how many cusps the valve has.

DOPPLER EVALUATION OF THE AORTIC VALVE

Aortic valve velocity reaches its peak in the first third of systole (average, 1 m per second; Fig. 10-6). The flow profile is often defined by opening and closing valve clicks generated by the highly reflective valve tissue passing through the Doppler beam. The interval from the opening click to the closing click represents left ventricular ejection time (LVET). The valve is usually studied from the apical position with the patient resting on the left side. The flow is away from the transducer. Should this view fail to provide an adequate velocity profile, the transducer can be placed in the second or third right intercostal space with the patient resting on the right side, in which case the direction of flow will be toward the transducer. Suprasternal notch and subcostal windows can also be used.

The patient positions required to evaluate aortic valve flow usually preclude the use of pulsed-waved Doppler. The valve is so far from the transducer that the Nyquist limit may force aliasing before flow through the valve reaches peak velocity. For this reason, continuous-wave Doppler is the preferred modality.

*Aortic Valve Stenosis.* Aortic stenosis (AS) is reduction of the size of the valve lumen due to a rheumatic, degenerative, or congenital disorder. Rheumatic aortic stenosis is characterized by adhesion and fusion of the commissures, with vasculariza-

201

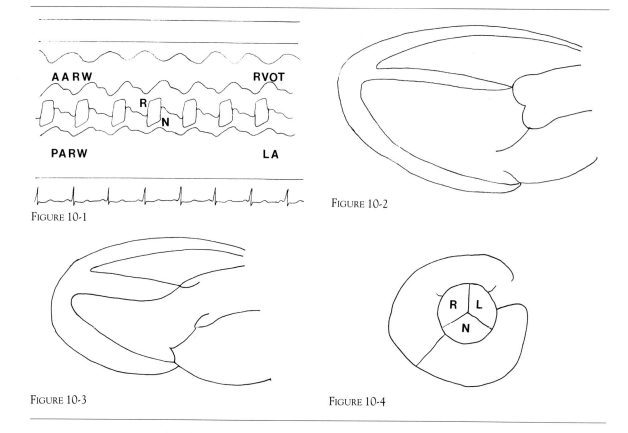

FIGURE 10-1

FIGURE 10-2

FIGURE 10-3

FIGURE 10-4

FIGURE 10-1. The normal M-mode diagram of the aortic valve shows the right coronary cusp opening toward the anterior aortic root wall (AARW) and the noncoronary cusp opening toward the posterior aortic root wall (PARW). (RVOT, right ventricular outflow tract, LA, left atrium; R, right coronary cusp; N, noncoronary cusp.)

FIGURE 10-3. Aortic valve in the open position during systole.

FIGURE 10-2. This parasternal long-axis diagram shows the position of the aortic cusps during diastole when the valve is closed.

FIGURE 10-4. Parasternal short-axis diagram of closed aortic valve with cusps labelled right coronary (R), left coronary (L), and noncoronary (N).

tion of the leaflets and valve ring. This results in shrinking and stiffening of the free borders and the formation of calcium deposits on both sides of the leaflets. The opening is usually round or triangular, and regurgitation is often present.

Degenerative (senile) calcific aortic stenosis results from formation of thick calcium deposits at the base of the cusps where they bend to open, which reduce motion. The commissures do not fuse. The most likely cause is accumulated tress of years of wear and tear on the valve. The

most common calcific aortic stenosis occurs secondary to a bicuspid valve in patients over 50 years of age. The bicuspid valve has one dominant leaflet where the commissures between two cusps do not separate. This resulting seam is called a raphe. When calcific aortic stenosis develops secondary to a bicuspid aortic valve, regurgitation usually develops too.

Congenital aortic stenosis is mentioned here only because the symptoms may not appear until the patient is an adult. A complete review of congenital aortic stenosis is covered in Part 5 of this book.

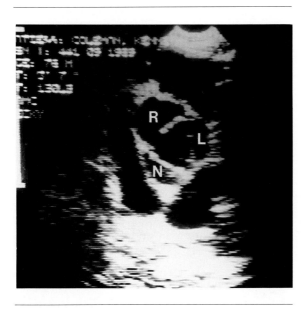

FIGURE 10-5. Picture of aortic cusp open, when the three cusps are clearly delineated. (R, right; L, left; N, noncoronary.)

*Clinical symptoms.* The gradual reduction of the aortic valve orifice (and increase in left ventricular outflow obstruction) is well compensated for by left ventricular hypertrophy, so symptoms of aortic stenosis may not develop until the sixth decade of life. The symptoms can develop earlier and do develop when the hypertrophy fails to keep up with the increased pressure demands placed on the ventricle by the stenotic valve. The most common symptoms are angina pectoris, syncope (fainting), and heart failure.

About two thirds of all patients with severe aortic stenosis have angina, and half have coronary artery obstruction.[8] Pain is usually brought on by exertion and relieved with rest. It is the result of increased oxygen demand from the hypertrophic myocardium, and slowed oxygen delivery through the compressed coronary arteries. Angina may also be due to coexisting coronary artery disease, or, rarely, calcium emboli of the coronary arteries.

Reduced cerebral blood flow that coincides with exercise causes syncope. The fixed cardiac output cannot respond to systemic vasodilatation when

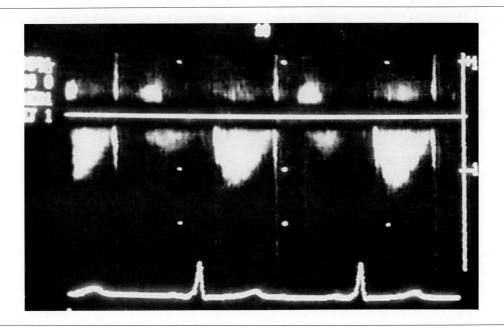

FIGURE 10-6. Normal aortic flow profile deflected negatively from baseline because the blood flow direction is away from the transducer when it is placed at the apex. The vertical line at the end of the flow profile is a valve click.

blood is diverted to the legs. The arterial pressure decreases, thereby reducing cerebral perfusion.

Symptoms of heart failure are seen later in the course of the disease. As left ventricular filling pressure rises, pulmonary venous hypertension develops. When the pressure is great enough, pulmonary edema precipitates exertional dyspnea (shortness of breath), orthopnea (difficulty breathing except in an upright position), and paroxysmal nocturnal dyspnea (sudden suffocation at night).

*Pathophysiology.* The left ventricle responds to the increasing pressure gradient across the gradually narrowing aortic valve by increasing myocardial thickness. The hypertrophic left ventricle can endure a hypertensive state for many years and maintain good cardiac output without showing dilatation, so symptoms become manifest later on in the disease. The increasing hypertrophy reduces ventricular compliance, so that atrial contraction plays an especially important role in ventricular filling.

Atrial fibrillation or atrioventricular (AV) dissociation (when atria and ventricles contract independently) may cause rapid clinical deterioration in a patient with severe AS. Cardiac output is normal at rest but cannot meet the demands of exercise. Later on in the disease, as cardiac output and stroke volume decline, the left ventricular-to-aortic pressure gradient reduces and pressure buildup is subsequently reflected in the left atrium, pulmonary veins, pulmonary capillaries, pulmonary artery, right ventricle (in systole and diastole), and right atrium. Late in the disease, as the left ventricle dilates mitral regurgitation may develop. With coexisting mitral regurgitation, the increase in left ventricular pressure exacerbates the mitral regurgitation.

*Physical examination.* The physical findings of mild AS may be overlooked, but findings of moderate or severe AS are easily detected. Typically, arterial pulses rise slowly and are weak and sustained. A carotid shudder can be readily felt, and is caused by systolic vibration of the cusps and anacrotic notch (abrupt reduction of early systolic flow). Delay in the carotid pulse is detected by palpating the cardiac impulse and the carotid artery simultaneously. The apical impulse is sustained when left ventricular failure is present. A systolic thrill can be felt in the second right and left intercostal

spaces, in the suprasternal notch, and often in the carotids. Reduced right ventricular compliance increases the A wave of the jugular venous pulse. Later, with pulmonary hypertension and right ventricular failure systolic pressure waves (CV waves) are felt from the carotid artery. Since the physical examination may be inconclusive or misleading, the diagnostic procedure of choice is the echocardiogram.

Auscultation reveals a systolic ejection murmur, which is best heard in the second right intercostal space, often peaking in midsystole as the aortic stenosis becomes more severe. The murmur radiates to the apex (often only the higher-frequency components of the murmur) and the carotids. The aortic component ($A_2$) of the second heart sound ($S_2$), (aortic closure) is softened and sometimes is not appreciated. The pulmonic component ($P_2$) of the second heart sound may be accentuated owing to pulmonary hypertension. A high-pitched decrescendo diastolic murmur of aortic insufficiency is often present.

*Laboratory tests.* The predominant electrocardiographic (ECG) change in patients with severe AS is left ventricular hypertrophy (85%). Left atrial enlargement appears in 80% of cases of severe isolated AS.[6]

In approximately 5% of patients, calcification from the aortic valve can infiltrate the conduction system, causing various forms and degrees of AV and intraventricular conduction delays or blocks.

Chest radiographs are usually normal until poststenotic dilatation of the ascending aorta develops. Cardiomegaly is seen with aortic regurgitation or left ventricular failure. Eventually, left atrial dilatation and pulmonary venous hypertension are seen. Fluoroscopy is preferred over radiography to exclude calcification of the aortic valve. Evaluation by angiographically guided cardiac catheterization is not recommended. Rapidly injecting large volumes of dye into a left ventricle that has elevated pressure is risky and is contraindicated in the presence of significant outflow tract obstruction or left ventricular failure.

Catheterization of the left side of the heart to measure internal chamber pressure is the gold standard for evaluating the severity of aortic stenosis (Table 10-1). Simultaneous pressure tracings from the left ventricle and aorta are recorded with the

Table 10-1. Parameters of aortic stenosis by catherization

| Degree of Stenosis | Peak Gradient (mm Hg) | Mean Gradient (mm Hg) | Aortic Valve Area (cm²) |
|---|---|---|---|
| None (normal) | 4 | ≤5 | 3 |
| Mild | ≤25 | ≤20 | 3.0–1.5 |
| Moderate | 25–60 | 20–50 | 1.5–0.8 |
| Severe | ≥60 | ≥50 | ≤0.8 |

ECG. The peak pressure gradient is the difference between the peak aortic pressure and peak ventricular pressure (termed peak-to-peak pressure). The mean gradient is the systolic area difference between the aortic pressure tracing and the left ventricular pressure tracing, recorded simultaneously, then divided by the systolic ejection period. The aortic valve area is derived by mathematic calculations, using Gorlin's equation,[7] which uses cardiac output and mean aortic pressure gradient values.

*Incidence, prognosis, and treatment.* AS, the most common of all valvular diseases, occurs more often in men than in women and is usually congenital or degenerative. Symptoms occur late in the course of the disease, and once symptoms of angina, syncope, and dyspnea appear the prognosis is poor. With optimal medical management the 5-year survival rate is 50%. Surgical replacement of the valve is often the only option for these patients, even if they are elderly or have poor left ventricular function (see Chapter 16). Replacing the valve as soon as symptoms develop dramatically improves the prognosis.

An investigational technique, dual balloon valvuloplasty, is gaining momentum as an alternative to surgical valve replacement.[9] In the catheterization laboratory a guide wire is introduced into the left ventricle and positioned in the stenotic aortic valve. Inflating a series of balloons along the guide wire can successfully separate fused commissures and fracture calcific nodules. Risk for embolization is low, but complications include those common to cardiac catheterization, cardiac tamponade, and vascular rupture. The cause of the AS is not eliminated, so stenosis can recur, but the results to date show remarkable clinical improvement for at least

6 months. The valve lumen is only slightly enlarged, so this method serves as a temporizing tactic until the valve can be replaced.

Another alternative replacement is debridement of the valve. A rapidly vibrating suction instrument frees the calcific nodules and restores mobility to the cusps.

*Echocardiographic features.* M-mode evaluation for AS can easily distinguish a thin, pliable, normal valve from the calcific valve of AS, but a spectrum of lesions between these two extremes complicate evaluation of the aortic valve, as do technical limitations. Doming of congenital aortic stenosis cannot be excluded by M-mode imaging.

Dedicated M-mode echocardiography can readily record increased echogenicity from the aortic valve (evidence of thickening) in systole, and often in diastole. Whether the thickening is focal (no restriction of leaflet motion) or is more general (immobile cusps) cannot be determined with confidence. When leaflet motion can be visualized, it is possible to conclude that one or two leaflets are mobile, but the left coronary cusp usually is not seen. Should that cusp be thickened and immobile, the evidence excludes only severe aortic stenosis. Multiple dense echoes from inside the aortic root with reduced leaflet excursion indicates that two cusps are thickened, and possibly immobile, but the third cusp may be normal, allowing for one third of the valve lumen to be patent.

A bicuspid aortic valve can be detected by recording its eccentric closure. During diastole, the aortic cusps are closed, appearing as a line in the center of the aortic root. If this closure line is displaced so that one third of the aortic root diameter is on one side of the line and two thirds are on the other side, a bicuspid aortic valve should be suspected.

Technical limitations arise when the beam is directed tangential to the largest diameter of the aortic root. The lateral wall of the aorta can appear as echoes inside the aortic root, mimicking thickened aortic cusps even though the cusps may be normal. Carefully sweeping medial and lateral to the long axis of the ascending aorta should reveal leaflet motion. The aortic root diameter (recorded with leaflet motion) should be the largest measurable diameter. Then the left ventricle should be evaluated for the degree of left ventricular hypertrophy. Imaging the pulmonic valve and seeking signs of pulmonary hypertension is also useful.

The properties of ultrasound limit evaluation of calcific AS. Reverberation from the calcium may produce multiple echoes with leaflet motion in systole, and thick bands of echoes in diastole. Measurements of the aortic valve are erroneous, as the echoes from inside the aortic root may actually represent reverberation and may not show the true position of the leaflet.

Two-dimensional echocardiography has eliminated some of the pitfalls of M-mode imaging. The parasternal long-axis view can distinguish normal leaflet opening from the doming motion of congenital AS. It is important *always* to look for aortic valve doming when evaluating for aortic stenosis or even for causes of systolic ejection murmur. Thickening of the valve can be visualized in this view (Fig. 10-7) but is seen better in the parasternal short-axis view.

In the short-axis view, focal aortic valve thickening can be differentiated from general, overall thickening. It is not possible to determine the cause of the stenosis. The leaflet motion and valve lumen are more easily assessed with 2-D echocardiography. It is tempting to assess the severity of the aortic stenosis, but several studies have found poor correlation with catheterization.[1,2,11] Again, left ventricular hypertrophy can be assessed, as can left ventricular function.

A bicuspid valve can be visualized in the parasternal long-axis view by the eccentric closure of the cusps. In the short-axis view the dominant (unseparated) leaflet is well visualized; occasionally the raphe is seen. Another benefit of 2-D echocardiography is the ability to assess aortic valve annulus size, which helps thoracic surgeons decide with what size and what kind of valve to replace the native valve. Some surgeons replace the pulmonic valve with porcine grafts or homografts and use the autologous pulmonic valve in the aortic position. For such procedures the diameter of the pulmonic valve annulus is important.

DOPPLER ULTRASOUND. Doppler ultrasound has significantly improved the assessment of the severity of AS (Fig. 10-8). The modified Bernoulli equation is used to determine the instantaneous peak pressure gradient across the aortic valve: (peak gradient = $4V^2$) where V represents the peak systolic

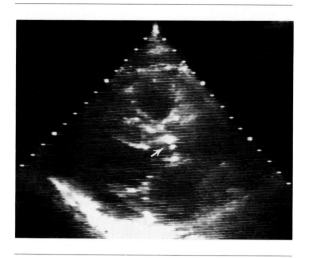

FIGURE 10-7. The arrow points to the thick, calcified aortic cusps. Just visible is the hypertrophied ventricular septum and posterior wall.

flow velocity. Doppler ultrasound can produce an erroneously low calculation of the gradient in the presence of left ventricular dysfunction and an erroneously high one when aortic regurgitation is present.

Because peak velocity can reach 4, 5, and even 6 m per second with aortic stenosis, continuous-wave Doppler examination is the most useful assessment. Pulsed-wave Doppler aliases at a much lower velocity, and high–pulse repetition frequency technique is not powerful enough to record these signals. The difficulty with this technique is in obtaining the peak velocity profile. Aortic stenosis jets are often eccentric and the lumen is small. It is sometimes necessary to evaluate the lesion not only from the apex but from the right parasternal border as well (with the patient lying on his right side), from the suprasternal notch or supraclavicular position or from the subcostal position. Even though the study is sometimes time consuming, lesions must be viewed from every possible window to obtain the best quality data.

In the Doppler profile the majority of the red blood cell targets should be moving at the same velocity, so that there is an outline (crust) to the profile. There is a larger proportion of high-frequency

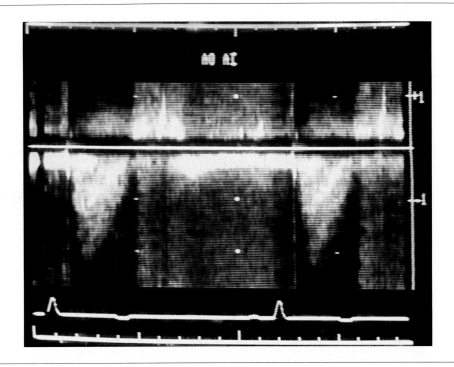

Figure 10-8. Doppler profile of mild aortic stenosis with velocities over 2 m per second.

sound in the audible signal. There should be little or no scattering of targets on the opposite side of the baseline.

Aortic stenosis is technically the most challenging lesion to record. Diligent searching and patience may be the only means of assessing severe aortic stenosis noninvasively. Once a good profile is obtained, it is easy to calculate the aortic valve peak instantaneous pressure gradient, but most catheterization laboratories report the difference between peak left ventricular pressure and peak aortic pressure. These two pressure curves peak at different times during systole, so they do not correlate with the instantaneous peak pressure gradient obtained by Doppler imaging. Many ultrasound units have the capability of determining the mean aortic gradient, which correlates well with the mean pressure gradients calculated in the catheterization laboratory (Fig. 10-9).

Aortic valve area can also be calculated noninvasively by using the continuity equation,[8] which is based on the fact that, for a given interval (in this case one cardiac cycle), the volume of flow through the left ventricular outflow tract (LVOT) must equal the volume of flow through the aortic valve. To determine the volume of flow through the LVOT in one cardiac cycle, the area of the LVOT (ALVOT), as measured by planimetry in the parasternal short-axis view, is multiplied by the peak blood flow velocity in the LVOT (VLVOT) obtained using pulsed-wave Doppler with the sample volume in the LVOT from the apical window. Blood flow velocity in aortic stenosis (VAO) can be assessed and aortic valve area calculated as follows:

$$(\text{ALVOT} \times \text{VLVOT}) - \text{VAO} = \text{AVA}$$

With experience, the procedure can be performed faster and is technically easier. To make the formula as accurate as possible, the values for LVOT area, LVOT velocity profile, and aortic velocity profile should be derived by averaging at least three

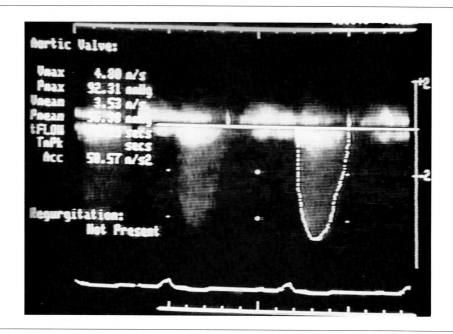

FIGURE 10-9. By tracing the profile, the ultrasound unit calculates the peak velocity at 4.8 m per second, the peak gradient at 92.31 mm Hg, and the mean gradient at 56.38 mm Hg.

measurements of each parameter. Averaging data from 10 beats is the best method to use when arrhythmias vary the profiles.

Another technique for calculating aortic valve area uses the same premise as the catheter laboratory equations.[3] The cardiac output is determined by means of an electrical bioimpedance study (noninvasive method for assessing cardiac output based on beat-to-beat variations in the body's electrical impedance). The mean gradient from the Doppler study and the data from the bioimpedance study are plugged into Gorlin's equation.

COLOR-FLOW ASSESSMENT OF AORTIC STENOSIS. Color-flow Doppler mapping can help align the Doppler beam parallel to the flow of the jet in the stenotic aorta valve. The transducer is then in the best position to obtain the peak velocity.

*Discussion.* Aortic stenosis (AS) can be the most difficult lesion for the echocardiographer to assess. Because cardiac catheterization is risky, expensive, and uncomfortable for the patient it is not a good procedure for ongoing evaluation of the valve.

Echocardiography can provide the physician with all the information necessary to decide if the patient must go to the catheter laboratory or surgery.

### AORTIC INSUFFICIENCY

Aortic insufficiency (AI) is leaking of blood back into the left ventricle during diastole. The regurgitation may be secondary to abnormal aortic cusps or dilatation of the aortic root or ascending aorta.

*Causes.* A common cause of chronic AI is rheumatic fever, which causes the cusps to become thickened, fibrotic, and shrunken. Because the leaflets no longer meet there is an opening in the center of the closed valve. Infective endocarditis may destroy or fenestrate (perforate) a cusp, causing it to leak, or a vegetation could interfere with normal closure, preventing the cusps from sealing. Trauma to the chest wall can tear a wall of the ascending aorta (aortic dissection) where it provides support for the aortic cusps, resulting in aortic valve prolapse and aortic insufficiency.

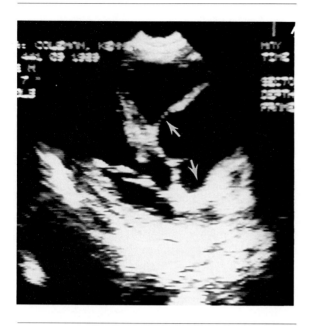

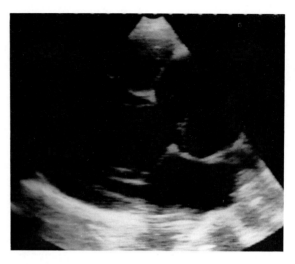

FIGURE 10-11. The ascending aorta is dilated to 6 cm in diameter immediately distal to the aortic annulus in this patient with Marfan's syndrome.

FIGURE 10-10. The arrows show the bulging of the dilated sinuses of Valsalva.

The most common cause of aortic regurgitation is aortic root dilatation, generally secondary to atherosclerotic disruption of the aorta or to the long-term effects of hypertension, or both (Fig. 10-10). Aortic root dilatation separates the aortic cusps so they do not coapt during diastole. Connective tissue diseases such as Marfan's syndrome commonly cause ascending aortic dilatation, as do inflammatory processes such as syphilitic aortitis (Fig. 10-11). Another common cause of ascending aortic dilatation and aneurysm is cystic medionecrosis.

*Symptoms.* Chronic AI is tolerated well, often not manifesting clinical symptoms until the fourth or fifth decade of life. The symptoms of left ventricular dysfunction may not occur for years after that. The first symptom of severe AI is exertional dyspnea, and when the heart rate slows with rest, angina (usually nocturnal) and diaphoresis develop, because of the very low diastolic pressure.

Patients may complain of an uncomfortable feeling of the heart beating (mostly when lying down) and chest pain from the heart pounding against the chest wall. Tachycardia from exertion or emotional stress may induce heart palpitations and head throbbing. Premature ventricular contractions cause alarm when postpremature beats eject a large amount of blood from the volume-overloaded left ventricle.

Acute aortic regurgitation presents as severe dyspnea, tachypnea, and orthopnea. The patient is usually weak and hypotensive. Angina is not a common complaint unless trauma is responsible for aortic dissection which is causing acute AI.

*Pathophysiology.* Chronic AI causes left ventricular dilatation, which accommodates the volume overload, and hyperdynamic function, which maintains normal effective forward stroke volume and ejection fraction. These ventricular end-diastolic volumes are the greatest of any form of heart disease, and evaluation of end-systolic volume is a sensitive index of contractility.

The left ventricular mass is greatly increased, often more than is seen in isolated aortic stenosis. With AS comes cardiac muscle hypertrophy, but the left ventricle chamber size remains normal or decreases. With AI the left ventricular cavity is so large that the muscle mass increase is not evident. This increased left ventricular mass allows the ventricle to compensate for the volume overload with little increase in filling pressures.

As the left ventricle decompensates, the aortic regurgitant volume remains the same but the left ventricular end-diastolic volume increases. The ejection fraction and stroke volume decrease; left ventricular emptying is impaired and end-systolic volume increases. Often, these changes occur before the patient reports any symptoms. The pressure elevation "backs up" into the left atrium, pulmonary veins, pulmonary capillaries, pulmonary artery, right ventricle, and right atrium. These pressures reduce the effective cardiac output with exercise—and eventually also at rest.

Acute AI does not allow the left ventricle time to adjust to the abrupt volume overload. Stroke volume cannot increase quickly enough, so left ventricular diastolic pressure rises rapidly to high levels and the left ventricle becomes less compliant. This high left ventricular pressure increases above left atrial pressure in early diastole so that the mitral valve closes early and protects the pulmonary venous bed. If the mitral valve fails to close completely, middiastolic mitral regurgitation develops. For the same degree of chronic regurgitation, the acute AI patient exhibits a lower effective forward output, a smaller left ventricular volume, and a faster heart rate.

*Physical Examination.* The characteristics of a bounding pulse are hallmarks of severe AI: waterhammer pulse, head bobbing, capillary pulsations, to name a few. Checking the blood pressure confirms a wide pulse pressure with systolic pressures elevated and diastolic pressures abnormally low (less than 50 mm Hg). This is due to the rapid pressure drop from the regurgitant blood flow into the left ventricle. Diastolic pressure can be difficult to determine as the pulse (Korotkoff sounds) can be heard at 0 mm Hg. A change in the pulse, a muffling, correlates with diastole and represents the diastolic blood pressure. As the heart begins to fail the arterial pulse pressure may rise owing to vasoconstriction. The apical impulse is displaced laterally and inferiorly, often with a palpable rapid ventricular filling wave. A systolic thrill may be felt at the base of the heart, at the suprasternal notch,

and in the carotids. A soft, high-frequency, diastolic, decrescendo murmur can usually be heard during auscultation. The murmur is best heard with the stethoscope at the apex when the patient is sitting up, leaning forward, and holding an expiration. An Austin Flint murmur (a middiastolic rumble) may also be heard, which is attributed to the AI jet hitting the mitral leaflets. Often the first heart sound $(S_1)$ is decreased in loudness or is absent.

With acute aortic regurgitation, auscultation still finds a diastolic murmur, but one shorter and lower pitched than that of chronic aortic regurgitation. The first heart sound may be soft or absent. A loud $P_2$ can be heard with pulmonary hypertension and often third and fourth heart sounds are present. Austin Flint murmurs, if audible, are short.

*Electrocardiography.* The electrocardiogram shows evidence for left ventricular diastolic volume overload in chronic aortic regurgitation. These signs eventually subside, but total QRS amplitude remains increased. T waves are usually inverted with ST-segment depression, but early in the course of the disease they may be tall and upright in the left precordial leads. Left ventricular dysfunction can cause intraventricular conduction defects. A prolonged PR interval suggests an inflammatory process causing the aortic insufficiency.

Acute aortic regurgitation commonly displays a nonspecific ST segment and T-wave changes. Signs of left ventricular hypertrophy may be present regardless of left ventricular failure.

*Echocardiographic Features.* The hallmark of chronic aortic insufficiency by M-mode echocardiography is the fluttering of the anterior, and occasionally posterior, mitral leaflet during diastole. If the regurgitant jet strikes the interventricular septum, diastolic fluttering can be seen involving this wall. If eccentric jets do not strike any surface the AI cannot be diagnosed. The left ventricular diastolic dimension increases, but the systolic dimension remains normal as long as the ventricle can compensate for the volume overload (hyperdynamic function). As the ventricle decompensates the hyperdynamic function decreases and the systolic dimension increases. At this point the patient must be followed closely. If valve replacement is delayed too long, left ventricular function may not improve significantly after surgery. Assessing left ventricular size and function by M-mode echocardiography was difficult because of technical limitations. The use of 2-D echocardiography has overcome these problems and has proved to be a reliable method for evaluating the left ventricle.

The echocardiographic findings for AI due to rheumatic processes may be difficult to assess if mitral stenosis is present. A thickened mitral valve leaflet may not demonstrate fine fluttering from the AI jet. M-mode echocardiographic findings of aortic insufficiency due to poor support for the cusps, such as connective tissue disease and aortic root dissections or aneurysms, may also demonstrate dilatation of the aortic root and intimal flaps of tissue in the aortic root from the dissection. It is important to image the pulmonic valve, to determine whether pulmonary hypertension is present.

Acute AI by M-mode echocardiography can show early closure of the mitral valve. The size and function of the ventricle can appear normal, as it cannot respond to the abrupt volume overload. If the acute AI is due to infective endocarditis, the vegetation, a "shaggy, echogenic mass," attached to an aortic cusp, may be seen in the LVOT during diastole and in the aortic root during systole. A ruptured valve may have the same appearance, so that entity should be included in the differential diagnosis. Nonmobile vegetations cannot be differentiated from focal aortic valve thickening.

Traumatic aortic root dissection, which causes acute AI, shows the characteristic double echoes of the aortic root walls. The dissection can bleed into the pericardial sac, causing a pericardial effusion, and even tamponade.

Two-dimensional echocardiography provides more detailed information about the hemodynamics and causes of chronic aortic insufficiency. The strong jets in aortic insufficiency can strike the anterior mitral leaflet, limiting its opening and interfering with ventricular filling. The parasternal short-axis view of the mitral valve can show the reduced leaflet excursion. Repeated pounding by the AI jet can form pockets in the ventricular walls that may also be visualized by 2-D echocardiography. Left ventricular size and function can be assessed more accurately with 2-D than with M-mode technique. Exercise echocardiography can evaluate

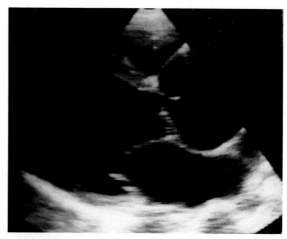

Figure 10-12

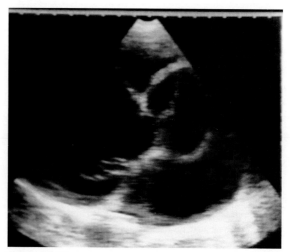

Figure 10-13

Figure 10-12. Prolapse of the noncoronary cusp in a patient with Marfan's syndrome.

Figure 10-13. The echo extending from the center of the aorta at the annulus up to the anterior aortic root wall is the flap of tissue involved in the dissection.

the effects of exercise on the left ventricle. Aortic valve prolapse is visualized readily, whether it is due to connective tissue disease or associated with ventricular septal defects (Fig. 10-12).

Aortic root dissections are nicely demonstrated by 2-D echocardiography (Fig. 10-13). The dissec-

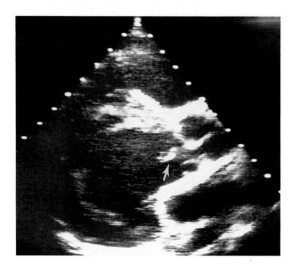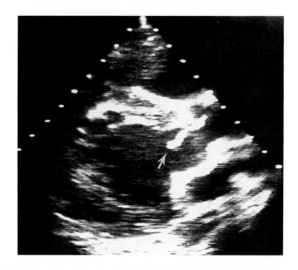

FIGURE 10-14. These echoes from the same patient demonstrate the vegetation (*arrow*) in the left ventricular outflow tract.

tion can be followed to the aortic arch and then down the descending thoracic aorta. Visualization of the ascending aorta can be achieved from either the left sternal border with the patient resting on the left side or the right sternal border with the patient resting on the right side. The suprasternal notch view allows for evaluation of the ascending aorta, aortic arch, and descending aorta. Apical views can record the descending aorta positioned posterior to the left atrium and left ventricle, whereas subcostal views can visualize the abdominal aorta.

Two-dimensional echocardiography demonstrates acute aortic regurgitation caused by infective endocarditis (Fig. 10-14) better than it does acute aortic regurgitation caused by aortic root dissection. Pericardial effusion caused by an aortic dissection can also be evaluated. Currently a ruptured aortic cusp cannot be differentiated from an aortic valve vegetation.

*Chest Radiography.* Chest radiographs in chronic aortic regurgitation usually show an enlarged cardiac silhouette, with enlargement directed caudad and to the left. Sometimes there is little change in the transverse heart diameter. Severe aneurysmal dilatation of the ascending aorta, possibly involving the aortic arch, suggests as a cause Marfan's syndrome, cystic medial necrosis, or other connective tissue disorders. If the walls of the ascending aorta display linear calcification, the diagnosis is probably syphilitic aortitis or a degenerative disease.

In acute aortic regurgitation left ventricular size may be normal or moderately increased on chest radiographs and pulmonary venous patterns may be redistributed to the upper lobes; pulmonary edema may also be noted. In severe chronic aortic regurgitation, resting and exercise nuclear ventriculograms are used to evaluate left ventricular function and end-systolic and end-diastolic volume.

Cardiac catheterization for aortography assesses aortic regurgitation. Dye is injected rapidly into the aorta, and regurgitant blood flow is rated in one of four grades:

1+ (mild regurgitation): A puff of dye is seen below the valve.

2+ (moderate regurgitation): The left ventricular cavity is faintly outlined.

3+ (moderately severe regurgitation): Dye is distributed equally between the aortic root and left ventricle and fills the left ventricle.

4+ (severe regurgitation): Dye immediately opacifies the left ventricular cavity but little remains in the aortic root.

*Incidence, Prognosis, and Treatment.* The incidence of aortic regurgitation is difficult to assess owing to its many causes. As a cause of AI, aortic root diseases (the incidence of which has been increasing) account for at least one third.[9] At the Oklahoma Medical Center, 12 to 16% of all echocardiograms and Doppler studies show some degree of aortic insufficiency, though many of these are mild cases. The prognosis for chronic aortic regurgitation is good. Symptoms usually develop in the fourth or fifth decade of life. Even after the diagnosis is made, of patients with severe or moderately severe chronic AI who do not receive medical treatment 75% will survive 5 years and 50%, 10 years. After symptoms appear, the patient's condition deteriorates rapidly. Patients usually die within about 4 years after angina develops if the valve is not replaced. Once ventricular failure begins the patient may survive 2 years without surgical intervention.

Acute aortic regurgitation carries a very poor prognosis if it is managed medically. Surgical intervention after a short period of stabilizing management usually results in a normal recovery. Even in the presence of active bacterial endocarditis, valve replacement is recommended if decompensation has begun.

Medical management of chronic AI—even if it is severe—is recommended for as long as the patient is without symptoms and has good left ventricular function and good exercise tolerance. For mild or moderate AI, prophylaxis for bacterial endocarditis is the only treatment necessary. Different causes suggest different drug therapies (e.g., a full course of penicillin for aortitis). Severe AI with left ventricular dilatation requires the addition of an inotropic agent (to increase contractility), salt restriction, and diuretics if the patient is in heart failure. Patients with evidence of heart failure should avoid vigorous or heavy exercise, even if they have no symptoms. Yearly follow-up tests are recommended to monitor left ventricular function and severity of the AI until the AI becomes severe, at which time semiannual evaluations are indicated.

It is most important that surgical intervention be undertaken before irreversible left ventricular dysfunction occurs. Left ventricular end-systolic volume is a particularly sensitive measure for monitoring this change. As long as the left ventricular end-systolic volume is normal (30 ml/m$^2$) the patient's chances of full recovery are excellent. If, however, the end-systolic volume is increased (90 ml/m$^2$) recovery is poor. When volume is between 30 and 90 ml/m$^2$ results vary.

Medical management is not recommended for acute aortic regurgitation. Death due to left ventricular failure is common if surgical intervention is delayed. Until the valve can be replaced, management with bed rest, diuretics, and reduction of systemic resistance (afterload) can help stabilize the patient.

*Doppler Studies.* Doppler technique has increased the sensitivity of echocardiography for diagnosing AI and has provided methods for assessing its severity.

Pulsed-wave Doppler differentiates diastolic aliasing signal by timing. An AI jet starts immediately on aortic valve closure and ends with aortic opening. The mitral flow velocity signal does not start until the end of isovolumic relaxation. The severity of AI can be assessed by mapping the area occupied by the aortic insufficiency jet. Then, using the parasternal long-axis or apical four- or five-chamber views, the sample volume is placed at the aortic valve on the ventricular side (Fig. 10-15). A signal mapped only in the LVOT is mild (1+). If it extends to the tips of the anterior mitral leaflet it is moderate (2+). AI beyond the tips of the mitral valve leaflets is considered severe: jets extending to the apex rate 4+ and jets extending up to half the distance from the tips of the leaflets to the apex rate 3+.

Another technique requires recording the flow velocities in the ascending aorta. Systolic aortic flow should be recorded above the baseline and the diastolic or regurgitant flow recorded below the

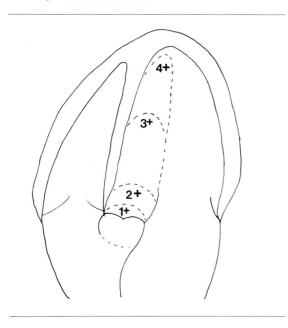

FIGURE 10-15. This apical five-chamber diagram shows the grading system used to assess the severity of aortic insufficiency by mapping with pulsed-wave Doppler.

baseline. A ratio of these two flow areas suggests the degree of aortic insufficiency. Some reverse flow in early diastole is normal, so regurgitation should be sustained throughout diastole before aortic insufficiency is diagnosed. This ratio cannot be used if aortic stenosis exists or when low-velocity signals are buried in baseline noise.

Continuous-wave Doppler studies provide another means of assessing the severity of aortic regurgitation. Just as mitral stenosis can be evaluated by the pressure half-time method, so also can AI.[10] From a clean profile the peak velocity and the slope of the decay are determined (Fig. 10-16). In the presence of arrhythmias, longer diastolic periods yield more accurate data. These numbers are plugged into an equation:

$$\frac{V_{max}}{slope} \times 0.293 = \text{Pressure half-time in seconds}$$

where $V_{max}$ is the maximum velocity obtained from the AI profile, and the slope is the rate of decay of the AI profile throughout diastole. The 0.4-second point was designated as the cutoff point between significant AI pressure half-times (<0.4 seconds;

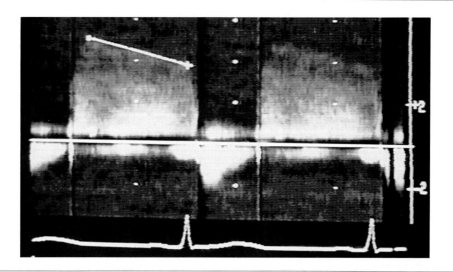

FIGURE 10-16. After a clear profile is obtained, the cursors are placed to determine peak velocity and the slope. The slow rate of decay indicates that this profile is from mild aortic insufficiency.

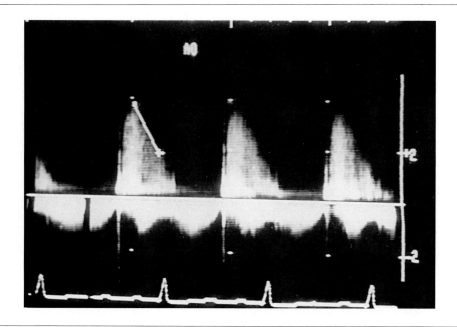

FIGURE 10-17. The steep slope, or rapid decay, of this aortic insufficiency flow profile demonstrates a severe lesion.

3+ and 4+); (Fig. 10-17) and mild aortic insufficiency pressure half-time ($\geq 0.4$ seconds; 1+ and 2+).

This simple range is very specific for AI. If left ventricular end-diastolic pressure is elevated, this method can overrate aortic insufficiency by one grade, as compared to results of aortography.

Again, as in evaluating aortic stenosis, a good AI profile must be obtained. No attempt should be made to measure pressure half-time if the peak velocity is not at least 4 m per second. The only exception is the well-defined velocity profile that while below 4 m per second is at least 3 m per second. As the pressure in the left ventricle rises very high and "backs up" through the left atrium, pulmonary veins, pulmonary capillaries, pulmonary artery, right ventricle, and right atrium, it is important to try to assess peak right ventricular systolic pressure. This is accomplished by determining peak tricuspid regurgitation velocity and calculating the pressure ($4V^2 + 13$).

Color-flow Doppler echocardiography can assess the severity of AI by determining the area of the left ventricle that is occupied by mosaic (aliased) signals. This is particularly useful when an adequate continuous-wave Doppler signal cannot be obtained, and the technique is much less time consuming than pulsed-wave Doppler mappings.

*Discussion.* Once AI is diagnosed, the patient must be followed to determine the optimal time for replacing the valve. Serial echocardiograms with Doppler, exercise nuclear ventriculograms or stress echocardiograms, and careful medical treatment and evaluation by the physician will ensure the best results.

## Pulmonary Valve

The pulmonary valve is a three-leaflet valve that allows blood to flow from the right ventricle into the pulmonary artery. At the beginning of systole, when the right ventricular pressure becomes higher than the pulmonary artery pressure, the valve opens; when pulmonary artery pressure rises above right ventricular pressure at the end of systole, the

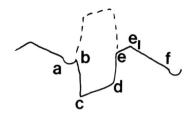

FIGURE 10-18. A normal M-mode diagram of a pulmonary valve shows the a wave and a dotted line indicating the motion of a seldom-seen leaflet.

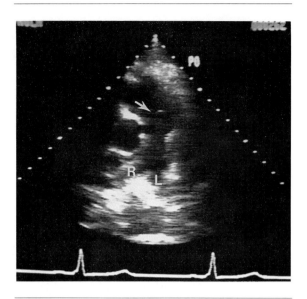

FIGURE 10-19. A nicely demonstrated bifurcation of the main pulmonary artery and one of the pulmonic leaflets (arrow). (PO, pulmonary outflow; R, right pulmonary artery; L, left pulmonary artery.)

valve closes. The pressures in the right ventricle and pulmonary artery are low—so low, that the transmitted pressure wave generated by the P wave to reopen the tricuspid valve (atrial kick) is reflected in the valve motion as a bulge called an A wave (Fig. 10-18). This presystolic wave plays an important role in echocardiography.

On M-mode echocardiography the pulmonic valve is usually a single line, the motion of which is determined by the pressures surrounding it. The A wave of the pulmonic valve is usually 3 to 5 mm deep. The valve is opened for systole b to e, and closed from e to f (Fig. 10-18).

Two-dimensional echocardiography routinely shows two pulmonic cusps, which are best seen in the parasternal short-axis view at the level of the aortic root. The cusps open to the extent of the pulmonary artery walls during systole and are closed throughout diastole. The presystolic wave is not seen.

Often the pulmonary artery can be seen, including its bifurcation into the left and right pulmonary arteries (Fig. 10-19). With the transducer in the parasternal short-axis view, the transducer is simply rotated a little clockwise and the probe is directed laterally or posteriorly. Sometimes the transducer must be moved more cephalad and then directed laterally or posteriorly. Patients with lung disease and athletes who routinely hyperinflate their lungs are difficult to examine, and usually it is impossible to image their pulmonary artery.

The Doppler flow profile from the pulmonic valve is recorded from the left lateral position with the transducer angled as when imaging the pulmonic valve; then fine tune the transducer angu-

lation until the peak velocity is obtained. Pulmonic flow is away from the transducer during systole and there is little or no noise on the opposite side of the baseline (Fig. 10-20). Pulmonic flow velocity peaks in midsystole (average 0.8 m per second). Blood flow velocity through the valve is slow enough that either pulsed- or continuous-wave Doppler can record a complete profile.

### PULMONIC VALVE STENOSIS

*Causes.* Most pulmonic stenosis is congenital (see Part 5). Causes of acquired disease include rheumatic and carcinoid processes, but these are rare. Rheumatic inflammation of the pulmonic valve is generally seen when other valves are affected and usually causes little deformity of the valve. Occasionally, carcinoid plaques constrict the pulmonic annulus and cause shrinking and fusion of the cusps. The result is pulmonic insufficiency. Cardiac tumors and aneurysms of the sinus of Valsalva can encroach into the area of the pulmonic valve, causing obstruction. Hypertrophic cardiomyopathies causing septal hypertrophy can obstruct the RVOT just as the same process can obstruct the LVOT.

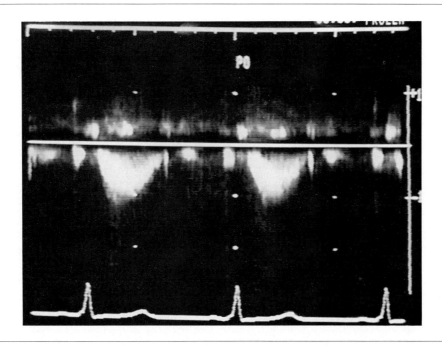

FIGURE 10-20. Notice the pulmonic flow profile peaks in midsystole and is marked by a valve click at the valve closure.

*Pulmonic Insufficiency.* Pulmonic insufficiency is commonly due to ring dilatation from pulmonary hypertension. Pulmonary artery dilatation also is common, whether idiopathic or secondary to connective tissue disease such as Marfan's syndrome. The second most common cause of pulmonic regurgitation is infective endocarditis, which can be due to surgical intervention for pulmonic stenosis or repair of tetralogy of Fallot. Rarely it is caused by chest trauma, syphilis, or placement of a catheter through the pulmonic valve.

*Symptoms.* Pulmonic regurgitation (PR) causes few problems, and symptoms do not develop until very late in the disease. If pulmonary hypertension is associated, right-sided heart failure develops. If the PR is due to pulmonic valve endocarditis, one complication can be septic embolization resulting in severe right-sided heart failure. Tricuspid valve vegetations may be the source of vegetations to the pulmonic valve or of septic emboli to the pulmonary beds (septic pulmonary embolization). Symp-

toms of right-sided heart failure are dyspnea on exertion and fluid retention. The dyspnea on exertion is caused by pulmonary hypertension; the fluid retention is manifested as ascites and peripheral or sacral edema.

*Pathophysiology.* Pulmonic regurgitation is usually not severe enough to cause significant hemodynamic changes. Pulmonic regurgitation caused by pulmonary hypertension results in right-sided heart failure. The constant pressure overload is tolerated by muscle hypertrophy until the ventricle begins to fail. Poor right-sided cardiac flow results in poor left-sided cardiac output (Starling's law, see Chapter 3). The body begins to retain fluid and sodium, which consequently boosts intravascular volume. There are also signs of increased central venous pressure, hepatomegaly, and hepatojugular reflux.

Septic pulmonary embolization does not cause right ventricular hypertrophy, as this process is more acute, but it does cause severe right ventricular failure, which then progresses through the same physiologic changes as if it were caused by pulmonary hypertension.

*Diagnosis.* The diagnosis of pulmonary insufficiency is usually incidental to the more dominant problems of right ventricular failure. The physical examination reveals signs of right ventricular volume overload. The right ventricle is hyperdynamic, so it can be felt along the left sternal border. Additionally, an enlarged pulmonary artery can be palpated in the second intercostal space. Pulmonic valve closure can be felt with pulmonary hypertension and pulmonic regurgitation.

Pulmonic regurgitation produces a low-pitched diastolic murmur heard best at the third and fourth intercostal spaces next to the sternum. The murmur starts after $P_2$ (pulmonic component of second heart sound) and peaks and diminishes before $S_1$ (the first sound). The murmur is louder with inspiration. Should the pulmonic regurgitation be secondary to pulmonary hypertension with systolic pressures higher than 70 mm Hg, Graham Steell's murmur can be heard. This murmur is high pitched and blowing, starting with $P_2$. It can be mistaken for the murmur of aortic insufficiency. A right-sided Austin Flint murmur can sometimes be heard, the low-frequency presystolic sounds originating from the tricuspid valve.

The electrocardiogram for pulmonic insufficiency shows configurations of right ventricular diastolic overload. If pulmonary hypertension is the cause of the PR, signs of right ventricular hypertrophy are evident.

Chest radiographs usually show an enlarged pulmonary artery and right ventricle. There may be evidence of pleural and pericardial effusions. Right-sided heart catheterization with injection of contrast into the main pulmonary artery detects pulmonic insufficiency. Simultaneous pressure recordings of the pulmonary artery and the right ventricle during mid- to late diastole can support the diagnosis.

Laboratory tests show evidence of right-sided heart failure with abnormal liver function. The results show a two- to ten-fold increase in transaminase levels (serum glutamic-oxaloacetic transaminase and serum glutamic-pyruvic transaminase),

elevated bilirubin, and prolonged prothrombin time. Signs of decreased renal perfusion yield low urinary sodium (<20 mEq/L) and two to three times the normal range for blood urea nitrogen.

Isolated pulmonic regurgitation is an insignificant finding that does not require treatment. Once right-sided heart failure develops from pulmonary hypertension it is treated, usually with cardiac glycosides to improve contractility. The cause of the pulmonary hypertension should also be addressed; if septic embolization is the cause, the infective endocarditis is treated. Surgical replacement of the valve is not common, but it may help improve symptoms of right heart failure.

*Echocardiographic Features.* The echocardiographic feature of pulmonic stenosis is an increased a wave of 7 to 10 mm. The transmitted pressure wave causing the presystolic bulge of the valve is amplified by the increased right ventricular pressure needed to open the stenotic valve. Thickening of the valve from rheumatic inflammation may be visualized.

Doppler imaging of the valve shows increased peak systolic velocity. Use of continuous-wave Doppler technique disposes of the problem of aliasing that may occur with pulsed-wave technique. Bernoulli's equation (pressure gradient = $4V^2$) provides the peak gradient across the valve.

Narrowing of the main pulmonary artery can be differentiated from pulmonic stenosis by placing the pulsed-wave sample volume gradually farther inside the pulmonary artery and then through the valve. Continuous-wave Doppler examination can then determine the degree of obstruction caused by narrowing.

Pulsed- or continuous-wave Doppler technique can record and assess RVOT obstruction. Infundibular pulmonic stenosis occurs in this same area (see Part 5).

Pulmonic insufficiency is recorded on Doppler studies as turbulent flow toward the probe during diastole, usually at a speed of less than 2 m per second. High velocities—on the order of 3 to 4 m per second—denote pulmonary hypertension (Fig. 10-21). No attempts have been made to assess the severity of pulmonic insufficiency.

Pulmonic insufficiency due to pulmonary hypertension is not determined by echocardiography,

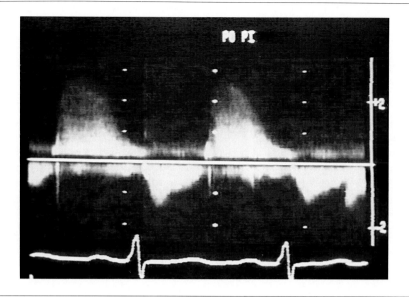

Figure 10-21. The pulmonic insufficiency profile seen here reaches a peak velocity close to 4 m per second, indicating coexisting pulmonary hypertension. (PO, pulmonary outflow; PI, pulmonary insufficiency.)

but signs of pulmonary hypertension can be diagnosed. M-mode recording of the posterior pulmonic cusp shows a flat or diminished a wave (<3 mm) and notching during systole. The increased pulmonary artery pressure reduces the presystolic bulge. The reason for the notching is not known. Two-dimensional echocardiography can visualize the systolic notching of the valve as well as the dilated pulmonary artery and enlarged right ventricle, and can evaluate right ventricular function. Right atrium size can be assessed and right ventricular compliance evaluated from the inferior vena cava. As seen from the subcostal view the inferior vena cava dilates in response to the increased pressure overload. During inspiration, the inferior vena cava narrows to half its normal size, but if right ventricular compliance is reduced, the size of the inferior vena cava does not change significantly.

Pulmonic insufficiency secondary to infective endocarditis may show the vegetations on the cusps as a shaggy mass by echocardiography. Doppler recordings of the pulmonic flow with pulmonary hypertension can show early peaking during systole. If peak tricuspid regurgitation velocities are obtained, peak right ventricular systolic pressure can be assessed.

## Acknowledgment

The author would like to thank Stephen M. Teague, M.D. for all of his help with and his critiques of this chapter. The research he has done in the area of aortic valve disease provided a rich resource from which to work.

## References

1. Braunwald E. Valvular heart disease. In: Braunwald E, ed. Heart Disease: A Textbook of Cardiovascular Medicine. Philadelphia: WB Saunders; 1980.
2. Chang A, Clements C. Aortic stenosis: Echocardiographic cusp separation and surgical description of aortic valve in 22 patients. Am J Cardiol. 1975; 39:499–504.
3. DeMaria AN, Bommer W, Joy J, et al. Value and limitations of cross-sectional echocardiography of the

aortic valve in the diagnosis and quantification of valvular aortic stenosis. Circulation. 1980; 62:304-312.

4. Feigenbaum H. Acquired valvular heart disease. In: Feigenbaum H. Echocardiography. 4th ed. Philadelphia: Lea & Febiger; 1986.

5. Goli V, Teague S, Prasad R, et al. Noninvasive evaluation of aortic stenosis severity utilizing Doppler ultrasound and electrical bioimpedance. J Am Coll Cardiol. 1988; 11:66-71.

6. Gooch AS, Calatagud JB, Rogers PA, et al. Analysis of the P wave in severe aortic stenosis. Dis Chest. 1966; 49:459.

7. Gorlin R, Gorlin S. Hydraulic formula for calculation of the area of the stenotic mitral valve, other cardiac valves, and central circulatory shunts. Am Heart J. 1951; 41:1-29.

8. Hakki AH, Kimbivis D, Iskandrian AS, et al. Angina pectoris and coronary artery disease in patients with severe aortic valvular disease. Am Heart J. 1980; 100:441.

9. Isner J, Salem D, Desnoyers M, et al. Dual balloon technique for valvuloplasty of aortic stenosis in adults. Am J Cardiol. 1988; 61:583-589.

10. Lewis JF, Kuo L, Nelson LG, et al. Pulsed Doppler echocardiographic determination of stroke volume and cardiac output: Clinical validation of two new methods using the apical window. Circulation. 1984; 70:425-431.

11. Olson LJ, Subramanian R, Edwards WD. Surgical pathology of pure aortic insufficiency: A study of 225 cases. Mayo Clin Proc. 1984; 59:835.

12. Teague S, Heinsemer J, Anderson J, et al. Quantification of aortic regurgitation utilizing continuous-wave Doppler ultrasound. J Am Coll Cardiol. 1986; 8:592-599.

13. Weyman AE, Feigenbaum H, Delton JC, et al. Cross-sectional echocardiography in assessing the severity of valvular aortic stenosis. Circulation. 1975; 52:828-834.

CHAPTER **11**

# Cardiomyopathies

JOHN C. POPE

Primary cardiomyopathy is a disease of the cardiac muscle of unknown cause. There are three distinct classes of cardiomyopathy—hypertrophic, dilated (congestive), and restrictive (infiltrative). Secondary cardiomyopathies—other diseases that affect the myocardium in a similar manner—are caused by viruses, ischemia, metabolic abnormalities, endocrinopathies, hypertension, and toxic reactions. In this chapter I describe the subjective and objective findings of patients with cardiomyopathies and review the echocardiographic criteria for establishing the diagnosis.

## Hypertrophic Cardiomyopathy

Hypertrophic cardiomyopathy (HCM) is a condition characterized by disproportionate hypertrophy of the left ventricle, and occasionally also of the right ventricle, which typically involves the interventricular septum more often than the left ventricular free wall but occasionally the left ventricular hypertrophy is concentric. Typically, the size and volume of the left ventricle are normal or reduced. Systolic pressure gradients across the left ventricular outflow tract (LVOT) are common. HCM is transmitted by an autosomal dominant gene with incomplete penetrance. Characteristic morphologic changes (e.g., muscle fiber disarray) usually are most severe in the interventricular septum.[4]

### CLINICAL PRESENTATION

The three major symptoms of HCM are dyspnea, angina, and syncope.[31] Symptoms usually develop in the second or third decade of life. Approximately 90% of patients with HCM experience dyspnea, but it is poorly correlated with the underlying dynamic outflow tract gradient. A proposed pathophysiologic mechanism for dyspnea is elevated left ventricular end-diastolic filling pressure and subsequent alteration of the volume-pressure relationship in that chamber. This increases left atrial pressure, which is transmitted to the pulmonary venous system, where it precipitates dyspnea.

Approximately 70% of HCM patients experience angina,[55] but only 25% of patients with HCM over 45 years of age have evidence of significant coronary artery disease on coronary arteriography.[55] The remainder of patients experience angina even though their extramural coronary arteries are normal. The pathophysiologic alterations proposed for producing angina are small-vessel coronary artery narrowing, intramyocardial compression of small arteries by the massive muscle hypertrophy, and abnormal diastolic filling dynamics resulting in an imbalance between oxygen supply and demand.[59]

Presyncope or syncope occurs in approximately 50% of patients with HCM.[54] The most common cause of such syncope is cardiac arrhythmias, which have been documented through Holter monitor recordings. Ventricular tachycardia has been seen in

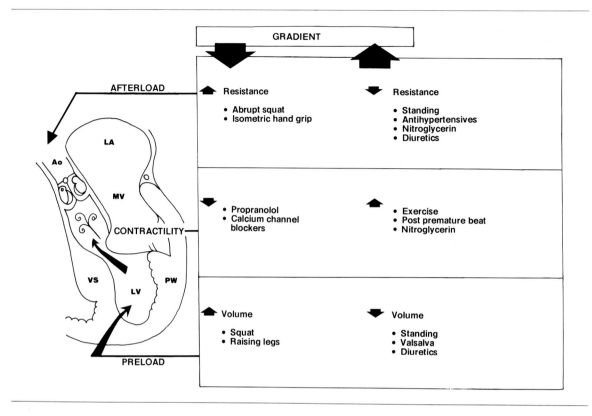

FIGURE 11-1. Various maneuvers and interventions that alter LVOT gradient. (LA, left atrium; Ao, aorta; MV, mitral valve; VS, ventricular septum; LV, left ventricle; PW, posterior wall.) (By permission of the American Society of Echocardiography.)

as many as 40% of these patients.[29] Congestive heart failure occurs in less than 10% of patients with HCM.

The physical examination findings in patients with HCM should be completely normal if there is no underlying outflow tract gradient. In contrast, physical findings are variable if a systolic gradient is present across the LVOT. Classic physical findings in patients with HCM and an LVOT gradient include a brisk carotid upstroke with a bifid contour (pulsus bisferiens) in a large majority of patients. This is related to exaggerated early systolic contraction and rapid early emptying of the left ventricle followed by midsystolic premature closure of the aortic valve that coincides with the systolic anterior motion of the mitral valve. The presence of a bifid pulse contour with a brisk upstroke is helpful in differentiating aortic stenosis in which there is a slow rate of rise of the carotid upstroke and a decrease in the amplitude of the carotid pulsation. On palpation, the apical impulse is usually prominent because of significant left ventricular hypertrophy. A presystolic apical impulse (palpable $S_4$) is common, whereas a pathognomonic "trident," or triple, impulse is noted in a small number of patients.

Provocations that decrease the left ventricular volume and reduce the outflow tract diameter, such as Valsalva's maneuver, amyl nitrite inhalation, and sudden assumption of an upright position, increase the subaortic gradient and thus increase the intensity of the heart murmur (Fig. 11-1). In contrast, maneuvers that increase left ventricular volume, such as sudden squatting, leg raising in a supine position, or phenylephrine infusion, decrease the subaortic gradient and produce a low-intensity murmur. It should be noted that the only other cardiac abnormality that responds similarly to these maneuvers is mitral valve prolapse, but this should be distinguishable by the presence of a nonejection systolic click and by the location and quality of the murmur.

In the majority of patients with HCM the electrocardiogram (ECG) is abnormal.[48] The most common resting ECG abnormalities are left ventricular hypertrophy, left atrial enlargement, and prominent Q waves in the inferior and lateral leads, which may simulate myocardial infarction.[48] Twenty-four–hour Holter monitor recordings have shown a high incidence of supraventricular arrhythmias (50%), multiform premature ventricular contractions (45%), and ventricular tachycardia (40%). Atrial fibrillation is also seen in a minority of patients. It may be associated with patients' clinical deterioration because of the loss of the atrial contribution to cardiac output. The patient's chest radiograph may be completely normal, but if it is abnormal, it usually displays mild to moderate enlargement of the cardiac silhouette. The left atrium is also enlarged (Fig. 11-2).

### ECHOCARDIOGRAPHIC FEATURES

Patients with HCM demonstrate three hallmarks of the disease: (1) asymmetric septal hypertrophy (ASH), (2) disorganization of septal myocardial cells, and (3) systolic anterior motion (SAM) of the mitral valve apparatus.[32] Figure 11-3 is an anatomic drawing that corresponds to a two-dimensional (2-D) echocardiographic parasternal long-axis view in a patient with an HCM. Note the significant abnormal thickness of the interventricular septum. In addition, the posterior wall of the ventricle is thickened and the papillary muscle is prominent. Note also that the LVOT is narrowed.

Normally, the anterior and posterior mitral valve leaflets remain together during systole and do not impinge on the interventricular septum. Figure 11-4 demonstrates SAM of the mitral valve. Note that the patient has evidence of ASH with a small left ventricular cavity. The mitral valve apparatus is noted to coapt with the interventricular septum. Figure 11-5 is an M-mode echocardiogram through the area of SAM of the mitral valve demonstrated on the 2-D examination. This shows evidence of SAM of the anterior mitral valve leaflet. Note that

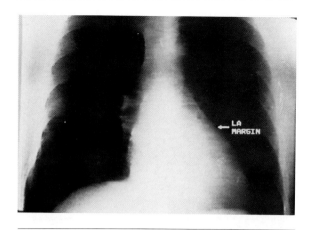

FIGURE 11-2. Posteroanterior chest film depicts cardiomegaly and left atrial enlargement (*arrow*).

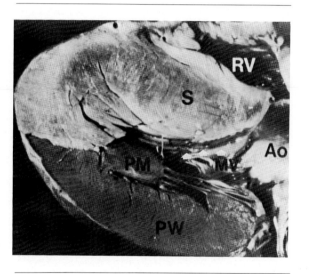

FIGURE 11-3. Anatomic view of a sectioned left ventricle shows abnormal thickness of the septum(S). The posterior wall (PW) is also hypertrophic. Note the narrow LVOT (*arrow*). (PM, papillary muscle; MV, mitral valve; AO, aorta.) (From Hagan AD, DiSessa TG, Bloor CM, et al. Two-Dimensional Echocardiography: Clinical-Pathological Correlations in Adult and Congenital Heart Disease. Boston: Little, Brown; 1983; 298.)

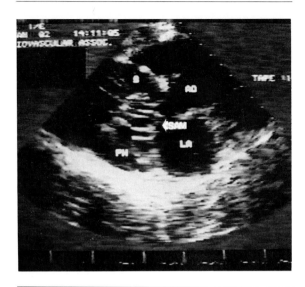

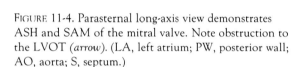

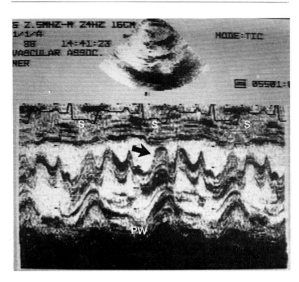

Figure 11-4. Parasternal long-axis view demonstrates ASH and SAM of the mitral valve. Note obstruction to the LVOT (*arrow*). (LA, left atrium; PW, posterior wall; AO, aorta; S, septum.)

Figure 11-5. M-mode panel shows SAM of the mitral valve (*arrow*). The septum (S) is thick, and the posterior wall (PW) is normal thickness.

the leaflet moves anteriorly to coapt with the interventricular septum. This obstructs blood flow in the subaortic area. In addition, the patient has evidence of ratio of interventricular septal thickness to posterior lateral wall thickness greater than 1.5 to 1.0. This is an additional echocardiographic feature of hypertrophic cardiomyopathy.

Reduction in contractility of the interventricular septum has been described and may be secondary to the muscle fiber disarray seen histologically in hypertrophic septa,[60] but this finding is not specific for HCM. In addition, investigators using 2-D echocardiography have pointed out that septal hypertrophy may extend uniformly or may be localized or exaggerated at various loci within the ventricle (e.g., in the basilar portion of the ventricle or nearer the apex).[34]

Although M-mode echocardiography is useful, results of the study may suggest an erroneous diagnosis of HCM if the M-mode cursor is misaligned at an oblique angle to the interventricular septum, making it appear thicker than it is. This alters the ratio of septum thickness to posterior wall thickness and produces the appearance of ASH. In addition, ASH may occur in a variety of conditions that are not related to HCM. Such conditions can be seen in athletes with physiologic cardiac hypertrophy,[28] right ventricular overload as in pulmonary atresia,[28] primary pulmonary hypertension,[15] hypertension,[3] aortic stenosis,[22] and aortic atresia.[22] Also, patients with a history of inferior wall myocardial infarction and thinning of the posterior wall with normal septal thickness may present with ASH.[20] ASH is a normal feature of embryonic life,[36] and a subset of infants born to diabetic mothers have benign ASH, which resolves in approximately 6 months.[17] ASH has also been reported in patients undergoing hemodialysis and in association with mural thrombus and with lymphoma.[7,46] ASH is not, therefore, pathognomonic for HCM.

An additional feature of HCM on 2-D echocardiography is a change in the acoustic property of the interventricular septal echo targets.[39] These findings are more prominent in the intramyocardial echoes from the interventricular septum and the posterior lateral ventricular walls, echoes that have been labelled as "speckling" (Fig. 11-6).

SAM of the mitral valve is said to be present

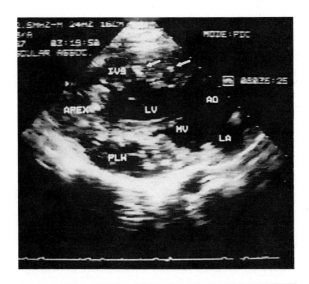

FIGURE 11-6. Parasternal long-axis 2-D echocardiogram of abnormal bright echoes (*arrow*) in the myocardium. (IVS, septum; PLW, posterior lateral wall; LV, left ventricle; AO, aorta; MV, mitral valve; LA, left atrium.)

when the mitral valve apparatus moves anteriorly toward the interventricular septum shortly after the onset of systole and then returns to its normal position just before the onset of ventricular diastole. This has been associated with systolic pressure gradients or obstructions across the LVOT (Fig. 11-7).[16] SAM concurrently involving the aortic posterior wall and the mitral valve has also been described. True SAM should return to the baseline prior to the onset of ventricular diastole. This can be sensitively illustrated with M-mode echocardiography (Fig. 11-8). SAM of the mitral valve is not specific for the diagnosis of HCM and may be seen in other conditions, such as transposition of the great vessels,[43] aortic regurgitation,[12] hypovolumic shock,[6] Pompe's disease,[49] and hypertension.

"Pseudosystolic anterior motion of the mitral valve" is seen in the presence of hyperdynamic left ventricular posterior walls, which produce parallel anterior motion of the mitral valve. This can be seen in atrial septal defect,[56] pericardial effusion,[19] and mitral valve prolapse.[35] Two-dimensional echocardiographic examination has proved that, if the M-mode beam is directed into the area of the mitral valve chords, the SAM, or buckling, that oc-

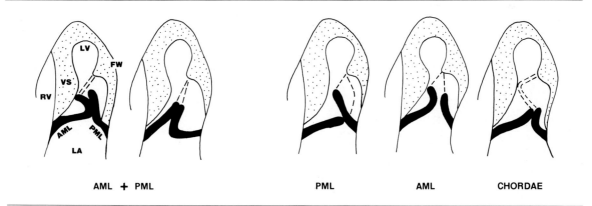

AML + PML          PML          AML          CHORDAE

FIGURE 11-7. Diagram demonstrates the various parts of the mitral valve apparatus that can encroach on the LVOT and possibly produce obstruction. (AML, anterior mitral leaflet; PML, posterior mitral leaflet; LV, left ventricle; VS, ventricular septum; RV, right ventricle; FW, left ventricular free wall; LA, left atrium.) (From Spirito R, Baron, BJ. Patterns of systolic anterior motion of the mitral valve in hypertrophic cardiomyopathy: Assessment by two-dimensional echocardiography. Am J Cardiol. 1984; 54:1039.)

curs is not true SAM. This condition may be seen in nonobstructive cardiomyopathy, hypertension, mitral valve prolapse, and in normal hearts. Other classic M-mode features associated with HCM include early systolic aortic valve closure and decreased rate of septal thickening.

Two-dimensional echocardiography has become the *diagnostic tool of choice* for patients suspected of having HCM. The primary technical advantage of the 2-D echocardiographic approach over M-mode method is the multiple windows of interrogation available on the former. It is imperative to use both parasternal long- and short-axis views to allow accurate measurement of the interventricular septum and posterior wall thickness and chamber sizes. The problem with abnormal tangential cuts of the interventricular septum with M-mode examination is eliminated because the entire interventricular septum may be visualized by the 2-D echocardiographic examination. Two-dimensional apical four- and two-chamber views are also very important for the identification of the left ventricular ejection fraction and eccentric areas of ventricular hypertrophy. Therefore, the 2-D examination has been able to identify the sites of prior myotomy or

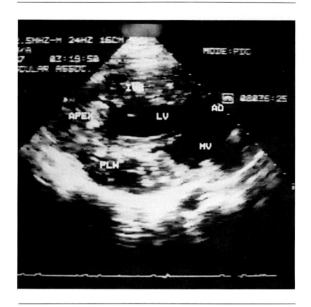

FIGURE 11-9. Parasternal long-axis 2-D echocardiogram of a patient with apical hypertrophic cardiomyopathy. Note apical hypertrophy. (IVS, interventricular septum; PLW, posterior lateral wall; LV, left ventricle; AO, aorta; MV, mitral valve.)

myectomy and to accurately evaluate the amount of tissue removed during the procedure.[54]

Two-dimensional echocardiography has also identified a subset of patients who have pronounced concentric hypertrophy located at the left ventricular apex, labelled apical hypertrophic cardiomyopathy.[37] Such a patient is presented in Figure 11-9. It should be noted that this patient does not have LVOT obstruction, though it is a common finding in patients with this variant of HCM. Most reports of this type of patient have been documented by Yamaguchi and associates.[62] It should be noted that the patient in Figure 11-9 has no evidence of SAM of the mitral valve or of septal hypertrophy in the basilar portion of the interventricular septum. Such patients are not typical in the United States, and apical hypertrophic cardiomyopathy is more common in Japan.

Doppler echocardiography also provides valuable information on abnormal flow patterns in the cardiac chambers and the great vessels. The primary hemodynamic problem with HCM is subaor-

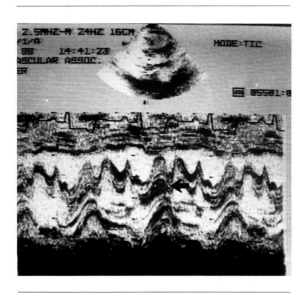

FIGURE 11-8. M-mode tracing of SAM of the mitral valve. Note complete return to baseline segment prior to opening of mitral valve (*arrow*).

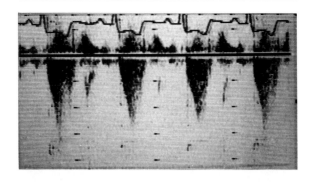

FIGURE 11-10. Continuous-wave Doppler tracing of abnormal increased velocity at 2.5 m per second in a patient with subaortic gradient.

tic obstruction or diastolic dysfunction due to increased left ventricular stiffness. Management of such a patient with HCM depends on which hemodynamic abnormality predominates in the patient's symptoms. The subaortic obstruction of HCM is dynamic and continuous-wave Doppler produces a unique spectral tracing (Fig. 11-10). Flow velocity increases gradually during early systole and peaks at late systole, creating a dagger-shaped Doppler display. Changes in flow velocity may be measured with a simplified version of Bernoulli's equation ($\Delta P = 4(V_2)^2$) where $V_2$ equals the velocity distal to an obstruction in cm/sec and $P$ equals pressure in mm/hg. This peak velocity can be converted into a subaortic pressure gradient.

Pulsed-wave (PW) Doppppler is useful in assessing diastolic function in HCM. A stiffened, hypertrophic ventricle has a prolonged relaxation time, so early left ventricular filling is compromised and pressure in the left atrium drops relatively slowly. The mitral valve velocity pattern by PW Doppler reflects the diastolic filling abnormality. The peak E wave is less than the peak A wave, and the mitral valve flow deceleration time is prolonged (Fig. 11-11). Color-flow imaging is also physiologically useful in timing the flow associated with HCM. It also aids in identifying mitral valve regurgitation, which may occur in as many as 50% of patients with HCM. The classic sequence of left ventricular

systole is ejection, obstruction, and regurgitation phenomenon. The regurgitation is variable, but usually correlates directly with the severity of obstruction to the LVOT.

The isovolumic relaxation time (IVRT) is the time required for the left ventricle to relax prior to mitral valve opening (i.e., beginning of early diastole). In HCM this period is frequently prolonged, permitting the differential relaxation of the left ventricle to become more apparent.[32]

Differential diagnosis of HCM includes patients with longstanding, moderate to severe hypertension whose echocardiogram may suggest HCM. In addition, there are patients with infiltrative diseases, such as amyloidosis and hemochromatosis, whose markedly thickened ventricles resemble those of HCM. Patients with other conditions, such as chronic renal failure, Friedreich's ataxia, cardiac sarcoma, and lymphoma, have been reported to produce disproportional septal thickening that simulates HCM.

HCM may occasionally cause obstruction of the RVOT. The echocardiogram shows evidence of

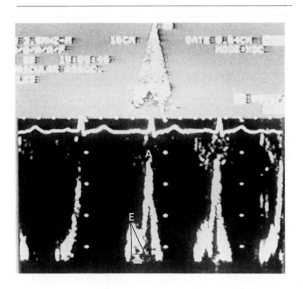

FIGURE 11-11. Pulsed-wave Doppler tracing of a patient with hypertrophic cardiomyopathy. Note reduction in early diastolic filling (E) and the increased velocity following atrial systole (A). The deceleration time is increased (arrows).

right ventricular hypertrophy with increased anterior right ventricular wall thickness. There is systolic anterior motion of the tricuspid valve, and midsystolic closure of the pulmonic valve may occur.[8]

Therapy for patients with HCM consists of either medical or surgical intervention. Medical management may include β-adrenergic receptor-blocking drugs, calcium channel–blocking drugs, antiarrhythmic agents, insertion of a permanent pacemaker, and prophylaxis for infective endocarditis. Surgical intervention consists of myotomy or myectomy.[38]

## Idiopathic Dilated Cardiomyopathy

Idiopathic dilated cardiomyopathy (IDC) is recognized by dilatation of unknown cause of one or both ventricles. Dilatation often becomes severe, and it is invariably accompanied by hypertrophy. Systolic ventricular function is impaired. Congestive heart failure may or may not supervene. Presentations with disturbances of ventricular or atrial rhythm are common, and death may occur at any stage.[4]

A careful history is of paramount importance in patients suspected of IDC. Patients should be questioned about their consumption of alcohol, possible exposure to toxic substances, and any history of infection, hypertension, and systemic illnesses, including rheumatic fever. It is usually difficult to separate IDC from "ischemic cardiomyopathy." Clues may be derived from a history of chest pain or heart attack or from the ECG or radionuclide imaging and echocardiographic studies.[10,11,51] Patients with IDC may have no symptoms and cardiomegaly on chest radiography may be the only clinical finding. They may have symptoms of subjective arrhythmias and problems with exertional dyspnea, orthopnea, paroxysmal nocturnal dyspnea, peripheral edema, or abdominal pain due to hepatic congestion. Less frequently, chest discomfort typical of angina pectoris or atypical chest discomfort may occur.[52]

Physical examination usually reveals an arterial pulse of small volume and increased venous pressures. Blood pressure may be normal or low. Palpation of the precordium often detects a diffuse lateral and inferiorly displaced left ventricular apex. There may also be a left parasternal lift or left ven-

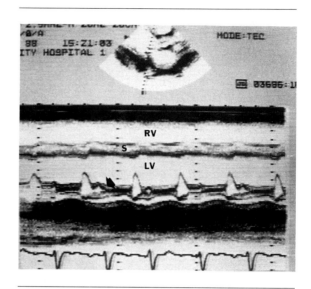

FIGURE 11-12. M-mode echocardiogram demonstrates right and left ventricular enlargement and poor contractility of both ventricles. The mitral valve shows a B notch (*arrow*). (RV, right ventricle; LV, left ventricle; S, septum.)

tricular heave. Auscultation reveals muffled heart sounds with paradoxical splitting of $S_2$ with an accentuated pulmonic component to it. An $S_4$ or $S_3$ gallop or a summation gallop may be present. Murmurs of tricuspid and mitral regurgitation are heard when there is atrioventricular valve annular dilatation. The patient's chest film shows generalized cardiomegaly without calcification of the valves or coronary arteries. There may be a large globular cardiac silhouette, in which case pericardial effusion should be expected. The patient's pulmonary vasculature may suggest increased pulmonary venous pressure. The ECG is almost always normal, but not specific. There may be Q waves suggestive of infarction, and any type of dysrhythmia may be present. Atrial fibrillation is seen in approximately 20% of these patients.[30] Ventricular arrhythmias are also common. On twenty-four hour holter monitoring, ventricular tachycardia was found in approximately 60% of patients.[21]

ECHOCARDIOGRAPHIC FEATURES
The echocardiographic findings on M-mode echocardiogram (Fig. 11-12) shows left and right ventricular enlargement with abnormal indices of left

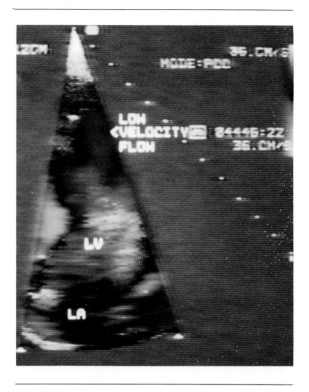

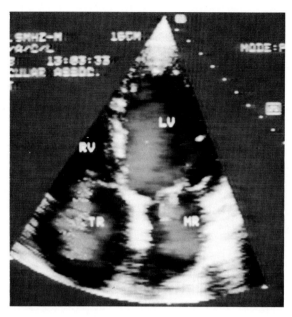

FIGURE 11-14. (See color insert.) Apical four-chamber 2-D echocardiogram with color-flow Doppler mapping. The patient has mitral (MR) and tricuspid (TR) valve regurgitation. (RV, right ventricle; LV, left ventricle.)

FIGURE 11-13. (See color insert.) Color-flow Doppler tracing of a patient with congestive cardiomyopathy. Note the low-velocity flow in the middle to distal left ventricle (LV). See arrow. (LA, left atrium.)

ventricular function (i.e., decreased ejection fraction and fractional shortening). The amplitude of separation of the mitral valve leaflets may be decreased and the mitral apparatus may be located posteriorly. So-called miniaturization of the mitral valve may be present, related to decreased cardiac output and decreased volumes flowing through the mitral valve during diastole. Abnormal closure of the mitral valve, as noted by a B notch, signifies elevated left ventricular end-diastolic filling pressure.[25] Pericardial effusion is commonly seen, and mural thrombi may be found.[11] The 2-D examination usually demonstrates a dilated left ventricle with evidence of poor left ventricular ejection fraction and of functional mitral and tricuspid valve regurgitation. There is also evidence of multiple chamber enlargement. In addition, the 2-D echocardiographic examination, compared to M-mode echocardiography, provides increased sensitivity in identifying mural thrombus and evaluating for segmental wall motion abnormalities, like those seen in patients with ischemic cardiomyopathies. The Doppler examination reveals reduced systolic function. The color-flow Doppler pattern, if the heart is examined from the cardiac apex, reveals a series of "puffs of smoke" during diastole (Fig. 11-13). This is related to the low cardiac output state. Most patients with dilated cardiomyopathy have associated atrioventricular valvular regurgitations of varying degrees. Color-flow Doppler imaging demonstrates mitral regurgitation as a bright blue or mosaic jet entering the left atrium (Fig. 11-14). Meese and colleagues[23] demonstrated a very high incidence of atrioventricular valvular regurgitations in patients with dilated cardiomyopathy. Mitral regurgitation was noted in all patients, and tricuspid regurgitation was present in 91%. Valvular regurgitation is usually mild to moderate. Semilunar valve regurgitation is less common. Meese's group found that approximately 23% of patients with IDC had aortic regurgitation and 58% had pulmonic regurgitation.[41]

Right ventricular pressures may be calculated with pulsed- or continuous-wave Doppler information by observing the peak tricuspid regurgitant velocity on a color flow–guided examination. This calculation may be made by adding the determined transtricuspid valve systolic gradient to the calculated or assumed right atrial pressure (see Chapter 12). Similarly, the peak end-diastolic pulmonary regurgitant velocity can be used to determine the pulmonary artery diastolic pressure.[23] Values for cardiac output calculated by Doppler method sampling the pulmonary artery or the LVOT are usually decreased.

Doppler-derived mitral flow velocities have proven useful in characterizing left ventricular filling patterns in patients with congestive cardiomyopathy. Takenaka and associates[57] analyzed the mitral flow velocity waveforms in patients with congestive cardiomyopathy and found a significantly lower peak velocity during rapid diastolic filling and reduced ratios of peak velocity during atrial systole to peak velocity during rapid diastolic filling. These findings suggest that atrial systole is responsible for the majority of diastolic filling of the ventricles. In the same study, peak velocities of patients with IDC and mitral regurgitation during rapid diastolic filling were similar to those of normal subjects. This observation probably reflects the increased flow from left atrium to left ventricle in diastole secondary to mitral valve regurgitation. Therefore the presence of mitral regurgitation falsely alters the ratio of peak E and A velocities in diastole.

ADDITIONAL CONSIDERATIONS FOR PATIENTS WITH IDIOPATHIC DILATED CARDIOMYOPATHY

Myocarditis should be considered in patients with a relatively short history of congestive heart failure, particularly if there was a prior febrile illness, in which case endomyocardial biopsy should be considered.[45] In addition, longstanding valvular heart disease may precipitate global left ventricular dysfunction. Color-flow Doppler imaging is important in the assessment of the severity of valvular lesions, and thereafter cardiac catheterization may be necessary to determine the appropriateness of surgical treatment for patients suspected of having left ventricular dysfunction as a result of a significant valvular regurgitation instead of IDC. Severe aortic stenosis with low-output states may masquerade as IDC. Again, Doppler examination is extremely important in evaluating this condition. The Doppler examination is sensitive enough to accurately assess the severity of the patient's aortic valve disease so that appropriate management can be instituted.

Treatment of patients with IDC consists of weight reduction, restriction of sodium, and abstinence from alcohol and tobacco. Diuretics, positive inotrophic agents, vasodilators, anticoagulants, and antiarrhythmics all are indicated at various points in the natural history of the disease. In addition, immunosuppressants have been used to treat a subset of patients determined by endomyocardial biopsy to have myocarditis. "Physiologic" dual-chambered pacing and cardiac transplantation have certainly decreased the morbidity and mortality associated with congestive cardiomyopathies.

## Other Congestive Cardiomyopathies

Other disorders associated with a clinical picture resembling IDC are abnormalities of the autoimmune system such as those seen in patients whose body has rejected a heart transplant. Isovolumic relaxation times are highly sensitive and specific for identifying patients who are rejecting cardiac transplants. There is a significant decrease in the isovolumic relaxation time during the acute process as compared to nonrejection phases.[47] Cardiac abnormalities have also been noted in patients with acquired immunodeficiency syndrome (AIDS); they usually include pericardial effusion, hypokinetic left ventricle, and secondary myocarditis.[13] Additional reported abnormal findings are segmental wall motion abnormalities, left ventricular enlargement, and abnormal left ventricular systolic function.

Chagas' disease is endemic to South America. It results from chronic parasitic infections caused by the protozoan *Trypanosoma cruzi* and produces severe left ventricular dysfunction and apical aneurysms with evidence of multiple segmental wall motion abnormalities.[9]

Some drugs may cause cardiac toxicity—Doxorubicin, cyclophosphamides, antiparasitic drugs, chloroquine, and psychotrophic drugs such as phenothiazines, tricyclic antidepressants, and lithium. Hypersensitivity myocarditis has been reported secondary to therapy with sulfonamides and methyldopa.[58] Cardiac toxicity has also been induced by chemicals such as hydrocarbons, carbon monoxide, arsenic, lead, phosphorus, mercury, and cobalt.[58] Physical agents such as radiation may precipitate congestive heart failure or pericardial disease. Connective tissue diseases such as systemic lupus erythematosus, Kawasaki's disease, periarteritis nodosa, and systemic giant cell arteritis have all been implicated in producing depressed left ventricular cardiac function. Additionally, patients who have chronic alcoholism may develop dilated cardiomyopathy.[3]

### Restrictive Cardiomyopathy

Restrictive cardiomyopathy is a condition that may exist with or without obliteration of the left ventricle and right ventricular cavity. Restrictive cardiomyopathies include such entities as myocardial fibrosis and Löeffler's cardiomyopathy. Endomyocardial scarring usually affects either one or both ventricles and restricts ventricular filling. Involvement of the atrioventricular valves is common, but the outflow tracts are spared. Cavity obliteration of the left ventricle is characteristic of advanced cases.[4] Another class of disease similar to restrictive cardiomyopathy and usually included with it is infiltrative cardiomyopathy. Their pathophysiology is essentially the same as that of restrictive cardiomyopathies, but their cause is known.

The most common clinical presentation of patients with restrictive cardiomyopathy is congestive heart failure. Other symptoms may be arrhythmia, anginalike chest discomfort, syncope, or sudden death. The patient's examination may reveal evidence of biventricular failure or elevated jugular venous pressure with prominent jugular vein distention. The patient's chest radiograph may be normal, but more frequently it shows an enlarged cardiac silhouette. The ECG may demonstrate rhythm disturbances consisting of sinus node dysfunction with evidence of sick sinus syndrome, various degrees of atrioventricular disease, or complete heart block. Sudden death has been reported in approximately 30% of patients with restrictive cardio-

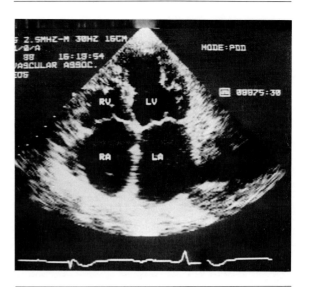

FIGURE 11-15. Apical four-chamber 2-D echocardiogram of a patient with severe biatrial enlargement and normal-sized ventricles. (RV, right ventricle; LV, left ventricle; RA, right atrium; LA, left atrium.)

myopathy; it is presumed to be related to disturbances in conduction and rhythm.

*Echocardiographic Features.* All restrictive cardiomyopathies (primary restrictive cardiomyopathy, Löeffler's endocarditis, and endomyocardial fibrosis) have similar pathophysiologic findings, typically, atrial enlargement out of proportion to the ventricular internal dimensions. This is primarily the result of reduced left ventricular compliance and subsequent atrial dilatation. Figure 11-15 is an apical four-chamber view of a patient with classic features of restrictive cardiomyopathy. There is evidence of normal left and right ventricular wall thickness and interventricular septal thickness, but there is also evidence of biatrial enlargement and abnormal elevated atrial pressures. Hemodynamic data from cardiac catheterization is consistent with abrupt elevation of early diastolic pressures at rest and with exercise and usually can be differentiated from that seen in constrictive pericardial disease.[40] Recent studies using Doppler interrogation provide evidence that restrictive and constrictive myocardial disease may be separated by evaluation of the

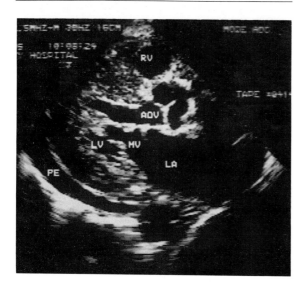

FIGURE 11-16. Parasternal long-axis 2-D echocardiogram shows severe left ventricular hypertrophy with a "granular, sparkling" appearance consistent with infiltrative cardiomyopathy. The valves are thickened, and there is a pericardial effusion (PE). Severe left atrial enlargement is present (LA). (RV, right ventricle; LV, left ventricle; MV, mitral valve; AOV, aortic valve.)

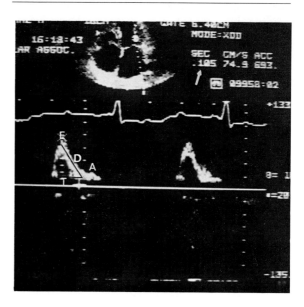

FIGURE 11-17. Pulsed-wave Doppler echocardiogram of a patient with abnormal diastolic filling. The deceleration time is significantly shortened (105 msec). (E, early rapid filling velocity; A, filling velocity following atrial systole; D, deceleration slope; T, time.)

flow through the atrioventricular valves.[1,18] Endomyocardial biopsies have not been helpful in defining the cause of restrictive cardiomyopathy, except in patients with amyloid heart disease.

The most commonly reviewed restrictive (infiltrative) cardiomyopathy is that secondary to amyloidosis (extracellular deposition of fibrous protein amyloid in one or more sites).[27] The primary form of amyloid has a predilection for mesenchymal structures, including the heart. In advanced forms, the 2-D echocardiographic examination identifies abnormal myocardial tissue characteristics, notably a hyperrefractile granular appearance of the myocardium.[53] Figure 11-16 is a 2-D parasternal long-axis view of a patient with classic features of this restrictive cardiomyopathy. There is evidence of hypertrophy of the left and right ventricular walls and the interventricular septum and evidence of a small left ventricular cavity with hypokinesia of all cardiac walls. There is also evidence of multiple valvular thickenings and pericardial effusion.

The primary hemodynamic abnormality seen in these patients is ventricular diastolic dysfunction. The unifying hemodynamic changes include rapid completion of early diastolic filling into a nonelastic ventricle resulting in ventricular filling being completed early in diastole with very little late diastolic flow.[24] A sensitive diagnostic Doppler echocardiographic feature is represented by a shortened deceleration time of the mitral and tricuspid velocity envelopes.[2] Figure 11-17 demonstrates the restrictive Doppler flow pattern seen on pulsed-wave examination.

The treatment and prognosis of patients with amyloid cardiomyopathy is currently unsatisfactory. To date, no mode of treatment has proved safe and effective in reversing, or even slowing the progress of, amyloid deposition. Mean survival among patients with primary amyloidosis, with or without heart disease, averages approximately 1 year from the time of diagnosis; survival beyond 2 years is unusual.[26]

*Other Restrictive Cardiomyopathies of Known Cause.*
Additional infiltrative cardiomyopathies include sarcoidosis and hemochromatosis. Sarcoidosis is a multisystem granulomatous disease that may involve the heart.[50] The incidence of heart involvement with sarcoidosis is low. Approximately 5% of patients may present with conduction system abnormalities, including complete heart block, ventricular dysrhythmias, sudden death, progressive heart failure, and recurrent pericardial effusions. These findings are most common in young or middle-aged adult patients. Echocardiographic features include abnormal ventricular wall thickness, pericardial effusions, and right ventricular dysfunction secondary to corpulmonale (which is caused by the pulmonary sarcoidosis).

Hemochromatosis is an iron-storage disease that affects multiple organs and tissue systems. There are primary and secondary forms.[5] Echocardiographic features (principally in the early stages) include nondilated, thickened left ventricular walls with preserved systolic function and diminished compliance. In later stages of hemochromatosis, the ventricular cavities become dilated with impaired systolic function and left atrial enlargement. The mortality rate of these patients is approximately 50%.[44] Doppler assessment reveals both restrictive and abnormal relaxation patterns. Secondary hemochromatosis has been identified in patients with anemia who require multiple transfusions. Their echocardiographic features have been described by Vaides-Cruz and coworkers.[61]

Other chemical storage disorders such as those of glycogen and of lipid have been identified, although few echocardiographic studies have been performed in these patients.[49]

## Acknowledgment

The author would like to acknowledge the review and critique of this chapter by Abdulla M. Abdulla, M.D.

## References

1. Appleton CP, Hatle LK, Popp RL. Central venous flow velocity patterns can differentiate constrictive pericarditis from restrictive cardiomyopathy (abstr.) J Am Coll Cardiol. 1987; 9:119.
2. Appleton CP, Hatle LK, Popp RL. Demonstration of restrictive ventricular physiology by Doppler echocardiography. J Am Coll Cardiol. 1988; 2(4):757–768.
3. Ballas M, Zoneraich S, Unis M, et al. Non-invasive cardiac evaluation in chronic alcoholic patients with alcohol withdrawal syndrome. Chest. 1982; 82:148–153.
4. Brandenburg RO, Chazov E, Cherian G, et al. Report of WHO/ISFC task force on definition and classification of cardiomyopathies. Circulation 1981; 64:437A–438A.
5. Buja LM, Roberts NC. Iron in the heart: Etiology and clinical significance. Am J Med. 1971; 51:209–221.
6. Bulkley BH, Fortuin NJ. Systolic anterior motion of the mitral valve without asymmetrical septal hypertrophy. Chest. 1976; 69:694–696.
7. Cabin HS, Costello RM, Vasudevan C, et al. Cardiac lymphoma mimicking hypertrophic cardiomyopathy. Am Heart J. 1981; 104:466–468.
8. Cardiel EA, Alonso M, Delcon JL, et al. Echocardiographic sign of right-sided hypertrophic obstructive cardiomyopathy. Br Heart J 1978; 40:1321–1325.
9. Oliveira JS, et al. Apical aneurysm of Chagas' heart disease. Br Heart J. 1981; 46:432–437.
10. Curtius JM, Freimuth M, Kuhn H, et al. Exercise echocardiography in dilated cardiomyopathy. Ztschr Kardiol. 1982; 71:727–730.
11. Demaria AN, Bommer W, Lee G, et al. Value and limitations of two-dimensional echocardiography in assessment of cardiomyopathy. Am J Cardiol. 1980; 46:1224–1231.
12. Feigenbaum H. Echocardiography. 3d ed. Philadelphia: Lea & Febiger; 1981:462.
13. Fink L, Reichele N, Sutton MGSJ. Cardiac abnormalities in acquired immune deficiency syndrome. Am J Cardiol. 1984; 54:1161–1163.
14. Frank S, Braunwald E. Idiopathic hypertrophic subaortic stenosis: Clinical analysis of 126 patients with emphasis on the natural history. Circulation. 1968; 37:759–788.
15. Goodman DJ, Harrison DC, Popp DC. Echocardiographic features of primary pulmonary hypertension. Am J Cardiol. 1974; 33:438–443.
16. Gustavson A, Liedholm H, Tylen U. Hypertrophic cardiomyopathy: A correlation between echocardiography, angiographic and hemodynamic findings. Ann Radiol (Paris). 1977; 20:419–430.
17. Gutgesell HP, Speer ME, Rosenberg HS. Characterization of the cardiomyopathy in infants of diabetic mothers. Circulation. 1980; 64:441–450.
18. Hatle LK, Appleton CP, Popp RL. Constrictive pericarditis and restrictive cardiomyopathy differentiation by Doppler according to atrioventricular flow velocities (abstr.) J Am Coll Cardiol. 1987; 9:178.

19. Hearne MJ, Sherber HS, deLeon AD. Asymmetric septal hypertrophy in acromegaly: An echocardiographic study. Circulation. 1975; 52(suppl 2):II-35 abstr 130.

20. Henning H, O'Rourke RA, Crawford MH, et al. Inferior myocardial infarction as a cause of asymmetric septal hypertrophy: An echocardiographic study. Am J Cardiol. 1978; 41:817-822.

21. Huang SK, Messer JV, Denes P. Significance of ventricular tachycardia in idiopathic dilated cardiomyopathy: Observations in 35 patients. Am J Cardiol. 1983; 51:507-512.

22. Kansac S, Roitman D, Sheffield LT. Interventricular septal thickness and left ventricular hypertrophy: An echocardiographic study. Circulation 1979; 60:1058-1065.

23. Kitabatake A, Kodama K, Masuyama T, et al. Continuous wave Doppler echocardiographic detection of pulmonary regurgitation and its application to non-invasive estimation of pulmonary artery pressure. Circulation. 1986; 74:484-492.

24. Klein AL, Luscher TF, Hatle LK, et al. Spectrum of diastolic function abnormalities in cardiac amyloidosis. Circulation. 1987; 76(suppl 4): 4-126 abstr 499.

25. Konecke LL, Feigenbaum H, Chang S, et al. Abnormal mitral valve motion in patients with elevated left ventricular diastolic pressures. Circulation. 1973; 47:989-996.

26. Kyle RA, Bayrd ED. Amyloidosis: Review of 236 cases. Medicine. 1975; 54:271-299.

27. Kyle RA, Greipp PR. Amyloidosis (AL): Clinical and laboratory features in 229 cases. Mayo Clin Proc. 1983; 58:665-683.

28. Larter WE, Allen HD, Sahn DJ, et al. The asymmetrically hypertrophied septum: Further differentiation of its causes. Circulation 1976; 53:19-27.

29. McKenna WJ, England D, Doi YL, et al. Arrhythmias in hypertrophic cardiomyopathy: I. Influence on prognosis. Br Heart J. 1981; 46:168-172.

30. Mann B, Ray R, Goldberger AL, et al. Atrial fibrillation in congestive cardiomyopathy: Echocardiographic and hemodynamic correlates. Cathet Cardiovasc Diagn. 1981; 7:387-395.

31. Maron BJ, Epstein SE. Clinical course of patients with hypertrophic cardiomyopathy. Cardiovasc Clin. 1971; 10(1):253-265.

32. Maron BJ, Epstein SE. Hypertrophic cardiomyopathy. Recent observations regarding the specificity of three hallmarks of the disease: Asymmetric septal hypertrophy, septal disorganization and systolic anterior motion of the anterior mitral leaflet. Am J Cardiol. 1980; 45:141-154.

33. Maron BJ, Edwards JE, Epstein SE. Disproportionate ventricular septal thickening in patients with systemic hypertension. Chest. 1978; 73:466-470.

34. Maron BJ, Gottdiener JS, Epstein SE. Patterns and significance of distribution of left ventricular hypertrophy in hypertrophic cardiomyopathy: A wide-angle, two-dimensional echocardiographic study of 125 patients. Am J Cardiol. 1981; 48:418-428.

35. Maron BJ, Gottdiener JS, Perry LW. Specificity of systolic anterior motion of anterior mitral leaflet for hypertrophic cardiomyopathy. Br Heart J. 1981; 45:206-216.

36. Maron BJ, Verter J, Kapur S. Disproportionate ventricular septal thickening in the developing normal human heart. Circulation. 1978; 57:520-526.

37. Maron BJ, Bonow RO, Seshagiri TNR, et al. Hypertrophic cardiomyopathy with ventricular septal hypertrophy localized to the apical region of the left ventricle (apical hypertrophic cardiomyopathy). Am J Cardiol. 1982; 49:1838-1848.

38. Maron BJ, Merrill WH, Freier PA, et al. Long-term clinical course and symptomatic status of patients after operation for hypertrophic subaortic stenosis. Circulation. 1978; 57:1205-1213.

39. Martin RP, Rakowski H, French J, et al. Idiopathic hypertrophic subaortic stenosis viewed by wide-angle, phased-array echocardiography. Circulation. 1979; 59:1206-1217.

40. Meaney E, Shabetai R, Bhargava V, et al. Cardiac amyloidosis, constrictive pericarditis and restrictive cardiomyopathy. Am J Cardiol. 1976; 38:547-556.

41. Meese R, Adams D, Kisslo J. Assessment of valvular regurgitation by conventional and color-flow Doppler in dilated cardiomyopathy. Echocardiography. 1987; 3(6):505-511.

42. Mills TJ, Seward JB, Khandheria BK, et al. Color-flow imaging in cardiomyopathies: observation and implications. Echocardiography. 1987; 4(6):527-535.

43. Nanda NC, Gramiak R, Manning JA, et al. Echocardiographic features of subpulmonic obstruction in dextrotransposition of the great vessels. Circulation. 1975; 51:515-521.

44. Olson LJ, Baldus WP, Tajik AJ. Cardiac involvement in idiopathic hemochromatosis: Echocardiographic and clinical correlations. Am J Cardiol. 1987; 60(10):885-889.

45. Parrillo JE, Aretz HT, Palacios I, et al. The results of transvenous endomyocardial biopsy can frequently be used to diagnose myocardial disease in patients with idiopathic heart failure: Endomyocardial biopsies in 100 consecutive patients revealed a substantial incidence of myocarditis. Circulation. 1984; 69:93-101.

46. Pollick C, Koilpillai C, Howard R, et al. Left ventric-

ular thrombus demonstrating canalization and mimicking asymmetrical septal hypertrophy on echocardiographic study. Am Heart J. 1982; 104:641–643.

47. Pope JC, Zumbro GL, Battey LL, et al. Isovolumic relaxation period as an indicator of cardiac allograft rejection. J Heart Transplant. 1986; 5(5):380 abstr.

48. Prescott R, Quinn JS, Littmann D. Electrocardiographic changes in hypertrophic subaortic stenosis which simulate myocardial infarction. Am Heart J. 1963; 66:42–48.

49. Rees A, Eibl F, Minhas K, et al. Echocardiographic evidence of outflow tract obstruction in Pompe's disease (glycogen storage disease of heart). Am J Cardiol. 1976; 27:1103–1106.

50. Roberts WC, Ferrans VJ. Pathologic anatomy of the cardiomyopathies: Idiopathic, dilated and hypertrophic types, infiltrative types and endomyocardial disease with and without eosinophilia. Hum Pathol. 1975; 6:287–342.

51. Saltissi A, Hockings B, Croft DN, et al. Thallium 209 myocardial imaging in patients with dilated and ischemic cardiomyopathy. Br Heart J. 1981; 46:209–295.

52. Segal JP, Stapleton JF, McClellan JR, et al. Idiopathic cardiomyopathy: Clinical features, prognosis and therapy. Curr Prob Cardiol. 1978; 3:1–48.

53. Sigueira-Filho AG, Cunha CL, Tajik AJ, et al. M-mode and two-dimensional echocardiographic features in cardiac amyloidosis. Circulation 1981; 63:188–196.

54. Spirito P, Maron BJ, Rosing DR. Morphologic determinants of hemodynamic state after ventricular septal myotomy-myectomy in patients with obstructive hypertrophic cardiomyopathy: M-mode and two-dimensional echocardiographic assessment. Circulation. 1984; 70:984–995.

55. Stewart S, Schreiner B. Co-existing idiopathic hypertrophic subaortic stenosis and coronary artery disease: Clinical implication and operative management. J Thorac Cardiovasc Surg. 1981; 82:278–280.

56. Tajik AJ, Gau GT, Schattenberg TT. Echocardiographic "pseudo IHSS" pattern in atrial septal defect. Chest. 1972; 62:324–325.

57. Takenaka K, Dabestani A, Gardin JM, et al. Pulsed Doppler echocardiographic study of left ventricular filling in dilated cardiomyopathy. Am J Cardiol. 1986; 58:143–147.

58. Taliereio CP, Olney BA, Lie JT. Myocarditis related to drug hypersensitivity. Mayo Clin Proc. 1985; 60:463–468.

59. TenCate FJ, Balakumaran K, McGhie J, et al. Angina pectoris in hypertrophic cardiomyopathy (HCM): Cause or consequence of disturbed relaxation? (abstr). Circulation 1980; 62(suppl 3):317.

60. TenCate FJ, Hugenholtz PG, VanDorp WG, et al. Prevalence of diagnostic abnormalities in patients with genetically transmitted asymmetric septal hypertrophy. Am J Cardiol. 1979; 43:731–737.

61. Vaides-Cruz LM, Reinecke C, Rutkowski M, et al. Preclinical abnormal segmental cardiac manifestations of thallassemia major in children on transfusion-chelation therapy: Echocardiographic alterations of left ventricular posterior wall contraction and relaxation patterns. Am Heart J. 1982; 103:505–511.

62. Yamaguchi H, Ishimura T, Nishyama S, et al. Hypertrophic non-obstructive cardiomyopathy with giant negative T waves (apical hypertrophy): Ventriculographic and echocardiographic features in 30 patients. Am J Cardiol. 1979; 44:401–412.

# CHAPTER 12

# Coronary Artery Disease

JOHN C. POPE, LOUIS L. BATTEY

**T**wo-dimensional (2-D) echocardiography is an essential technique for the detection of coronary artery disease and its complications, acute myocardial infarction, congestive heart failure, and acute valve dysfunction. Because of superior spatial resolution, a tomographic investigation (imaging an organ in multiple planes or layers) of both ischemic and infarcted myocardial segments and myocardial performance may be accurately assessed.[36] Complications of myocardial infarction such as papillary muscle dysfunction, ventricular septal rupture, left ventricular aneurysm, and thrombus all may be visualized by 2-D examination. This ultrasound technique is tremendously versatile, inexpensive, portable, and very accurate, making it an important modality when planning interventional therapy for patients with suspected coronary artery disease. M-mode echocardiographic examination is still useful in evaluating systolic wall thickening, valve function, and the pericardium, but it lacks spatial resolution, making it inappropriate for evaluation of global left ventricular function. Additionally, cardiac Doppler examination, with pulsed-wave, continuous-wave, and color-flow imaging, has contributed to our understanding of normal and abnormal myocardial function. In this chapter we review the current diagnostic applications of 2-D, M-mode, and Doppler-flow echocardiography in coronary artery disease.

## Anatomy

Three major coronary arteries and their tributaries supply the myocardium—the right coronary artery, the left anterior descending coronary artery, and the circumflex coronary artery. The ventricular muscle supplied by these vessels can be correlated with anatomic sections obtained with 2-D scanning. Figure 12-1 shows four anatomic views: the parasternal long-axis and short-axis views and the apical two-chamber and four-chamber views. The parasternal long-axis view visualizes the interventricular septum and the posterior lateral wall of the left ventricle. The basilar, middle, and distal interventricular septum are usually perfused by the left anterior descending artery. The proximal basilar portion of the interventricular septum is perfused by numerous branches of the left anterior descending artery called septal perforators. A wall motion abnormality that appears distal to the basilar septum is related to a lesion distal to the first septal perforator. The posterior lateral wall of the left ventricle in the parasternal long-axis view is perfused by the left circumflex coronary artery. Short-axis views afford circumferential visualization of the left and right ventricles. The left anterior descending coronary artery is located in the anterior sulcus between the right and left ventricular walls. This artery supplies the anterior wall of the left ventricle and the anterior portion of the

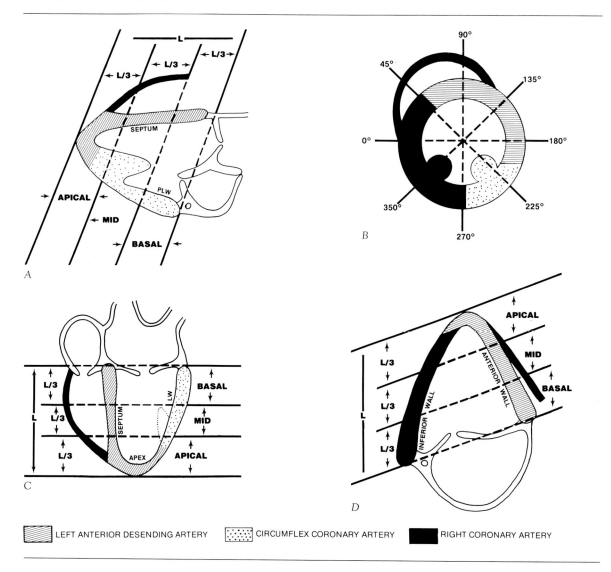

FIGURE 12-1. Two-dimensional echocardiographic planes of (A) parasternal long-axis, (B) parasternal short-axis, (C) apical four-chamber, and (D) apical two-chamber views. (Modified by permission of the American Society of Echocardiography. Nomenclature and Standards: Identification of Myocardial Wall Segments, November, 1982.)

interventricular septum. The right coronary artery, with its posterior descending branch, is located in the posterior groove between the right and left ventricular walls. This artery supplies blood to the postero-medial portion of the left ventricle and to the posterior half of the interventricular septum.

The circumflex vessel and its branches, consisting of obtuse marginals, usually supply the posterolateral portions of the myocardium.

The two-chamber apical view visualizes the anterior, apical, and inferior walls of the myocardium. Therefore, the artery that supplies the anterior wall is the left anterior descending vessel and the right coronary artery supplies the inferior wall. The apex of the heart is usually supplied by the left anterior descending artery. In the four-chamber apical view, the interventricular septum in its proximal, middle, and distal portions, is supplied by the left anterior descending coronary artery. The lateral free wall is supplied by branches of the circumflex artery, usually obtuse marginal branches.

This distribution of coronary artery vascularization is a generalization and there are individual variations. Nevertheless, because of the reproducible distribution of the coronary arteries, depiction of this pattern is useful in clinical circumstances.

## Myocardial Physiology

The basal metabolic need of the myocardium, without regard to the contraction process, is approximately 2 ml/min/100 g of left ventricle, or about 20% of the oxygen needs of the normal beating heart under basal conditions. The remaining 8 to 15 ml (or more) of oxygen (per minute per 100 g) consumed by the beating heart is the energy consumed by contraction. With left ventricular hypertrophy, hypertension, or tachycardia the ventricular work per minute increases substantially, causing increased demand for oxygen delivery to the cardiac muscle. Therefore, changes in oxygen requirements are an essential determinant of myocardial performance. Because the myocardium consumes a great deal of energy it is imperative that the coronary arteries that nourish it be without significant atherosclerotic obstructive plaque. Therefore, if oxygen demand exceeds supply, myocardial dysfunction follows.

Symptoms (dyspnea and angina) and signs (hypotension and pallor) develop as a consequence of hypoxia caused by significant coronary artery stenosis. This anatomic abnormality precipitates the myocardial pathophysiology of both diastolic and systolic myocardial dysfunction. These cardiac conditions may be investigated with echocardiography.

It has been shown that resting blood flow to the myocardium must be decreased by approximately 40% to produce significant ventricular wall motion abnormalities. At least 20% of the entire thickness of the muscle wall must be involved by ischemia or

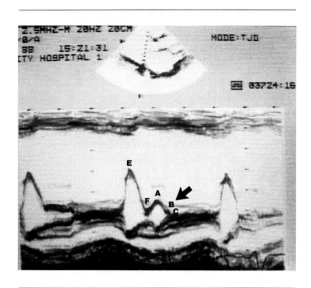

FIGURE 12-2. B notch (*arrow*) is noted between points A and C on the mitral valve diagram. This indicates possible elevated left ventricular end-diastolic filling pressures.

infarction to produce ventricular wall motion abnormalities on 2-D scanning.[17,24]

### ECHOCARDIOGRAPHIC EVALUATION OF DIASTOLIC AND SYSTOLIC FUNCTION

Abnormal diastolic ventricular function may be analyzed by M-mode echocardiography by observing a B notch on the mitral valve waveform (Fig. 12-2). The B notch signifies prolonged closure of the valve following electrical atrial systole (P wave on ECG). This finding may indicate elevated left ventricular end-diastolic filling pressure. The PRAC interval measurement evaluates the temporal aspect of mitral valve closure in reference to the PR interval on an ECG performed simultaneously. When the AC interval on the M-mode strip is subtracted from the PR interval on ECG, a value of less than 60 msec indicates an abnormality, possibly related to elevated left ventricular diastolic filling pressure.[11,33] The presence of a B notch between the AC interval of the mitral valve tracing is the more reliable indicator of elevated diastolic filling pressures. Pulsed-wave Doppler investigation allows assessment of blood flow through the tricuspid and mitral valves during diastole. In the event of ischemia, the relaxation of the ventricle is decreased, which in turn increases its stiffness and decreases its contraction. This may elevate the left ventricular end-diastolic filling pressures and decrease stroke volume, left ventricular filling, and, subsequently, coronary artery perfusion.

Doppler parameters used to assess ventricular diastolic function are peak early diastolic velocity (E point), peak atrial contraction velocity (A point), peak E–peak A ratio, and rate of middiastolic closure (deceleration time; Fig. 12-3). With reduction in early ventricular dynamics as seen in a stiffened (noncompliant) ventricle (e.g., in hypertension, coronary artery disease, or cardiomyopathy), the peak E–peak A ratio is less than <0.9 (normal ≥ 1.0).[8]

A recent study by Channer[12] showed a significant linear relationship between the peak E–peak A peak ratio as the left ventricular diastolic pressure increases. This was due principally to a reduction in the atrial component of filling in patients with elevated ventricular pressures. A peak E–peak A ratio greater than 2 was associated with left ventricular end-diastolic pressures greater than 20 mm Hg (found in patients with ischemic heart disease and left ventricular diastolic dysfunction). Although this appears promising, further investigation is needed into this aspect of Doppler echocardiography. It does appear that assessment of ventricular diastolic function by Doppler echocardiographic examination will become an integral part of the echocardiographic examination.

Systolic ventricular function may be divided into global and segmental indices. Examples of global measures are ventricular ejection fraction, stroke volume, and wall motion. In addition, E to septal separation, mean circumferential fiber shortening rate, and percent fractional shortening are useful M-mode measurements of ventricular function. Segmental indices include M-mode quantitative examination (percentage of wall thickening in systole; <30% systolic thickening is abnormal) and qualitative assessment of wall motion by describing subjectively hypokinesia, akinesia, and dyskinesia.

A wall motion scoring system, which has been used by a variety of centers,[19,22] includes visual and mathematical determination of systolic thickening

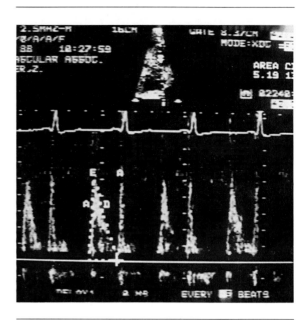

FIGURE 12-3. Normal Doppler flow velocity profile through the mitral valve, illustrating E and A points with normal E-to-A ratio of 1.0. (E, peak early velocity; A, peak atrial velocity; A, acceleration slope; D, decleration slope.)

of each left ventricular segment. After each segment is examined from as many different views as possible, a wall motion score is assigned for each segment. A score of 1 indicates normal contractility; 2, mild to moderate hypokinesia, 3, severe hypokinesia; 4, dyskinesia; and 5 indicates a scarred area with aneurysm formation. If varying degrees of contractility are present in a single segment, the number assigned corresponds to the worst contraction pattern. The wall motion score is the average of the scores of all segments visualized (normal = 1; Fig. 12-4). A newer method of quantifying left ventricular wall motion is the center line technique. End-diastolic and end-systolic contours are outlined, and a computer generates a line midway between the two (center line), from which a predefined number of perpendicular chords are drawn, generating a chordal percent shortening index. Applied to long-axis echocardiographic views this method is accurate in identifying wall motion abnormalities.[14]

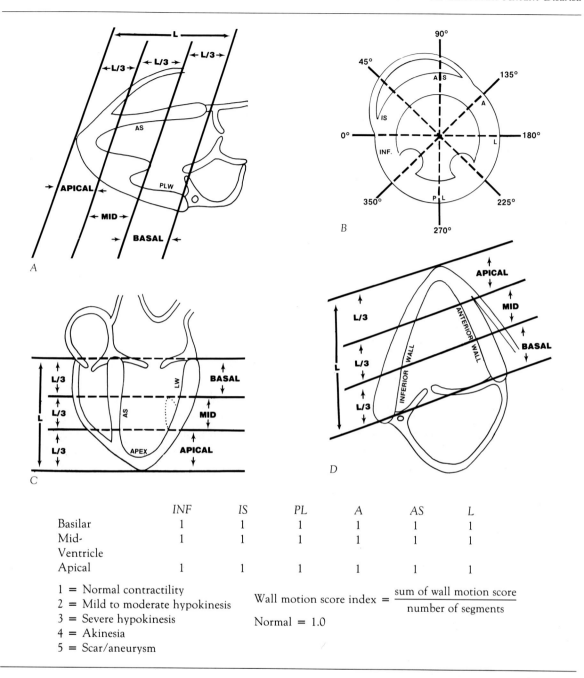

|  | INF | IS | PL | A | AS | L |
|---|---|---|---|---|---|---|
| Basilar | 1 | 1 | 1 | 1 | 1 | 1 |
| Mid-Ventricle | 1 | 1 | 1 | 1 | 1 | 1 |
| Apical | 1 | 1 | 1 | 1 | 1 | 1 |

1 = Normal contractility
2 = Mild to moderate hypokinesis
3 = Severe hypokinesis
4 = Akinesia
5 = Scar/aneurysm

$$\text{Wall motion score index} = \frac{\text{sum of wall motion score}}{\text{number of segments}}$$

$$\text{Normal} = 1.0$$

FIGURE 12-4. Two-dimensional echocardiographic planes of (A) parasternal long-axis, (B) parasternal short-axis, (C) apical four-chamber, and (D) apical two-chamber views. (INF, inferior wall; IS, inferior septum; PL, posterolateral wall; A, anterior wall; L, lateral wall; AS, anteroseptal wall.) (Modified by permission of the American Society of Echocardiography. Nomenclature and Standards: Identification of Myocardial Wall Segments. November, 1982.)

Generally, a distance greater than 10 mm between E point on the mitral valve and the interventricular septum on an M-mode tracing would indicate abnormal systolic ejection fraction, in the range of 40% or less.[28] Left ventricular ejection fraction may be calculated by a variety of geometric methods, but because abnormal ventricles usually have abnormal shapes, we currently use two formulas. Simpson's rule and a fractional shortening method[32] have proven to be reliable and reproducible. Simpson's rule states:

$$V = \frac{L}{4}\left(AM + AM + AP_1 + \frac{AP_1 + AP_2}{2} + 1/3\, AP_2\right)$$

where V equals volume, L equals longest length from apical four chamber view, AM equals the area of the left ventricle in short axis at the mitral valve level; $AP_1$ equals the area of the left ventricle at the high papillary muscle area and $AP_2$ equals the area of short axis at the low papillary muscle level. The ejection fraction equals the diastolic volume minus the systolic volume divided by the diastolic volume.

The fractional shortening method states:

Ejection fraction = $(\%\Delta D^2) + \{(1 - \%\Delta D^2)(\%\Delta L)\}$

where $\%\Delta D$ equals (diameter of the left ventricle in end-diastole squared minus the diameter of the left ventricle in end-systole squared divided by the diameter of the left ventricle in end-diastole squared and $\%\Delta L$ is the fractional shortening of the long axis of the left ventricle estimated from apical contraction. A value of 0.15 represents normal apical motion; 0.05, apical hypokinesis; 0, apical akinesis; and −0.05 apical dyskinesis. These calculations may be performed via microcomputer if the appropriate software is included in the echocardiographic unit or on an off-line quantitative computer system.

## Determination of Prognosis by Echocardiographically Derived Ventricular Function Indices

Several studies[1,6,23] have validated the prognostic value of wall motion indices after myocardial infarction. Nishimura and coworkers[31] studied 61 consecutive myocardial infarction patients. Twenty-four of twenty-seven (89%) patients with an initial wall motion score of 2 or more developed one or more complications of myocardial infarction (pump failure, malignant arrhythmia, death). For patients with a wall motion score of less than 2 the prevalence of these complications was 18%. Similar to these results are reports from the University of Virginia involving 47 patients whose disease was rated Killup class I (normal heart size, no evidence of pulmonary congestion, no gallop) at the time of admission. This group included 14 patients with a wall motion index greater than 2.0; 11 (79%) developed serious myocardial complications. Conversely, only 6 of the 33 whose wall motion index was less than 2 developed complications.[6]

Long-term prognosis has been evaluated in relationship to 2-D echocardiographic findings in patients with myocardial infarction. The value of a predischarge 2-D echocardiogram has been studied by researchers at the Mayo Clinic in 46 patients followed 15 to 28 months after discharge.[29] The wall motion score based on predischarge 2-D echocardiograms was significantly higher (more than 2.0) in patients who subsequently died, suffered recurrent myocardial infarction, or developed significant congestive heart failure or recurrent angina. A wall motion score below 2.0 was not associated with these complications.

## Clinical Indications for Echocardiographic Evaluation of Coronary Artery Disease

Indications for obtaining an echocardiographic study are (1) chest discomfort evaluation, (2) determination of myocardial performance, (3) evaluation of acute or chronic ischemic conditions such as unstable angina or ischemic cardiomyopathies, and (4) complications of myocardial infarction, including congestive heart failure, papillary muscle dysfunction or rupture of the interventricular septum, and infarct expansion, extension, or reinfarction.

Patients with chest discomfort syndrome usually are evaluated in an outpatient setting. Typical angina is a heavy oppressive anterior precordial chest pressure, usually precipitated by exercise and relieved with rest or nitroglycerin. The patient's history is of the utmost importance for determining the probability of significant underlying coronary artery disease. Atypical discomfort is sharp, stabbing, precordial pain or chronic, vague left arm pain (with no precipitating factors or pattern). These atypical pains may be related to underlying valve abnormalities such as mitral valve prolapse, cardiomyopathies, or pericardial disease. Two-dimensional echocardiography is well-suited for evaluating cardiac performance and valvular abnormalities such as mitral prolapse. Patients with cardiomyopathies may have no physical findings to suggest the underlying anatomic abnormality. Patients with mitral valve prolapse usually do have a systolic click or murmur, which suggests the condition.

Most patients with angina and positive ECG (Q waves) findings will have abnormal wall motion scores assessed with echocardiography, although others who have true angina without ECG changes or a history of previous myocardial infarction usually have normal echocardiographic findings. Another subset of patients have transient abnormalities based on silent ischemia (defective warning system in patients who have ischemia but no chest pain) such as diabetes patients who have altered sympathetic nervous system receptors. For such patients and for those with historical evidence of true angina but normal resting ECG tracings exercise echocardiography is useful for evaluating abnormal wall motion (i.e., ischemia) precipitated by exercise.

Patients with prior myocardial infarction and symptoms of left ventricular dysfunction (shortness of breath, poor exercise tolerance, paroxysmal nocturnal dyspnea, peripheral edema) may be evaluated with echocardiography to determine resting left ventricular ejection fraction, wall motion score, and diastolic function. Furthermore, this type of information is very helpful in selecting therapeutic agents to improve an ischemic, dysfunctioning myocardium. Positive inotropic agents and preload and afterload therapy are very helpful in alleviating symptoms and may improve left ventricular ejection fraction and wall motion indices.

Evaluation of acute or chronic ischemic conditions may also be accomplished with 2-D echocardiography. Progressive worsening of ventricular segmental wall motion signals the possibility of acute, prolonged ischemia; 2-D imaging is important for staging patients prior to interventions such as thrombolytic therapy or percutaneous transluminal coronary angioplasty (PTCA) or for determining how extensive therapy should be. Certainly, patients with chronic ischemic conditions and very poor myocardial performance are less likely to benefit from thrombolytic therapy or PTCA. In contrast, patients with adequate left ventricular function and more viable myocardium at risk are more likely to benefit from thrombolytic therapy or PTCA.

Complications of myocardial infarction can be evaluated accurately with 2-D and Doppler-flow examinations. These techniques allow direct visualization of mitral valve regurgitation, ruptured interventricular septum, and left ventricular dysfunction. Color-flow Doppler imaging is particularly useful in quickly assessing the location and quantifying the extent of abnormal blood flow. Anatomic information may be obtained through direct visualization of the mitral valve and papillary muscle network. Patients with papillary muscle dysfunction usually show insignificant mitral regurgitation, but patients with papillary muscle rupture may show evidence of severe mitral regurgitation on Doppler examination and evidence of abnormal left ventricular performance consistent with acute ventricular volume overload.

Infarct expansion and extension are also serious short- and long-term consequences of myocardial infarction. (Infarct expansion is disproportionate thinning or dilatation of the infarct segment, which probably begins within hours of acute infarction and usually reaches a peak within 7 to 14 days.) Infarct expansion occurs in approximately 35 to 45% of patients with anterior transmural myocardial infarction, and less frequently with infarctions at other sites. The prognosis is poor, and patients generally have limited exercise tolerance, more congestive heart failure symptoms, and higher mortality rates, early and late, than those who do not suffer infarct expansion. Infarct extension, another serious complication of myocardial infarction, is reinfarction in an already infarcted area. Its prevalence in patients with myocardial infarction is approximately 20%, and these patients have a high incidence of congestive heart failure, arrhythmias, cardiogenic shock, and death. Recurrent myocardial infarction occurs in an area remote from the initial lesion in 10 to 20% of patients.

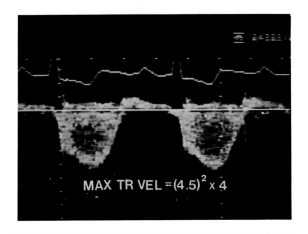

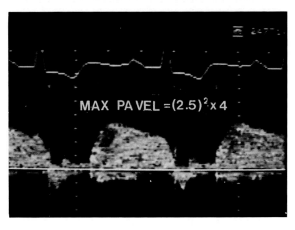

FIGURE 12-5. Calculation of right ventricular (RV) or pulmonary artery (PA) (without pulmonic stenosis) systolic pressure from continuous-wave Doppler tracing:
Maximum tricuspid regurgitation velocity (MAX TR VEL) = 4.5 m/s.
Transvalvular pressure gradient = $4(4.5)^2$ = mm Hg.
PA systolic pressure = $4 \times (4.5)^2$ + Right atrial pressure = 81 mm Hg + 20 mm Hg (approximately) = 101 mm Hg.
Numerical assignment of right atrial pressure (in millimeters of mercury) is subjective and based on chamber sizes of the right ventricle and right atrium and/or the presence of dilated inferior vena cava or jugular venous distention.[16]

FIGURE 12-6. Calculating pulmonary artery (PA) diastolic pressure from continuous-wave Doppler tracing.
Maximum pulmonary artery velocity at end diastole (MAX PA VEL) = 2.5 m/s
Transvalvular pressure gradient = $4 (2.5)^2$ = 25 mm Hg
PA diastolic pressure = 25 mm Hg + right atrial pressure = 25 mm Hg + 10 mm Hg = 35 mm Hg.
Numerical values of pressure (in millimeters of mercury) within the right atrium are subjective, based on the chamber size of the right ventricle and right atrium and presence of jugular venous or inferior vena cava distention.[16]

Therefore, the extent of myocardial necrosis is the principal determinant of prognosis.

In patients with myocardial infarction, additional information is provided by Doppler flow investigation, particularly pulsed-wave and continuous-wave studies. These techniques assess myocardial hemodynamics. The ability to accurately assign these values hinges on recording all the Doppler velocity envelopes (mitral, tricuspid, pulmonic, and aortic valve regurgitation). An example of Doppler derived pulmonary artery systolic pressure is seen in Figure 12-5. Additional information may be gained through assessment of the pulmonary artery diastolic pressure by observing the velocity shift at end-diastole on the pulmonic regurgitant velocity intergral[25] (Fig. 12-6). A V wave of

mitral regurgitation may be calculated from observing the velocity shift through the mitral valve (in systole) and subtracting this peak calculated pressure from the systolic blood pressure. We have found these formulas to be extremely useful for managing patients with changing hemodynamic abnormalities; they also help identify patients who require continuous monitoring via Swan-Ganz catheter.

Although the ECG is a sensitive indicator of myocardial abnormalities, it is not nearly as specific, so relying solely on them leads to errors in the diagnosis of ischemia and myocardial infarction. Echocardiography plays an important role in situations where patient history does not correlate with objective data (ECG, chest x-rays). Evaluation of such patients allows assessment of left ventricular wall motion and function. In addition, these patients infrequently have unrecognized cardiomyopathies that are discovered on echocardiographic investigation. Chest radiographs provide detailed information on pulmonary vasculature and heart size, although patients in heart failure may have a fairly normal-looking cardiac silhouette and very little evidence of pulmonary congestion. Again, assessment of such patients with 2-D echocardiography and Doppler-flow mapping provides ventricular wall motion analysis, ejection fractions, and important hemodynamic data. Blanke and coworkers[7] have shown that if ECG alone is used to identify patients for acute interventional therapy some who are candidates for interventions will be overlooked because of the low specificity of ECGs.

We are now in the era of thrombolytic therapy for acute myocardial infarction. Current estimates suggest that the administration of streptokinase or tissue plasminogen activator (tPA) should produce reperfusion in approximately 80% of patients. In two European studies now in progress it has been shown that thrombolytic treatment of acute myocardial infarction limits infarct size by 30%.[35] Left ventricular function is preserved and the 1-year survival rate is improved when patients admitted within 4 hours after the onset of symptoms are treated with intracoronary injection of streptokinase. At present, investigators believe that thrombolysis with such agents should be followed by early angioplasty or bypass surgery. Final data of ongoing studies in this area are not available at this time. It certainly appears, however, that systemic or intracoronary interventions with chemical agents followed by mechanical interventions such as PTCA or surgery early after acute ischemia decrease morbidity and mortality rates.

## Echocardiographic Abnormalities That Demonstrate Ischemic Changes and Complications of Myocardial Infarction

Two-dimensional echocardiography is an excellent technique for documenting both ischemic changes and complications of myocardial infarction. Although M-mode echocardiography continues to have a place in the investigation of these lesions,

its usefulness is limited owing to its poor spatial resolution. For this reason most of the illustrations in this section are from 2-D and Doppler-flow studies.

Echocardiography plays an important role in planning acute interventional treatment of myocardial ischemia. Data from the Timi study performed at the Mayo Clinic demonstrated evidence of reversibility of wall motion abnormalities following thrombolytic therapy or acute PTCA. These wall motion changes occurred as early as 72 hours and were best appreciated 10 days after therapy. Figure 12-7 illustrates abnormal anterior wall motion before therapy and evidence of acceptable motion with a normal left ventricular ejection fraction after therapy. Right ventricular myocardial infarction may occur in the presence of right coronary artery occlusion. Figure 12-8 reveals a right ventricular infarction showing evidence of right ventricular enlargement and poor wall motion. The patient also has evidence of an inferior myocardial wall infarction involving the left ventricle.

As Blanke and coworkers[7] noted, ECG alone does not provide evidence of diagnostic changes in all patients with unstable angina or acute myocardial infarction. Because of its ability to visualize wall motion in an acute process, echocardiography has proved useful in selecting patients for emergency interventional therapy. Figure 12-9 is an echocardiogram of a patient who had posterior wall myocardial infarction despite a normal resting ECG.

Serial echocardiographic studies are extremely useful and readily available for assessing complications of myocardial infarction. These complications include left ventricular aneurysm with left ventricular thrombus formation, rupture of the papillary muscle, and postinfarction ventricular septal defects. Likewise, postinfarction pericarditis with subsequent development of pericardial effusion is easily demonstrated. Doppler modalities, particularly color-flow and pulsed-wave imaging, permit the detection of atrioventricular valve regurgitations and monitoring of diastolic and systolic left ventricular function.

The most frequent complication of myocardial infarction visualized by echocardiography is left ventricular aneurysm. Most aneurysms occur at the apex and are therefore best seen from the apical or subcostal position. The most easily appreciated

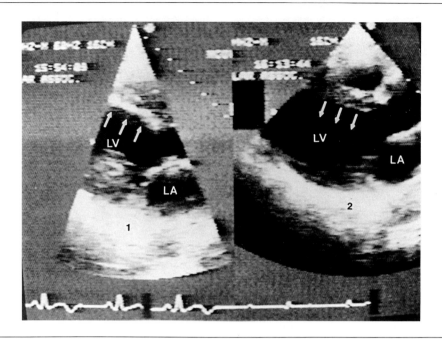

FIGURE 12-7. Split-screen 2-D parasternal long-axis views demonstrate dyskinesia of the anteroseptal wall in image 1. After therapy the anteroseptal wall shows improved motion with normal posterior motion during systole. (LV, left ventricle; LA, left atrium; AIVS, anterointerventricular septal wall.)

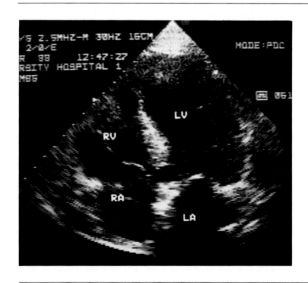

FIGURE 12-8. Two-dimensional apical four-chamber view demonstrates right ventricular enlargement and systolic fractional shortening consistent with right ventricular myocardial infarction. (RA, right atrium; RV, right ventricle; LV, left ventricle; LA, left atrium.)

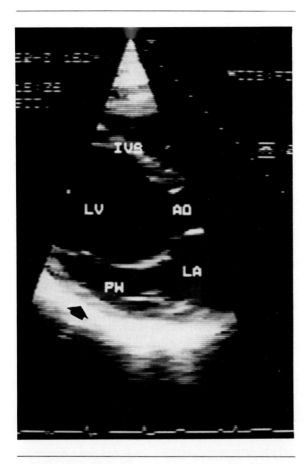

FIGURE 12-9. Parasternal long-axis view shows increased density of posterior wall (*arrow*) consistent with myocardial scarring. (IVS, interventricular septum; LV, left ventricle; AO, aorta; LA, left atrium; PW, posterior wall.)

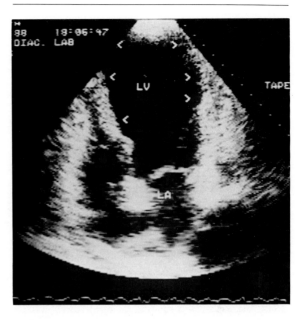

FIGURE 12-10. Apical four-chamber view shows large anteroapical aneurysm. No thrombus is present. (LV, left ventricle; LA, left atrium; arrowheads indicate systolic expansion.)

form of aneurysm is one in a well-demarcated apical segment showing dyskinesia or systolic expansion during ventricular systole (Fig. 12-10). Often akinesia rather than actual systolic expansion can be observed. Inferior and posterior aneurysms have been described, but they are less common than apical ones. When such aneurysms do occur, they can be demonstrated by parasternal long- or short-axis imaging (Fig.12-11). When left ventricular thrombus occurs, it is usually associated with anterior wall myocardial infarction and is positioned in the left ventricular apex. Clots have also been seen in

nonischemic ventricles (e.g., dilated cardiomyopathy), though they are less common.

Figure 12-12 shows evidence of a large apical thrombus. This particular patient had evidence of a cerebral vascular accident, and the thrombus was considered the probable source of that embolism. The ability to visualize a thrombus within the apex is critically dependent on the thrombus' size. A thrombus any smaller than 0.6 cm diameter[3] may be undetectable by 2-D scanning. Because the apex is the principal area for visualizing thrombus, artifacts also may complicate the picture. Certain features help distinguish true thrombi from artifacts: (1) Abnormal wall motion or evidence of aneurysm in this area is one. (2) A thrombus usually is not seen posterior to a bright reflector (e.g., chest wall reflector). (3) An ill-defined artifact (Fig. 12-13) usually moves quite mechanically with the apex of the heart. Generally, high-frequency transducers (i.e., 5 MHz with better near-field resolution) tend to overcome these problems. It must be remembered that a true thrombus is a well-defined structure that usually projects into the left ventric-

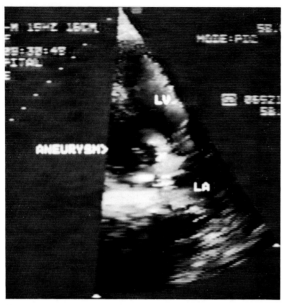

*A*

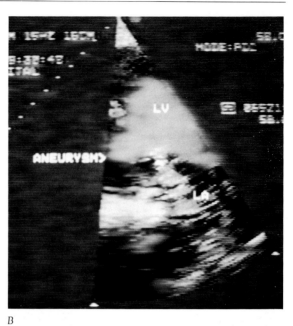

*B*

FIGURE 12-11. (See color insert.) (*A*) Parasternal long-axis view and (*B*) color-flow Doppler shows posteroinferior wall aneurysm. The abnormal flow into the aneurysm is displayed in blue. (LV, left ventricle; MV, mitral valve; LA, left atrium.)

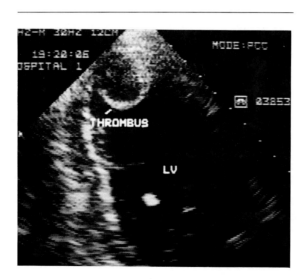

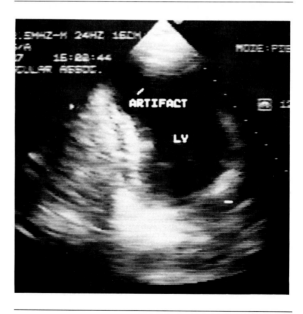

FIGURE 12-12. Zoom apical view shows large apical thrombus. (LV, left ventricle.)

FIGURE 12-13. Apical two-chamber view shows artifact at the apex. (LV, left ventricle.)

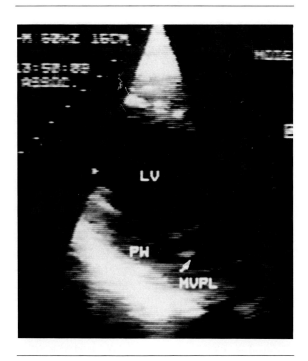

FIGURE 12-14. Parasternal long-axis view with flail posterior leaflet (MVPL). The LV is enlarged and the posterior wall appears thin. (LV, left ventricle; PW, posterior wall; MVPL, mitral valve posterior leaflet.)

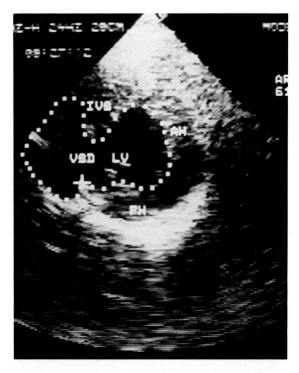

FIGURE 12-15. On this parasternal short-axis view there is evidence of a ruptured interventricular septum as a result of septal infarction. (IVS, interventricular septum; VSD, ventricular septal defect; LV, left ventricle.)

ular cavity. Embolization from an intracardiac thrombus is a significant cause of morbidity and mortality in patients recovering from myocardial infarction. The embolic potential of intracardiac thrombi has been evaluated, and it appears that the risk of embolization is greatest within the first 3 months after a thrombus forms. Therefore, anticoagulation is probably a reasonable treatment for these patients. The highest incidence of embolization is associated with thrombi that either protrude into the ventricular cavity or are mobile.

Rupture of the papillary muscle is an uncommon complication of myocardial infarction, but when it occurs, it is frequently a catastrophic event causing immediate clinical deterioration that progresses to pulmonary edema and shock. Heger and colleagues[21] found that 6 of 23 patients with acute myocardial infarction had either acute mitral regurgitation or complications of ventricular septal

rupture. The echocardiographic appearance of a ruptured papillary muscle is an atypical hypermobile, severely prolapsed mitral valve leaflet (Fig. 12-14) that clearly breaks the plane of the atrioventricular annulus. Doppler interrogation usually documents severe (4+) mitral regurgitation. A less serious complication of inferior wall myocardial infarction is papillary muscle dysfunction. Patients with this finding show abnormal closure of the mitral valve leaflets or restricted or retracted motion. Mitral regurgitation is usually mild.

Postinfarction ventricular septal defect also has been thoroughly described.[9,34] Patients so affected show evidence of abnormal systolic bulging of the interventricular septum with rupture (Fig. 12-15), commonly in the area of infarct, creating a left-to-right shunt. Doppler examination is extremely useful in the assessment of left-to-right shunting. Both color-flow and pulsed-wave Doppler examination allow identification of the level of the intracardiac shunt and provide a semiquantitative method of measuring the amount of flow by determining the cardiac output from the left and right ventricles. This is accomplished by measuring the velocity flow integral in the area of the aortic root annulus and computing the area of the outflow tract. Pulmonic flow is calculated in similar fashion. The ratio of pulmonic to systemic flow volume is then determined. Patients with Dressler's syndrome (post-myocardial infarction pericarditis) can also be evaluated with echocardiography. Typically they show evidence of a pericardial effusion, which can be followed serially to monitor for the possible development of cardiac tamponade. Pseudoaneurysms may be detected by 2-D echocardiography, although mortality rate after myocardial rupture is very high because of massive blood loss and illustrations of such are rare.

## Stress Echocardiography

Stress echocardiography is now a feasible modality for screening patients with suspected coronary artery disease. It also provides functional information on myocardial performance during exercise or immediately thereafter. Modern echocardiographic equipment has a 95% success rate for adequately visualizing the ventricular endocardium during or after exercise. By comparing resting wall motion or ejection fraction to exercise wall motion value or ejection fraction an assessment may be made in diagnosing the presence of obstructive coronary artery disease. A number of forms of stress testing have been devised, including upright and supine bicycle pedaling,[10] treadmill,[4] dipyridamole testing,[16] and atrial pacing.[13] It has been demonstrated that stress echocardiography is as accurate as thallium chloride scintillation scanning in diagnosing ischemic heart disease. In patients with prior myocardial infarction, Feigenbaum and associates[3] demonstrated the sensitivity of stress echocardiography to be 100% for detecting single-vessel disease and 97% for multivessel disease. For patients without prior myocardial infarction, the sensitivities are 90% for multivessel disease and approximately 75%

for single-vessel disease. Consequently, the majority of false negative results occur in studies of patients with single–coronary artery disease without prior myocardial infarction. Many studies validate this observation[5,27] At our institution, we have undertaken the task of comparing results of stress echocardiography with those of single-photon emission computed tomographic (SPECT) thallium scanning and coronary angiography (when performed). The patient is imaged at rest, with parasternal long-axis and short-axis and apical two-chamber and four-chamber views in the left lateral decubitus position. During this study a mark is placed on the precordium to allow the examination plane to be reproduced. Then the heart is imaged immediately after exercise, usually within 30 seconds after the patient steps down from the treadmill repeating the resting imaging planes. The data are entered into an off-line computer (Digisonics) with which we produce a quad screen format to analyze and compare the images taken at rest to those made after exercise. Wall motion and fractional shortening or ejection fraction are analyzed throughout diastole and systole, and the images are stored on floppy disk.

Thus far we have compared information gained from stress echocardiography and SPECT scanning to cardiac catheterization in 46 patients. The data so far reveal that the sensitivity and specificity of echocardiography in comparison to cardiac catheterization data are 85 and 95%, respectively. This makes the predictive value of a positive test 95%. Results of echocardiography agree with those of SPECT thallium scanning 85% of the time. The specificity and sensitivity of SPECT thallium scanning are approximately 80 and 95%, respectively, so the data show that stress echocardiography is a valuable adjunctive technique for screening selected patients suspected of having coronary artery disease.

## Future Directions

Investigators are exploring the possibility of expanding the applications of echocardiography to tissue characterization and myocardial perfusion determinations. The purpose of tissue characterization is to study the acoustic properties of the myocardium. Sophisticated techniques analyze reflected ultrasound frequencies and assign different radio frequency values to tissues involved by acute and chronic ischemia. This investigational area holds great promise. Myocardial perfusion determination through contrast echocardiography is an exciting area that allows visualization of normally perfused myocardium and poorly perfused myocardium. With computer analysis of time intensity curves, an estimate of coronary flow can be obtained.[20] The material used in this technique is sonicated radiographic contrast material or specially prepared albumin microbubbles (microcavitation). The contrast medium injected into the aortic root or infused into the coronary artery via catheters increases the sonodensity of the myocardium. The absence of contrast implies significant coronary atherosclerotic disease, whereas a uniformly bright, dense myocardium implies normal myocardial perfusion. This technique is still investigational, but numerous reports,[2,18] allude to its clinical usefulness in studying collateral flow distribution prior to PTCA procedures.

## Summary

Two-dimensional and Doppler echocardiography play essential roles in the evaluation of patients with known or suspected coronary artery disease. The 2-D examination allows immediate evaluation of abnormal anatomy and physiology, provides prognostic indicators, and helps the practitioner select appropriate therapeutic agents to improve myocardial performance. Serial examinations are used to evaluate the effects of therapy on hemodynamics and myocardial performance. Detection of complications of myocardial infarction such as thrombus formation, valvular dysfunction, aneurysm, ventricular failure, and infarct expansion or extension are also possible. Exercise echocardiography not only reveals the presence of coronary artery disease but is also useful for evaluating myocardial performance with exercise. Newer applications of echocardiography—tissue characterization and myocardial perfusion—and of Doppler techniques—left ventricular diastolic and systolic function parameters—may have a substantial impact on the clinical management of CAD patients in the near future.

## Acknowledgment

The authors wish to thank Rebecca Weathers, who created the line illustrations for this chapter.

## References

1. Alyusuf AR, Bhatnagar SK, Moussa MA. The role of prehospital discharge two-dimensional echocardiography in determining the prognosis of survivors in first myocardial infarction. Am Heart J. 1985; 109:472–477.
2. Armstrong WF, Dillon JC, Feigenbaum H. Assessment of myocardial perfusion using contrast-enhanced echocardiography: Initial human experience (abstr). Clin Res. 1985; 33:166A.
3. Armstrong WF, Feigenbaum H, O'Donnell T. Exercise echocardiography: Effect of prior myocardial infarction and extent of coronary disease on accuracy of exercise echocardiography. J Am Coll Cardiol. 1987; 10:531–538.
4. Armstrong WF, Feigenbaum H, Robertson WS, et al. Exercise echocardiography: A clinically practical addition in the evaluation of coronary artery disease. J Am Coll Cardiol. 1983; 2:1085–1091.
5. Armstrong WF, Vasey CG, West SR, et al. Comparison of continuous loop exercise echocardiography and thallium scintigraphy for detection of coronary artery disease (abstr). Circulation. 1985; 72 (suppl 3):III–58.
6. Bishop HL, Gibson RS, Stamm RB, et al. Value of early two-dimensional echocardiography in patients with acute myocardial infarction. Am J Cardiol. 1982; 49:1110–1119.
7. Blanke H, Cohen M, Schlueter GU, et al. Electrocardiographic and coronary arteriographic correlations during acute myocardial infarction. Am J Cardiol. 1984; 54:249–255.
8. Bonow RO, Maron BJ, Spirito P. Non-invasive assessment of left ventricular diastolic function: Comparative analysis of Doppler echocardiography and digitized M-mode echocardiography. Am J Cardiol. 1986; 58:837–843.
9. Borsante L, Farcot JC, Rigaud M, et al. Two-dimensional echocardiographic visualization of ventricular septal rupture after acute anterior myocardial infarction. Am J Cardiol. 1980; 45:370–377.
10. Brizendine M, Conant R, Ginzton LE, et al. Exercise subcostal two-dimensional echocardiography: A new method of segmental wall motion analysis. Am J Cardiol. 1984; 53:805–811.
11. Chang S, Feigenbaum H, Konecke LL, et al. Abnormal mitral valve motion in patients with elevated left

ventricular diastolic pressures. Circulation. 1973; 47:989–996.

12. Channer KS, Culling W, Wilde P, et al. Estimation of left ventricular end-diastolic pressure by pulsed Doppler ultrasound. Lancet. 1986; 1:1005–1006.

13. Chapman PD, Doyle TP, Troup PJ, et al. Stress echocardiography with transesophageal atrial pacing: Preliminary report of a new method for detection of ischemic wall motion abnormalities. Circulation. 1984; 70:445–450.

14. Cleman M, Highman HA, Wohlgelernter D, et al. Regional myocardial dysfunction during coronary angioplasty: Evaluation by two-dimensional echocardiography and 12-lead electrocardiography. J Am Coll Cardiol. 1986; 7:1245–1254.

15. Collins SM, Nichols J, Skorton DJ, et al. Quantitative texture analysis in two-dimensional echocardiography: Application to diagnosis of experimental myocardium contusion. Circulation. 1983; 68:217–223.

16. Disante A, Picano E, Masini M, et al. Dipyridamole-echocardiography test in effort angina pectoris. Am J Cardiol. 1985; 56:452–456.

17. Ellis SC, Henschke CI, Sandor T, et al. Relation between the transmural extent of acute myocardial infarction and associated myocardial contractility two weeks after infarction. Am J Cardiol. 1985; 55:1412–1416.

18. Feinstein SB, Feldman T., Lang RM, et al. Contrast echocardiography for evaluation of myocardial perfusion: Effects of coronary angioplasty. J Am Coll Cardiol. 1986; 8:232–235.

19. Feldman CL, Moynihan PF, Paris AF. Quantitative detection of regional left ventricular contraction abnormalities by two-dimensional echocardiography: I. Analysis of methods. Circulation. 1981; 63:752–760.

20. Force T, Kember AJ, Kloner R, et al. Contrast echocardiographic estimation of regional myocardial blood flow after acute coronary occlusion. Circulation. 1985; 72:1115–1124.

21. Heger J, Noble R, Weyman AE, et al. An analysis of site, extent and hemodynamic consequences of acute myocardial infarction by cross-sectional echocardiography (abstr). Circulation. 1977; 56(suppl 3):III-152.

22. Heger JJ, Wann LS, Weyman AE, et al. Cross-sectional echocardiographic analysis of the extent of left ventricular asynergy in acute myocardial infarction. Circulation. 1980; 61:1113–1118.

23. Horowitz RS, Morganroth J. Immediate detection of early high-risk patients with acute myocardial infarction using two-dimensional echocardiographic evaluation of left ventricular regional wall motion abnormalities. Am Heart J. 1982; 103:814–822.

24. Jugdutt BI, Liegerman AN, Weiss JL, et al. Two-dimensional echocardiography and infarct size: Relationship of regional wall motion and thickening to the extent of myocardial infarction in the dog. Circulation. 1981; 63:739–746.

25. Kitabatake A, Kodama K, Masuyama T, et al. Continuous-wave Doppler echocardiographic detection of pulmonary regurgitation and its application to non-invasive estimation of pulmonary artery pressure. Circulation. 1986; 74:484–492.

26. Knoebel SB, Lovelace DE, Rasmussen S, et al. Echocardiographic detection of ischemic and infarcted myocardium. J Am Coll Cardiol. 1984; 3:733–743.

27. Limachen MC, Poliner LR, Quinones MA, et al. Detection of coronary artery disease with exercise two-dimensional echocardiography. Circulation. 1983; 67:1211–1218.

28. Massie BM, Ratshin RA, Schiller NB, et al. Mitral-septal separation: New echocardiographic index of left ventricular function. Am J Cardiol. 1977; 39:1008.

29. Miller FA, Nishimura RA, Reeder GS, et al. Prognostic value of predischarge two-dimensional echocardiogram after acute myocardial infarction. Am J Cardiol. 1984; 53:429–432.

30. Miller JG, Mimbs JW, Yuhas DE, et al. Detection of myocardial infarction in vitro based on altered attenuation of ultrasound. Circ Res. 1977; 41:192–198.

31. Nishimura RA, Shub C, Tajik AJ, et al. Role of two-dimensional echocardiography in the prediction of in hospital complications after acute myocardial infarction. J Am Coll Cardiol. 1984; 4:1080–1087.

32. Quinones MA, Reduto LA, Waggoner AD, et al. A new, simplified and accurate method for determining ejection fraction with two-dimensional echocardiography. Circulation. 1981; 64:744.

33. Saito T. Non-invasive assessment of left ventricular function and prognosis in acute myocardial infarction: Clinical significance of B-"B" step of the mitral valve in M-mode echocardiography. Jpn Circ J. 1982; 46:1045–1049.

34. Scanlon JG, Seward JB, Tajik AJ. Visualization of ventricular septal rupture utilizing wide-angle two-dimensional echocardiography. Mayo Clin Proc. 1979; 54:381.

35. Serruys PW, Simoons ML, Vandenbrand M, et al. Early thrombolysis in acute myocardial infarction: Limitation of infarct size and improved survival. J Am Coll Cardiol. 1986; 7:717–728.

36. Vatner SF. Correlation between acute reductions in myocardial blood flow and function in conscious dogs. Circ Res. 1980; 47:201–207.

# CHAPTER 13

# Pericardial Disease

RAMESH C. BANSAL, MARIE DE LANGE, HOLLY RACKER

The normal pericardium is composed of an outer fibrous layer and an inner layer of serous membrane. The inner serous membrane consists of a single layer of mesothelial cells and is in intimate contact with the myocardium and epicardial fat to form the visceral pericardium, or epicardium. The epicardium extends a short distance over the great vessels and then reflects back on itself to line the outer fibrous layer and form the parietal pericardium. The space between the serosal surfaces of visceral and parietal pericardia is the pericardial cavity, which normally contains up to 20 ml of clear fluid. Under pathologic states, collection of an abnormal quantity of fluid in this potential space causes pericardial effusion. Behind the left atrium as the visceral pericardium is reflected from the back of the left atrium onto the pulmonary veins, a recess called the oblique sinus of the pericardium is formed. Under special circumstances, pericardial fluid may accumulate in this oblique sinus. Another similar recess, called the transverse sinus, lies posterior to the great arteries and anterior to the atria and superior vena cava. The fibrous parietal pericardium has ligamentous attachments anteriorly to the sternum, posteriorly to the vertebral column, and inferiorly to the diaphragm.[28,37] The normal pericardium may play a role in (1) fixing the heart to avoid excessive motion; (2) preventing spread of infection and malignancy from contiguous structures; (3) preventing cardiac distension under volume-loading states; and (4) the phenomenon of diastolic ventricular interdependence (i.e., distension of one ventricle affects the distensibility of the other).

If an excessive quantity of fluid collects in the pericardial space, pericardial effusion develops. Accumulation of pericardial fluid under pressure limits filling of the heart during diastole and causes cardiac tamponade. Fibrosis, thickening, and eventually calcification may lead to fusion of the visceral and parietal layers of pericardium and restriction of diastolic filling of the heart, as is seen in constrictive pericarditis. In this chapter we discuss briefly the causes, pathophysiology, and clinical findings of the various disorders of the pericardium and emphasize the uses, limitations, and pitfalls of echocardiography in the evaluation of such problems. A few comments will be made about the rare anomalies of congenital absence of the pericardium and pericardial cysts.

## Pericardial Effusion

A variety of disorders may cause an excess of pericardial fluid to accumulate and cause pericardial effusion; the condition can also be idiopathic, or primary.

## Causes of Pericardial Effusion

A. Idiopathic or primary
B. Infection
   1. Viruses: Coxsackieviruses A and B, echoviruses, adenoviruses, mumps, varicella, hepatitis B, and Epstein-Barr virus
   2. Bacteria: *Staphylococcus, Streptococcus, Pneumococcus, Meningococcus, Gonococcus,* and *Legionella* species
   3. Mycobacteria: Tuberculosis
   4. Fungi: Coccidioidomycosis, histoplasmosis, candidiasis, and blastomyocosis
   5. Parasites: Amebiasis, echinococcosis, toxoplasmosis
   6. Spirochetes: Lyme disease
C. Congestive heart failure
D. Acute myocardial infarction
E. Uremia
F. Connective tissue and autoimmune disorders
   1. Systemic lupus erythematosus
   2. Rheumatoid arthritis
   3. Periarteritis nodosa
   4. Scleroderma
   5. Acute rheumatic fever
   6. Postmyocardial infarction syndrome or Dressler's syndrome
   7. Postpericardiotomy syndrome
G. Metastatic neoplasms
   1. Lung cancer
   2. Breast cancer
   3. Leukemia, lymphoma, melanoma, etc.
H. Chest trauma
 I. Mediastinal irradiation
J. Dissecting aortic aneurysm
K. Chylopericardium
L. Myxedema

## Clinical Features

Small pericardial effusion or slowly accumulating large effusions without elevation of intrapericardial pressure usually produce no symptoms. They are usually discovered when a routine chest radiograph demonstrates an unexpectedly large cardiac silhouette. If the pericardial effusion is due to pericarditis, typical clinical features of acute pericarditis develop—pleuropericarditic chest pain (retrosternal pain that increases with coughing and breathing and is relieved by sitting up), cough, dyspnea, and fever. The physical findings depend on the cause and quantity of the effusion, and on how rapidly it accumulates in the pericardium. Three-component pericardial friction rub is the classic finding in acute pericarditis. Large pericardial effusions may muffle the heart sounds and cause compression of the left lower lobe of the lung, producing an area of dullness to percussion, or positive Ewart's sign.

## Diagnostic Tests

*Electrocardiography.* The ECG shows diffuse ST segment elevation with an upward concave contour in acute pericarditis. Several days later ST changes return to normal and are followed by T-wave inversion. In a large pericardial effusion, QRS voltage may be reduced.

*Radiography.* Chest films may reveal an enlarged cardiac silhouette, but the heart size may appear normal when the volume of pericardial fluid is less than 250 ml.

*Echocardiography.* Prior to the development of echocardiography, the clinical diagnosis of pericardial effusion was often difficult and imprecise. Edler first reported on the use of echocardiography in the detection of pericardial effusion in the 1950s.[12] In the mid 1960s, Feigenbaum and associates[15-17] established echocardiography as the procedure of choice in the diagnosis and follow-up of patients with pericardial effusion.

M-mode echocardiography is adequate for the diagnosis of pericardial effusion in the majority of patients. Two-dimensional (2-D) echocardiography provides additional help when the findings on M-mode echocardiogram are confusing or uncertain. Proper recording techniques are extremely important for detecting pericardial effusion. The patient is placed in the left lateral decubitus position, and the trunk is elevated 20 to 30 degrees to encourage redistribution of pericardial fluid toward the apex. M-mode sweep is then performed from the left ventricular apex to the aortic root. Clear recording of the anterior right ventricular wall and of the left ventricular posterior wall is obtained by careful adjustment of the gain, reject, and damping controls. All components of the posterior left ventricular wall (endocardium, epicardium, parietal pericardium) are identified by careful adjustment of the gain control. The intensity of the recording is grad-

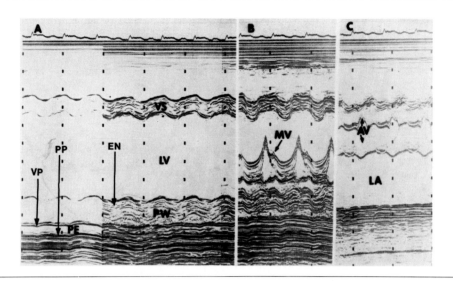

FIGURE 13-1. M-mode echocardiogram from a patient with myocarditis and a small pericardial effusion. (A) A nondilated left ventricle (LV) is producing poor contractions. A small sonolucent space noted behind the posterior LV wall represents a small pericardial effusion (PE). The overall gain was gradually reduced to visualize the parietal pericardium (PP), pericardial effusion, visceral pericardium (VP). The gain was then gradually increased to record the endocardium (EN) of the posterior left ventricular wall (PW). (B) Mitral valve (MV). (C) Systolic convergence of the aortic valve (AV) is due to poor cardiac output. There is no fluid behind the left atrium (LA). Calibration marks are 1 cm apart.

ually reduced to optimize the strong posterior pericardial echo, which normally moves anteriorly during systole. After the parietal pericardium is defined, the intensity is increased gradually to record epicardial and endocardial echoes (Fig. 13-1). In current practice, these M-mode scans are obtained quickly by moving the M-mode cursor line through the 2-D image from parasternal long- or short-axis position. Normal epicardium and parietal pericardium are apposed throughout most of the cardiac cycle, so only a potential space is available for accumulation of fluid. Occasionally, in normal subjects, a small sonolucent space may appear between the chest wall and the anterior right ventricular wall; this is believed to represent epicardial fat. Minimal separation of the two layers of pericardium posteriorly only during systole is not considered to be pathologic and probably represents normal pericardial fluid.

The echocardiographic hallmarks of pericardial effusion are the presence of a sonolucent space posterior to the heart and absence of motion of the parietal pericardium. The pericardial fluid appears first in the region of the posterior atrioventricular groove, the most dependent portion of the pericardial cavity. Two-dimensional echocardiography also reveals that some collection of fluid around the right atrium is not uncommon, even with small effusions. The parietal pericardium becomes motionless in the presence of pericardial effusion because the fluid acts as an insulator and minimizes transmission of posterior left ventricular wall motion to the pericardium. Precise quantitation of pericardial fluid volume is not extremely accurate; most laboratories[15,37] describe effusions as trivial, small, medium, and large. With a trivial pericardial effusion there is a slight sonolucent space between the posterior wall epicardium and the parietal peri-

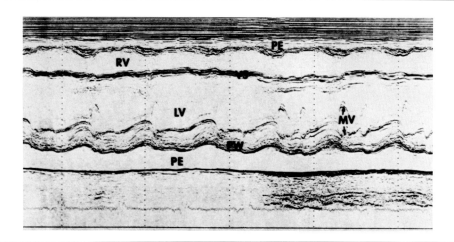

Figure 13-2. M-mode echocardiogram from a patient with anteroseptal myocardial infarction and Dressler's syndrome shows a moderately large pericardial effusion (PE). A small anterior sonolucent space in front of the right ventricle (RV) and a moderately large posterior sonolucent space behind the posterior left ventricular wall represent a moderately large pericardial effusion. Note the lack of motion of the parietal pericardium. Ventricular septum (VS) is thin, dense, and akinetic, owing to infarction. Calibration marks are 0.5 cm apart. (LV, left ventricle; PW, posterior wall; MV, mitral valve.)

cardium throughout systole and part of diastole. A small posterior sonolucent space visible throughout systole and diastole indicates the presence of a small effusion (Fig. 13-1). With moderate pericardial effusion there is a moderate posterior sonolucent space and a trivial anterior one (Fig. 13-2). With large effusions the anterior and posterior echofree spaces enlarge further and the fluid may appear behind the left atrium in the oblique sinus (Fig. 13-3). With the large anterior and posterior pericardial effusions, the heart may move freely within the pericardial cavity.[17] This type of motion tends to occur in large effusions associated with malignant neoplasms and has been called swinging heart syndrome (Fig. 13-3). The heart is suspended by the great vessels and swings freely within the pericardial cavity, causing the anterior and posterior walls of the heart to move synchronously (anteriorly during systole and posteriorly during diastole, or vice versa). The swinging may cause the phenomenon of electrical alternans. As the heart swings forward during systole, abnormal anterior motion of the septum and pseudosystolic anterior motion (SAM) of the mitral valve may be recorded.[6] As the heart swings backward, pseudomitral and tricuspid valve prolapse motion patterns may be recorded (see Fig. 13-3).

*Apparent motion pattern in swinging heart syndrome*
1. Systolic anterior motion of the mitral valve (SAM)
2. Apparent mitral valve prolapse
3. Apparent tricuspid valve prolapse
4. Paradoxical motion of ventricular septum
5. Midsystolic closure of aortic valve
6. Midsystolic notch of the pulmonic valve.

The echocardiographer must be familiar with the technical and anatomic pitfalls in the diagnosis of pericardial effusion. Most false positive and false negative results of echocardiographic studies are due to faulty technique, but some entities are difficult and confusing to evaluate sonographically.

*Pitfalls in the diagnosis of pericardial effusion*
A. Technical errors
    1. Gain setting too high or too low
    2. Excessive medial angulation of the transducer

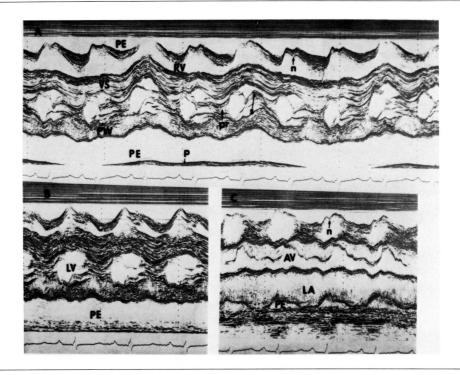

FIGURE 13-3. M-mode echocardiogram from a patient with a large pericardial effusion and swinging heart. (A) Large echo-free spaces in front of the right ventricular wall and posterior to the left ventricular wall indicate a large effusion. Normal thickness of the parietal pericardium (P) is noted. The tracing shows the swinging motion pattern of the entire heart. During the anterior swing, there is pseudosystolic (s) anterior motion of the mitral valve. When the heart swings posteriorly, pseudoprolapse (pr) of the mitral valve is noted. Abnormal septal motion due to swing is also clearly visible. The anterior right ventricular wall is hyperkinetic and shows a notch (n) during the isometric contraction phase, a sign of cardiac tamponade. (B) When the subject holds the breath the swinging motion is lost. (C) On the M-mode echocardiogram of the aortic valve a small sonolucent space is noted behind the left atrium, which indicates collection of pericardial fluid in the oblique sinus. Calibration marks are 0.5 cm apart. (VS, ventricular septum; PW, posterior wall; PE, pericardial effusion; RV, right ventricle.)

B. Structures that mimic pericardial effusion
   1. Left pleural effusion
   2. Mitral annulus calcification
   3. Descending thoracic aorta
   4. Dilated coronary sinus
   5. Giant left atrium
   6. Left ventricular pseudoaneurysm
   7. Foramen of Morgagni hernia
   8. Hiatus hernia
   9. Pericardial cyst
   10. Epicardial fat.

High gain settings can obscure a sonolucent space and produce a false negative result. Excessive medial angulation of the transducer from a parasternal recording position may image the coronary sinus, pulmonary vein, or other mediastinal structures and produce a misdiagnosis of effusion. Vari-

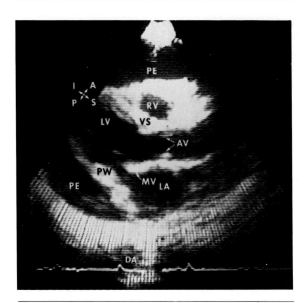

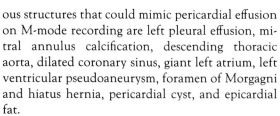

FIGURE 13-4. Parasternal long-axis view of the 2-D echocardiogram from a patient with a large pericardial effusion (PE). A large sonolucent space is noted anterior to the right ventricle (RV) and posterior to the left ventricle (LV), indicating a large pericardial effusion. The heart is suspended by the great arteries in this large effusion and shows a swinging motion pattern on real-time imaging. The descending thoracic aorta (DA) is imaged in its short axis and is displaced posteriorly by this large pericardial effusion. (This does not happen with pleural effusion.) (A, anterior; I, inferior; P, posterior; S, superior; PW, posterior wall; VS, ventricular septum; MV, mitral valve; AV, aortic valve; MV, mitral valve; LA, left atrium.)

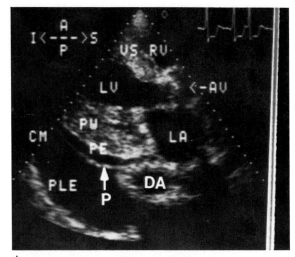

A

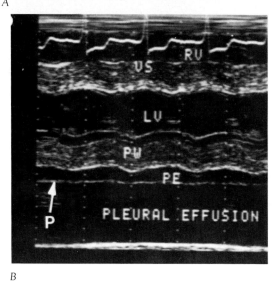

B

FIGURE 13-5. Two-dimensional parasternal long-axis (A) and M-mode (B) echocardiograms from a patient with severe aortic stenosis, left ventricular hypertrophy, a small pericardial effusion (PE), and a large left pleural effusion (PLE). Normal thickness of parietal pericardium (P) is clearly seen, both on 2-D and M-mode studies. The parietal pericardium is sandwiched between a small pericardial effusion and a large pleural effusion. The descending thoracic aorta (DA) is behind the small pericardial effusion but anterior to the pleural effusion. This sign is helpful in differentiating pericardial from pleural effusions.

ous structures that could mimic pericardial effusion on M-mode recording are left pleural effusion, mitral annulus calcification, descending thoracic aorta, dilated coronary sinus, giant left atrium, left ventricular pseudoaneurysm, foramen of Morgagni and hiatus hernia, pericardial cyst, and epicardial fat.

Continuous M-mode sweep from the left ventricular apex to the base of the heart directed cephalad shows that the pericardial effusion gradually disappears at the level of the atrioventricular groove whereas pleural effusion will extend behind

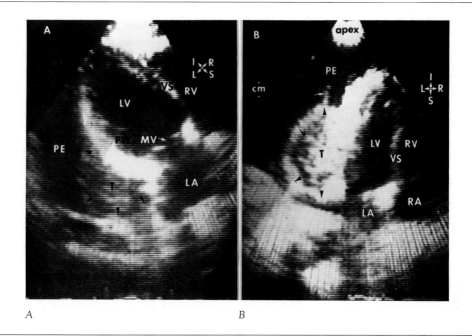

*A*    *B*

FIGURE 13-6. Two-dimensional subcostal four-chamber view (A) and apical four-chamber view (B) show a large pericardial effusion (PE) and a big tumor mass (T) in the pericardial effusion. A few fibrinous strands (*arrow*) project from the surface of the tumor mass in this patient with history of breast carcinoma. (RA, right atrium; R, right; L, left; I, inferior; S, superior; LV, left ventricle; PW, posterior wall; VS, ventricular septum; MV, mitral valve; RV, right ventricle; LA, left atrium.)

the left atrium. Also a large posterior collection of fluid without an anterior sonolucent space is more likely to be pleural in origin. Two-dimensional echocardiography helps tremendously in achieving more precise and accurate diagnosis of pericardial effusion and in differentiating it from left pleural effusion and from other anatomic structures (Fig. 13-4). Normally, the descending thoracic aorta is imaged in its short axis, behind the posterior atrioventricular groove from the parasternal long-axis view. Most large pericardial effusions cause posterior displacement of the descending thoracic aorta, but this posterior displacement is not seen with pleural effusion (Fig. 13-5).

Two-dimensional echocardiography provides better spatial orientation and helps in the diagnosis of anterior and posterior loculated effusions, which sometimes occur after open heart surgery. By im-

aging multiple tomographic sections, the operator can get a precise idea of the distribution of pericardial fluid[29] and of the safest approach (apical, subcostal, parasternal) for pericardiocentesis.[5] Two-dimensional echocardiography can reveal metastatic lesions and "fibrinous strands" in the pericardial fluid (Fig. 13-6). Some investigators find 2-D echocardiography uesful in positioning the needle[6] or pigtail catheter in the pericardial sac[5] during pericardiocentesis. After the needle is placed in the pericardial fluid, 5 to 10 ml of saline solution can be injected through the needle, and the appearance of microbubbles in the pericardium confirms correct positioning of the needle. Two-dimensional echocardiography also helps identify loculation and extensive adhesions; pericardiocentesis should be avoided in these patients because of the high risk of complications.

## Cardiac Tamponade

There is no satisfactory definition of cardiac tamponade, which probably should be defined in hemodynamic and clinical terms. Cardiac tamponade is an abnormal hemodynamic state resulting from impaired diastolic filling of the heart due to collection of pericardial fluid under pressure.[31] The hemodynamic spectrum of tamponade varies from minimal hemodynamic abnormality to severe hypotension and collapse. In early or mild, and even in moderate tamponade of gradual onset, the abnormality may be limited to abnormal hemodynamics and classic clinical signs of tamponade may be absent. In severe tamponade the clinical signs become apparent.

PATHOPHYSIOLOGY

The normal intrapericardial and intrapleural pressures are very closely related. The mean intrapericardial pressure is 0 mm Hg, and it drops during inspiration to $-2$ to $-3$ mm Hg and increases during expiration up to 5 mm Hg.[30] The intrapericardial pressure increases slightly during the atrial contraction and slow-filling phase, and decreases during ventricular systole or ejection and rapid-filling phase.[30] The pericardial space normally contains approximately 20 ml of fluid and accumulation of excessive quantities of fluid may lead to an elevation of intrapericardial pressure. The degree of intrapericardial pressure elevation depends on the rapidity of fluid accumulation, the quantity of fluid, the compliance of the pericardium, and the size of the heart.[28] In a normal unstretched pericardium, if 150 ml of fluid is added precipitously, intrapericardial pressure rises markedly. On the other hand, if the fluid accumulates slowly, the pericardium stretches and becomes more compliant and is able to accommodate up to 1 L of fluid without significant elevation of intrapericardial pressure (IPP). Normal intracardiac pressures are as follows: right atrial (RA) mean pressure, 5 mm Hg or less; right ventricular end-diastolic pressure (RVEDP), 5 mm Hg or less; left atrial (LA) mean pressure or pulmonary artery wedge (PAW), 12 mm Hg or less; left ventricular end-diastolic pressure (LVEDP), 12 mm Hg or less. As the fluid accumulates in the pericardial sac, the intrapericardial pressure rises and becomes equal to right atrial and right ventricular end-diastolic pressure. This rise in intrapericardial pressure can cause collapse of the right atrium at end-diastole and during early ventricular systole, when right atrial volume is at its lowest. Right ventricular collapse occurs during early diastole, when right ventricular volume and pressure are at their lowest.

Further accumulation of fluid elevates the intrapericardial pressure to the level of LA and LVEDP. At this stage it is in the range of 10 to 15 mm Hg, and diastolic filling is impaired in all four cardiac chambers. Left atrial collapse may develop at this stage. Systemic venous pressure will be elevated, left ventricular stroke volume decreased, and systemic blood pressure decreased during inspiration more than 10% below that during expiration (pulsus paradoxus). If the intrapericardial pressure keeps rising, eventually there will be hypotension, shock, and hemodynamic collapse. Thus, in mild to moderate hemodynamic tamponade, the intrapericardial pressure is elevated abnormally owing to accumulation of pericardial fluid (5 to 10 mm Hg) and is equal to right atrial and right ventricular end-diastolic pressure. In moderately severe tamponade intrapericardial pressure is 10 to 15 mm Hg and in severe tamponade it is more than 15 to 20 mm Hg. Features of moderate to severe tamponade are as follows:

1. Abnormal accumulation of pericardial fluid
2. Near equalization of diastolic intracardiac pressures so that IPP = RA = RVEDP = PAW = LA = LVEDP
3. Decreased stroke volume and pulsus paradoxus.

CAUSES

Acute cardiac tamponade may develop after cardiac trauma and intrapericardial bleeding; the subacute form may develop in association with almost any cause of pericarditis.

Causes of acute or subacute pericardial effusion that can lead to tamponade are malignant neoplasm, idiopathic pericarditis, uremic pericarditis, bacterial pericarditis, systemic lupus erythematosus, tuberculous pericarditis, myxedema, radiation, and postpericardiotomy syndrome. Intrapericardial bleeding, another precipitant of cardiac tamponade, can result from dissecting aortic aneurysm (type A), anticoagulant therapy for acute myocardial infarction, myocardial rupture, and cardiac surgery. Tamponade can also be a sequela of trauma to the heart, penetrating (knife blade, ice

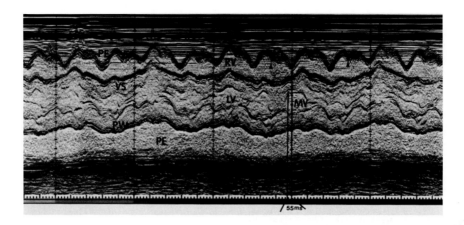

FIGURE 13-7. M-mode echocardiogram from a patient with cardiac tamponade shows swinging heart motion pattern, right ventricular epicardial notch (*arrowhead*) during the isometric contraction phase, and right ventricular collapse during early diastole. Note that the anterior right ventricular wall continues to move downward during early diastole, even after the mitral valve (MV) opens for 55 msec after the E point, which suggests presence of early diastolic right ventricular (RV) compression and tamponade. (PE, pericardial effusion; VS, ventricular septum; PW, posterior wall; LV, left ventricle; MV, mitral valve; ms, milliseconds.)

pick, bullet, cardiac catheterization, or pacemaker placement) or blunt (steering wheel contusion or severe blow to the chest).

### CLINICAL FEATURES

The classic Beck's triad—increased venous pressure, decreased systemic blood pressure, and quiet heart—occurs in acute tamponade due to intrapericardial bleeding. The symptoms and physical findings in more slowly developing tamponade depend on the cause and hemodynamic stage of tamponade. The findings are further modified in rare situations of low-pressure and regional, or localized, tamponade.[28] The common symptoms include dyspnea, chest pain, and fatigue. The physical findings in moderately severe hemodynamic tamponade include elevated jugular venous pressure, pulsus paradoxus, pericardial friction rub, heart sounds of decreased intensity, tachycardia, tachypnea, and hypotension.

### DIAGNOSTIC TESTS

*Electrocardiography.* The ECG may show ST abnormalities such as those seen in pericarditis. Electrical alternans of QRS complexes in the presence of pericardial effusion is a reliable indicator of tamponade. Total electrical alternans of P, QRS, and T waves is rare and is specific for extreme tamponade.

*Radiography.* The chest films may show enlargement of the heart with clear lung fields. Fluoroscopy shows decreased cardiac pulsations.

*Cardiac Catheterization.* The hemodynamic findings depend on the stage of tamponade and are described in the section on pathophysiology of tamponade.

*Echocardiography.* A variety of M-mode, 2-D, and Doppler echocardiographic findings have been reported in tamponade.[3,4,8,9,14,17,20,33,34,36,37,39]

Vignola and coworkers[39] described a notch on the epicardial surface of the right ventricle during isometric contraction and also noted coarse oscillations of the left ventricular posterior wall in patients with cardiac tamponade (Fig. 13-7). These observations were not confirmed by other studies.

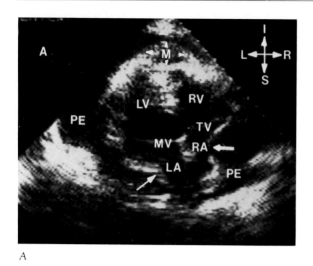

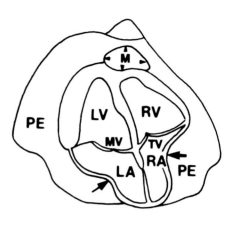

A                                                                    B

FIGURE 13-8. Two-dimensional apical four-chamber view (A) and a corresponding schematic diagram (B) show a large pericardial effusion (PE) and a tumor mass (M) in a patient with lung carcinoma. It shows marked collapse of the right atrium (*thick arrow*) and left atrium (*thin arrow*) during early systole. (TV, tricuspid valve; LV, RV, left and right ventricles; MV, mitral valve; LA, RA, left and right atria.)

The swinging heart motion pattern[17,37] occurs in large pericardial effusions and frequently suggests the presence of tamponade (Fig. 13-7). Right atrial collapse is seen on the 2-D echocardiogram in apical or subcostal four-chamber views (Fig. 13-8). It is a highly sensitive sign of tamponade that occurs when intrapericardial pressure transiently exceeds the right atrial pressure in end-diastole and early systole.[36] Right ventricular collapse can be seen by parasternal long- and short-axis and apical or subcostal four-chamber views (Fig. 13-9). It occurs in early diastole when right ventricular volume and pressure are at their lowest.[36] Engel and coworkers[14] showed the early diastolic collapse of the right ventricle on M-mode recordings. They showed abnormal posterior motion of the right ventricular wall during early diastole, which persisted more than 0.05 seconds after opening of the mitral valve in patients with cardiac tamponade (Fig. 13-7). Schiller and colleagues[33] described compression of the right ventricle throughout the cardiac cycle and suggested that a right ventricular end-diastolic dimension, at end-expiration, of 2 mm or less was indicative of tamponade. High right atrial pressure

leads to dilatation of the inferior vena cava (IVC) that prevents inspiratory collapse.[20] Left atrial collapse in late diastole to early systole (Fig. 13-8) occurs at a later stage in the development of cardiac tamponade.[8] Reciprocal variations in the internal dimension of the left and right heart during different phases of respiration were described by D'Cruz[9] and confirmed by other investigators.[34] During inspiration, owing to negative intrathoracic pressure, there is a slight decrease in intrapericardial pressure and blood flows from the superior and inferior vena cava into the right atrium and right ventricle. In cardiac tamponade, there is competition between right and left ventricle for space in the distended and taut pericardial sac. This increased right ventricular filling during inspiration causes the ventricular septum to shift to the left, so that the dimension of the RV increases during inspiration and there is reciprocal decrease in the dimension and filling of the left ventricle.[34] Therefore, during inspiration, M-mode echocardiography shows increased right ventricular internal dimension (RVID), increased tricuspid valve (TV) opening, decreased left ventricular internal dimension

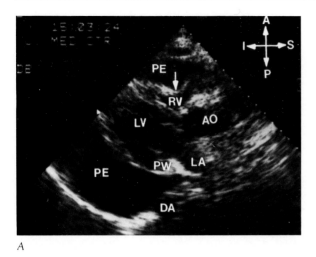
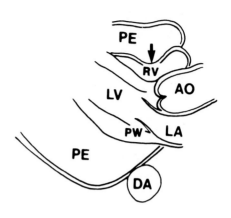

*A*                                    *B*

FIGURE 13-9. Two-dimensional parasternal long-axis view (A) and its schematic diagram (B) from a patient with cardiac tamponade show collapse of the right ventricle (RV, *arrow*) during early diastole. (AO, aorta; DA, descending aorta; PE, pericardial effusion; PW, posterior wall; LA, left atrium.)

(LVID), and decreased mitral valve (MV) opening, and aortic valve (AV) opening. During expiration these changes are reversed (Figs. 13-10 to 13-12). Minor changes in ventricular diameter can occur in normal subjects and in persons with cor pulmonale with pulsus paradoxus.

Recent Doppler studies[3,4] have confirmed these M-mode echocardiographic findings. Doppler studies show that normally during inspiration there is a slight increase in diastolic tricuspid valve flow (TVF) and systolic pulmonic valve flow (PVF), and a slight decrease in diastolic mitral valve flow (MVF) and systolic aortic valve flow (AVF). These changes in flow velocities are reversed during expiration. This change in flow between the different phases of respiration is less than 5% in the aortic valve, 5 to 10% in the mitral valve, 10 to 15% in the pulmonic valve, and less than 25% in the tricuspid valve.[3] In tamponade, these changes become exaggerated and lead to excessive reduction of systolic aortic flow and stroke volume (SV) during inspiration (Figs. 13-13, 13-14). This causes excessive reduction of systolic blood pressure during inspiration (pulsus paradoxus). Left ventricular ejection time (LVET) and left ventricular isovolumic relax-

ation time (LVIVRT), which normally show no significant changes between the different phases of respiration, also become abnormal.

*M-mode, 2-D, and Doppler echocardiographic findings in tamponade*

1. Right ventricular epicardial notch during isometric contraction
2. "Swinging heart" motion pattern
3. Right atrial collapse in late diastole and early systole
4. Right ventricular collapse in early diastole
5. Right ventricular cavity compression
6. Dilated inferior vena cava (IVC) and no inspiratory collapse
7. Left atrial collapse in late diastole and early systole
8. Reciprocal respiratory variation in RVID and LVID (M-mode)*
   a. Inspiration: ↑ RVID, ↑ TV opening, ↓ LVID, ↓ MV opening, and ↓ AV opening
   b. Expiration: ↓ RVID, ↓ TV opening, ↑ LVID, ↑ MV opening, and ↑ AV opening

*Note: ↑ = increased; ↓ = decreased.

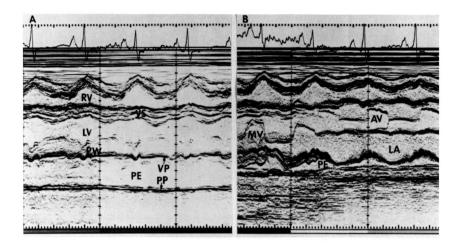

FIGURE 13-10. M-mode echocardiogram from a patient with lung carcinoma, large pericardial effusion (PE), and cardiac tamponade. (A) A large posterior and a small anterior echo-free space are consistent with a large pericardial effusion. The thickness of the parietal pericardium (PP) is normal, but the visceral pericardium (VP) appears denser than usual. Some oscillations of the posterior left ventricular (LV) wall (PW) in the region of visceral pericardium are also noted. (B) Pericardial effusion extends behind the left atrium (LA). Calibration marks are 1 cm apart. (MV, mitral valve; AV, aortic valve; VS, ventricular septum.)

9. Reciprocal respiratory variation in transvalvular right- and left-sided flows velocities by Doppler
   a. Inspiration: ↑ TVF, ↑ PVF, ↓ MVF, ↓ AVF, ↓ SV, ↓ LVET, ↑ LVIVRT
   b. Expiration: ↓ TVF, ↓ PVF, ↑ MVF, ↑ AVF, ↑ SV, ↑ LVET, ↓ LVIVRT
10. Hepatic venous flow-pattern abnormalities (Doppler)
   a. Marked decrease in diastolic forward flow on expiration
   b. Marked reversal of flow in late diastole on expiration.

The normal hepatic vein Doppler flow profile shows a biphasic forward flow pattern toward the right atrium with a systolic forward flow peak slightly larger than the diastolic one. Both peaks show a slight increase during inspiration and a slight decrease during expiration. There is a slight reversal of flow (away from the right atrium) following the atrial contraction, called atrial contrac-

tion-related reversed flow or AR. The reverse flow is less during inspiration and greater during expiration. The ratio of reverse to total forward flow is less than 15% during inspiration and less than 25% during expiration in normal subjects. In tamponade the forward diastolic flow is very small during inspiration and almost disappears during expiration. The increase in systolic flow during inspiration is also less than normal. There is marked reversal of flow in late diastole and at the time of atrial contraction during expiration; ratio of reverse flow to total forward flow is over 100%.[4]

Although cardiac tamponade is a hemodynamic and clinical diagnosis, all of these Doppler echocardiographic criteria are extremely valuable in alerting the clinician to the possibility of tamponade.

MANAGEMENT

The definitive therapy for tamponade is pericardiocentesis or surgical drainage. With malignant effu-

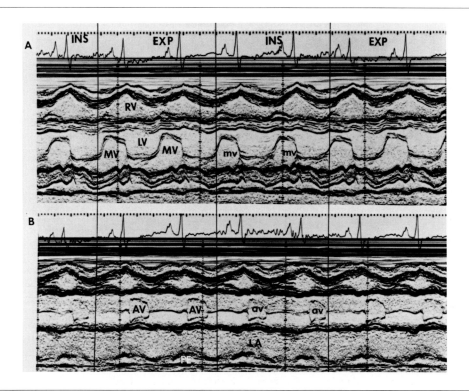

FIGURE 13-11. M-mode echocardiograms from a patient with a large pericardial effusion and tamponade, as shown in Figure 13-10. (A) Opening of the mitral valve; (B) opening of the aortic valve during different phases of respiration. Although these recordings were not obtained simultaneously, by rough approximation of heart rate, RR interval, and respiration, they have been mounted together to show the effect of respiration on the opening of these valves in tamponade. During expiration (EXP), the opening of the mitral valve is larger (MV). At the same time during expiration, the opening of the aortic valve (AV) is larger, indicating greater stroke volume. The duration of aortic valve opening, or left ventricular ejection time, is also longer, but during inspiration (INS), the opening of mitral valve is smaller (mv). The opening of the aortic valve (av) is also smaller. Aortic valve echo also shows systolic convergence and reduced left ventricular (LV) ejection time during inspiration, which is consistent with lower stroke volume. These findings would explain the phenomenon of pulsus paradoxus. (RV, right ventricle.)

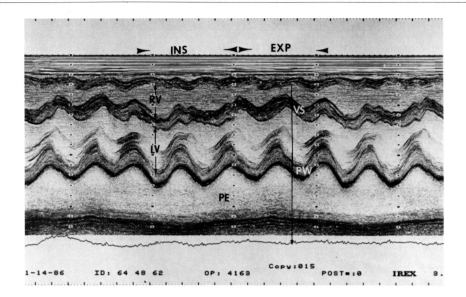

FIGURE 13-12. M-mode echocardiogram from a heart transplant recipient who developed a large pericardial effusion (PE), mainly posteriorly. This recording shows the swinging heart motion pattern. The increase in the dimension of the right ventricle (RV) and the decrease in the dimension of the left ventricle (LV) during inspiration (INS) probably are due to a leftward septal shift during inspiration. During expiration (EXP) the changes are reversed and there is a decrease in the dimension of RV and an increase in the dimension of LV. The long arrow indicates the abnormal ventricular septal (VS) motion during systole.

FIGURE 13-13. Transmitral flow velocity is recorded in the patient shown in Figure 13-12 using pulsed Doppler technique from the apical four-chamber view. Mitral flow occurs predominantly in early diastole at E point, and the velocity shows marked phasic variation during the different phases of respiration. It is higher during expiration (EXP) and much lower during inspiration (INS). This finding indicates a larger mitral valve opening and higher flow through the mitral orifice during expiration, which will produce higher stroke volume during expiration and lower stroke volume during inspiration and explains the phenomenon of pulsus paradoxus. Calibrations are at intervals of 0.2 m per second.

FIGURE 13-14. Pulsed Doppler echocardiograms show transmitral flow (A) and aortic flow (B) in a patient with a large pericardial effusion due to malignancy and tamponade. These tracings were not obtained simultaneously, but by approximate matching of heart rate, RR interval, and phases of respiration they have been mounted together to show the effects of respiration on transmitral (MV) and transaortic (AV) flow. During expiration (EXP), transmitral flow (MV) is much higher (0.6 m/sec) than during inspiration (INS) (0.4 m/sec). (B) During expiration, aortic valve (AV) flow is 1 m/sec, which is significantly higher than the 0.5-m/sec (av) flow during inspiration. In the presence of pericardial effusion, these Doppler features indicate cardiac tamponade.

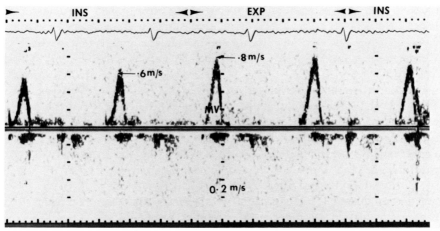

FIGURE 13-13

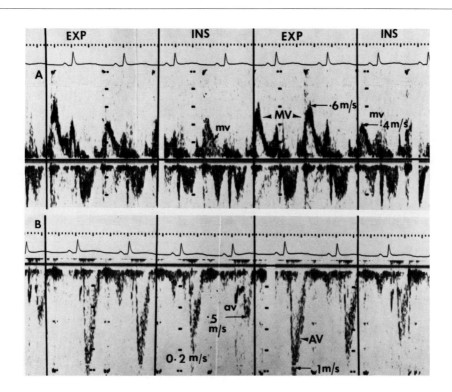

FIGURE 13-14

sions, after pericardial fluid is evacuated, tetracycline can be injected into the pericardium to produce its sclerosis.[35]

## Constrictive Pericarditis

In pericardial constriction there is thickening, fibrosis, and calcification of the pericardium with fusion of the epicardium and parietal pericardium. This rigid, fibrotic pericardial sac restricts diastolic filling of all chambers of the heart.[28] In effusive constrictive pericarditis the two layers are not fused. The epicardium is thickened and adherent to the myocardium and produces visceral constriction. The thickened parietal pericardium is not fused with thickened epicardium but is separated by 100 to 500 ml of pericardial fluid under tension.[18]

### PATHOPHYSIOLOGY

Since diastolic expansion is restricted by the rigid pericardium, the right-sided diastolic pressures are elevated and are equal to the left-sided diastolic pressures. Mean right atrial (RA) pressure may be elevated in excess of 15 mm Hg and may be equal to the elevated right ventricular end-diastolic pressure (RVEDP) and pulmonary artery diastolic pressure (PAD). These elevated right-side diastolic pressures are equal to, or within 5 mm of, the left-sided filling pressures (mean pulmonary artery wedge, mean left atrial, and left ventricular end-diastolic pressures). Thus, there is near equalization of the intracardiac diastolic pressures so that RA = RVEDP = PAD = PAW = LA = LVEDP. During early diastole, there is no restriction to filling and early diastolic filling is more rapid than normal, producing the characteristic square root–sign ($\sqrt{\phantom{x}}$) or dip-and-plateau configuration of the diastolic pressure wave form.[18,28]

### CAUSES

Most cases of constrictive pericarditis probably start as acute pericarditis with exudation of fluid into the pericardial cavity. The fluid is eventually reabsorbed and the visceral and parietal pericardial layers undergo fibrotic thickening, calcification, and fusion. Causes of constrictive pericarditis[21] include Mulibrey nanism (a hereditary disorder, most common in Finland); bacterial, tuberculosis,

fungal, viral, or parasitic infection; uremia; connective tissue diseases such as rheumatoid arthritis, systemic lupus erythematosus, periarteritis nodosa, and rheumatic fever; radiation therapy; lymphoma and pericardial metastases; intrapericardial bleeding; cardiac surgery; and methysergide therapy. Causes of effusive-constrictive pericarditis include neoplasms; radiation therapy; uremia; rheumatoid arthritis; tuberculosis; and cardiac surgery. Both types of pericarditis can also arise when no other disorder (idiopathic or primary) is present.

### CLINICAL FEATURES

Symptoms—dyspnea, ankle edema, abdominal distension, weakness, fatigue, weight loss, muscle wasting—may be present for months. The patient may appear chronically ill with reduced muscle mass, jugular vein distension, edema, hepatomegaly and splenomegaly, and ascites. Heart sounds may be distant. A loud and early third heart sound, or pericardial knock, is characteristic of constrictive pericarditis.

### DIAGNOSTIC STUDIES

*Electrocardiography.* The ECG may show decreased QRS voltage, T-wave changes, and atrial fibrillation in up to 25% of patients. A pattern of right ventricular hypertrophy and right axis deviation is noted in a minority of patients.

*Chest Radiography.* Pericardial calcification is seen in 30 to 60% of cases. Pleural effusions are present in up to 50%. Heart size is normal or slightly enlarged.

*Cardiac Catheterization.* Cardiac catheterization reveals classic hemodynamic features of constrictive pericarditis, dip-and-plateau configuration of ventricular diastolic pressure tracings and near equalization of diastolic intracardiac pressures so that RA = RVEDP = PAD = PAW = LVEDP.

*Computed Tomography (CT) and Magnetic Resonance Imaging (MRI) of the Thorax.* Chest CT and MRI are excellent tools to detect pericardial thickening.

*Echocardiography.* A technically adequate M-mode echocardiographic scan from aorta to apex should be obtained by carefully varying the gain settings.

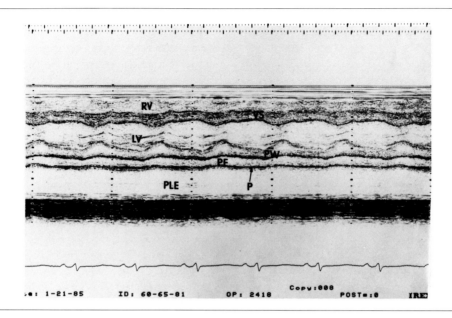

FIGURE 13-15. M-mode echocardiogram from a patient with a small pericardial (PE) and a large left pleural effusion (PLE). By damping the gain control, the precise thickness of the parietal pericardium (P) can be demonstrated very well. The parietal pericardium is sandwiched between the two effusions and its thickness is normal in this case. (RV, LV, right and left ventricles; VS, ventricular septum; PW, posterior wall.)

A high index of suspicion is needed to diagnose pericardial thickening. The echocardiographer must be cautious not to diagnose pericardial thickening unless a technically satisfactory tracing is obtained. In the presence of both pericardial and left pleural effusion, pericardial thickness can be measured (Fig. 13-15). Echocardiographic features of constrictive pericarditis are as follows[1,7,10,11,13,19,22,23,27,38,40,41]:

A. On M-mode echocardiography
 1. Pericardial thickening
 2. Increased depth of A wave on pulmonary valve
 3. Premature diastolic opening of pulmonary valve
 4. Rapid early and flat middiastolic motion of posterior left ventricular wall
 5. Rapid early and flat middiastolic motion of posterior aortic root
 6. Posterior atrial systolic notch on septum
 7. Abnormal (abrupt anterior or posterior) early diastolic ventricular septal motion
 8. Abnormal septal motion in systole
B. On 2-D echocardiography
 1. Dense, rigid shell of pericardium
 2. Normal-sized left ventricle, mildly enlarged atria
 3. Atrial and ventricular septal bulge to left during inspiration
 4. Rapid early diastolic filling followed by prominent halt
 5. Dilated IVC and hepatic vein, and spontaneous contrast effect
 6. Enlarged liver and spleen; ascites
C. On Doppler studies
 1. Excessive decrease in peak mitral flow velocity in inspiration
 2. Marked decrease in forward diastolic flow and increase in reverse flow during expiration in hepatic veins.

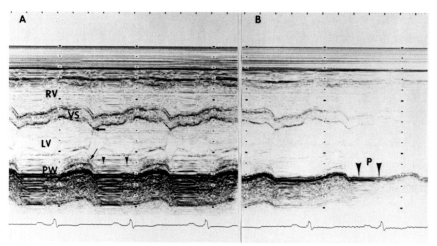

FIGURE 13-16

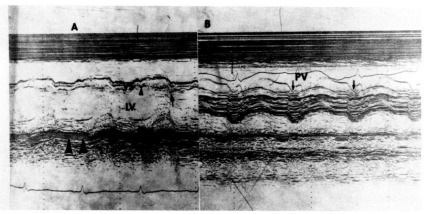

FIGURE 13-17

FIGURE 13-16. M-mode echocardiogram from a patient with constrictive pericarditis. Recording *B* was taken after damping the gain control to its lowest level. Large arrowheads indicate thickened, dense, and calcified pericardium. (*A*) The rapid early diastolic descent or dip in the endocardial motion of the posterior left ventricular wall (*thin arrow*) is visible. The endocardial motion is flat in middle to late diastole (*thin arrowheads*). The ventricular septal (VS) motion is flat during systole, and there is early diastolic posterior motion of the septum (*thick arrow*).

FIGURE 13-17. M-mode echocardiogram from a patient with constrictive pericarditis. (*A*) Notable features are thickened calcified pericardium (*thick arrowheads*), probable atrial systolic notch (*thin arrowhead*), and early diastolic posterior motion of the ventricular septum (VS, *arrow*). (*B*) A large atrial "kick" on the pulmonary valve echo in this patient with constrictive pericarditis probably indicates upward motion of the pulmonic valve (PV) due to high right ventricular pressure following atrial contraction. Calibration marks are 0.5 cm apart. (PW, posterior wall; LV, left ventricle.)

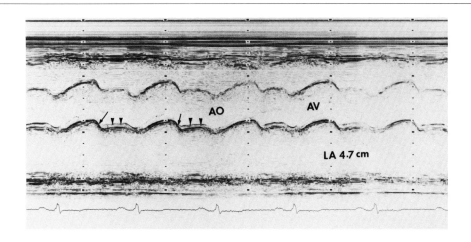

FIGURE 13-18. M-mode echocardiogram of the aortic root (AO) from a patient with constrictive pericarditis. The posterior aortic root motion shows rapid early diastolic descent (*arrow*) and flat motion of the posterior aortic wall during middle to late diastole (*arrowheads*), reflecting the physiology of constriction. Calibration marks are 1 cm apart. The left atrium (LA) is slightly enlarged. (AV, aortic valve.)

The echocardiographic patterns of a thickened pericardium (Figs. 13-16, 13-17) are well-described.[23] In chronic fibrocalcific constrictive pericarditis there are parallel dense and thick echoes separated by a small clear space that may be filled by multiple lines. In effusive-constrictive pericarditis thick echoes are reflected from the epicardium. A small pericardial effusion and flat motion of the thickened parietal pericardium occur.

The elevated right ventricular middiastolic pressure may cause premature opening of the pulmonic valve.[41] Contraction of the right atrium in the presence of high right ventricular diastolic pressure may produce an extremely large a wave on the pulmonic valve (Fig. 13-17), particularly during inspiration.[10] These findings are not specific for constrictive pericarditis and have been reported in Uhl's anomaly, sinus of Valsalva aneurysm rupture into the right atrium, right ventricular infarction, Löffler's endocarditis, pulmonary regurgitation, and after tricuspid valvulectomy.[10,11,41] The hemodynamic phenomenon of dip-and-plateau pattern in the left ventricle is reflected in the diastolic motion of the endocardium of the posterior left ventricular wall[40] and posterior aortic root.[7] There is rapid early diastolic descent of the posterior left ventricular wall followed by a flat motion (i.e., motion of less than 1 mm during mid to late diastole).[40] Although it is not specific, this is one of the most common and reliable signs of constrictive pericarditis (see Fig. 13-16).

The posterior aortic root (Fig. 13-18) similarly shows rapid motion in early diastole and little or no motion in middle to late diastole.[7] Since filling of both ventricles is restricted by a rigid pericardium, there is a greater ventricular interdependence and the transseptal pressure gradient at the time of the P wave may cause an abrupt posterior notch on the ventricular septum during atrial contraction (see Fig. 13-17), the so-called atrial systolic notch.[38] Abrupt anterior or posterior early diastolic septal motion (see Figs. 13-16, 13-17) may be seen; these patterns reflect the direction of transseptal pressure gradients in different patients with constrictive pericarditis.[13] Septal motion during systole is also frequently abnormal in patients with constrictive pericarditis (see Figs. 13-16, 13-17), and it varies from hypokinesis to paradoxical motion.[13]

Systolic septal motion abnormalities are nonspecific and are also seen in right ventricular volume overload, after cardiac surgery, with congenital absence of pericardium, and with coronary artery disease and left bundle branch block.[13] Although ventricular size is normal, the atria show mild enlargement in the majority of patients with constrictive pericarditis.[13] Engel and colleagues[13] reviewed these M-mode features in 40 patients with constrictive pericarditis and concluded that many were seen in most patients but no single feature was diagnostic.

Two-dimensional echocardiographic features of constrictive pericarditis include normal-sized ventricles and some enlargement of the atria, thick pericardium, atrial and ventricular septal bulge to left during inspiration, rapid filling in early diastole followed by a prominent halt,[27] dilated inferior vena cava and hepatic veins with spontaneous contrast effect,[22] enlargement of liver and spleen, and ascites. Characteristic Doppler features differentiate constrictive pericarditis from restrictive cardiomyopathy.[1,2,19,26] In constrictive pericarditis there is an extraordinary decrease in the peak mitral flow velocity during inspiration.[19] The hepatic vein Doppler flow profile shows a biphasic flow pattern. Both systolic and diastolic velocities increase during inspiration, as in normal persons, but during expiration there is a marked decrease in diastolic forward flow and an increase in reverse flow in late diastole and at the time of the atrial contraction.[1] In contrast, in restrictive cardiomyopathy, the ratio of the mitral flow at the time of E wave to that of A wave (E-A ratio) is more than 2.5, mitral deceleration time is short (<150 msec), and hepatic venous flow velocity is decreased in systole.[2,26]

The echocardiographer must have a high index of suspicion and utilize the various M-mode, 2-D, and Doppler echocardiographic features to make the diagnosis of constrictive pericarditis.

TREATMENT

Definitive treatment for constrictive pericarditis is surgical resection of the pericardium (pericardiectomy).

## Congenital Absence of Pericardium

Total absence of the pericardium is a rare congenital anomaly and usually produces no symptoms.

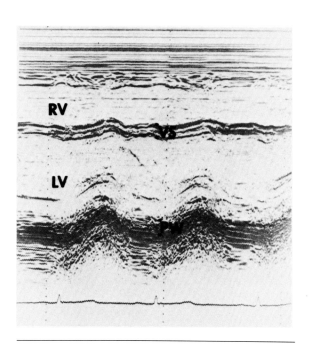

FIGURE 13-19. M-mode echocardiogram from a patient with congenital absence of the pericardium. It reveals paradoxical septal motion but otherwise is normal. Chest films showed typical abnormalities of this condition. Calibration marks are 0.5 cm apart. (RV, LV, right and left ventricles; VS, ventricular septum; PW, posterior wall.)

Most patients seek medical attention because of heart murmur, abnormal cardiac silhouette on chest radiographs, and abnormal ECG findings. Chest films show marked leftward displacement of the heart and a prominent pulmonary artery. ECG abnormalities include an incomplete right bundle branch block, right axis deviation, or poor R-wave progression. M-mode and 2-D echocardiography show features of right ventricular volume overload (Fig. 13-19), but Doppler echocardiography excludes atrial septal defect and any significant valvular lesions.[25,28] To record the 2-D apical four-chamber view, the transducer must be placed on the chest beyond the anterior axillary line because of the abnormal levoposition, but the echocardiographic images do not reveal any significant chamber enlargement. This finding with typical radiographic and ECG abnormalities should suggest a diagnosis of congenital absence of pericardium. In partial absence of left-sided pericardium, a left atrial appendage can herniate through the pericardial defect. Marked enlargement of a left atrial appendage has been observed on the parasternal short-axis view.[32]

## Pericardial Cyst

Pericardial cysts are rare developmental anomalies that usually produce no symptoms and typically are located at the right costophrenic angle. They can be diagnosed accurately by 2-D echocardiography[24] and CT of the chest.

## References

1. Appleton CP, Hatle LK, Popp RL. Central venous flow velocity patterns can differentiate constrictive pericarditis from restrictive cardiomyopathy (abstr). J Am Coll Cardiol. 1987; 9(2):119A.
2. Appleton, CP, Hatle LK, Popp RL. Demonstration of restrictive ventricular physiology by Doppler echocardiography. J Am Coll Cardiol. 1988; 11:757–768.
3. Appleton CP, Hatle LK, Popp RL. Cardiac tamponade and pericardial effusion: Respiratory variation in transvalvular flow velocities studied by Doppler echocardiography. J Am Coll Cardiol. 1988; 11:1020–1030.
4. Burstow DJ, Oh JK, Seward JB, Tajik AJ. et al. Cardiac tamponade: Pulsed-wave Doppler findings (abstr). J Am Coll Cardiol. 1988; 11(2):75A.
5. Callahan JA, Seward JB, Nishimura RA, et al. Two-dimensional echocardiographically guided pericardiocentesis: Experience in 117 consecutive patients. Am J Cardiol. 1985; 55:476–479.
6. Chandraratna PAN. Uses and limitations of echocardiography in the evaluation of pericardial disease. Echocardiography. 1984; 1:55–74.
7. Chandraratna PAN, Aronow WS, Imaizumi T. Role of echocardiography in detecting anatomic and physiologic abnormalities of constrictive pericarditis. Am J Med Sci. 1982; 383:141–146.
8. D'Cruz I, Callaghan W, Arensman F, et al. Left atrial compression: A neglected sign of tamponade (abstr). J Am Coll Cardiol. 1988; 11(2):84A.
9. D'Cruz IA, Cohen HC, Prabhu R, et al. Diagnosis of cardiac tamponade by echocardiography: Changes in mitral valve motion and ventricular dimensions, with special reference to paradoxical pulse. Circulation. 1975; 52:460–465.
10. Doi YL, Sugiura T, Spodick D. Motion of pulmonic valve and constrictive pericarditis. Chest. 1981; 80:513–515.
11. Doyle T, Troup PJ, Wann LS. Mid-diastolic opening of the pulmonary valve after right ventricular infarction. J Am Coll Cardiol. 1985; 5:366–368.
12. Edler I. Diagnostic use of ultrasound in heart disease. Acta Med Scand. 1955; 152(suppl 308):32.
13. Engel PJ, Fowler NO, Tei C, et al. M-mode echocardiography in constrictive pericarditis. J Am Coll Cardiol. 1985; 6:471–474.
14. Engel PJ, Hon H, Fowler NO, et al. Echocardiographic study of right ventricular wall motion in cardiac tamponade. Am J Cardiol. 1982; 50:1018–1021.
15. Feigenbaum H. Echocardiography. 4th ed. Philadelphia: Lea & Febiger; 1986; 548–578.
16. Feigenbaum H, Waldhausen JA, Hyde LP. Ultrasound diagnosis of pericardial effusion. JAMA. 1965; 191:711–714.
17. Feigenbaum H, Zaky A, Grabhorn LL. Cardiac motion in patients with pericardial effusion: A study using reflected ultrasound. Circulation. 1966; 34:611–614.
18. Hancock EW. Subacute effusive-constrictive pericarditis. Circulation. 1971; 43:183–192.
19. Hatle LK, Appleton CP, Popp RL. Constrictive pericarditis and restrictive cardiomyopathy: Differentiation by Doppler recording of atrioventricular flow velocities (abstr). J Am Coll Cardiol. 1987; 9(2):17A.
20. Himelman RB, Kircher B, Schiller NB. Lack of inspiratory vena caval collapse in pericardial effusion: A sign of hemodynamic compromise (abstr). J Am Coll Cardiol. 1988; 11(2):84A.
21. Hirschmann JV. Pericardial constriction. Am Heart J. 1978; 96:110–122.
22. Hjemdahl-Monson CE, Daniels J, Kaufman D, et al. Spontaneous contrast in the inferior vena cava in a patient with constrictive pericarditis. J Am Coll Cardiol. 1984; 4:165–166.
23. Horowitz MS, Rossen R, Harrison DC. Echocardiographic diagnosis of pericardial disease. Am Heart J. 1979; 97:420–427.
24. Hynes JK, Tajik AJ, Osborn MJ, et al. Two-dimensional echocardiographic diagnosis of pericardial cyst. Mayo Clin Proc. 1983; 58:60–63.
25. Kansal S, Roitman D, et al. Two-dimensional echocardiography of congenital absence of pericardium. Am Heart J. 1985; 109:912–914.
26. Klein AL, Oh JK, Miller FA, et al. Two-dimensional and Doppler echocardiographic assessment of infiltrative cardiomyopathy. J Am Soc Echocardiogr. 1988; 1:48–59.
27. Lewis BS. Real-time two-dimensional echocardiography in constrictive pericarditis. Am J Cardiol. 1982; 49:1789–1793.
28. Lorell BYH, Braunwald E. Pericardial disease. In: Braunwald E, ed. Heart Disease. Philadelphia: WB Saunders; 1988: 1484–1534.

29. Martin RP, Rakowski H, Popp RL. Localization of pericardial effusion with wide angle phased array echocardiography. Am J Cardiol. 1978; 42:904–912.

30. Morgan BC, Guntheroth WG, Dillard DH. Relationship of pericardial to pleural pressure during quiet respiration and cardiac tamponade. Circ Res. 1965; 41:493–498.

31. Reddy PS, Curtiss EI, O'Toole JD, et al. Cardiac tamponade: Hemodynamic observations in man. Circulation. 1978; 58:265–272.

32. Ruys F, Paulus W, et al. Expansion of left atrial appendage is a distinctive echocardiographic feature of congenital defect of the pericardium. Eur Heart J. 1983; 4:738–740.

33. Schiller NB, Botvinick EH. Right ventricular compression as a sign of cardiac tamponade: An analysis of echocardiographic ventricular dimensions and their clinical implications. Circulation. 1977; 56:774–779.

34. Settle HP, Adolph RJ, Fowler NO, et al. Echocardiographic study of cardiac tamponade. Circulation. 1977; 56:951–959.

35. Shepherd FA, Morgan C, Evans WK, et al. Medical management of malignant pericardial effusion by tetracycline sclerosis. Am J Cardiol. 1987; 60:1161–1166.

36. Singh S, Wann LS, Schuchard GH, et al. Right ventricular and right atrial collapse in patients with cardiac tamponade: A combined echocardiographic and hemodynamic study. Circulation. 1984; 70:966–971.

37. Tajik AJ. Echocardiography in pericardial effusion. Am J Med. 1977; 63:29–40.

38. Tei C, Child JS, Tanaka H, et al. Atrial systolic notch on the interventricular septal echogram: An echocardiographic sign of constrictive pericarditis. J Am Coll Cardiol. 1983; 1:907–912.

39. Vignola PA, Pohost GM, Curfman GE, et al. Correlation of echocardiographic and clinical findings in patients with pericardial effusion. Am J Cardiol. 1976; 37:701–707.

40. Voelkel AG, Pietro DA, Folland ED, et al. Echocardiographic features of constrictive pericarditis. Circulation. 1978; 58:871–875.

41. Wann LS, Weyman AE, Dillon JC, et al. Premature pulmonary valve opening. Circulation. 1977; 55:128–133.

# CHAPTER 14

# Inflammatory, Neoplastic, and Thrombotic Disease

BARBARA A. NICHOLS

Intracardiac masses may result from infective endocarditis, cardiac neoplasms, or cardiac thrombosis. Echocardiography is a noninvasive means of assessing the presence and monitoring the progression of such masses. In the latter half of the 1950s, shortly after its introduction into clinical practice, echocardiography was able to provide the information needed to establish a diagnosis of atrial myxoma.[10,11] By that time, M-mode echocardiography had been accepted as a clinical tool for intracardiac assessment. Ultrasonography technology has advanced dramatically since then. For several years, real-time two-dimensional (2-D) imaging has been the diagnostic procedure of choice for cardiac evaluation when a cardiac neoplasm is suspected.[15] Transesophageal echocardiography[48] and ultrasonic tissue characterization[20] currently show great promise for this application. As technology continues to be refined the capabilities of echocardiography also improve.

## Infective Endocarditis

Infective endocarditis is a serious infection of the endocardium, the endothelial tissue that lines the internal structures of the heart. Infective endocarditis most often involves the valves. Mural endocardium, ventricular septal defects, and areas of the great arteries also may be involved.

In the 1920s, the majority of cases of infective endocarditis were diagnosed in persons less than 30 years of age.[54] With the introduction of antibiotics in the 1940s, the average age of infective endocarditis patients gradually increased until, in 1980, it was approximately 50 years.[18] This shift may be partly a result of the fact that the age of peak incidence of certain diseases associated with infective endocarditis is increasing.[59]

One form of cardiac disease commonly associated with infective endocarditis is rheumatic heart disease, a complication of rheumatic fever,[25] a disease that most often strikes children and teenagers. Although treatment of streptococcal pharyngitis with pencillin has decreased the number of cases of rheumatic fever each year, some strains have become resistant to antibiotics.[17]

Certain forms of congenital disease are found in a significant portion of persons with infective endocarditis.[25] Bicuspid aortic valve is the most common, but patent ductus arteriosus, ventricular septal defect, tetralogy of Fallot, coarctation of the aorta, and pulmonary stenosis are also seen. Thanks to current medical and surgical treatment, a greater percentage of persons with congenital heart defects are surviving to adulthood.

Mitral valve prolapse and degenerative valve disease have also been recognized as preexisting valve abnormalities associated with infective endocarditis.[34,47] Redundancy and calcification of the valve tissue seem to place a person at greater risk. If a valve of this type is significantly damaged by endocarditis, it may be replaced with a prosthetic valve. Ironically, endocarditis also represents a more serious complication of prosthetic valve implantation.

Which cardiac valve is affected by the endocarditis depends on the underlying disease, but it appears that valves in the left side of the heart are most often involved.[37] The tricuspid and pulmonary valves generally are involved only in persons who are intravenous drug abusers. Therefore, the incidence of right-sided endocarditis is likely to vary with the number of intravenous drug users.

*Streptococcus viridans* and Enterococcus species are microorganisms of low virulence capable of causing infective endocarditis in the presence of a cardiac abnormality.[60] If the infection is caused by a highly virulent microorganism (usually *Staphylococcus aureus*) preexisting cardiac disease need not be present.[59]

PATHOPHYSIOLOGY
The events leading to infection of *abnormal* cardiac valves differ from those leading to infection of *normal* cardiac valves. Factors involved in the development of infective endocarditis of *abnormal* valves include hemodynamic and thrombotic factors, transient bacteremia, and immunologic factors.[59]

*Hemodynamic Factors.* Characteristically, the surfaces of the leaflets downstream to the regurgitant blood flow are involved, typically the atrial side of the atrioventricular valves and the ventricular side of semilunar valves. Rodbard demonstrated that an infected fluid flowing at a high velocity from an area of high pressure to one of lower pressure will consistently deposit microorganisms in the same location.[44] The great turbulence created by a small orifice, such as a regurgitant valve, sets the stage for optimal growth of microorganisms.

*Thrombotic Factors.* Regurgitant valves eventually are traumatized by the turbulent high-velocity jet. A combination of platelets and fibrin then adheres to the damaged valve; this is the thrombus of nonbacterial thrombotic endocarditis.

*Transient Bacteremia.* Microorganisms seem to enter the bloodstream in many ways.[12] Often, the oral cavity is involved. Dental procedures, oral infections, even chewing hard candy can lead to bacter-

emia. Microorganisms have also been known to enter the blood during urologic, gastrointestinal, and gynecologic procedures. Open heart surgery or the skin trauma associated with burns and with open heart surgery may also allow for entry of microorganisms capable of causing infective endocarditis. Once in the bloodstream, the microorganisms reach the heart valves rapidly through the venous system.

*Immunological Factors.* The mechanism by which microorganisms adhere to the traumatized valve is very complex and incompletely understood. Dextran, a polymer of glucose produced by certain microorganisms, apparently increases their ability to adhere to the valve.[59] Another important factor seems to be platelet aggregation.[7] Regardless of the mechanism, once colonization takes place, the bacteria are protected from the body's defense mechanisms. Many clumped bacteria are found within the protected platelet aggregation.

*Normal Valves.* The exact pathophysiologic factors that lead to the development of infective endocarditis on a *normal* cardiac valve are unknown. The pathogenesis appears most likely to be related to the virulence and the number of circulating microorganisms.[59]

SYMPTOMS AND COMPLICATIONS
Symptoms of infective endocarditis generally appear within 2 to 3 weeks of the onset of bacteremia. Several areas of the body may be involved. The overall infection generally produces either a low-grade fever (<103°F), when associated with streptococci, or a high fever, when associated with *S. aureus*. Other symptoms, such as night sweats, chills, aching, loss of appetite, weight loss, fatigue, and weakness, may occur.

The bacteria in the vegetations are capable of invading the valves. Destruction of valve tissue or valve ring abscess may result. Vegetations may be small (millimeters) or large (centimeters), single or multiple. Cardiac involvement is manifested in a cardiac murmur, the quality of which may change from day to day, depending on the progression of the infection on the valve. Should valve leaflet perforation or ring abscess occur, severe regurgitation and subsequent congestive heart failure will result.

Additional complications may include rupture of the chordae tendineae, papillary muscle, or ventricular septum, and aneurysm formation of the sinuses of Valsalva.

Because the lesions are friable, fragments of the vegetation commonly embolize, and when they do, symptoms associated with impaired organ function may result. Intracardiac embolus may lead to coronary artery obstruction, and subsequently to myocardial infarction.[47] Other structures at risk with left-sided endocarditis include the spleen, kidneys, gastrointestinal tract, brain, and extremities. Right-sided lesions may embolize to the pulmonary circulation and cause pulmonary infarction. Myocarditis and pericarditis may also occur.

### RELATED DIAGNOSTIC PROCEDURES

*Blood Cultures.* The principal diagnostic test for infective endocarditis is the isolation of the causative organism or organisms from cultures of the blood. Blood samples generally are drawn over a 36- to 48-hour period. Most bacteria are isolated within a week, although some take 3 weeks or more.

*Electrocardiography.* Electrocardiography can provide nonspecific information in the presence of uncomplicated infective endocarditis. Development of atrioventricular block or bundle branch block may result from abscess formation. Premature ventricular contractions and T-wave changes may also be seen.

*Echocardiography.* The echocardiographic examination has tremendous value in the diagnosis and follow-up of persons suspected to have endocarditis.[32] Although M-mode echocardiography plays a role, the 2-D technique is the preferred approach for the detection of an intracardiac vegetation. Its increased scanning area affords more complete visualization of the cardiac structures and more detailed assessment of the size, location, and degree of mobility of the vegetation. Because of the resolution of the technique, tiny valve vegetations (<2 to 3 mm) may not be seen. This should not be a crucial limitation, as the incidence of complications in patients without echocardiographic evidence of vegetation is much lower than in patients in whom a vegetation has been identified.[52]

*Echocardiographic findings.* The primary echocardiographic finding in the presence of a cardiac vegetation is an area of shaggy, irregular echoes on the valvular endocardium (Fig. 14-1).[32] The appearance of the mass may vary. It may appear flat, echo-dense, and sessile (short pedicle) or globular, pedunculated, and mobile. Vegetations may be localized to a small area of the valve surface or may involve the entire cusp or leaflet. Generally, valve vegetations do not interfere with the opening motion of the valve and move in unison with blood flow, unless the vegetation becomes large or the valve is destroyed, in which case motion may become erratic and independent of blood flow.

The size of the vegetation is influenced by such things as the infecting microorganism, the progression of the infection, and the adequacy of antimicrobial therapy. To optimally assess the size of the vegetation, proper utilization of gain and reject controls is essential. With unnecessarily high gain settings, a vegetation will appear larger than it is. Conversely, vegetations may appear smaller than they are or may be missed entirely if the gain settings are too low or the reject is set too high.

Echocardiographic detection of valvular vegetations may be more difficult in the presence of degenerative heart disease. Care must be taken to avoid confusing areas of valve thickening associated with calcification or myxomatous degeneration with vegetations. In general, the distinction can be made on the basis of valve mobility and the phase of the cardiac cycle during which the density is seen. If the thickened area can be visualized in both systole and diastole and if valve opening is impaired, it most likely represents calcification. If the density is seen better during diastole and does not impair valve excursion, endocarditis should be suspected. In either case, it is best to give a description rather than a diagnosis. Regardless of whether other valve pathology is present, vegetations greater than 3 mm should be readily detectable. Smaller vegetations may be detected if the examiner scans the entire valve surface in multiple scan planes from all available echocardiographic windows. In experienced hands, echocardiography is able to accurately detect cardiac vegetations in 60 to 80% of infected patients.[52]

A valve vegetation may be accompanied by a flail segment of the valve. Echocardiographically, this appears as coarse, erratic fluttering of the leaf-

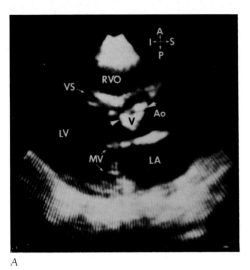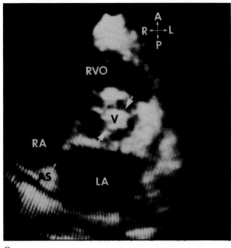

FIGURE 14-1. Parasternal long-axis (A) and short-axis (B) 2-D views of a patient who presented with bacteremia and acute aortic insufficiency. Note the large irregular, sonodense mass on the aortic cusps. In this clinical setting, a valvular vegetation was suspected. (LV, left ventricle; MV, mitral valve; LA, left atrium; Ao, aorta; V, vegetation; VS, ventricular septum; RVO, right ventricular outflow tract; AS, atrial septum; RA, right atrium.) (From Pohost G, O'Rourke RA, eds. Cardiac Imaging. Boston: Little, Brown; 1989.)

let. Portions of a flail segment of the mitral valve may be visualized in the left atrium and may produce multiple echoes adjacent to the leaflet. Rupture of the chordae tendineae or ventricular septum may also occur. In the presence of a valve ring abscess, areas of echogenicity and of echolucency are noted around the abscess cavity. An eccentric aortic insufficiency jet may cause diastolic fluttering of the mitral valve and the ventricular septum. If the aortic insufficiency is acute, premature mitral valve closure may also be noted (Fig. 14-2). Cardiac chamber enlargement is a common secondary finding and is frequently accompanied by a left ventricular volume overload pattern.

Although the echocardiographic assessment of infective endocarditis revolves around the 2-D technique, the Doppler examination can be a useful adjunct. With this modality, details about the valvular regurgitation (degree, direction, origin) may be obtained.

## Neoplastic Disease

Defined simply, a neoplasm—a mass caused by neoplastic disease—is any new tissue growth that serves no physiologic function.

### Related Diagnostic Procedures

Sometimes chest radiography, fluoroscopy, radionuclide imaging, and angiography reveal the presence of a cardiac tumor.[8,38,49] At present, echocardiography is the technique of choice for the diagnosis of cardiac tumors.[15] Computed tomography (CT) and magnetic resonance imaging (MRI) are also being used to assess intracardiac masses in selected cases.[1,19] Unfortunately, CT involves the injection of contrast medium and exposure to ionizing radiation and MRI is costly. Echocardiography provides a noninvasive, inexpensive way to detect cardiac dysfunction due to neoplastic infiltration.

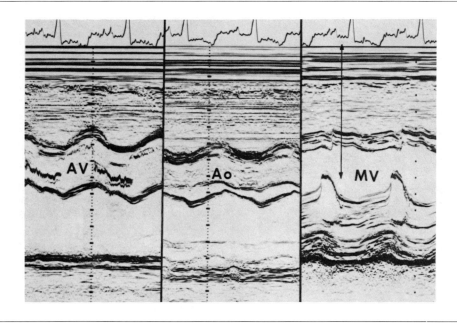

FIGURE 14-2. M-mode echocardiograms of a patient with an aortic root abscess secondary to infective endocarditis. The rapid fluttering of the aortic cusps (AV) suggests the presence of a vegetation. Note the sonolucent area within the aortic root (Ao) demonstrating the abscess cavity. Premature closure of the mitral valve (MV) is also present secondary to the acute aortic insufficiency.

## PRIMARY BENIGN CARDIAC TUMORS

Primary cardiac tumors—neoplasms that originate in the heart—are extremely rare, and, fortunately, most are benign.[27] Occasionally, they may cause life-threatening complications if they cause obstruction or compression. Systemic and pulmonary emboli, fever, cachexia, malaise, and arthralgia, as well as rash, clubbing, and Raynaud's phenomenon, are reported noncardiac manifestations of cardiac tumors.[21,33,46] Primary tumors may also produce cardiac complications. Common ones are chest pain, syncope, and congestive heart failure. Additionally, valvular stenosis with or without insufficiency, constrictive pericarditis, pericardial effusion, arrhythmia, heart block, and intracardiac shunt may be seen.[21]

Characteristically, benign tumors grow slowly by enlarging and expanding. Because they are almost always encapsulated and do not infiltrate into surrounding tissues benign tumors are often surgically resectable.

### ATRIAL TUMORS

*Myxoma.* The most common benign primary cardiac tumor is myxoma. Most myxomas occur in women and in persons between 30 and 60 years of age, although they have been found in persons aged 3 to 83 years.[5] More than 90% of myxomas are found in the atria. The left atrium is the most common site, but biatrial, ventricular, and combined left atrial and left ventricular myxomas have been reported.[9,31,61] Myxomas in unusual locations may be related to a condition of children known as syndrome myxoma. This syndrome is characterized by diffuse freckling, peripheral myxoid tumors, and endocrine neoplasms.[56] The tumors tend to be multiple and recurrent.

Grossly, the myxoma is approximately 2 to 8 cm

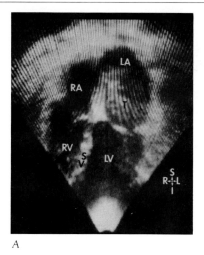
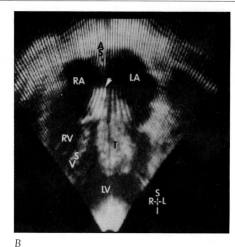

A

B

FIGURE 14-3. Apical four-chamber 2-D echocardiogram in systole (A) and diastole (B) of a patient with a large pedunculated left atrial myxoma (T). The gelatinous mass is attached to the left atrium (LA) in the area of the fossa ovalis membrane (*arrow*). During systole the mass is visualized within the left atrium; it "plops" into the left ventricle (LV) during diastole. (RA, right atrium; RV, right ventricle; VS, ventricular septum; AS, atrial septum.)

in diameter. It is generally pedunculated but may be sessile (short stalked), and has a fibrovascular stalk, which usually is attached to the left atrial wall in the area of the fossa ovalis membrane. Most myxomas are pale, gelatinous, and friable, which may account for their propensity toward embolization.[28]

*Echocardiographic findings.* Echocardiographically, an atrial myxoma appears as an oval, echogenic mass within the atrial chamber that moves in unison with intracardiac blood flow (Figs. 14-3, 14-4). If the myxoma is pedunculated, the mass moves appreciably with each cardiac cycle. Not uncommonly, the myxoma is seen "plopping" through the mitral valve orifice during diastole and moving back into the left atrium during systole. In contrast, sessile myxomas often remain relatively fixed throughout both systole and diastole. Sparkling, echodense areas can often be seen within the capsule of the myxoma. The calcium deposits often found in myxomas may account for this phenomenon.

The myxoma usually is attached near the area of the fossa ovalis membrane. It is important for the

sonographer to identify the point of attachment (Fig. 14-5). A mass attached to the fossa ovalis membrane can be confidently identified as a myxoma, but if the attachment point is not the atrial septum, the sonographer must be aware of other possible sources for the atrial mass, such as another type of tumor (Fig. 14-6) or a thrombus.

Additionally, cardiac chamber enlargement may be present, in which case the Doppler examination would aid in the assessment of valvular regurgitation or outflow obstruction.

*Lipoma of the Atrial Septum.* Lipoma is another mass that involves the atrial septum. This disorder is characterized by an excessive accumulation of fetal fat cells, which form a mass that may bulge into the right atrium. Often, the fossa ovalis membrane is not infiltrated, but fat is deposited in the remainder of the atrial septum. Prior to echocardiography, lipomatous hypertrophy of the atrial septum was detected only at autopsy,[36] that is to say, this entity commonly goes unrecognized. On occasion, it has been associated clinically with supraventricular arrhythmias and sudden death.[24]

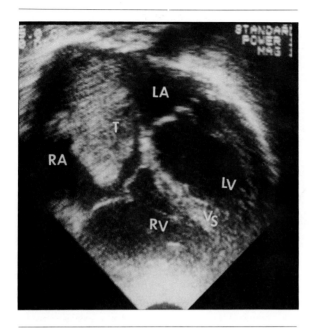

FIGURE 14-4. Modified apical four-chamber view of the heart of a patient with a myxoma (T) in the right atrium (RA). Myxomas are found less commonly in the right atrium. The attachment point must be identified to exclude thrombus or metastasis of a malignant tumor as the source. (LA, left atrium; LV, left ventricle; VS, ventricular septum; RV, right ventricle.) (From Pohost G, O'Rourke RA, eds. Cardiac Imaging. Boston: Little, Brown; 1989.)

*Echocardiographic findings.* On 2-D echocardiography, lipomatous infiltration of the atrial septum often has a dumbbell shape (Fig. 14-7).[16] From the subcostal window, which is the optimal scanning plane, sonodense thickening in the areas of the atrial septum can be seen superior and inferior to the fossa ovalis membrane. The atrial septal thickness must be at least 15 mm if the diagnosis of lipoma of the atrial septum is to be made.[16]

## VENTRICULAR TUMORS

*Lipoma.* Other areas of the heart may be subject to lipomatous infiltration. These lipomas, unlike lipoma of the atrial septum, are true neoplasms composed of mature fat cells. Lipomas occur at any age and affect males and females equally.[8] They are located either beneath the endocardium or epicar-

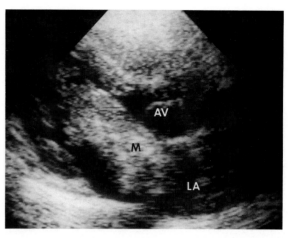

FIGURE 14-5. Parasternal long-axis echocardiographic view in a patient who presented with a right-sided cerebrovascular accident and a history of osteogenic sarcoma. The large left atrial mass (M) prolapses into the left ventricle during diastole. No connection with the atrial septum could be made. Although the mass appeared to be a left atrial myxoma, it was actually metastatic sarcoma. (LA, left atrium; AV, aortic valve.)

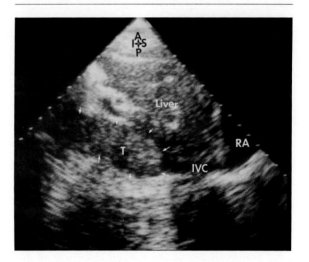

FIGURE 14-6. Subcostal 2-D echocardiogram concentrating on the inferior vena cava (IVC). A hypernephroma (carcinoma of the kidney) fills the inferior vena cava and extends into the right atrium (RA). (From Pohost G, O'Rourke RA, eds. Cardiac Imaging. Boston: Little, Brown; 1989.)

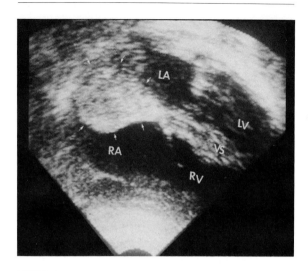

FIGURE 14-7. Subcostal four-chamber view demonstrates the typical dumbbell appearance of lipomatous infiltration of the atrial septum *(arrows)*. The area of infiltration is highly refractile and measures more than 15 mm. (LA, left atrium; LV, left ventricle; RV, right ventricle; RA, right atrium; VS, ventricular septum.) (From Applegate PA, Tajik AJ, Ehman RL, et al. Two-dimensional echocardiographic and magnetic resonance imaging observations in massive lipomatous hypertrophy of the atrial septum. Cardiol. 1987; 59:489–491.)

dium or within the myocardium, usually in the left ventricle or right atrium. If a cardiac lipoma extends into the pericardial space, it may result in cardiac compression; if located within the myocardium or endocardium, it may cause obstruction or conduction abnormalities. Fortunately, most are small and do not result in symptoms or in life-threatening complications.

*Rhabdomyoma.* More than half of the benign primary cardiac tumors found in children are rhabdomyomas.[6] Frequently they are seen in conjunction with a disease known as tuberous sclerosis.[3] Tuberous sclerosis is a familial disease characterized by tumors and sclerotic patches on the surface of the brain, which lead to convulsions and mental retardation. Skin lesions and widely disseminated tumorlike nodules also occur.

Rhabdomyomas commonly are multiple, and usually intramyocardial. They are most often found in the ventricles; left and right ventricle are affected with equal frequency. Rhabdomyomas may be small (1 mm) and asymptomatic. Large ones (20 mm) can project into a cardiac chamber or outflow tract and cause a variety of symptoms. Cardiomegaly, heart failure, murmurs, and arrhythmias may be seen. Fortunately, rhabdomyomas commonly have a benign course and have been known to regress spontaneously.[2] Occasionally, they must be excised to relieve symptoms caused by obstruction.

*Fibroma.* Fibromas are another type of mass located within the cardiac ventricles. They most often affect children but have been seen in males and females of all ages.[2,58] The most common locations for cardiac fibromas are within the myocardium of the interventricular septum and the left ventricular anterior wall.[39] Occasionally, they may be located in the left ventricular posterior wall or the right ventricle.[22] Fibromas are composed of fibroblasts within fibrous tissue. These well-circumscribed, nonencapsulated tumors are generally solitary and smaller than 7 cm.[45] Like lipomas and rhabdomyomas, fibromas do not cause symptoms unless they obstruct blood flow, or impair ventricular function, or alter conduction.

*Echocardiographic Findings of Ventricular Tumors.* Primary benign cardiac tumors that are commonly located within the ventricles have similar echocardiographic appearances. Each appears as a density embedded in the myocardium, endocardium, or epicardium (Fig. 14-8). With the exception of the rhabdomyoma (Fig. 14-9) most are single. The mass has a different acoustic impedance from the ventricular myocardium, and therefore it generally appears brighter. For this reason, with a complete echocardiographic examination that uses all available imaging windows the mass should be readily detectable.

Cardiac chamber enlargement and outflow tract obstruction is commonly seen. In this setting, Doppler examination allows assessment of the degree to which the tumor is obstructing blood flow, the amount of valvular regurgitation, and the intracardiac pressures.

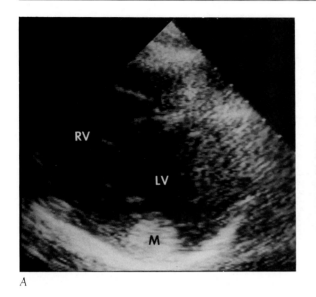

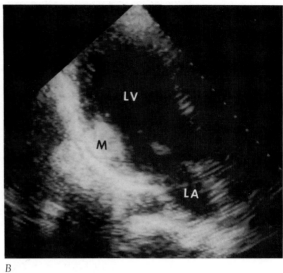

A                                    B

FIGURE 14-8. Parasternal short-axis view (A) of the left ventricle at the level of the papillary muscles shows a highly refractile, well-circumscribed mass (M) in the inferior wall. The mass, a fibroma, was also imaged in the apical long-axis view (B). The difference in acoustic impedance between the mass and the normal myocardium allows easy detection of the mass. (LV, left ventricle; LA, left atrium; RV, right ventricle.)

FIGURE 14-9. Parasternal long-axis 2-D echocardiogram of a patient with tuberous sclerosis. Multiple echogenic masses (M) are embedded in the myocardium of the left and right ventricles. These masses are rhabdomyomas, the benign tumors associated with tuberous sclerosis. (LV, left ventricle; RV, right ventricle; LA, left atrium.)

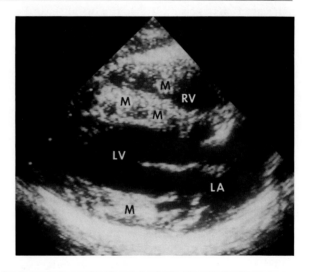

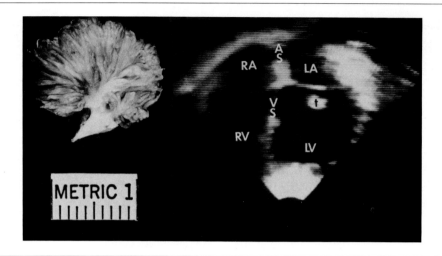

FIGURE 14-10. Pathologic specimen of a papillary fibroelastoma that was surgically removed from a patient's mitral valve. This benign tumor is demonstrated well on the apical four-chamber 2-D echocardiogram. The real-time examination revealed a highly mobile, pedunculated, 1-cm × 1-cm mass attached to the ventricular surface of the anterior leaflet of the mitral valve. (RA, RV, right atrium and ventricle; AS, VS, atrial and ventricular septa; LA, LV, left atrium and ventricle.) (From Shub C, Tajik AJ, Seward JB, et al. Cardiac papillary fibroelastomas: Two-dimensional echocardiographic recognition. Mayo Clin Proc. 1981; 56:629–633.)

### VALVULAR TUMORS

*Papillary Fibroelastoma.* Cardiac tumors also can be found on the valves or chordae tendineae. One such tumor, papillary fibroelastomas, or papilloma, has a frondlike appearance and may interfere with valve function. In most cases, however, papillomas do not cause symptoms and are incidental findings at surgery or autopsy. Characteristically, they are less than 1 cm in diameter and most often are found on the aortic valve in adults and on the tricuspid valve in children.[53]

*Echocardiographic findings.* Echocardiographically, a papillary fibroelastoma appears as a highly mobile, pedunculated mass resembling a pom-pom and attached to the surface of the valve (Fig. 14-10). As one might imagine, the echocardiographic features of a papilloma and a valvular vegetation are nearly identical (Fig. 14-11), so when a valvular mass is identified, the overall clinical picture becomes very important in the final diagnosis.

### PRIMARY MALIGNANT CARDIAC TUMORS

Approximately 25% of all primary cardiac tumors are found to be malignant.[41] Unlike benign tumors, malignant neoplasms tend to proliferate rapidly, and because they are not encapsulated, they easily infiltrate surrounding tissue. Most malignant neoplasms metastasize to areas of the body far from where they originate.[50] For this reason, they are more difficult to treat surgically. Treaments of primary malignant cardiac tumors include radiation and chemotherapy, but such treatments are palliative rather than curative.

Primary malignant cardiac tumors are classified as sarcomas. They arise from such mesenchymal tissues as blood vessels, lymphatics, and nerve tissue. They may occur at any age but are most common in persons between the ages of 30 and 50 years.[8] Angiosarcoma, the most common malignant tumor, occurs most often in the right atrium (Fig. 14-12).[45] Rhabdomyosarcomas and fibrosarcomas have no predilection for any cardiac chamber. Fre-

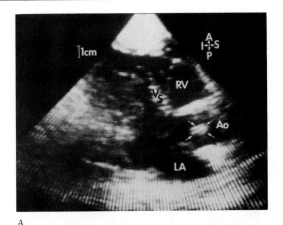
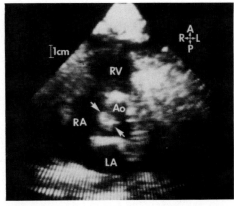

A                                    B

Figure 14-11. Parasternal long-axis (A) and short-axis (B) views demonstrate a pedunculated papilloma on the noncoronary cusp of the aortic valve (*arrows*). Although its appearance is nearly identical to that of a valvular vegetation, in the absence of a history of infective endocarditis the mass was correctly diagnosed as a papilloma. (Ao, aorta; LA, left atrium; RA, right atrium; RV, right ventricle; VS, ventricular septum.) (From Shub C, Tajik AJ, Seward JB, et al. Cardiac papillary fibroelastomas. Mayo Clin Proc. 1981; 56:629–633.)

Figure 14-12. Apical four-chamber echocardiogram of a patient with angiosarcoma. The laminated mass (T, *arrows*) is seen along the lateral wall of the right atrium (RA). (RV, right ventricle; LA, left atrium; LV, left ventricle; VS, ventricular septum.) (From Pohost G, O'Rourke RA, eds. Cardiac Imaging. Boston: Little, Brown; 1989.)

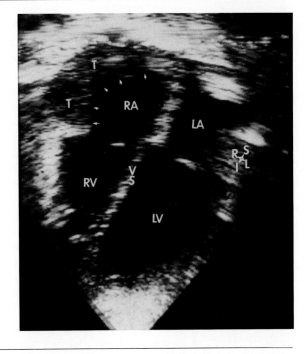

quently, sarcomas cause valvular obstruction and myocardial dysfunction. With time, heart failure occurs. As the tumor extends into the pericardium it causes a bloody pericardial effusion that may produce cardiac tamponade.

### Secondary Malignant Cardiac Tumors

Secondary tumors of the heart are much more common than primary tumors.[41] Any malignant primary tumor can metastasize to the heart. Bronchogenic carcinoma, leukemia, lymphoma, and carcinoma of the breast are the most common secondary tumors.[51] Interestingly, however, more than half of persons with malignant melanoma will have metastasis to the heart.[51] A tumor may spread to the heart by direct extension, through the lymphatic system, or through the venous system.[51]

Cardiac metastases are mostly small, multiple, discrete nodules found in the pericardium or endocardium. Clinical findings, then, relate to the area of metastasis. Pericardial effusion, together with signs of cardiac tamponade or constrictive pericarditis, may be found. Additional findings include conduction abnormalities, cardiac chamber enlargement, and congestive heart failure. It is not uncommon for early cardiac metastasis to be asymptomatic.

*Echocardiographic Findings.* Malignant cardiac tumors occur most frequently in the ventricles. Unlike benign tumors, malignant tumors commonly cause myocardial dysfunction by compressing or invading the ventricle (Fig. 14-13). Initially, regional wall motion abnormalities may be seen on the echocardiogram. Later, ventricular dilatation may result from progressive heart failure. Myocardium that has been infiltrated by a primary malignant tumor usually has a different acoustic impedance from the surrounding tissue. With careful observation, the sonographer should be able to delineate the extent of tumor involvement and its overall effects on cardiac function. Frequently, valvular regurgitation and intracardiac pressure elevation are found on the Doppler examination.

Another finding often associated with metastatic disease is malignant pericardial effusion, and enough fluid frequently accumulates to cause cardiac tamponade. Doppler examination, particularly pulsed-wave Doppler, affords early recognition of impending tamponade.

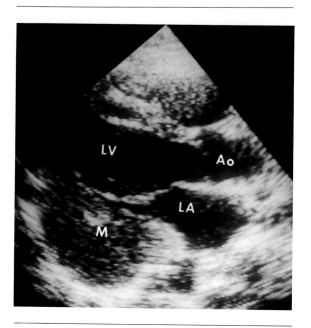

Figure 14-13. Parasternal long-axis echocardiogram demonstrates malignant melanoma of the left ventricular inferior wall. The large infiltrating mass (M) is well-circumscribed and appears to impinge slightly on the left ventricle (LV) and left atrium (LA). (Ao, aorta.)

## Thrombotic Disease

Intracardiac thrombi may occur for many reasons. Myocardial and valvular disease are responsible for the majority of thrombus formation. In addition, the presence of any foreign body (e.g., prosthetic valve, infusion catheter, hemodynamic monitoring catheter) may lead to thrombus formation.

### Pathophysiology

The exact mechanism of thrombus formation is not totally understood, but certain conditions are prerequisite.[26] First, the normally smooth endothelial surface must be damaged (roughened). Second, the flow of blood past the damaged surface must be very slow. Finally, the viscosity and coagulability of the blood must increase. Once the stage is set, intact and ruptured platelets are deposited on the rough, inflamed endocardial surface, to which they adhere. This adhesion leads to the formation of a fibrin net, which creates a foundation for the additional accumulation of various blood elements, thereby creating a mural thrombus.

LOCATION

Left ventricular mural thrombus is a common complication of ventricular dysfunction secondary to dilated cardiomyopathy, acute myocardial infarction, or ventricular aneurysm.[42,43] In these situations, blood stasis takes place in the areas of akinesia or dyskinesia. Ventricular thrombus is located in the apex in the majority of cases.

Ventricular dysfunction may also lead to thrombus formation in one of the atrial appendages. Ordinarily, however, thrombus in the appendage occurs in the presence of atrial fibrillation secondary to long-standing mitral or tricuspid disease. Infusion and monitoring catheters and central venous lines have also been associated with atrial thrombus formation.[29,53]

Thrombus may form in the right ventricle following a right ventricular myocardial infarction or, more commonly, after trauma to the heart (Fig. 14-14).[30] An example of this type of trauma is chest contusion by the steering wheel in an automobile accident. The predominant location for thrombus formation of this type is the right ventricular apex. The thrombus is usually laminar but may be mobile and pedunculated.

Although they are rare, diseases do exist in which thrombus forms when there is no underlying wall motion abnormality or chamber dilatation.[13] One such disease, eosinophilic endomyocardial fibrosis, can be caused by leukemia, parasitic infestation, asthma, or drug reactions, to name a few. In this disease, the endocardium develops fibrotic areas that become covered with a layer of thrombus. The inflow areas of the ventricles, the ventricular apices, the papillary muscles, and the chordae tendineae are most often affected (Fig. 14-15).

RELATED DIAGNOSTIC PROCEDURES

The most commonly utilized modality for the assessment of intracardiac thrombi is 2-D echocardiography. Because it allows visualization of many areas within the cardiac chambers, particularly the left ventricular apex, from a variety of angles, it has proven to be a sensitive technique for the detection of left ventricular thrombi. Whereas the predictive accuracy of angiography in detecting ventricular thrombi is, at best, 57%, the predictive accuracy of

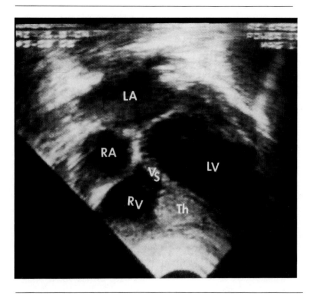

FIGURE 14-14. Subcostal four-chamber echocardiogram of a child following cardiac resuscitation. The chest trauma has led to thrombus formation (Th) in the right ventricular apex (RV). (VS, ventricular septum; LV, left ventricle; LA, left atrium; RA, right atrium.) (From Pohost G, O'Rourke RA, eds. Cardiac Imaging. Boston: Little, Brown; 1989.)

echocardiography is 79%. Unlike computed tomography and magnetic resonance imaging, echocardiography is inexpensive, noninvasive, and uses no ionizing radiation.

*Echocardiographic Findings.* An apical left ventricular thrombus may be flat and contiguous with the ventricular wall or sessile and protruding into the cavity (Fig. 14-16). Distinguishing the margin between the thrombus and the myocardium generally is not difficult. Thrombi often appear granular, whereas the myocardium has a darker and more uniform appearance. The prerequisite for thrombus formation is the presence of an underlying regional wall motion abnormality. As the ventricular wall moves in an akinetic or dyskinetic fashion, the thrombi move synchronously with the wall. At times, portions of a thrombus may be pedunculated and so may not move in unison with the wall. Most large thrombi can be visualized in the apical four-chamber view, but those that are very small and laminar may be missed. The apical short-axis

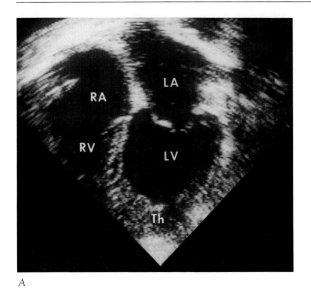

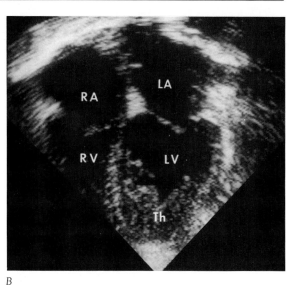

*A*                                                    *B*

FIGURE 14-15. Apical four-chamber view in diastole (*A*) and systole (*B*). Laminated thrombus (Th) can be seen in the apex of the left ventricle (LV). In systole, nearly half of the ventricle is obliterated. This thrombus was the result of eosinophilic endomyocardial fibrosis. In the real-time examination, no regional wall motion abnormalities were present, reinforcing the suspicion of a nonischemic cause of the thrombus formation. (LA, left atrium; RV, right ventricle; RA, right atrium.)

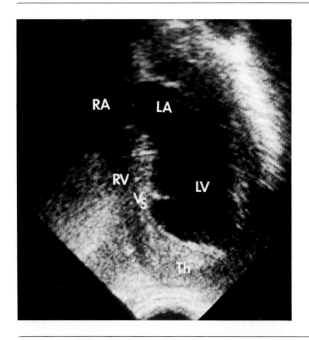

FIGURE 14-16. Apical four-chamber view in a patient who had had an extensive inferoapical and anteroapical myocardial infarction. A large, laminar thrombus (Th) can be seen within the left ventricular apex. On the real-time image, the thrombus was flat and contiguous with the ventricular wall and moved in a dyskinetic fashion. (RA, RV, right atrium and ventricle; LA, LV, left atrium and ventricle; VS, ventricular septum.) (From Pohost G, O'Rourke RA, eds. Cardiac Imaging. Boston: Little, Brown; 1989.)

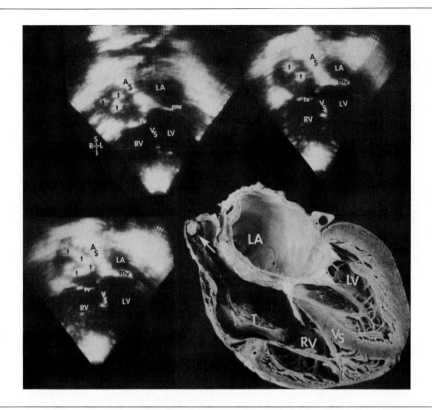

FIGURE 14-17. Multiple four-chamber echocardiograms in a patient with a right atrial thrombus (t) secondary to a right atrial catheter. Within the right atrium, a popcornlike mass can be seen moving in an erratic fashion. The pathologic specimen from the same patient verifies the presence of the thrombus and identifies the attachment point near the superior vena cava. (AS, atrial septum; LA, left atrium; mv, mitral valve; tv, tricuspid valve; VS, ventricular septum; LV, left ventricle; RV, right ventricle.) (From Pohost G, O'Rourke RA, eds. Cardiac Imaging. Boston: Little, Brown; 1989.)

view provides optimal visualization of the true apex. In this view, the smaller thrombi can be more easily distinguished from the ventricular myocardium, and wall motion may be more thoroughly assessed. This scanning plane is achieved with clockwise rotation and anterior and lateral beam angulation from the position used for the apical two-chamber view. At times, the paraapical position is superior to the true apical position for visualizing the entire apex.

As with left ventricular thrombi, 2-D echocardiography is highly sensitive for visualizing thrombi within the body of the left or right atrium.

While free-floating thrombi may be seen in the left atrium with long-standing mitral stenosis, they are more common in the right atrial cavity. The source of right atrial thrombi is generally either an infusion catheter or a central venous line (Fig. 14-17). Thrombi originating in the inferior vena cava may also travel to the right atrium. The echocardiographic appearance of right atrial thrombi is similar to that of popcorn on a string, moving erratically during diastole (Fig. 14-18). Portions of thrombus occasionally may be seen moving to and fro through the tricuspid valve orifice.

Unfortunately, conventional 2-D echocardiog-

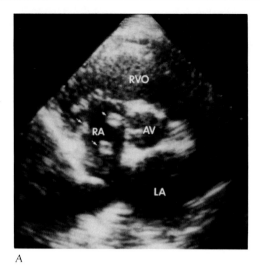
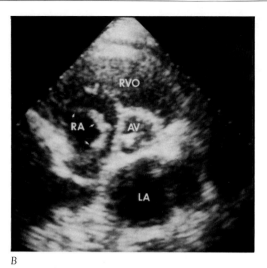

A   B

FIGURE 14-18. Parasternal short-axis echocardiograms at the level of the aortic valve (AV) demonstrate a mobile right atrial thrombus. During different phases of the cardiac cycle, the echogenic mass can be seen moving erratically within the right atrial cavity (RA). Occasionally, the thrombus moved through the tricuspid valve orifice into the right ventricle. This patient was thought to have had a pulmonary embolism. (LA, left atrium; AV, aortic valve; RVO, right ventricular outflow tract.) (From Pohost G, O'Rourke RA, eds. Cardiac Imaging. Boston: Little, Brown; 1989.)

raphy has proven to be less sensitive in its ability to visualize thrombus in the atrial appendages. Often the left atrial appendage may be visualized by using a nonstandard imaging position, such as a high, left parasternal window (Fig. 14-19). At present, the optimal modality for the assessment of atrial thrombi appears to be transesophageal echocardiography. This technique affords complete visualization of both left and right atrial appendages and should be performed as an adjunct to the 2-D echocardiogram.

## Echocardiographic Pitfalls

Certain structures, both extracardiac and intracardiac, may give the appearance on the echocardiogram of a cardiac tumor. Sonographers must be familiar with these structures to avoid misinterpreting them. Sonographers investigating intracardiac masses or source of emboli often pay close attention to extraneous echoes that normally would be overlooked.

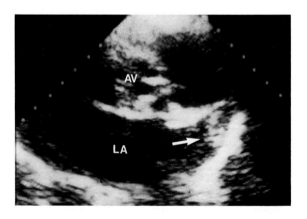

FIGURE 14-19. Parasternal short-axis scan at the aortic valve level. A sonodense area can be seen within the left atrial appendage. Because most thrombi within the appendages are small and laminar they are often difficult to image echocardiographically. In this case the thrombus was found by using a high left parasternal imaging window.

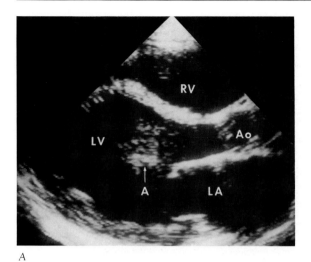
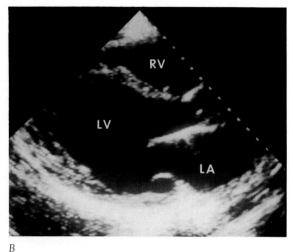

A

B

FIGURE 14-20. (A) Two-dimensional echocardiogram demonstrating an artifact (*arrow*) within the left ventricle (LV). Changing the depth of the scan eliminated the artifact (B). An alternate method is to introduce a pulsed-wave Doppler sample volume into the 2-D image, which also increases the frame rate. (RV, right ventricle; Ao, aorta; LA, left atrium.)

The acoustic beam itself has the potential to create misleading echoes. Side lobe artifacts—extraneous echoes produced by the elements of the transducer—commonly produce confusion. Echoes generated by objects outside the scanning plane may be received and displayed by the echocardiographic system (Fig. 14-20A). Fortunately, these echoes generally are weaker than the majority of received echoes generated from the cardiac structures. The source of these echoes can be identified by changing the frame rate of image acquisition. This may be accomplished in several ways. Changing the depth range of the scan or using simultaneous imaging (2-D and M-mode or 2-D and Doppler) are two simple methods. As the frame rate is altered, the extraneous echoes generally are eliminated (Fig. 14-20B).

Reverberation, or shadowing, another important ultrasound artifact, can be created when the ultrasound beam strikes an unusually dense or mobile structure at a right angle. An example is often seen in the subcostal four-chamber image. A tumorlike structure may be visualized moving within the left atrial chamber. With careful observation, the structure can be associated with the area of the tricuspid valve annulus, near the right atrioventricular groove. In actuality, then, the "mass" is simply a reverberation. When the beam direction is altered the mass appears to change location. Because no point of attachment can be found it is unlikely to represent an intracardiac mass.

Structures adjacent to the heart may be misinterpreted as intracardiac masses. The descending thoracic aorta, which lies close to the left atrium, normally appears as a circular echofree space posterior to the left atrioventricular groove. If enlarged, it may appear to impinge on the left atrial free wall (Fig. 14-21). With improper gain settings, it may look exactly like an intracardiac tumor. Angulating the beam more superiorly and inferiorly and readjusting the gain settings will demonstrate the sonolucent aorta.

Noncardiac structures may be mistaken for cardiac masses. In addition to fibrinous strands, portions of a collapsed lung may be seen in a pleural effusion. When imaged from the subcostal window

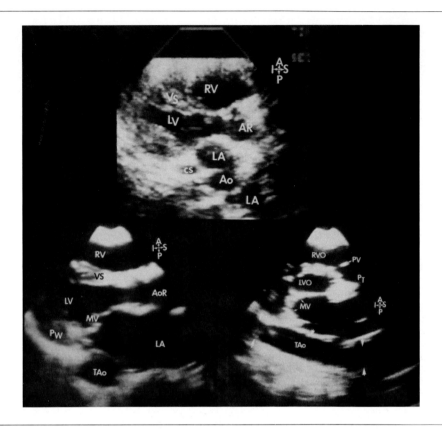

FIGURE 14-21. (A, B) Parasternal long-axis view in a patient with obstructive lung disease. The thoracic aorta (Ao) appears as a sonolucent structure within the left atrium (LA). Rotating the transducer clockwise toward the right ventricular outflow tract view (C) verifies the origin of this sonolucent structure. The thoracic aorta (TAo) will be imaged longitudinally posteriorly to the left atrium. (RV, right ventricle; VS, ventricular septum; AR/AoR, aortic root; cs, coronary sinus; MV, mitral valve; PW, posterior wall; LVO, left ventricular outflow tract; PV, pulmonary valve; PT, pulmonary trunk.) (From Pohost G, O'Rourke RA, eds. Cardiac Imaging. Boston: Little, Brown; 1989.)

the lung may appear to be an extracardiac tumor (Fig. 14-22). A diaphragmatic hernia may appear to be a left atrial mass (Fig. 14-23).[35] Most often, this structure is visualized in the parasternal and apical views. With certain beam angles the left atrium may appear to be obliterated. Confusion may often be eliminated simply by directing the beam slightly anteriorly. If the mass disappears completely, an extracardiac structure should be suspected. An alternate method is to image the area while the patient swallows a liquid. Visualizing this liquid mov-

ing within the "mass" confirms the diagnosis of diaphragmatic hernia.

Several common anatomic variants in the normal heart have been misinterpreted as pathologic structures. Two such structures, the eustachian valve and the Chiari network,[60] are located in the right atrium. Neither has any clinical significance. Echocardiographically, both may appear as long, thin, rapidly moving echoes near the junction of the inferior vena cava and the right atrium (Fig. 14-24). Occasionally, these structures may become un-

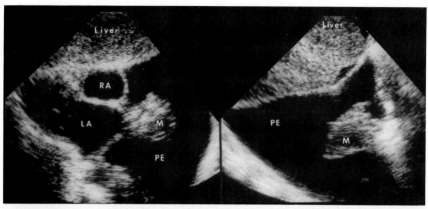

FIGURE 14-22

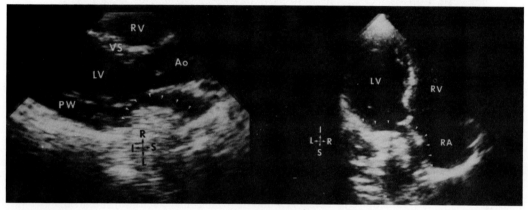

FIGURE 14-23A                    FIGURE 14-23B

FIGURE 14-22. Subcostal four-chamber view in a patient with a collapsed lung. The lung appears as an extracardiac mass (M) within the pleural effusion (PE). Rotating the transducer clockwise into a short-axis scanning plane gives the mass the more characteristic appearance of a collapsed lung. (RA, right atrium; LA, left atrium.)

FIGURE 14-23. Parasternal short-axis (A) and four-chamber (B) echocardiograms of a patient with a diaphragmatic hernia. The large, sonodense mass (*arrows*) appears to protrude into the left atrial cavity. After the patient swallowed some water, swirling echoes were noted within the mass. Without careful observation, this extracardiac structure might be misinterpreted as an atrial mass. (PW, posterior wall; LV, left ventricle; VS, ventricular septum; RV, right ventricle; Ao, aorta; RA, right atrium.) (From Nishimura RA, Tajik AJ, Schattenberg TT, et al. Diaphragmatic hernia mimicking an atrial mass: A two-dimensional echocardiographic pitfall. J Am Coll Cardiol. 1985; 5(4):992–995.)

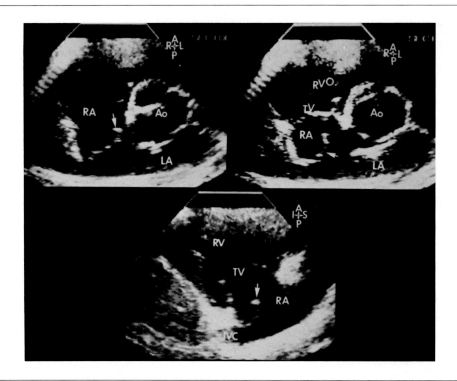

Figure 14-24. Parasternal short-axis (A, B) and right ventricular inflow (C) views reveal a thin, highly mobile, echogenic structure (A, B) (*arrows*) traversing the right atrium (C) (RA). The insertion point of the structure at the entrance of the inferior vena cava (IVC) into the right atrium confirms that it is simply a redundant eustachian valve. (LA, left atrium; Ao, aorta; RVO, right ventricular outflow tract; TV, tricuspid valve; RV, right ventricle.) (From Seward JB, Edwards WD, Tajik AJ, et al, eds. Two-Dimensional Echocardiographic Atlas of Congenital Heart Disease. Berlin: Springer-Verlag; 1987; 143.)

usually redundant and display a whiplike motion. They should not be confused with mobile thrombi or intracardiac masses. Imaging from the parasternal short-axis and subcostal windows affords optimal visualization of the right atrium, and correct identification can then be made.

Normal cardiac variants are also found in the ventricles. False tendons, also known as anomalous chordae tendineae, may occur in the left ventricle.[4] These fine, filamentous structures may traverse the ventricle in a variety of locations (Fig. 14-25). When located near the apex they may be difficult to diagnose. Differentiating false tendons from apical thrombi is often difficult. The apical cross-sec-

tional view may provide the necessary information to make an accurate diagnosis. Often the false tendon can be identified from this view as a separate structure independent of the apical myocardium. Regional wall motion may also be assessed.

Another source of confusion with regards to ventricular thrombi is the moderator band (Fig. 14-26). The moderator band, located in the apical third of the right ventricle, is one of the four muscular bands that separate the inflow tract from the outflow tract. The inflow tract is normally heavily trabeculated. If the right ventricle becomes hypertrophic, as it does in pulmonary hypertension, the trabeculae become thickened. The moderator band

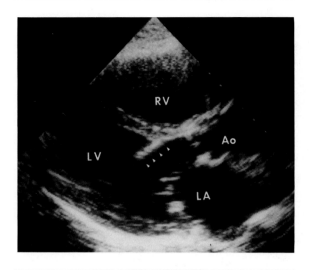

FIGURE 14-25. Parasternal long-axis view demonstrates a highly refractile structure (*arrows*) within the left ventricle (LV) near the outflow tract. It was found to be an anomalous chorda tendineae traversing the ventricle from the ventricular septum to the papillary muscle. Such echoes may be confusing and must not be mistaken for intracardiac masses. (RV, right ventricle; Ao, aorta; LA, left atrium.)

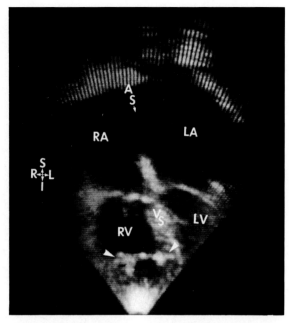

FIGURE 14-26. Apical four-chamber 2-D echocardiogram of a patient with a thickened, echogenic moderator band (*arrows*). Care must be taken to avoid misinterpreting this normal structure as a right ventricular thrombus. (RA, right atrium; RV, right ventricle; LV, left ventricle; VS, ventricular septum; AS, atrial septum; LA, left atrium.) (From: Lundstrom N-R, ed. Pediatric Echocardiography—Cross Sectional, M-Mode and Doppler. New York: Elsevier North-Holland Biomedical Press; 1980; 105–120.)

may also become hypertrophic. If this is kept in mind, right ventricular apical thrombus should not be misdiagnosed.

## Summary

In the hands of experienced, knowledgeable, and conscientious medical and paramedical personnel, echocardiography provides diagnostic information. In most instances, whether a cardiac mass is secondary to infective endocarditis or is a neoplasm or a thrombus, the echocardiogram is able to provide an accurate assessment of its size, shape, and location. In addition, information on the overall effect of the mass on cardiac function and intracardiac blood flow can be obtained. Echocardiography will likely continue to be the technique of choice for the assessment of intracardiac masses.

## Acknowledgments

The author would like to express sincerest gratitude to Dr. A. J. Tajik for his helpful suggestions in the preparation of this manuscript and for his continued support and encouragement; and to Drs. J. B. Seward and B. K. Khandheria for their assistance in obtaining the echocardiographic illustrations.

## References

1. Amparo EG, Higgins CB, Farmer D, et al. Gated MRI of cardiac and paracardiac massess: Initial experience. AJR. 1980; 44:143–149.
2. Arciniegas E, Hakimi M, Farooki ZQ, et al. Primary

cardiac tumors in children. J Thorac Cardiovasc Surg. 1980; 79:582–591.

3. Bass JL, Breningstall GN, Swaiman KF. Echocardiographic incidence of cardiac rhabdomyoma in tuberous sclerosis. Am J Cardiol. 1985; 55:1379–1382.

4. Boyd MT, Seward JB, Tajik AJ, et al. Frequency and location of prominent left ventricular trabeculations at autopsy in 474 normal human hearts: Implications for evaluation of mural thrombi by two-dimensional echocardiography. J Am Coll Cardiol. 1987; 9:323–326.

5. Bulkey BH, Hutchins GM. Atrial myxomas: A fifty-year review. Am Heart J. 1979; 97:639–643.

6. Chan HS, Sonley MJ, Moes CA, et al. Primary and secondary tumors of childhood involving the heart, pericardium, and great vessels: A report of 75 cases and review of the literature. Cancer. 1985; 56:825–836.

7. Clawson CC, Rao GHR, White JG. Platelet interaction with bacteria: IV. Stimulation of the release reaction. Am J Pathol. 1975; 81:411–419.

8. Colucci WS, Braunwald E. Primary tumors of the heart. In: Braunwald E (ed). A Textbook of Cardiovascular Medicine. 2d ed. Philadelphia: WB Saunders; 1984.

9. Dashkoff N, Boersma RB, Nanda NC, et al. Bilateral atrial myxomas: Echocardiographic considerations. Am J Med. 1978; 65:361–366.

10. Edler I. Cardiac studies by ultrasound. In: Luisada AA, ed. Cardiology: An Encyclopedia of the Cardiovascular System. New York: McGraw-Hill; 1962; 2:410-424.

11. Effert S, Domanig E. The diagnosis of intra-atrial tumours and thrombi by ultrasonic echo method. Ger Med Mon. 1959; 4:1–3.

12. Everett ED, Hirschmann JV. Transient bacteremia and endocarditis prophylaxis: A review. Medicine. 1977; 56:61–77.

13. Fauci AS, Harley JB, Roberts WC, et al. NIH conference: The idiopathic hypereosinophilic syndrome: Clinical, pathophysiologic, and therapeutic considerations. Ann Intern Med. 1982; 97:78–92.

14. Fenoglio JJ Jr, McAllister HA Jr, Ferrans VJ. Cardiac rhabdomyoma: A clinicopathologic and electron microscopic study. Am J Cardiol. 1976; 38:241–251.

15. Fyke FE III, Seward JB, Edwards WD, et al. Primary cardiac tumors: Experience with 30 consecutive patients since the introduction of two-dimensional echocardiography. J Am Coll Cardiol. 1983; 5:1465–1473.

16. Fyke FE III, Tajik AJ, Edwards WD, et al. Diagnosis of lipomatous hypertrophy of the atrial septum by two-dimensional echocardiography. J Am Coll Cardiol. 1983; 1:1352–1357.

17. Gantz NM, Gleckman RA, Brown RB, et al. Surgery in active infective endocarditis. In: Gantz NM, Gleckman RA, Brown RB, et al (eds). Manual of Clinical Problems in Infectious Disease. 2nd ed. Boston: Little, Brown; 1986.

18. Garvey GJ, Neu HC. Infective endocarditis: An evolving disease. Medicine. 1978; 57:105–127.

19. Godwin JD, Axel L, Adams JR, et al. Computed tomography: A new method for diagnosing tumor of the heart. Circulation. 1981; 63:448–451.

20. Green SE, Joynt LF, Fitzgerald PJ, et al. In vivo ultrasonic tissue characterization of human intracardiac masses. Am J Cardiol. 1983; 51:231–236.

21. Harvey WP. Clinical aspects of cardiac tumors. Am J Cardiol. 1968; 21:328–343.

22. Heath D. Pathology of cardiac tumors. Am J Cardiol. 1968; 21:315–327.

23. Houser S, Forbes N, Stewart S. Rhabdomyoma of the heart: A diagnostic and therapeutic challenge. Ann Thorac Surg. 1980; 29:373–377.

24. Hutter AM Jr, Page DL. Atrial arrhythmias and lipomatous hypertrophy of the cardiac interatrial septum. Am Heart J. 1971; 82:16–21.

25. Kaye D. Definitions and demographic characteristics. In: Kaye D, ed. Infective Endocarditis. Baltimore: University Park Press; 1976.

26. Luckmann J, Sorensen KC. Abnormalities of cardiac structure and function: An overview. In: Luckmann J, Sorensen KC, eds. Medical-Surgical Nursing: A Psychophysiologic Approach. 2nd ed. Philadelphia: WB Saunders; 1980.

27. McAllister HA Jr. Primary tumors and cysts of the heart and pericardium. In: Harvey WP, ed. Current Problems in Cardiology. Chicago: Year Book Medical Publishers; 1979; 4.

28. McAllister HA Jr, Fenoglio JJ Jr. Tumors of the cardiovascular system. In: Hartmann W, Cowan WR, eds. Atlas of Tumor Pathology. Fascicle 15, 2nd series. Washington: US Armed Forces Institute of Pathology; 1978.

29. McQuiston DJ. Hickman catheter complications: A three-year retrospective analysis. Proc Oncol Nurs Soc. 1983; 61–65.

30. Miller FA, Seward JB, Gersh BJ. Two-dimensional echocardiographic findings in cardiac trauma. Am J Cardiol. 1982; 50:1022–1027.

31. Morgan DL, Palazola J, Reed W, et al. Left heart myxomas. Am J Cardiol. 1977; 40:611–614.

32. Narenthiran S. Echocardiography in subacute bacterial endocarditis. Ceylon Med J. 1985; 30:125–129.

33. Nasser WK, Davis RH, Dillon JC, et al. Atrial myxoma: I. Clinical and pathologic features in nine cases. Am Heart J. 1972; 83:694–704.

34. Nishimura RA, McGoon MD, Shub C, et al. Echo-

cardiographically documented mitral valve prolapse: Long-term follow-up of 237 patients. N Engl J Med. 1985; 313:1305–1309.

35. Nishimura RA, Tajik AJ, Schattenberg TT, et al. Diaphragmatic hernia mimicking an atrial mass: A two-dimensional echocardiographic pitfall. J Am Coll Cardiol. 1985; 5:992–995.

36. Page DL. Lipomatous hypertrophy of the atrial septum: Its development and probable clinical significance. Hum Pathol. 1970; 1:151–163.

37. Pelletier LL, Petersdorf RG. Infective endocarditis: A review of 125 cases from the University of Washington Hospitals, 1963–72. Medicine. 1977; 56:287–313.

38. Peters MN, Hall RJ, Cooley DA, et al. The clinical syndrome of atrial myxoma. JAMA. 1974; 230:694–701.

39. Piehler JM, Lie JT, Guiliani ER. Tumors of the heart. In: Brandenberg RO, Fuster V, Guiliani ER, et al. eds. Cardiology: Fundamentals and Practice. Chicago: Year Book Medical Publishers; 1981.

40. Pohost GM, Pastore JO, McKusick KA, et al. Detection of left atrial myxomas by gated radionuclide cardiac imaging. Circulation. 1977; 55:88–92.

41. Prichard RW. Tumors of the heart: Review of the subject and report of one hundred and fifty cases. Arch Pathol. 1951; 51:98–128.

42. Reeder GS, Lengyel M, Tajik AJ, et al. Mural thrombus in left ventricular aneurysm: Incidence, role of angiography, and relation between anticoagulation and embolization. Mayo Clin Proc. 1981; 56:77–81.

43. Reeder GS, Tajik AJ, Seward JB. Left ventricular mural thrombus: two-dimensional echocardiographic diagnosis. Mayo Clin Proc. 1981; 56:82–86.

44. Rodbard S. Blood velocity and endocarditis. Circulation. 1963; 27:18–28.

45. Rossi NP, Koichos JM, Aschenbrener CA, et al. Primary angiosarcoma of the heart. Cancer. 1976; 37:891–894.

46. St John Sutton MG, Mercier L-A, Guiliani ER, et al. Atrial myxomas: A review of clinical experience in 40 patients. Mayo Clin Proc. 1980; 55:371–376.

47. Scheld WM, Sande MA. Endocarditis and intravascular infections. In: Mandell GL, Douglas RG Jr, Bennett JE, eds. Principles and Practice of Infectious Diseases. 2nd ed. New York: Wiley; 1985.

48. Seward JB, Khandheria BK, Oh JK, et al. Transesophageal echocardiography: Technique, anatomic correlation, implementation, and clinical applications. Mayo Clinic Proc. 1988; 63:649–680.

49. Sharratt GP, Grover ML, Monro JL. Calcified left atrial myxoma with floppy mitral valve. Br Heart J. 1979; 42:608–610.

50. Silverman NA. Primary cardiac tumors. Ann Surg. 1980; 191:127–138.

51. Smith LH. Secondary tumors of the heart. Rev Surg. 1976; 33:223–231.

52. Stewart JA, Silimperi D, Harris P, et al. Echocardiographic documentation of vegetative lesions in infective endocarditis: Clinical implications. Circulation. 1980; 61:374–380.

53. Swan HJ. Techniques of monitoring the seriously ill patient with heart disease (including use of Swan-Ganz catheter). In: Hurst JW, ed. The Heart: Arteries and Veins. 6th ed. New York: McGraw-Hill; 1985.

54. Thayer WS. Studies on bacterial (infective) endocarditis. Johns Hopkins Hosp Rep. 1926; 22:1–185.

55. Urba WJ, Longo DL. Primary solid tumors of the heart. In: Kapoor AS, ed. Cancer and the Heart. New York: Springer-Verlag; 1986.

56. Vidaillet HJ, Seward JB, Su WPD, et al. "Syndrome myxoma": A subset of patients with cardiac myxoma associated with pigmented skin lesions and peripheral and endocrine neoplasms. Br Heart J. 1987; 57:247–255.

57. Werner JA, Cheitlin MD, Gross BW, et al. Echocardiographic appearance of the Chiari network: Differentiation from right-heart pathology. Circulation. 1981; 63:1104–1109.

58. Williams DB, Danielson GK, McGoon DC, et al. Cardiac fibroma: Long-term survival after excision. J Thorac Cardiovasc Surg. 1982; 84:230–236.

59. Wilson WR, Geraci JE, Giuliani ER. Infective endocarditis. In: Brandenberg RO, Fuster V, Giuliani ER, et al., eds. Cardiology: Fundamentals and Practice. Chicago: Year Book Medical Publishers; 1987.

60. Wilson WR, Washington JA II. Infective endocarditis: A changing spectrum? (editorial). Mayo Clin Proc. 1977; 52:254–255.

61. Wold LE, Lie JT. Cardiac myxomas: A clinicopathologic profile. Am J Pathol. 1980; 101:219–240.

CHAPTER **15**

# Cardiac Trauma

HENNY J. WASSER, ALVIN GREENGART, JUDAH A. CHARNOFF

Chest trauma has become increasingly common in the past few decades, owing to the increased incidence of high-speed motor vehicle accidents[45] and violent crime.[2] Cardiac injury resulting from chest trauma may initially go unnoticed as attention is directed to more obvious injuries.[4] Recognition of cardiac injury is crucial, as it may alter the management of patients with chest injuries.[13]

The large constellation of possible cardiac abnormalities that can result from trauma make detection of cardiac injury a challenge. Diagnosis is usually based on clinical findings and on results of procedures such as radiography, electrocardiography, and cardiac enzyme studies.[4] Owing to the wide range of possible anatomic abnormalities resulting from cardiac trauma, echocardiography can contribute important diagnostic information, though the examination may be hampered by the serious physical condition of the patient or by bandages or other injuries.[38]

The incidence of iatrogenic cardiac injuries is rising as a result of the increasing use of catheters (penetrating injury) and of cardiopulmonary resuscitation (blunt injury).[9] Blunt thoracic injuries are more common than penetrating injuries.[4] The two major life-threatening consequences of cardiac trauma are exsanguinating hemorrhage and cardiac tamponade. Effective treatment has resulted in an increasing number of immediate survivors, and later sequelae—including myocardial infarction, aneurysm, pseudoaneurysm, ventricular septal de-

fects, valve damage, recurrent pericarditis, and constrictive pericarditis—are becoming far more common.[9] In this chapter the common injuries resulting from cardiac trauma are discussed and the role of echocardiography in its diagnosis and management is described.

## Nonpenetrating Chest Trauma

Blunt chest trauma accounts for one fourth of all traumatic deaths annually in the United States.[29] The most common cause of blunt chest injury is motor vehicle accidents; damage to the heart most often results from steering wheel contusion. The violent decelerative force of impact can damage the heart and great vessels even if the chest wall is not punctured (Fig. 15-1). Other causes include sports injuries, falls from heights, blows from blunt objects, and closed chest massage during cardiopulmonary resuscitation.[9,45]

Cardiac damage can result from direct compression of the sternum against the heart or from increased intrathoracic pressure transmitted from a blow to the chest or abdomen.[45]

Cardiac injury due to trauma covers a wide spectrum of anatomic and physiologic abnormalities. Injury can occur immediately or it can develop gradually. Table 15-1 lists the different forms of injury that blunt chest trauma produces.[9] It is important to obtain the details of the traumatic event, as a steering wheel injury sustained in a high-speed

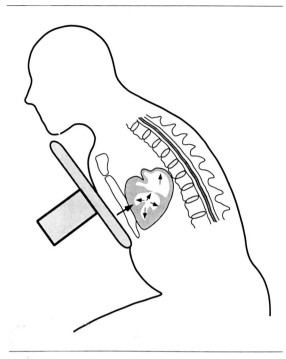

FIGURE 15-1. Decelerative impact forces of steering wheel injury. Reprinted by permission. (Illustration by Greg Lawrence.)

TABLE 15-1. Types of cardiac injury from blunt trauma

Myocardium
   Contusion
   Laceration
   Rupture
   Septal perforation
   Aneurysm, pseudoaneurysm
   Hemopericardium, tamponade
   Thrombosis, systemic embolism
Pericardium
   Pericarditis
   Postpericardiotomy syndrome
   Constrictive pericarditis
   Pericardial laceration
   Hemorrhage
   Cardiac herniation
Endocardial structures
   Rupture of papillary muscle
   Rupture of chordae tendineae
   Rupture of atrioventricular and semilunar valves
Coronary artery
   Thrombosis
   Laceration
   Fistula

(From Jackson DH, Murphy GW. Nonpenetrating cardiac trauma. Mod Conc Cardiovas Dis. 1976; 45:123. By permission of the American Heart Association, Inc.)

motor vehicle accident has different effects on the heart than does striking the chest during a minor fall.[7]

Fractures of the ribs, clavicle, or sternum are the hallmarks of chest trauma. The associated pain often masks underlying cardiac injury and may make diagnosis difficult. Cardiac trauma may be present even in the absence of fractures and may be more severe in this setting, if the heart absorbs most of the energy of impact.[5,40,45]

With severe or massive cardiac injury, death occurs immediately. If damage is less severe, patients may reach an emergency room, where prompt diagnosis and treatment is received if they are to survive. The myocardium may be injured by fragments of bone driven into the heart or from compression of the heart between the sternum and the spine or against the chest wall.[7] When time and the patient's condition permit, echocardiography is a valuable screening tool for the evaluation of cardiac involvement following blunt chest trauma.[6]

PERICARDIAL EFFUSION

Pericardial effusion often follows blunt chest trauma, and usually indicates that the heart has been injured. Pericardial effusion rarely appears as a solitary lesion; usually it is found in association with cardiac contusion or great vessel or myocardial tears. Effusions due to trauma frequently are bloody; they may accumulate rapidly or take a week or more to develop. The major sequela of pericardial effusion due to trauma—cardiac tamponade—can develop immediately or several days or weeks after the traumatic event.[1] A possible long-term complication of a bloody pericardial effusion is constrictive pericarditis.[8,9,13]

Echocardiography is the method of choice for detecting pericardial effusion. Bloody effusions and clots usually are more echogenic than serous fluid.[14] Traumatic effusions may be loculated if pericardial adhesions develop following cardiac injury. Multiple echocardiographic views may be needed to delineate a loculated effusion. For example, a loculated effusion near the right atrium would not be detected by M-mode or by most 2-D views. An apical or subcostal four-chamber view would be necessary to make the diagnosis.[26] Tamponade can be detected on the 2-D examination by noting small right-sided chambers and diastolic collapse of the right ventricular or right atrial wall. The role of echocardiographic diagnosis is more prominent if the patient's hemodynamics are stable. With unstable patients suspected of having cardiac tamponade, emergency chest surgery and exploration are usually performed. In addition to the initial echocardiographic work-up, patients with pericardial effusion should have follow-up studies to determine whether the effusion is resolving and to detect complications such as pericardial constriction.[38]

Pneumothorax (air within the pleural space) is a frequent complication of rib fractures due to trauma.[40] Pneumothorax may cause the heart to shift position and can make echocardiographic scanning difficult.

## CARDIAC CONTUSION

Cardiac contusion can be conceptualized as a bruise to the myocardium. Histologic examination reveals cellular injury, hemorrhage, and resulting necrosis of myocardial fibers. Cardiac contusion is similar to myocardial infarction, except that damage is usually patchy instead of discrete and cardiac contusion rarely leads to severe heart failure unless complications arise.[9,43,45] In addition, patients with contusion generally are young, with normal coronary arteries and no evidence of underlying heart disease.[9] The most common cause of this injury is compression of the sternum against the steering wheel in vehicular accidents.

The extent of myocardial injury varies greatly, depending on the degree of trauma. In severe cases the myocardium may rupture. Because the right ventricle is the most anterior cardiac structure, it is the most susceptible to injury. The interventricular septum is also vulnerable. It tends to rupture near the apex. Myocardial contusion or rupture can also result from closed-chest massage during cardiopulmonary resuscitation.[9,45]

Complications of contusion include atrial and ventricular arrhythmias, hemopericardium with possibility of tamponade, and thrombus formation.[30] Ventricular aneurysms and pseudoaneurysms may occur as late sequelae.[45]

Clinical manifestations of patients with contu-sion are variable, depending on the degree of injury and the presence of associated injuries. The most common complaint is angina-type chest pain that is not relieved by vasodilator drugs.

Until recently the clinical diagnosis of cardiac contusion was based primarily on serial electrocardiographic changes, but these are often nonspecific and unreliable.[30] Most contusions occur on the right side of the heart, and a standard electrocardiogram is relatively insensitive to right ventricular abnormalities.[45] Electrocardiography can detect conduction defects and arrhythmias, both of which are common following cardiac contusion.[4]

Chest radiography is generally of little value for detecting cardiac contusion, although associated findings such as rib fractures can alert the physician to the possibility of its presence.[25] More recently, the presence of contusion has been determined by noting an elevated level of creatine phosphokinase isoenzyme (CPK-MB) in the blood following trauma.[27,30] Although CPK-MB level appears to be a fairly sensitive test for the diagnosis of myocardial contusion, it is relatively nonspecific, and a normal CPK-MB level does not rule out contusion.[45]

The current consensus appears to be that 2-D echocardiography coupled with serial electrocardiographic and CPK-MB determinations offer the best chance of detecting cardiac contusion.[4,15,38,45]

Pandian and coworkers produced myocardial contusion in dogs and were able to note characteristic echo patterns: increased echogenicity of the contused area, sonolucencies where intramural hematomas were present (Fig. 15-2), increased wall thickness at end-diastole, and impaired regional systolic function.[35,42]

Several clinical studies have reported the usefulness of 2-D echocardiography in the diagnosis of cardiac contusion. Characteristic findings include chamber enlargement (usually the right ventricle), mural thrombi, wall motion abnormalities ranging from hypokinesis to aneurysm formation, sonodense myocardial areas, and pericardial effusion.[4,12,25] An added advantage of echocardiography is its ability to distinguish between right and left ventricular contusion and to differentiate right ventricular contusion from pericardial effusion, a distinction that has important therapeutic implications.[30,45]

Control

Trauma

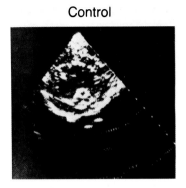 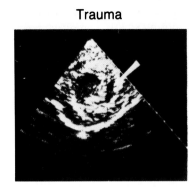 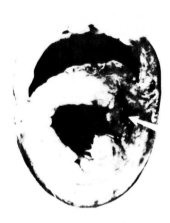

FIGURE 15-2. Short-axis 2-D echocardiographic recordings from a dog at the level of the papillary muscles before (A) and 15 minutes after (B) left-sided chest trauma. Wall thickness is increased in the contused area. Within the bright sonodense area, a discrete, linear, sonolucent zone is seen, representing an intramural hematoma (arrow). A transverse cut section of the pathologic specimen of the same dog shows the contusion (dark area) and the hematoma (arrow). (From Pandian NC, Skorton PJ, Doty DB, et al. Immediate diagnosis of acute myocardial contusion by two-dimensional echocardiography. J Am. Coll Cardiol. 1983; 2:488–496.)

## VALVE INJURY

The prevalence of valve injury in patients with blunt chest injury is in the range of 9%.[9] Owing to the higher pressures on the left side of the heart, the aortic and mitral valves appear to be more susceptible to damage than the right-sided valves.[45] Preexisting valve disease and the presence of a prosthetic valve[8] both tend to predispose to injury during trauma.[38] Valve injury is usually associated with other cardiac abnormalities, as any trauma severe enough to cause valve injury would affect other areas of the heart as well.[10,11] Patients with valve injury generally develop new, loud, musical murmurs.[9] In addition, these patients usually present with varying degrees of congestive heart failure.[10] Echocardiography is very useful for assessing valve injury, as it allows visualization of the valves and supporting structures, and for determining severity of regurgitation and degree of cardiac function. Severe regurgitation may be seen acutely following trauma or may take several weeks to months to develop. Because a small laceration may develop into a larger tear owing to hemodynamic stress on the valve, patients with suspected valve disruption probably should be followed with serial echocardiography.[16]

*Aortic Valve.* Because most aortic injuries due to blunt trauma result from rapid deceleration with shearing stress at points of relative fixation, tears usually are found near the insertion of the valve to the annulus.[8]

There appears to be a relationship between timing of the chest wall trauma and the cardiac cycle.[8] The aortic valve is probably most vulnerable to damage early in diastole, when the ventricle and aorta are nearly full.[9]

In a case report of a young child who fell from a tree, the echocardiogram detected rupture of the left coronary aortic valve cusp. The echocardiographic findings included dilatation of the left ventricle, diastolic aortic flutter, posterior motion of the left coronary cusp in diastole, and unusually wide excursion of the valve in systole. Owing to the absence of valve thickening and dilatation of the aortic root, other causes of aortic insufficiency, such as endocarditis, were ruled out.[16] Pulsed-wave and Doppler color-flow mapping would have further aided in the diagnosis of aortic insufficiency in this patient, or in any patient with suspected aortic insufficiency.

*Mitral Valve.* Traumatic disruption of the mitral valve can occur at the level of the annulus, leaflets, chordae tendineae, or papillary muscle; the latter two are more common.[10,11] Damage is most likely to develop if trauma occurs during diastole, when left ventricular outflow is obstructed.[9,10] Papillary muscle dysfunction may occur acutely as a result of direct laceration at the moment of impact, or it may develop as a sequela to myocardial contusion.[10]

Two-dimensional echocardiography allows detailed analysis of the mitral valve apparatus. A flail mitral leaflet can be identified by the presence of the tip of the leaflet in the left atrium during diastole.[10] Pulsed-wave and color-flow Doppler studies can be instrumental in determining the presence and degree of mitral insufficiency. Scarring of the injured valve can lead to stenosis,[10] in which case continuous-wave Doppler technique may be utilized as well.

*Tricuspid Valve.* Nonpenetrating traumatic injury to the tricuspid valve is often found in association with rupture of the right ventricular free wall.[11] As with the mitral valve, disruption can occur at the various levels of the tricuspid valve apparatus.[13]

M-mode findings of ruptured tricuspid valve chordae tendineae have included wide diastolic excursion with coarse, erratic diastolic fluttering and paradoxical septal motion.[22] Two-dimensional findings have included motion of the flail tricuspid leaflet into the right atrium during systole and loss of the normal coaptation point.[47] Doppler investigation allows further assessment of ensuing regurgitation.

GREAT VESSEL INJURY

Aortic laceration, a common complication of blunt chest trauma,[9] unfortunately is usually fatal. The diagnosis is made at postmortem examination.[40] In a study by Parmley, only 20% of patients with aortic rupture survived more than an hour after trauma.[36] Pulmonary artery laceration is less common, but is also usually fatal.[21] If the patient survives, great vessel injury can be detected on a chest radiograph by noting a widened mediastinum. The next diagnostic step is usually angiography.[40] Emergency surgery must be performed to repair a tear.[7] CT or MRI may be used to diagnose great vessel injury if the patient's condition is stable enough. Echocardiography does not have a significant role in the diagnosis of traumatic great vessel rupture as the views of the great vessels are limited.

## Penetrating Trauma

Most penetrating cardiac trauma results from injury due to knives, bullets, or other projectiles; ballistics cause more extensive cell destruction. Penetrating wounds to the heart most often are associated with injury to the precordium, but they may be seen in conjunction with wounds elsewhere in the chest, neck, or upper abdomen. The frequency of injury to the various cardiac structures correlates with the area of exposure on the anterior chest wall. Thus, the cardiac chamber most often injured is the right ventricle, then in decreasing order of frequency, the left ventricle, right atrium, and left atrium.[43] Perforation of one or more chambers of the heart, the cardiac valves and their support structures, and the interventricular and interatrial septa may occur.[16,31,41]

The management of suspected acute cardiac trauma depends on the clinical condition of the patient. Most patients with penetrating cardiac wounds die shortly after the injury as a result of cardiac tamponade or of massive bleeding. Rarely is there time for diagnostic procedures. The management of those who survive consists primarily of thoracotomy and surgical exploration. First, however, the patient's condition must be stabilized by administering fluids or blood and by placing a chest tube, if indicated. Pericardiocentesis for evaluation and stabilization of patients with suspected cardiac tamponade prior to arrangements for thoracotomy is somewhat controversial.[9]

Most of the literature on echocardiography and penetrating injury to the heart discusses its role after initial repair of the injury and stabilization of the patient's condition. Patients with penetrating cardiac wounds may have multiple cardiac defects, but only the most superficial wounds are usually recognized upon initial evaluation as requiring surgical repair. Several studies in the literature address the utility of echocardiography in evaluating patients postoperatively for the presence of residual injury.[18,19,24,32,41] Mattox and coworkers[28] reported on follow-up 2-D and Doppler echocardiographic studies in 32 patients who survived cardiac injury and operative repair. The abnormalities noted on 2-D included pericardial effusion, abnormal wall motion, chamber enlargement, and an intracardiac retained missile fragment. In addition, Doppler examination revealed ventricular septal defects, tricuspid insufficiency, and arteriovenous fistulas. The study concluded that patients who had an abnormal electrocardiogram, chest radiograph, or auscultory finding postoperatively should undergo 2-D and Doppler echocardiography.

The echocardiographic findings in this setting can be quite dramatic. Figure 15-3 illustrates a large ventricular septal defect with ragged edges, the result of an icepick wound to the heart. The patient originally underwent emergency surgical repair of a hole in the anterior wall of the right ventricle. Postoperatively, the symptoms of congestive heart failure developed and a systolic murmur was detected. Echocardiographic demonstration of the residual ventricular septal defect promoted reoperation and repair of the defect.

Cardiac defects caused by penetrating injury usually are more irregular and complex than congenital or naturally acquired lesions. They are often multiple and may be situated in unusual locations. A cursory 2-D echocardiographic examination may miss some of these lesions, so Doppler echocardiography has become important for detecting them. Doppler examination can detect even small lesions and can prompt the echocardiographer to obtain nonstandard 2-D views to better demonstrate the abnormalities.[24] Color-flow Doppler mapping in particular should provide rapid detection of shunts and valvular lesions, resulting in more prompt repair of these defects.

### LOCALIZATION OF FOREIGN BODIES WITH SONOGRAPHY

Echocardiography has been used extensively in the management of patients with penetrating missile wounds of the heart.[20,39] The dangers of fragments retained in the myocardium are migration, embolization, and erosion into adjacent structures. They also may serve as a locus for endocarditis. Symbas and colleagues[44] suggested that foreign objects should be surgically removed only if they protrude

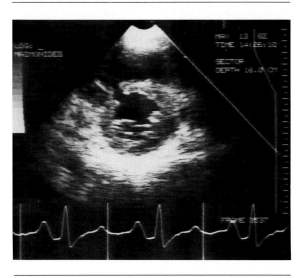

FIGURE 15-3. Two-dimensional short-axis view demonstrates a ventricular septal defect in the anterior septum acquired due to ice pick injury.

into the ventricular cavity. Fragments embedded in the myocardium tend to become encased in fibrin and generally do not pose a threat to the patient.[43] Although chest radiography and cardiac fluoroscopy may reveal the metal fragments in the heart, echocardiography is the most effective tool for identifying the exact location of such retained fragments and may be useful in guiding surgical intervention.[20]

Hassett and associates[20] reported on nine patients with penetrating missile wounds of the heart, all of whom were correctly diagnosed by echocardiography as having retained missile fragments. Retained fragments were defined echocardiographically as bright targets with multiple reverberations seen in at least two views (Fig. 15-4). Low gain and minimal reject settings were used to distinguish the metallic particles from cardiac tissue. In this series, the patients who required surgery for removal of the missile particles were evaluated during the operation by echocardiography. Intraoperative echocardiograms were found to be very useful as they provided immediate localization of the fragments and, so, shortened the operative procedure and minimized potential tissue damage.[20]

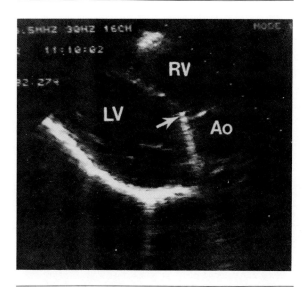

FIGURE 15-4. Stop-frame, 2-D echocardiographic image in the left parasternal long-axis view. A bullet fragment (*arrow*) is located high in the interventricular septum and has the typical appearance of such missiles, with dense trailing reverberations. (Ao, aortic root; LV, left ventricle; RV, right ventricle.) (From Hassett A, Moran J, Sabiston DC, et al. Utility of echocardiography in the management of patients with penetrating missile wounds of the head. J Am Coll Cardiol. 1986; 1151–1156. Reprinted with permission from the American College of Cardiology.)

## Iatrogenic Injury

Another increasingly common source of cardiac trauma is invasive diagnostic and therapeutic procedures. Techniques such as cardiac catheterization, pericardiocentesis, and pacemaker implantation are not without risk, and prompt recognition of complications is imperative to prevent further damage.[23] The role of echocardiography in most cases of suspected iatrogenic injury is to evaluate for the presence of pericardial effusion. Occasionally, however, echocardiography can also be useful for locating intracardiac or pericardial catheters.

### CATHETERIZATION

Major advances in the application of cardiac catheterization have recently been made. Cardiac cath-

eterization has been a useful diagnostic tool for assessing the extent of coronary artery disease, for determining cardiac hemodynamics, and for evaluating wall motion and valve function. With the advent of coronary angioplasty and balloon valvuloplasty, cardiac catheterization has become a therapeutic tool as well. The manipulation of wires within the heart and great vessels can lead to complications, among them perforation of the coronary arteries, dissection of the aorta, perforation of the cardiac chambers, and injury to the cardiac valves. Many of these complications are recognized during the catheterization procedure and are attended to immediately. Echocardiography is useful in detecting pericardial effusions and possible signs of tamponade when perforation is suspected. In the rare event of aortic dissection due to the passage of catheters within the aorta, precordial and/or transesophogeal echocardiography can be useful in identifying an intimal flap (Fig. 15-5).[23]

During coronary angiography or angioplasty, perforation or dissection of a coronary artery can cause ischemia in the area of the myocardium normally supplied by the vessel and wall motion abnormalities may ensue. Visualization of the coronary arteries currently is not reliable with conventional echocardiographic techniques, but it can be used to evaluate changes in regional wall motion that may occur with ischemia.

Both right- and left-sided heart catheterization can lead to atrial or ventricular perforation, but right-sided catheterization is more likely to cause perforation because the walls of the right atrium and right ventricle are thinner. Stiffer catheters, such as those used for cardiac catheterization, pose more of a problem than the soft, flexible Swan-Ganz catheters used for hemodynamic monitoring in critically ill patients. Perforation can lead to the formation of a pericardial effusion, and occasionally to pericardial tamponade, which can be evaluated rapidly and noninvasively by echocardiography.

The technique of balloon valvuloplasty involves multiple guidewires and catheters of fairly large diameter; as a consequence the incidence of associated complications is higher. Valvuloplasty increases the size of the valve orifice but may also cause regurgitation. Echocardiography is used routinely to monitor the improvement in valve function of these patients and to determine the pres-

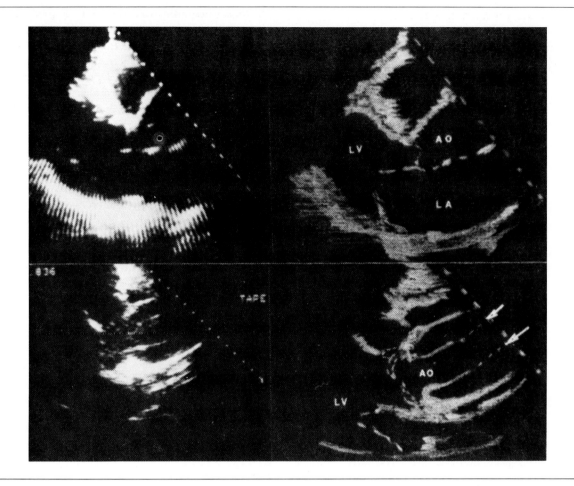

FIGURE 15-5. Precordial long-axis view of the ascending aorta before *(upper panels)* and after *(lower panels)* cardiac catheterization. In the examination performed after cardiac catheterization, 2-D echocardiography revealed the presence of two additional fluttering linear echoes *(arrows)* in the aortic lumen, parallel to the aortic walls. These echoes were not present in the examination performed the day before the invasive study. (AO, aorta; LA, left atrium; LV, left ventricle.) (From Iliceto S, Gianfranco A, Sorino M, et al. Two-dimensional echocardiographic recognition of complications of cardiac invasive procedures. Am J Coll Cardiol. 1984; 53:847. Reprinted with permission from the American College of Cardiology.)

ence and degree of valvular insufficiency. Mitral valvuloplasty is achieved by passing the catheter through the interatrial septum to gain entry into the left atrium and mitral valve orifice. This technique causes a small defect in the interatrial septum, which usually has no clinical significance. Such atrial septal defects were thought to disappear with time, but Doppler color-flow evaluation has shown that they persist several months after the procedure.[33] Given the complexity of the mitral valve apparatus, another complication of mitral valvuloplasty is rupture of the chordae tendineae.[34] Two-dimensional and Doppler echocardiography allow careful analysis of this region. As valvuloplasty becomes more routine and more widely available the need to recognize potential complications will increase rapidly. Echocardiography is certainly suitable for this purpose, as it provides immediate information noninvasively.[23]

Another complication of intravenous or right-sided heart catheterization occurs when the catheter fractures and a piece migrates into the right atrium, right ventricle, or pulmonary artery. Such fragments most often are detected with fluoroscopy because they are composed of a radiopaque material. Echocardiography can also be used to locate such fragments and guide their removal.

PERICARDIOCENTESIS

Pericardiocentesis is a procedure used to drain pericardial effusions for diagnostic or therapeutic purposes. The needle can puncture the heart and damage the myocardium. During the procedure, an echocardiogram can be performed to help guide the needle.

The pericardiocentesis needle is usually inserted in the subxyphoid region under sterile technique. The echocardiographic transducer is then placed at the cardiac apex, outside the sterile field. If an apical approach is chosen for pericardiocentesis, the subcostal echocardiographic view can be used. The echocardiographic plane may have to be modified so that the beam is aligned parallel to the needle to allow better visualization during the procedure.[37]

CARDIAC PACEMAKERS

When the cardiac conduction system fails to supply impulses at the proper intervals to ensure regular myocardial contraction, an electrical device is often needed to provide this stimulus. A pacemaker may be required on a temporary basis or a permanent pacing system may be implanted. A transvenous pacing electrode is inserted in either case. With a temporary pacemaker the electrode is attached to an external battery source; with a permanent pacemaker, the battery is implanted subcutaneously in the chest wall.

The transvenous pacemaker electrode is usually placed into the apex of the right ventricle for ventricular pacing, or if sequential activation of the atrium and ventricle is required, two pacemaker electrodes are placed, one in the right atrial appendage and one in the right ventricular apex. Again, atrial or ventricular perforation is a potential problem because of the relatively thin right atrial and right ventricular walls. If the free wall of these chambers is perforated, pericardial effusion will result—and perhaps cardiac tamponade.

Echocardiography can be used to guide lead placement and to check for possible misplacement of leads. In addition to perforation of the right ventricular free wall, perforation can occur through the interatrial or interventricular septum.[45] The exact location of the electrode may be difficult to determine fluoroscopically, whereas the 2-D echocardiographic technique can better trace the course of the pacing catheter. Echocardiographically, a catheter generally appears as a bright linear echo coursing through the right side of the heart. Figure 15-6 shows a subcostal echocardiographic view obtained when a change in the QRS configuration was noted on the electrocardiogram after a temporary pacemaker was inserted. The catheter is clearly seen crossing the interventricular septum, with the tip touching the lateral left ventricular wall.

MYOCARDIAL BIOPSY

Occasionally, an exact cardiac diagnosis cannot be made with the usual clinical, electrocardiographic, and imaging techniques that are currently available, and histologic diagnosis requires a sample of tissue from the heart. This biopsy technique has been developed mainly to evaluate heart transplant recipients for signs of rejection, to follow patients undergoing chemotherapy with cardiotoxic drugs, and to check for possible inflammatory and infiltrative diseases of the heart. The biopsy is performed with a bioptome, a stiff catheter with steel jaws attached to its end. The bioptome is usually guided via the internal jugular vein into the right ventricle, where a sample of myocardial tissue is obtained. Localization of the catheter is most often performed by fluoroscopy, but it can be confirmed with echocardiography. Because this technique involves removal of a piece of tissue, there is a risk of perforation of the right ventricular wall. In the event of such a mishap echocardiography may be used to detect the presence of hemopericardium.

CARDIAC SURGERY

Cardiac surgery is a form of cardiac trauma. Echocardiographically, it is not unusual to note some degree of pericardial effusion or pneumomediastinum in patients who have undergone uncomplicated open-heart surgery. Pericardial effusions are frequently loculated, owing to the adhesions of the pericardium that often occur postoperatively. Oc-

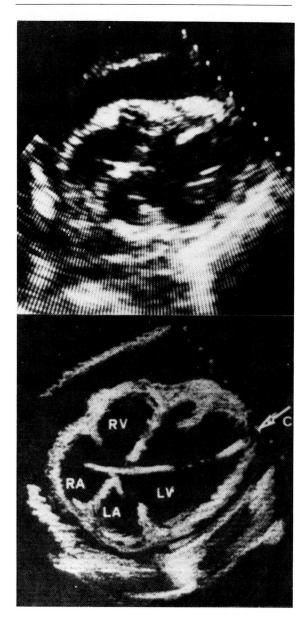

FIGURE 15-6. Two-dimensional echocardiogram from the subcostal approach. The catheter (c) imaged as a bright band of echoes is seen entering the left ventricle (LV) through the ventricular septum. (LA, left atrium; RA, right atrium; RV, right ventricle.) (From Iliceto S, Gianfranco A, Sorino M, et al. Two-dimensional echocardiographic recognition of complications of cardiac invasive procedures. Am J Coll Cardiol. 1984; 53:847. Reprinted with permission from the American College of Cardiology.)

casionally, uncontrolled bleeding following cardiac surgery may result in cardiac tamponade. Large blood clots compressing the right side of the heart can also cause tamponade (Fig. 15-7). The echocardiographic examination should therefore include a thorough investigation of the area adjacent to the heart.

The placement of prosthetic cardiac valves can lead to unusual complications. Echocardiographic detection of pseudoaneurysm formation following mitral valve replacement has been reported. The diagnosis was made by noting myocardial discontinuity and a sonolucent space posteriorly, adjacent to the prosthetic valve (Fig. 15-8).

## CARDIAC RESUSCITATION

The technique of external cardiac massage for cardiopulmonary resuscitation has become widespread. The procedure itself can cause serious complications. Fracture of the sternum or ribs during compression can cause laceration to the heart.[9] Right ventricular papillary muscle rupture, as well as rupture of the atria and aorta, have been reported following closed chest massage.[3,17] If the patient survives the resuscitative efforts and if signs or symptoms of cardiac injury are present, echocardiography may be employed to assess the extent of the cardiac damage.

## Summary

For patients who survive the initial event, echocardiography can be a useful technique for the investigation of cardiac trauma. As opposed to MRI and CT, which are time consuming and require the patient to remain still for prolonged periods, echocardiography can be performed relatively quickly at the patient's bedside.

The most common echocardiographic finding after trauma is pericardial effusion, which indicates that some degree of cardiac injury has occurred. A full echocardiographic work-up is then indicated to determine the extent of cardiac injury.

While echocardiography can be used in the immediate care of trauma patients, its most important role appears to be in the evaluation of the long-term sequelae in patients who survive the initial insult.

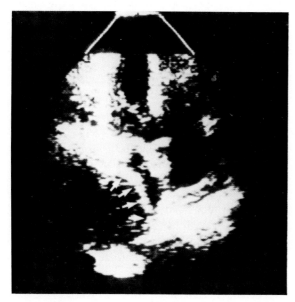

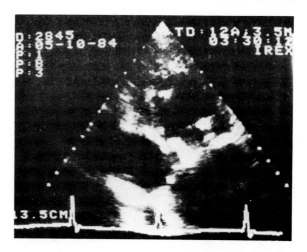

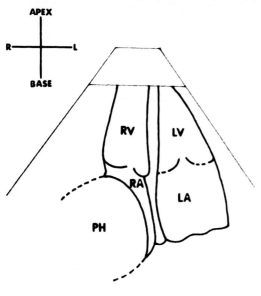

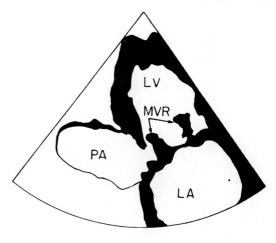

FIGURE 15-7. Apical four-chamber view of 2-D echocardiogram showing a large pericardial hematoma (PH) compressing the right side of the right atrial wall (*arrows*). Note the slitlike appearance of the right atrial cavity (RA). (L, left; LA, left atrium; LV, left ventricle; R, right; RV, right ventricle.) (From Kronzon I, Cohen ML, Winer HE. Cardiac tamponade by loculated pericardial hematoma: Limitations of M-mode echocardiography. J Am Coll Cardiol. 1983; 1:913–915. Reprinted with permission from the American College of Cardiology.)

FIGURE 15-8. Echocardiographic apical two-chamber view of a patient with a prosthetic mitral valve and pseudoaneurysm (A) and diagrammatic representation of the same patient (B). Myocardial discontinuity is demonstrated between the prosthetic valve and the pseudoaneurysm. (LA, left atrium; LV, left ventricle; MVR, Ionescu-Shiley mitral valve prosthesis; PA, pseudoaneuryms.) (From Lichtenberg GS, Greengart A, Wasser H, et al. Echocardiographic demonstration of pseudoaneurysm after mitral valve replacement. Am Heart J. 1986; 112(a):417.)

# References

1. Allen MN, Nanna M, Lichtenberg GS, et at. Blunt trauma causing delayed cardiac tamponade: Echocardiographic diagnosis. J Diagn Med Sonogr. 1988; 4:269–273.

2. Baillot R, Dontigny L, Verdant A, et al. Penetrating chest trauma: A 20-year experience. J Trauma. 1987; 27:994–997.

3. Baker PB, Keyhani-Rofagha S, Graham RL, et al. Dissecting hematoma (aneurysm) of coronary arteries. Am J Med. 1986; 80:317–319.

4. Beggs CW, Helling TS, Evans LL, et al. Early evaluation of cardiac injury by two-dimensional echocardiography in patients suffering blunt chest trauma. Ann Emerg Med. 1987; 16:542–545.

5. Beresky R, Klinger R, Peake J. Myocardial contusion: When does it have clinical significance? J Trauma. 1988; 28:64–68.

6. Berkery W, Hare C, Warner RA, et al. Nonpenetrating traumatic rupture of the tricuspid valve. Chest. 1987; 91:778–780.

7. Boyd AD. Nonpenetrating thoracic injuries. Hosp Med. 1988; 24:25–48.

8. Brady PW, Deal CW. An unusual cause of mitral incompetence: Post-traumatic paraprosthetic mitral incompetence. J Trauma. 1988; 28:259–261.

9. Cohn PF, Braunwald E. Traumatic heart disease. In: Braunwald E, ed. Heart Disease: A Textbook of Cardiovascular Medicine. 3rd ed. Philadelphia: WB Saunders; 1988.

10. Cuadros LC, Hutchinson JE III, Mogtader AH. Laceration of a mitral papillary muscle and the aortic root as a result of blunt trauma to the chest. J Thorac Cardiovasc Surg. 1984; 88:134–140.

11. Dodd DA, Johns JA, Graham TP Jr. Transient severe mitral and tricuspid regurgitation following blunt chest trauma. Am Heart J. 1987; 114:652–654.

12. Eisenach JC, Nugent M, Miller FA Jr, et al. Echocardiographic evaluation of patients with blunt chest injury: Correlation with perioperative hypotension. Anesthesiology. 1986; 64:364–366.

13. Fabian TC, Mangiante EC, Patterson RC, et al. Myocardial contusion in blunt trauma: Clinical characteristics, means of diagnosis, and implications for patient management. J Trauma. 1988; 28:50–58.

14. Feigenbaum H. Pericardial disease. In: Feigenbaum H, ed. Echocardiography. 4th ed. Philadelphia: Lea & Febiger; 1986.

15. Frazee RC, Mucha P, Farnell MB, et al. Objective evaluation of blunt cardiac trauma. J Trauma. 1986; 26:510–518.

16. Gay JA, Gottdiener JS, Gomes MN, et al. Echocardiographic features of traumatic disruption of the aortic valve. Chest. 1983; 1:150–151.

17. Gerry JL, Bulkley BH, Hutchins GM. Rupture of the papillary muscle of the tricuspid valve: A complication of cardiopulmonary resuscitation and a rare cause of tricuspid regurgitation. Am J Cardiol. 1977; 40:825–828.

18. Goldberg SE, Parameswaran R, Nakhjavan FK, et al. Echocardiographic diagnosis of traumatic ventricular septal defect. Am Heart J. 1984; 107:416–417.

19. Goldman AP, Kotler MN, Goldberg SE, et al. The uses of two-dimensional Doppler echocardiographic techniques preoperatively and postoperatively in a ventricular septal defect caused by penetrating trauma. Ann Thorac Surg. 1985; 40:625–627.

20. Hassett A, Moran J, Sabiston DC, et al. Utility of echocardiography in the management of patients with penetrating missile wounds of the heart. J Am Coll Cardiol. 1986; 7:1151–1156.

21. Hawkins ML, Carraway RP, Ross SE, et al. Pulmonary artery disruption from blunt thoracic trauma. Am Surg. 1988; 54:148–152.

22. Ichikawa T, Okudaira S, Yoshioka J, et al. A case of isolated tricuspid insufficiency. J Cardiogr. 1977; 6:635.

23. Iliceto S, Antonelli G, Sorino M, et al. Two-dimensional echocardiographic recognition of complications of cardiac invasive procedures. Am J Cardiol. 1984; 53:846–848.

24. Jacoby SS, Gilliam LD, Pandian NG, et al. Two-dimensional and Doppler echocardiography in the evaluation of penetrating cardiac injury. Chest. 1985; 88:922–924.

25. King MR, Mucha P, Seward JB, et al. Cardiac contusion: A new diagnostic approach utilizing two-dimensional echocardiography. J Trauma. 1983; 23:614–620.

26. Kronzon I, Cohen ML, Winer HE. Cardiac tamponade by loculated pericardial hematoma; Limitations of M-mode echocardiography. J Am Coll Cardiol. 1983; 1:913–915.

27. Lindsey D, Navin R, Finley PR. Transient elevation of serum activity of MB isoenzyme of creatine phosphokinase in drivers involved in automobile accidents. Chest. 1978; 74:15–18.

28. Mattox KL, Limacher MC, Feliciano DV, et al. Cardiac evaluation following heart injury. J Trauma. 1985; 25:758–765.

29. Mayfield W, Hurley EJ. Blunt cardiac trauma. Am J Surg. 1984; 148:162–167.

30. Miller FA Jr, Seward JB, Gersh BJ, et al. Two-dimensional echocardiographic findings in cardiac trauma. Am J Cardiol. 1982; 50:1022–1027.

31. Miller JT, Richards KL, Miller JF, et al. Doppler echocardiographic determination of the cause of a systolic murmur following penetrating chest trauma.

Am Heart J. 1985; 111:988–990.

32. Missri J, Sverrisson J. Doppler echocardiographic detection of traumatic ventricular septal defect: A case report. J Vasc Dis. 1987; 785–787.

33. O'Shea JP, Abascal VM, Marshall JE, et al. Long-term persistence of atrial septal defect following percutaneous mitral valvuloplasty: A Doppler-echocardiographic follow-up study. Circulation. 1988; 78(suppl II):II-1.

34. O'Shea JP, Abascal VM, Wilkins GT, et al. Unusual sequelae of percutaneous mitral valvuloplasty: A Doppler-echocardiographic study. Circulation. 1988; 78(suppl II): II-32.

35. Pandian NG, Skorton DJ, Doty DB, et al. Immediate diagnosis of acute myocardial contusion by two-dimensional echocardiography: Studies in a canine model of blunt chest trauma. J Am Coll Cardiol. 1983; 2:488–493.

36. Parmley LF. Non-penetrating traumatic injury to the aorta. Circulation. 1958; 17:1086.

37. Preis HK, Taylor GJ, Martin RP. Two-dimensional echocardiographic visualization of an unfortunate event. Arch Intern Med 1982; 142:2327–2329.

38. Reid CL, Kawanishi DT, Rahimtoola SH. Chest trauma: Evaluation by two-dimensional echocardiography. Am Heart J. 1987; 113:971–976.

39. Roehm EF, Eilen SD, Crawford MH. Two-dimensional echocardiographic demonstration of a bullet in the heart. Am Heart J. 1985; 110:910–912.

40. Shorr RM, Crittenden M, Indeck M, et al. Blunt thoracic trauma. Ann Surg. 1987; 206:200–205.

41. Sklar J, Clarke D, Campbell D, et al. Traumatic ventricular septal defect and lacerated mitral leaflet. Chest. 1982; 2:247–249.

42. Skorton DJ, Collins SM, Nichols J, et al. Qualitative texture analysis of two-dimensional echocardiography: Application to the diagnosis of experimental myocardial contusion. Circulation 1983; 6:211–223.

43. Symbas PN. Traumatic heart disease. In: Harvey WP, O'Rourke RA, eds. Current Problems in Cardiology. Chicago: Year Book Medical Publishers; 1982.

44. Symbas PN, DiOrio DA, Tyras DH, et al. Penetrating cardiac wounds: Significant residual and delayed sequelae. J Thorac Cardiovasc Surg. 1973; 66:526–532.

45. Tenzer ML. The spectrum of myocardial contusion: A review. J Trauma. 1985; 25:620–627.

46. Villanueva FS, Heinsimer JA, Burkmsan MH, et al. Echocardiographic detection of perforation of the cardiac ventricular septum by a permanent pacemaker lead. J Am Coll Cardiol. 1987; 59:370–371.

47. Watanabe T, Katsume H, Matsukubo H, et al. Ruptured chordae tendineae of the tricuspid valve due to nonpenetrating trauma. Chest. 1981; 80:751–753.

# CHAPTER 16

# Prosthetic Heart Valves

EVALIE DUMARS

The last two decades have witnessed enormous and rapid growth in the development and surgical implantation of prostheses for diseased heart valves. With this development came the need to evaluate the function of prosthetic valves in situ. Traditionally, invasive methods similar to those employed in cardiac catheterization were used. However, a noninvasive method of evaluating prosthetic valves was clearly desirable, so phonocardiography and echocardiography were used adjunctively.

The development of Doppler echocardiography offered a powerful tool for noninvasive evaluation of valves. Now structural data and spatial and quantitative information on flow characteristics across the valves can be obtained easily. Doppler studies have proved to be reliable and their results, reproducible.

The sonographer confronted with such patients must identify valve types and obtain useful, technically accurate, and concise information on valve function. In this chapter, the most commonly encountered prosthetic heart valves are presented through picture descriptions, radiographs, echocardiographic (M-mode and two-dimensional), and flow (Doppler) characteristics. A systematic imaging approach is also suggested. This may be one of the most challenging applications of current echo-

cardiography and of Doppler echocardiographic techniques.

It is important that each patient who is to be examined be questioned about pertinent medical history, symptoms, and current medications. Often these data are recorded in the patient's charts. Most patients who have undergone heart valve replacement receive an identification card from the manufacturer of the prosthesis, which should be carried at all times. Such a card identifies the valve type and its diameter, which is important for velocity comparisons.

Auscultation is an important and useful adjunct to the echocardiographic study for determining the valve type, presence of murmurs, and valve sounds. The sounds produced by valve prostheses vary depending upon location, manner of opening and closing, and valve composition (plastic, steel, or biological tissue). In general, the metal ball used in the ball-and-cage valves, like the Starr-Edwards, produces the loudest, most distinctive sounds on both opening and closing. The tilting-disc valves, like the Bjork-Shiley, the Lillehei-Kaster, and the St. Jude Medical, produce loud, crisp sounds on closing but little or no sound on opening. The bioprosthetic valves are not associated with such sounds. Examination of chest radiographs can also be useful to identify the specific valve type.

## Types of Prosthetic Valves

(Only those valves currently in use and most commonly seen will be fully presented. The reader is referred to the bibliography section for more detailed historical information.)

The two principal types of valves are the mechanical and the bioprosthetic. The mechanical valves consist entirely of man-made materials while the bioprosthetic valves incorporate tissue mounted on metallic frame stents (Table 16-1).

### Mechanical

*Ball-and-Cage Valves.* Ball-and-cage valves consist of a ball, or poppet, enclosed in a cage (Figs. 16-1 to 16-9). At closure, the ball sits in the sewing ring (base) and moves to the apex of the cage at opening position. The motion plane is superior-inferior. Because the ball-and-cage is an old design, the clinical experience is considerable. The cage is quite visible on radiographs (x-ray) and is highly echogenic on two-dimensional (2-D) echocardiography. The increased echogenicity of the cage material can make poppet excursion difficult to identify (especially if the acoustic beam is directed closer to right angles to the valve) making determination of thrombus formation less reliable.

The appearance of a ball-and-cage valve is similar on M-mode and 2-D echocardiography. To study ball motion and poppet excursion, and to obtain velocity determinants, the echo beam should be directed parallel to the valve plane. For valves in the mitral position, the transducer is best placed at the cardiac apex (apical portion) with the beam directed up toward the left atrium. Those valves in the aortic position are best studied from the high right sternal border with the beam angled inferior and to the left and from the cardiac apex with the beam directed medial and cephalad (in this view, the excursion pattern will be reversed). It is also recommended to run the M-mode recordings at 75 or 100mm/sec for easier evaluation of rapid signals.

*Central Occluder Valves.* This mechanical valve presents a lower profile (is less bulky) than ball-and-cage valves and utilizes a disc occluder, which moves in a noneccentric nontilting manner parallel to the sewing ring throughout its excursion (Figs. 16-10 to 16-13). The Cross-Jones variety has an open-ended titanium cage with a Silastic disc[52];

TABLE 16-1. Classification of prosthetic heart valves

Mechanical
  Ball-and-cage
    Starr-Edwards
    Smeloff-Cutter
    Braunwald-Cutter
    Harken*
    Magovern-Cromie*
  Central occluder, caged disc, noneccentric nontilting
    Beall-Surgitool
    Kay-Shiley*
    Cross-Jones*
    Starr-Edwards*
  Tilting (eccentric) disc
    Bjork-Shiley
    Lillehei-Kaster
    Wada-Cutter*
    Medtronic-Hall
  Bi-leaflet
    St. Jude Medical
Bioprosthetic (tissue)
  Heterografts (xenografts)
    Hancock (porcine)
    Carpentier-Edwards (porcine)
    Ionescu-Shiley (pericardial)
  Homografts (allografts)
    Stented (aortic)*
    Unstented (aortic)*
    Dura mater*
  Autografts
    Fascia lata*

*Valves marked with an asterisk are rarely seen and not all are presented in this chapter.

the Starr-Edwards valve uses a hollow metallic disc[52]; and the Beall valve has a pyrolite carbon disc.[52] The Kay-Shiley valve also uses a Silastic disc.[52] These valve designs were used extensively in the early 1970s.[52] Their echocardiographic appearance is similar to that of caged ball valves but reflects a lower profile and smaller disc excursion.

*Tilting-Disc (Eccentric) Valves.* The Bjork-Shiley and the Lillehei-Kaster represent the most commonly encountered valves of this design used in the 1970s into the 1980s. These valves incorporate a disc poppet that tilts open approximately 60 degrees in the manner of a swinging door (Figs. 16-14 to 16-21). The amount of excursion varies with the size of the prosthesis. Since the opening of the disc is eccentric, it produces different echo patterns with different beam angles. Special care should be taken to demonstrate maximal excursion.

*(Text continues on page 328.)*

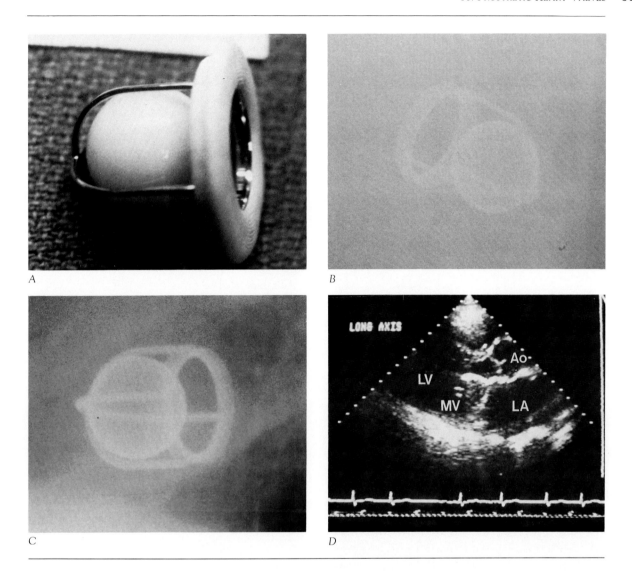

FIGURE 16-1. (A) Unlike other ball-and-cage designs, the Starr-Edwards ball and cage is closed at the apex. Blood flows around the central flow occluder (ball). (B, C) Radiographs display the cage and the ball poppet of the Starr-Edwards valve. (D) Two-dimensional long-axis echocardiograph scan of a Starr-Edwards mitral valve prosthesis in place for 11 years. Note the high profile of the cage as it projects into the left ventricle. (LV, left ventricle; MV, mitral ball-and-cage prosthesis; Ao, aorta; LA, left atrium.)

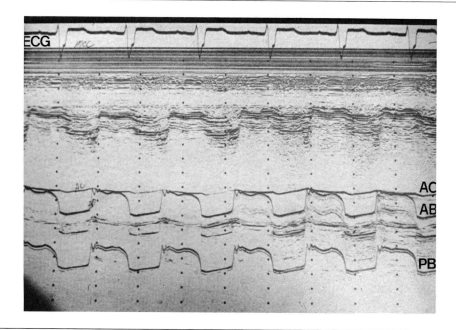

FIGURE 16-2. M-mode tracing (apical approach) of a ball-and-cage prosthesis that has been in the mitral valve 9 years. This approach is recommended to obtain the best recordings of the ball or poppet in mitral prostheses.

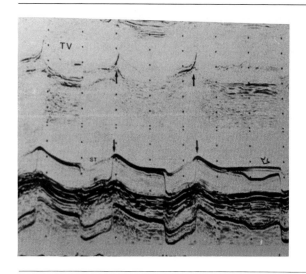

FIGURE 16-3. M-mode tracing of a ball-and-cage prosthesis (normal), in a patient with atrial fibrillation. Long RR intervals normally can result in prolonged separation between poppet and strut. (From Salcedo E. Atlas of Echocardiography, 2nd ed. Philadelphia: W.B. Saunders; 1987; 183.)

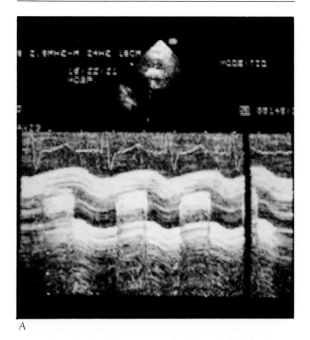

*A*

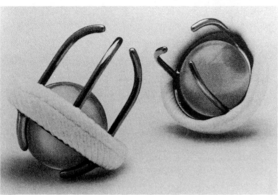

*B*

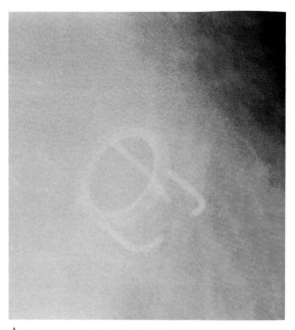

*A*

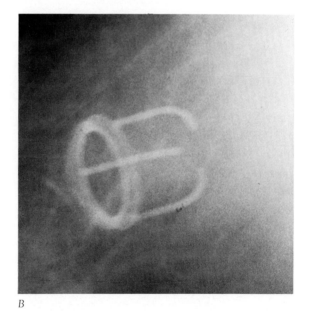

*B*

FIGURE 16-4. (A) M-mode tracing from a patient with an aortic Smeloff-Cutter ball-and-cage valve prosthesis. The short-axis view demonstrates the dense, columnar echo pattern. Apical or high right sternal placement is the best approach for imaging valves in the aortic position. (B) Smeloff-Cutter ball-and-cage prosthesis. (From Davey HB, Smeloff EA. Med Instrumen. 1977; 11: 95.)

FIGURE 16-5. Two radiographs of a Braunwald-Cutter ball-and-cage prosthesis. Note the cage is open at the apex.

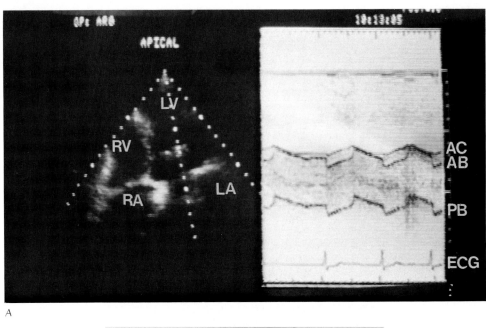

A

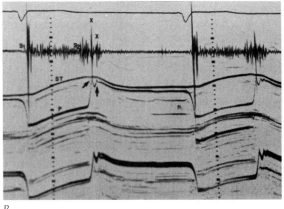

B

Figure 16-6. (A) Combined 2-D and M-mode echocardiographs of a Smeloff-Cutter ball-and-cage valve. This apical view is best for demonstrating the cage echo lines and excursions of the ball or poppet in the mitral valve. (LV, left ventricle; RV, right ventricle; RA, right atrium; LA, left atrium; AC, anterior cage; AB, anterior ball; PB, posterior ball.) (B) Normal M-mode and phonocardiographic tracings of a Smeloff-Cutter prosthesis in the mitral valve. Two opening clicks (x) are recorded as the poppet hits the strut (st) in early diastole. The closing click coincides with the first heart sound ($S_1$), at which time the poppet (p) moves away from the strut toward the suture ring. (B from Salcedo E. Atlas of Echocardiography, 2nd ed. Philadelphia: W.B. Saunders; 1987; 185.)

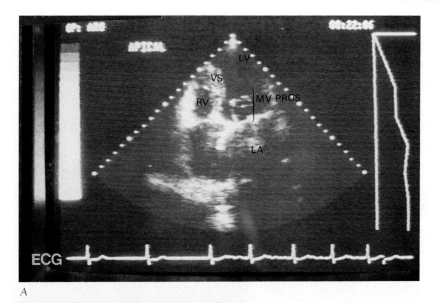

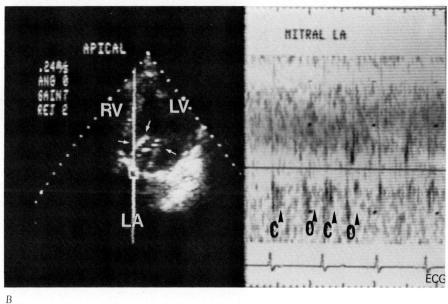

Figure 16-7. (A) Two-dimensional echocardiogram (apical approach) of a Braunwald-Cutter ball-and-cage prosthesis in the mitral position. (B) Two-dimensional echocardiogram and pulsed-wave Doppler scan of a patient with a Braunwald-Cutter ball-and-cage prosthesis in the mitral position. Note the distinct closing and opening sounds (C, O). It is important to map the area around the valve ring as well as behind the valve, to identify leaks. (LV, left ventricle; RV, right ventricle; LA, left atrium; VS, ventricular septum.)

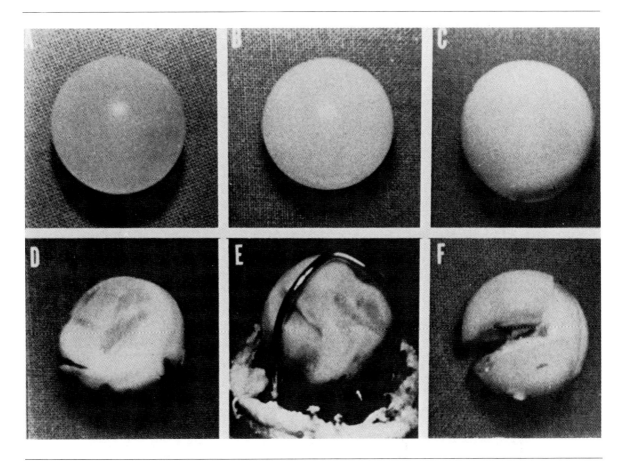

Figure 16-8. Examples of ball variance: (A) Normal Silastic poppet, 1½ years after implantation. (B) Opaque ball after 3 years in situ. (C) Slightly eccentric and grooved ball, removed after 3 years. (D) Grooved poppet. (E) Grooved poppet stuck in the open position. (F) Cracked ball removed 4 years after insertion. (From Hylen JC. Ball Variance. Circulation. 1968; American Heart Assoc. 38: 90–106. Reproduced by permission of the American Heart Association, Inc.)

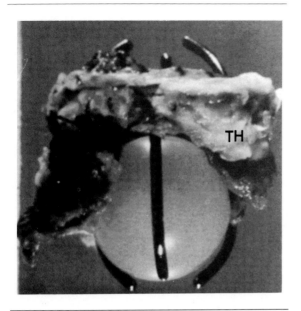

FIGURE 16-9. Excised Smeloff-Cutter ball-and-cage valve. Note the large thrombus (Th) around the poppet. (From Salcedo E. Atlas of Echocardiography, 2nd ed. Philadelphia: W.B. Saunders; 1987; 185.)

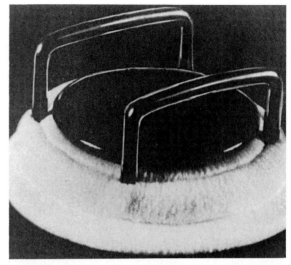

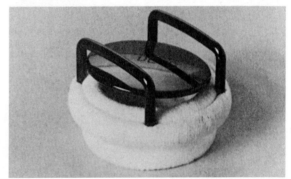

FIGURE 16-10. A Beall-Surgitool valve with pyrolite carbon-coated struts and a pyrolite carbon disc. A standard sewing ring lies above and a turtleneck ring below. (Courtesy of Travenol Laboratories, Deerfield, IL.)

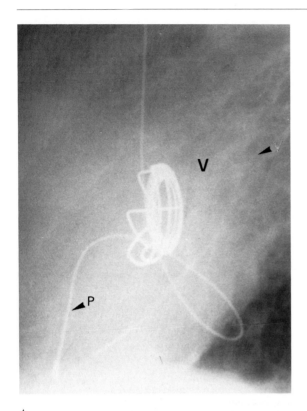

A

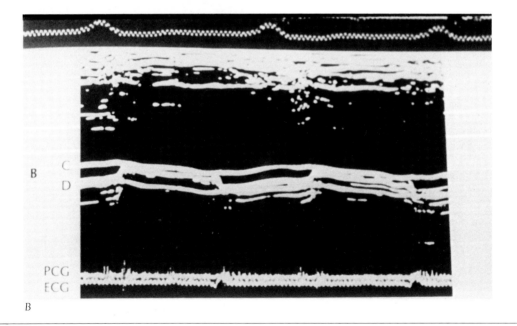

B

Figure 16-11. (A) Radiograph of a Beall valve prosthesis. This valve is a low-profile, noneccentric central occluder. (B) M-mode tracing of a noneccentric central occluder disc valve.

FIGURE 16-12. An early model of the Beall-Surgitool disc prosthesis with a Teflon disc. (From Lefrak EA, Starr A, et al. Cardiac Valve Prostheses. New York: Appleton-Century-Crofts; 1982; 187.)

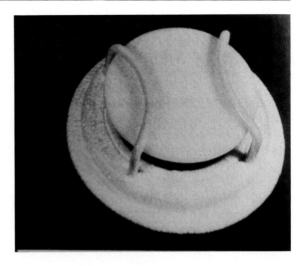

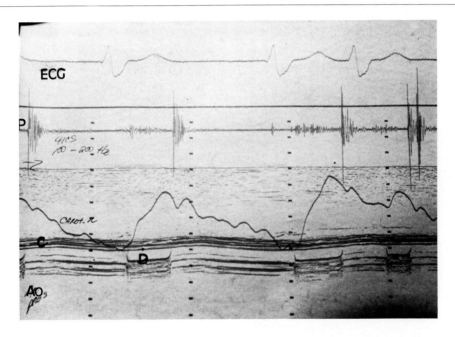

FIGURE 16-13. M-mode and phonocardiographic tracings from a patient with an aortic disc prosthesis.

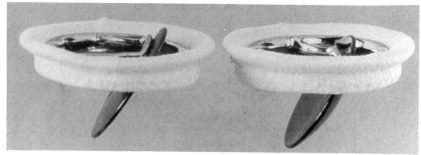

A

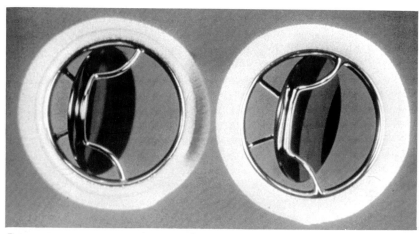

B

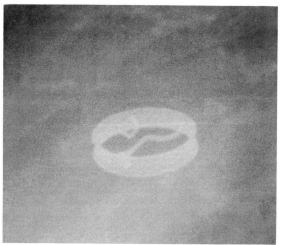

C

FIGURE 16-14. (A) Side and (B) top views of two Bjork-Shiley valves with concave and convex disc designs. (C) Radiograph of a Bjork-Shiley valve. (A, B courtesy of Shiley Laboratories, Irvine, CA.)

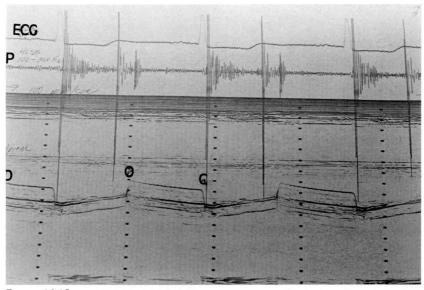

FIGURE 16-15

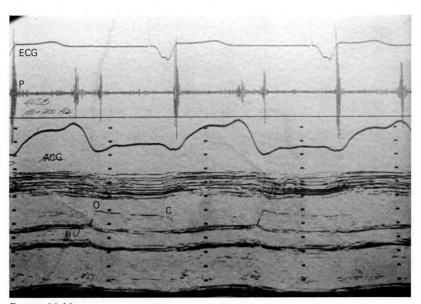

FIGURE 16-16

FIGURE 16-15. M-mode and phonocardiographic tracings of a Bjork-Shiley valve prosthesis in a mitral position. (Normal findings.)

FIGURE 16-16. M-mode and phonocardiographic tracings and an apex cardiogram from a patient with a Bjork-Shiley valve prosthesis in the mitral position. Note the paced rhythm.

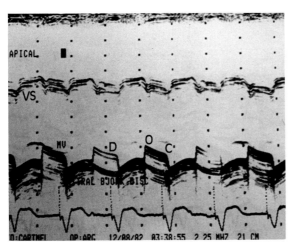

FIGURE 16-17

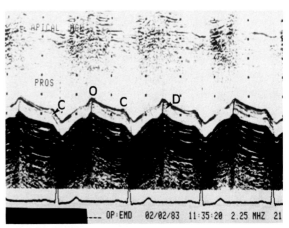

FIGURE 16-19A

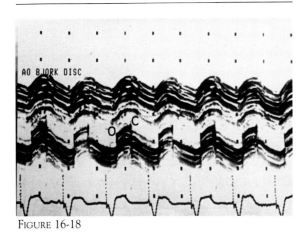

FIGURE 16-18

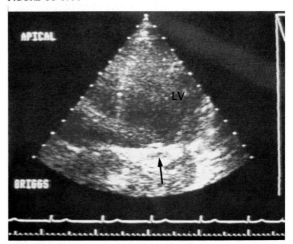

FIGURE 16-19B

FIGURE 16-17. M-mode tracing of a Bjork-Shiley valve prosthesis in the mitral position.

FIGURE 16-18. M-mode tracing of a Bjork-Shiley valve in the aortic position.

FIGURE 16-19. (A) M-mode tracing (apical approach) of a Bjork-Shiley valve prosthesis in the mitral position. (B) Two-dimensional echocardiogram (apical view) of a patient with a Bjork-Shiley valve in the mitral position. Note the highly echogenic reflections (arrow) from these valves. (C) Pulsed-wave mapping of the left atrium in a patient with a Bjork-Shiley valve prosthesis in the mitral position. Note the prominent opening and closing sounds (O, C).

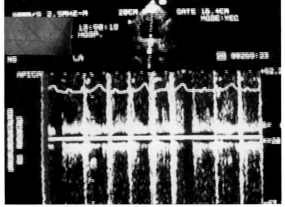

FIGURE 16-19C

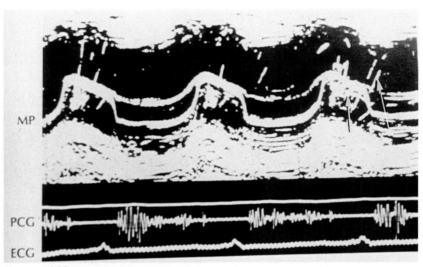

FIGURE 16-20

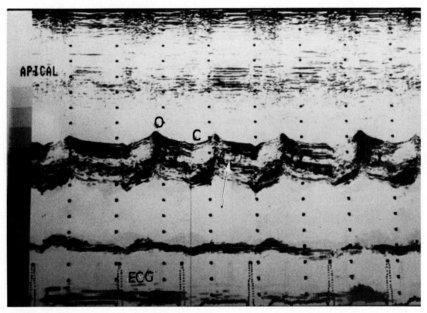

FIGURE 16-21

FIGURE 16-20. M-mode and phonocardiographic tracings of an abnormal Bjork-Shiley valve prosthesis. The increased echogenicity and erratic linear echoes indicate thrombus formation.

FIGURE 16-21. M-mode tracing of a Bjork-Shiley valve prosthesis. The appearance is abnormal, owing to the presence of increased density, reflectivity, and erratic linear echoes.

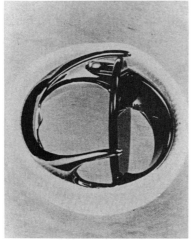

A

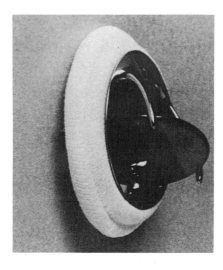

FIGURE 16-22. (A) A Lillehei-Kaster disc prosthesis. (B) Radiograph of a Lillehei-Kaster valve prosthesis. Although the image is slightly blurred, the spiky projections of the valve can be seen. (A from: Lefrak EA, Starr A. Cardiac Valve Prostheses. New York: Appleton-Century-Crofts; 1982: 251, 256.)

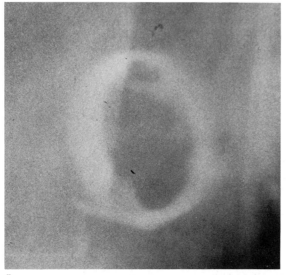

B

(Text continues from page 314.)

It is especially important to obtain baseline echocardiograms from patients with prosthetic valves so that changes in flow dynamics or valve excursion can be recognized.

*Lillehei-Kaster Tilting-Disc Valve.* This mechanical tilting-disc valve is similar echocardiographically to the Bjork-Shiley valve but unlike the Bjork design has two spinelike projections as part of the cage support (Figs. 16-22 to 16-24). M-mode recordings of mitral tilting-disc valves reveal disc excursion of 7 to 12 mm. Echophonocardiography has helped to identify the association between the opening of the valve prosthesis and the aortic component of the second heart sound (opening follows $A_2$ by 0.05 to 0.09 seconds).[29,40,72,81]

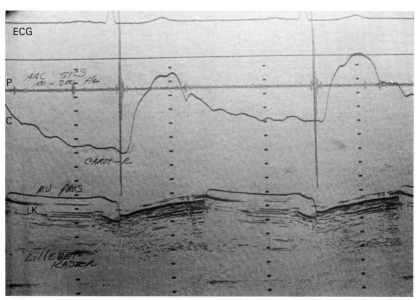

FIGURE 16-23

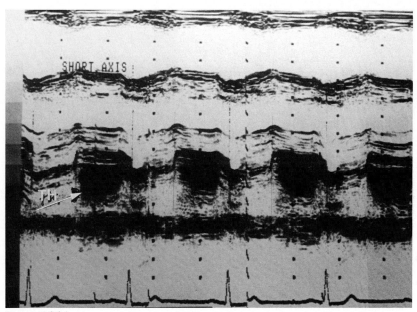

FIGURE 16-24

FIGURE 16-23. M-mode, carotid, and phonocardiographic tracings of a Lillehei-Kaster valve prosthesis in the mitral position that has been in situ for 7 years.

FIGURE 16-24. M-mode tracing of a Lillehei-Kaster valve prosthesis containing thrombus. Note the abnormal density behind the valve. A large thrombus was removed at surgery.

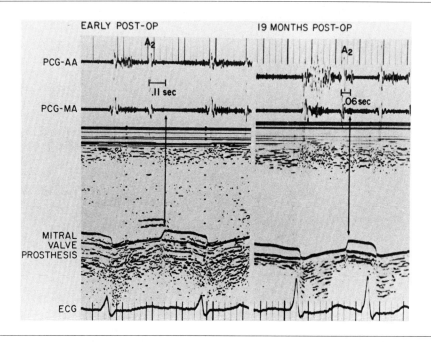

FIGURE 16-25. Comparative M-mode and phonocardiographic tracings of a patient with a Lillehei-Kaster valve in the mitral position. In the early postoperative study the interval between $A_2$ and valve opening was normal (0.11 sec). Nineteen months later, the prosthesis became obstructed by thrombus and the interval was decreased to 0.06 sec. (From Brodie BR, et al. Diagnosis of prosthetic mitral valve malfunction with combined echo-phonocardiography. Circulation. 1976; 53:93–100.)

*Bi-leaflet Tilting-Disc Valve.* A current example of this design is the St. Jude Medical valve. The St. Jude bi-leaflet disc prosthesis consist of two centrally hinged semi-circular disc leaflets of equal size (Fig. 16-25). These low-profile valves are made entirely of biologically inert pyrolite carbon which cannot be imaged radiographically (Figs. 16-26 to 16-27). Their flow pattern is more central and not occluded. M-mode recordings through the open St. Jude bi-leaflet valve demonstrate four parallel lines reflecting from both leaflets and from the anterior and posterior aspects of the valve ring. The appearance resembles the capital letter H. Longer RR intervals can result in leaflet flutter (Figs. 16-27 to 16-32).

Two-dimensional examination is helpful to assess ring motion, leaflet motion, and valvular position-orientation in the heart. Phonocardiography reveals an opening sound $60 \pm 12$ msec after the onset of the ventricular (QRS) complex on the electrocardiogram (ECG).[22,38,83]

*(Text continues on page 334.)*

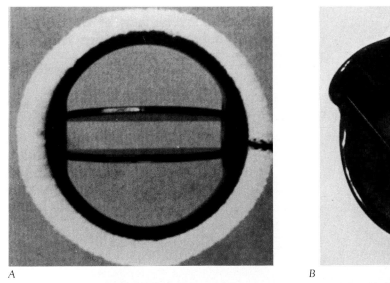

A

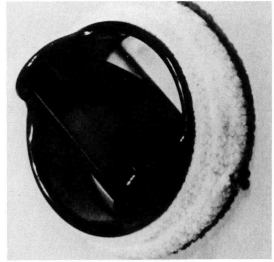

B

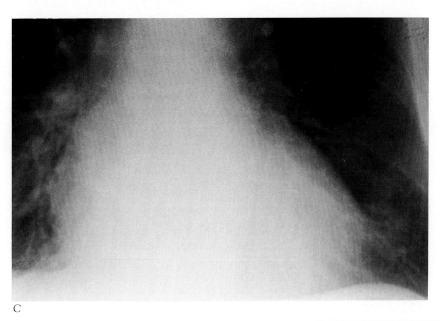

C

Figure 16-26. (A, B) St. Jude bi-leaflet valves. (C) Radiograph of a St. Jude bi-leaflet valve in situ. By composition, St. Jude valves are radiolucent. (A from Salcedo E. Atlas of Echocardiography, 2nd ed. W.B. Saunders; 1987; 180; B from Amann F, Burckhardt D, Hasse J, et al. St. Jude valve prothesis. Am Heart J. 1981; 101:45–51.)

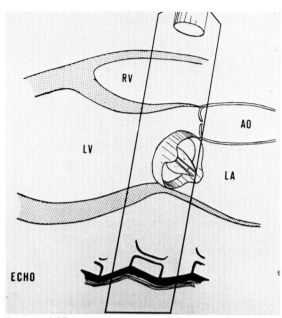

FIGURE 16-27

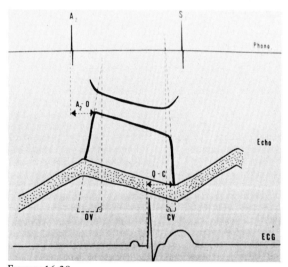

FIGURE 16-28

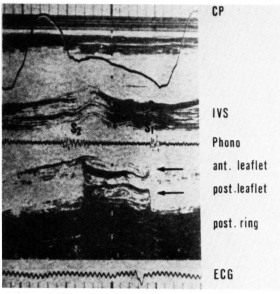

FIGURE 16-29A

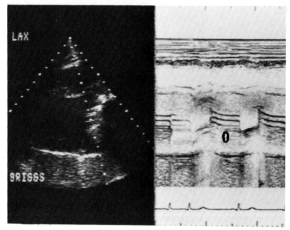

FIGURE 16-29B

FIGURE 16-27. Schematic representation of the St. Jude bi-leaflet prosthesis in the mitral position, demonstrating beam and the resulting M-mode recording. (From Amann F, Burckhardt D, Hasse J, et al. St. Jude valve prothesis. Am Heart J. 1981; 101:45–51.)

FIGURE 16-28. Schematic M-mode and phonocardiographic tracing of a St. Jude valve prosthesis in the mitral position. (From Amann F, Burckhardt D, Hasse J, et al. St. Jude valve prothesis. Am Heart J. 1981; 101:45–51.)

FIGURE 16-29. (A) Normal M-mode and phonocardiographic tracings of a St. Jude bi-leaflet valve prosthesis in the mitral position. (B) Two-dimensional scan and M-mode recording of a St. Jude bi-leaflet valve prosthesis in the mitral position. Note the four parallel lines on the long axis 2-D scan and the multiple lines at the open phase on the M-mode tracing. (A from Amann F, Burckhardt D, Hasse J, et al. St. Jude valve prothesis. Am Heart J. 1981; 101:45–51.)

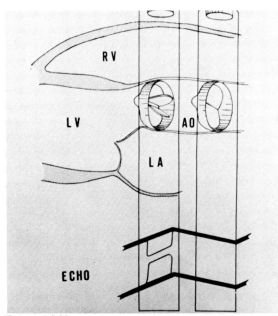

FIGURE 16-30

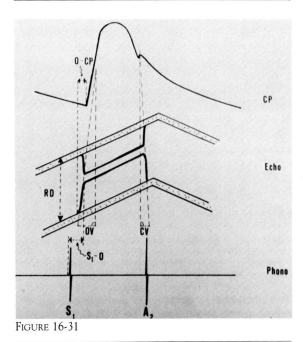

FIGURE 16-31

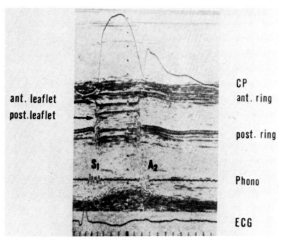

FIGURE 16-32A

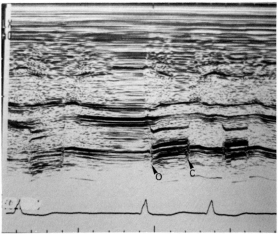

FIGURE 16-32B

FIGURE 16-31. Schematic drawing of a St. Jude bi-leaflet valve prosthesis in the aortic position. (From Amann F, Burckhardt D, Hasse J, et al. St. Jude valve prothesis. Am Heart J. 1981; 101:45–51.)

FIGURE 16-32. (A) M-mode and phonocardiographic tracings and carotid recordings from a patient with a St. Jude bi-leaflet valve in the aortic position. (B) M-mode tracing of a patient with a normal St. Jude bi-leaflet valve prosthesis in the aortic position. (From Amann F, Burckhardt D, Hasse J, et al. St. Jude valve prothesis. Am Heart J. 1981; 101:45–51.)

FIGURE 16-30. Schematic drawing of a St. Jude bi-leaflet valve in the aortic position, showing beam direction and the resulting M-mode recording at systole and diastole. (From Amann F, Burckhardt D, Hasse J, et al. St. Jude valve prothesis. Am Heart J. 1981; 101:45–51.)

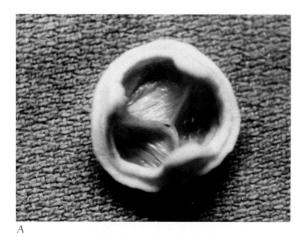

A

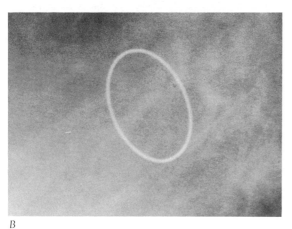

B

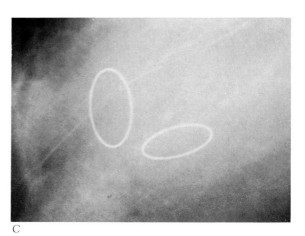

C

FIGURE 16-33. (A) Hancock porcine xenograft (top view). Radiographs show a Hancock porcine xenograft in (B) mitral and (C) mitral and aortic positions.

(Text continues from page 330.)

BIOPROSTHETIC VALVES

*Heterografts (Xenografts)*

*Hancock and Carpentier-Edwards.* The most common heterografts (grafts incorporating tissue from a nonhuman species) are the Hancock and the Carpentier-Edwards valves, which consist of a porcine aortic valve covered with woven Dacron mounted in a cage (Figs. 16-33 to 16-46). The Hancock xenograft has three flexible polypropylene stents sup-

ported on a stellite ring (Fig. 16-53). Until it is implanted, the porcine tissue is preserved with glutaraldehyde solution.[52] In the Carpentier-Edwards valve, the xenograft is mounted on an Elgiloy frame (Fig. 16-41).

These valves are also lower profile or less bulky in size as compared with the ball-and-cage types and offer more central flow and reduced turbulence. The incidence of associated thromboembolism is lower than with mechanical valves.[52]

(Text continues on page 341.)

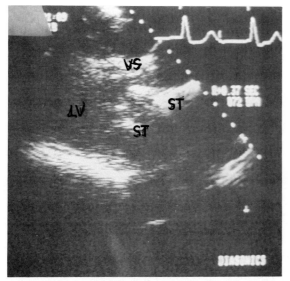

FIGURE 16-34A

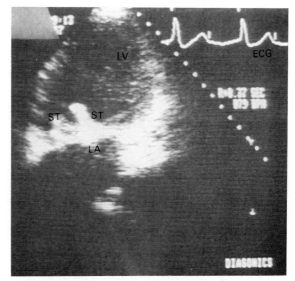

FIGURE 16-34B

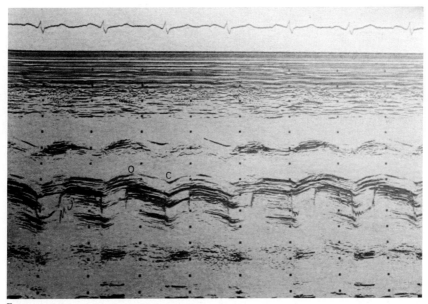

FIGURE 16-35

FIGURE 16-34. (A) Two-dimensional (long-axis) scan of a Hancock porcine xenograft in the mitral position. The two parallel stents look like a horseshoe. (B) Apical 2-D scan of a Hancock porcine xenograft in the mitral position. (LV, left ventricle; LA, left atrium; St, stent of graft.)

FIGURE 16-35. M-mode tracing of a patient with a Hancock valve in the mitral position. An apical scanning approach was used.

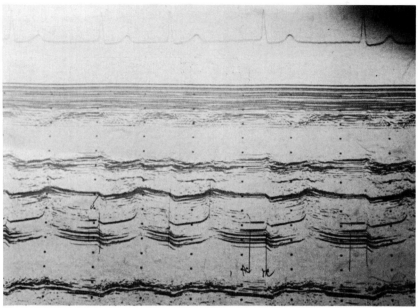

FIGURE 16-36

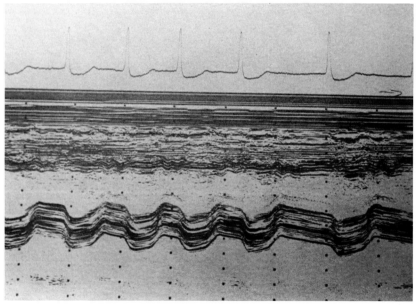

FIGURE 16-37

FIGURE 16-36. M-mode tracing from a patient with a Hancock porcine xenograft in the mitral position. Note the early closure pattern with longer RR intervals (atrial fibrillation).

FIGURE 16-37. M-mode tracing from a patient with a 3-year-old Hancock porcine xenograft in the mitral position. The valve has recalcified and appears similar to native calcific mitral valve stenosis.

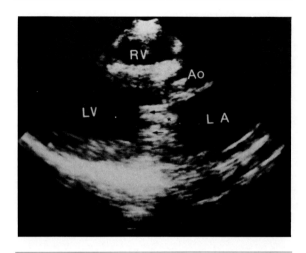

FIGURE 16-38. Two-dimensional scan of a patient with mitral and aortic Hancock porcine xenografts. A large vegetation (*) is seen in the mitral prosthesis, behind the anterior stent. (From Salcedo E. Atlas of Echocardiography, 2nd ed. Philadelphia: W.B. Saunders; 1987; 189.)

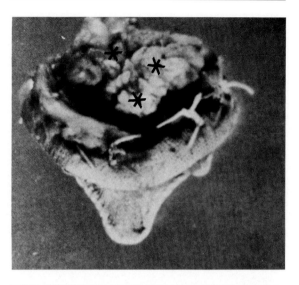

FIGURE 16-39. Porcine valve with vegetation. (From Salcedo E. Atlas of Echocardiography, 2nd ed. Philadelphia: W.B. Saunders; 1987; 194.)

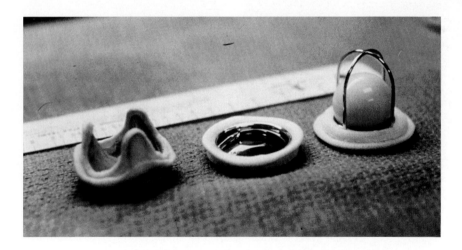

FIGURE 16-40. Carpentier-Edwards porcine xenograft (left); Bjork-Shiley disc prosthesis (center); and Starr-Edwards ball and cage prosthesis (right). Note the profile variances.

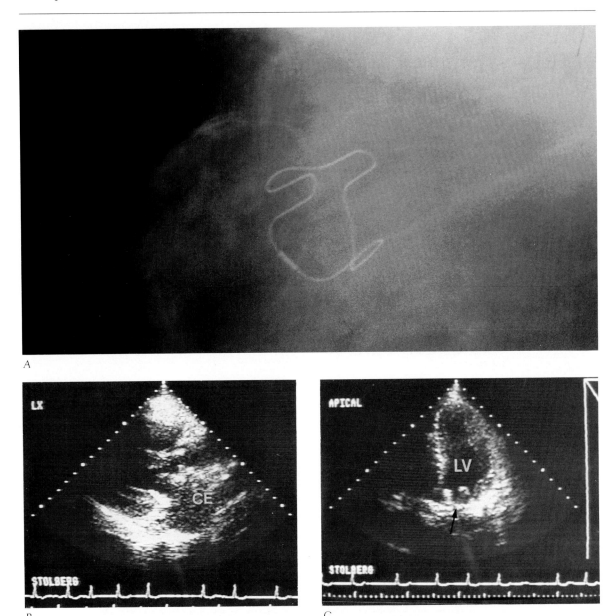

FIGURE 16-41. (A) Radiograph of a Carpentier-Edwards porcine xenograft. Note the distinct appearance of its frame. (B) Two-dimensional scan (long-axis view) of a Carpentier-Edwards porcine xenograft (CE) in the mitral position. Like other bioprosthetic valves, it resembles a horseshoe. (C) Two-dimensional scan (apical view) of a Carpentier-Edwards porcine xenograft in the mitral position. (LV, left ventricle.)

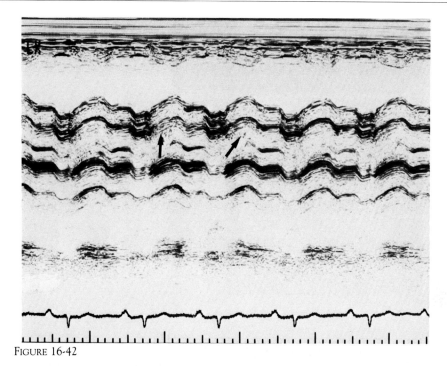

FIGURE 16-42

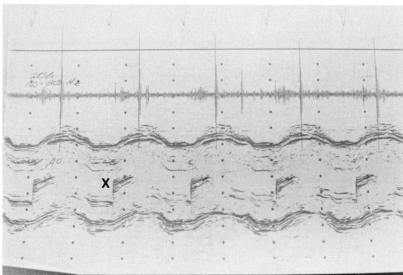

FIGURE 16-43

FIGURE 16-42. M-mode tracing (long-axis view) of a 2-year-old Carpentier-Edwards porcine xenograft in the aortic position. Note the systolic flutter (*arrows*).

FIGURE 16-43. M-mode tracing of a 4-year-old Carpentier-Edwards porcine xenograft in the aortic position. The cusps exhibit increased density and reflectivity and appeared less mobile on both 2-D and M-mode studies.

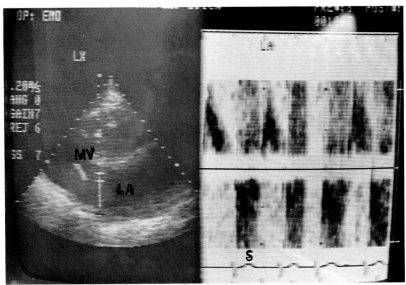

FIGURE 16-44

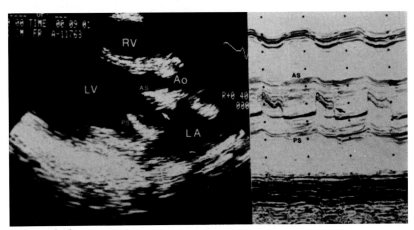

FIGURE 16-45

FIGURE 16-44. Two-dimensional (long-axis) scan and pulsed-wave left atrial Doppler studies of a patient with a Carpentier-Edwards porcine xenograft in the mitral position.

FIGURE 16-45. Porcine mitral valve studies (2-D long-axis and M-mode) in a 60-year-old patient with a No. 33 Carpentier-Edwards prosthesis. Note the similarity in appearance to the Hancock prosthesis. The arrows point to the leaflets. (LV, left ventricule; RV, right ventricle; Ao, aorta; LA, left atrium; AS, PS, anterior and posterior septum.) (From Salcedo E. Atlas of Echocardiography, 2nd ed. Philadelphia: W.B. Saunders; 1987; 192.)

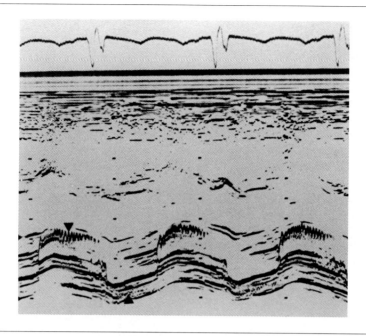

FIGURE 16-46. M-mode tracing demonstrating diastolic and systolic fluttering of a porcine valve in the mitral position, in the presence of mitral regurgitation. (S, interventricular septum; ST, stents.) (From Feigenbaum H. Echocardiography. Philadelphia: Lea & Febiger; 1986; 4: 340.)

(Text continues from page 334.)

*Ionescu-Shiley pericardial valve.* The Ionescu-Shiley bioprosthetic valve incorporates bovine pericardium which is mounted on an Elgiloy frame with three struts (Figs. 16-47 to 16-51). This too is a central-flow, nonoccluding, low-profile valve. Generally, it is seen clearly on standard 2-D and M-mode echocardiograms.

*Homografts.* Homografts, or allografts, contain tissue from another human. To make heart valve allografts, human dura mater is mounted in the outer surface of the stents. The normal echocardio-graphic appearance resembles that of native aortic valve.

*Autografts.* Autografts contain tissue from the person who is to receive the prosthesis. This design uses fascia lata mounted in a stent and has been evaluated in the mitral position.

*Carpentier Ring.* This flexible ring is used in the AV valve positions for support annuloplasty procedures. Its echocardiographic appearance is similar to that of a calcified AV valve annulus (Figs. 16-52–16-54).

(Text continues on page 346.)

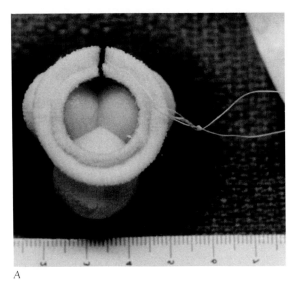

A

FIGURE 16-47. (A) Ionescu-Shiley bioprosthetic (bovine) valve. (B) Radiograph of an Ionescu-Shiley valve in the mitral position. Note the distinct cage design. (C) Radiograph of an Ionescu-Shiley valve prosthesis viewed from apex to base.

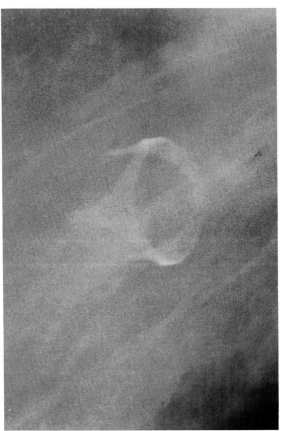

B

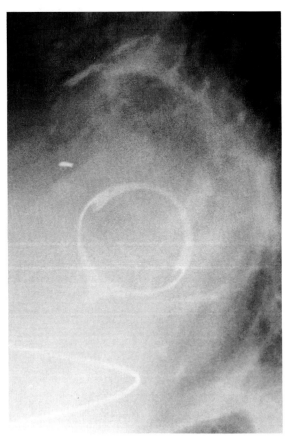

C

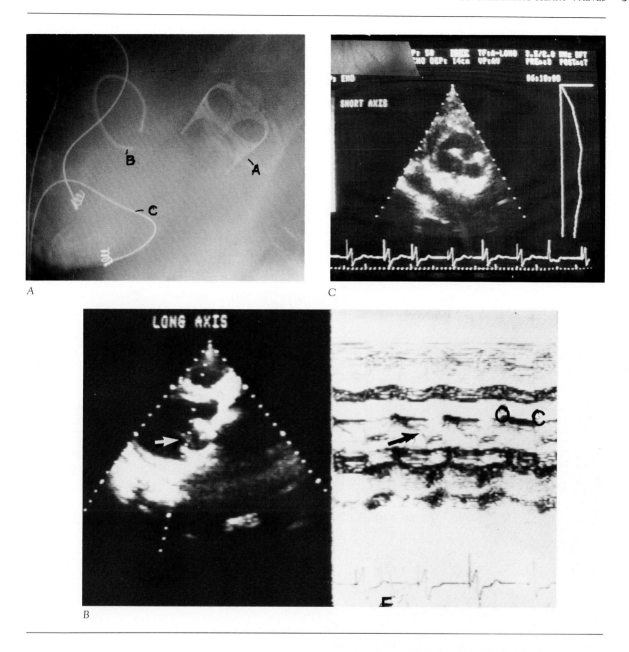

Figure 16-48. (A) Radiograph of an Ionescu-Shiley valve in the mitral position, and a Carpentier-Edwards annuloplasty ring in the tricuspid position. (B) Two-dimensional long-axis scan and an M-mode tracing from a patient with an Ionescu-Shiley valve in the mitral position. The tissue of this valve generally is quite echogenic. (C) Two-dimensional short-axis view of an Ionescu-Shiley prosthesis in the mitral position.

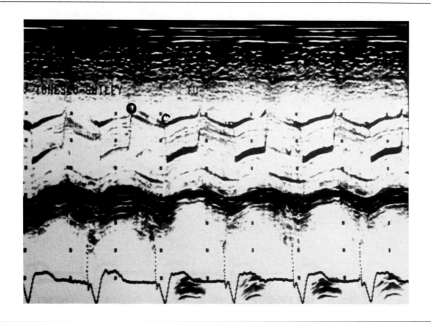

FIGURE 16-49. M-mode tracing in a patient with an Ionescu-Shiley valve prosthesis in the tricuspid position clearly demonstrates cusp opening and closing patterns.

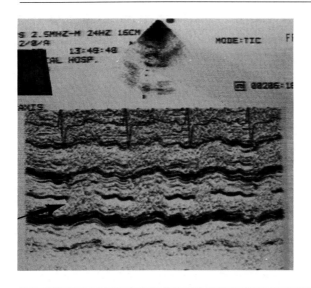

FIGURE 16-50. M-mode tracing (short-axis plane) of a patient with an Ionescu-Shiley prosthesis in the aortic position.

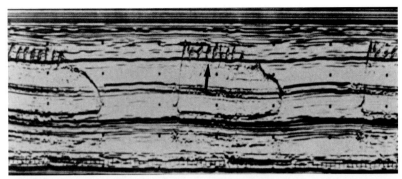

FIGURE 16-51

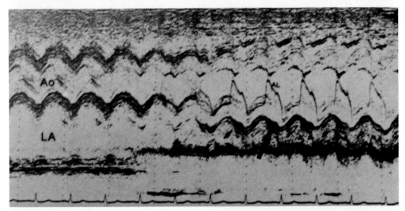

FIGURE 16-52

FIGURE 16-51. M-mode echocardiogram shows fluttering of a pericardial tissue valve secondary to degeneration of the valve and resultant regurgitation. (From Feigenbaum H. Echocardiography. Philadelphia: Lea & Febiger, 1986; 4: 340.)

FIGURE 16-52. M-mode recording from a patient with a Carpentier ring in the mitral position. The M-mode scan from the aorta to the left ventricle demonstrates an echodense structure simulating mitral annulus calcification behind the mitral valve. (From Salcedo E. Atlas of Echocardiography, 2nd ed. Philadelphia: W.B. Saunders; 1987, 196.)

FIGURE 16-53. Two-dimensional long-axis view of a Carpentier ring. Note the linear echo recorded at the level of the mitral annulus (arrows). Somewhat elongated anterior (AL) and posterior (PL) mitral valve leaflets are seen in the left ventricle (LV). (Ao, aorta; LA, left atrium.) (From Salcedo E. Atlas of Echocardiography, 2nd ed. Philadelphia: W.B. Saunders, 1987; 196.)

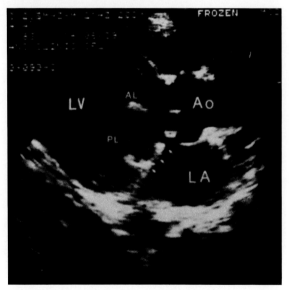

FIGURE 16-53

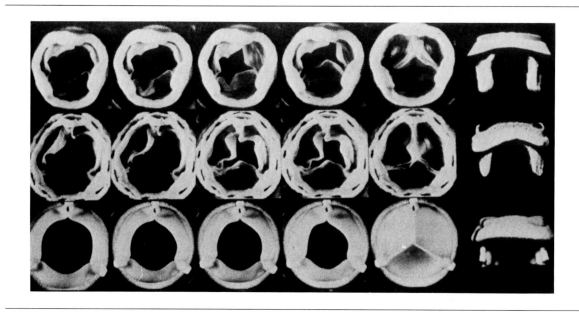

FIGURE 16-54. Comparison of orifice openings (which vary flow levels) in three types of valves: *(Top)* Hancock porcine; *(Middle)* Carpentier-Edwards porcine; *(Bottom)* Ionescu-Shiley bovine. (Courtesy of Edwards Laboratories, Irvine, CA.)

*(Text continues from page 341.)*

## Complications of Prosthetic Valves

### BALL OR DISC VARIANCE

Ball or disc variance refers to changes in the Silastic disc or poppet, probably due to abrasion and deposits of blood lipid. As a result, the disc or poppet increases in size or its normal contour is distorted. Any such alteration results in uneven stress, cracking, tearing, or grooving of the prosthesis which could eventually lead to valve incompetence or malfunction of the ball, disc, or poppet. Metallic prostheses do not have these problems.

### THROMBUS FORMATION OR BACTERIAL VEGETATION

In the presence of a thrombus the normal function of the poppet or disc is altered. It may fail to open and close completely, may obstruct blood flow, or stick in one position.

Bacterial endocarditis can involve a bioprosthetic valve and compromise valve function so it is important to determine the presence of thrombi or vegetations to prevent valve complications and peripheral embolism. Small thrombi or areas of bacterial vegetations can be difficult to image in the vicinity of the highly echogenic cage material.

### PERIVALVULAR LEAK AND DEHISCENCE OF SUTURE RING

Bacterial vegetations, thrombus, or suture failure can cause the valve prosthesis to loosen or separate from the sewing ring, in which case it will leak at the site of attachment and the valve will rock. Such flow abnormalities and spatial aberrations can be easily visualized with Doppler and 2-D echocardiography.

### HEMOLYSIS

Hemolysis—damage to red blood cells and platelets—occurs to some extent in all prosthetic valves. It is due to abnormal shear stress, turbulence, and collision of blood cells with foreign surfaces.[14,62,71]

Factors that contribute to red cell trauma include ball variance, perivalvular leakage, pressure gradients across the valve, valve ball-poppet materials, discs and sewing rings, and the position and number of valve prostheses.[14]

Because central flow-type valves (Bjork-Shiley,[8] St. Jude, homograft, xenograft[70,87]) produce less turbulence, hemolysis is mild. With bioprosthetic xenograft valves hemolysis is related to the Dacron covering. Hemolysis decreases over time as endothelial cells grow into the cloth and mechanical trauma to the red cells is reduced.[70]

### REDUCED OR COMPROMISED CARDIAC OUTPUT

Low cardiac output can result from impeded blood flow if the valvular prosthesis is too large for the left ventricle or aorta. Aortic regurgitation can result from distortion and misalignment of the leaflets in the presence of a large mitral prosthesis. If undue stress is applied to the suture ring, perivalvular leakage or dishiscence can occur. Cardiac arrhythmias also can occur with a large valvular prosthesis cage in a ventricular wall.

### CLINICAL ASPECTS OF PROSTHETIC VALVE FUNCTION

During diastole, the disc or ball of the mitral or tricuspid device is directed toward the apex of the cage as blood flow moves from the atrium to the ventricle. In systole, the disc or ball is forced against the base of the prosthesis, thus preventing regurgitation of the blood into the atria. The poppet or ball in the aortic valve position moves toward the apex of the cage in systole, allowing forward flow into the aorta (systemic circulation) and coapts with the base of the cage in diastole, preventing regurgitation into the ventricle.

Audible sounds (clicks) are produced by the impact of the poppet or disc against the apex or base of the cage in the open or closed positions.[68] Low-fidelity murmurs due to a small pressure gradient are often heard with these valve prostheses.[4,6,25] Some aortic poppets strike the apex of the cage several times during systole, producing several clicks. With valve dysfunction, these clicks may become muffled or intermittently disappear.[6,68] Eccentric valves produce fainter clicks than do ball-and-cage prostheses.[23,25,29] Paravalvular leaks may produce significant murmurs, which can become softer or even disappear in the presence of severe regurgitation or low cardiac output states.[17,32]

## Role of Echocardiography in the Evaluation of Prosthetic Valves

Standard or transthoracic echocardiography with Doppler evaluation has proved valuable in assessing valve prostheses in situ. Doppler velocity quantitation for determining pressure gradients and valve areas has become a standard technique in most echo labs and is a valuable reference guide to valve function over time and a fairly reliable indicator of valve dysfunction. For a current comparative analysis of pressure gradients and valve areas from various investigators, see Tables 16-2 and 16-3. The mitral valve data was obtained by Doppler evaluation of LV inflow velocities obtained from the apical approach. The aortic valve data was obtained from both the apical LV outflow tract and the high right sternal border approach.

However, transthoracic echocardiography can be limited by a number of factors: high echogenicity of valve materials, which can make visualization difficult; shadowing created by the prosthetic valve material, which can mask abnormal flow patterns; difficult to image valves in some patients due to girth; existing lung disease; or presentation (postoperative, supine position, and patients on ventilator assist).

Transesophageal echocardiography (TEE) now can be used to examine conscious or unconscious patients. A maneuverable transducer is placed on the tip of a modified endoscope, which is introduced through the esophagus to a position behind the heart, where it affords an unobstructed view of the left atrium and other cardiac structures. It is particularly superior for the evaluation of left atrial abnormalities, aortic root dissection, and mitral, aortic, and tricuspid valve abnormalities and vegetations and for monitoring segmental wall motion changes in high-risk patients during surgery.

TEE will play an important role in the future of echocardiography and will soon become a routine adjunctive technique.

Table 16-2. Current echocardiographic values for mitral valve prostheses

| Valve | Size (mm) | Peak Gradient (mm Hg) | Mean Gradient (mm Hg) | Effective Valve Area EOA (cm²) | References |
|---|---|---|---|---|---|
| Ball-and-cage | | | | | |
| Starr-Edwards | Not reported | 13–20 | 5±2 | 1.95–2.1 | 71, 79, 9, 93, 15, 29 |
| Disc | | | | | |
| Bjork-Shiley | Not reported | 11±3 | 3–11 | | Personal experience, 9 cases |
| | Not reported | 10±3 | 5±2 | 2.2±0.4 | 71 |
| | Not reported | 10±3 | | 2.5±0.8 | 93 |
| | Not reported | 6.4±3.3 | 2.0±1.6 | 2.14±0.3 | 81 |
| | Not reported | 9.8±2.8 | 2.5±1.4 | 2.14±0.3 | 15 |
| | 27 | | 2–4 | 1.7–2.3 | 43 |
| | 29 | | 2–4 | 1.8–2.3 | 41 |
| | 31 | | 2–4 | 1.65–2.5 | 35, 38 |
| Lillehei-Kaster | Not reported | 13.5 | 3.35 | 1.88±0.56 | 15 |
| | 18 | | | 1.4–1.6 | 41 |
| | 20 | | | 1.38–1.44 | 61 |
| St. Jude | Not reported | 7.6±3.6 | 2.3±0.9 | 3.6±0.9 | 90 |
| | Not reported | 11±4.0 | 5.0±2 | 3.0±0.6 | 71 |
| | Not reported | 10.6±3.5 | 2.3±1.1 | 2.9±0.6 | 15 |
| | Not reported | 12.0±4.4 | 5.6±2.1 | 3.1±0.8 | 16 |
| | Not reported | 7.8±3.6 | 3.3±1.1 | 2.6±0.6 | 50 |
| | Not reported | 8–12 | | | Personal experience, 4 cases |
| Bioprosthetic | | | | | |
| Hancock | Not reported | | 3.5–8 | | 40 |
| | 27 | | 5–7 | 1.03–1.43 | 40 |
| | Not reported | 15–20 | | 1.18–2.3 | 40, Personal experience, 27 cases |
| | 29 | | | 1.03–1.8 | 41 |
| | 31 | | | 1.7–2.2 | 40, 41 |
| | Not reported | | 6.5±1.4 | 1.4±0.6 | 41 |
| | Not reported | | | 1.54–0.3 | 24 |
| | Not reported | 14 | | 2.4 | 79 |
| | Not reported | 5.8±2.5 | 2.4±1.2 | 1.56–0.3 | 81 |
| | Not reported | 7.6±2.7 | | 1.6±0.3 | 80 |
| | 29, 31 | 5–7 | | | 35, 38 |
| Carpentier-Edwards | 33 | 15–20 | | | 35, 38 |
| | Not reported | 10.2±2.4 | | 2.4±0.4 | 28 |
| | Not reported | 17.3±0.2 | 7.5±0.2 | 2.6±0.7 | 16 |
| | Not reported | 9.6±1.9 | 4.4±1.9 | 2.2±0.4 | 60 |
| | Not reported | 10–16 | | | Personal experience, 11 cases |
| Ionescu-Shiley | Not reported | 7.7±2.0 | 3.5±0.8 | 2.3±0.8 | 60 |
| | Not reported | 9.7±3.4 | 2.9±1.6 | 2.4±0.7 | 15 |
| | Not reported | 10±3 | | | Personal experience, 6 cases |

Table 16-3. Current echocardiographic values for aortic valves prostheses

| Valve | Size (mm) | Peak Gradient (mm Hg) | Mean Gradient (mm Hg) | References |
|---|---|---|---|---|
| **Ball-and-cage** | | | | |
| Starr-Edwards | Not reported | 29.3 ± 13.3 | 12.1 ± 6.6 | 93 |
| | Not reported | 40.0 ± 3.0 | 24 ± 4.0 | 71 |
| | Not reported | 45 ± 12 | | 73 |
| | Not reported | 40.0 | | 79 |
| | Not reported | 28–35 | | Personal experience, 8 cases |
| Bjork-Shiley | Not reported | 30 ± 9 | 16 ± 5 | 48 |
| | Not reported | 21.5 ± 3.0 | | 93 |
| | Not reported | 18.8 ± 7.0 | | 73 |
| | Not reported | 22 ± 5.3 | | 81 |
| | 19 | | 21 ± 7.0 | 48 |
| | 21 | 30.5 ± 19.9 | | 73 |
| | 23 | | 16 | 48 |
| | 23 | 27.2 ± 8.7 | | 81, 73 |
| | 25 | 18.4 ± 5.3 | | 81, 73 |
| | 25 | | 13.3 ± 2.5 | 81, 48 |
| | Not reported | 22–31 | | Personal experience, 14 cases |
| | 27 | 14.6 ± 3.1 | | 81, 73 |
| | 27 | | 16 ± .2 | 81, 48 |
| | 29 | 14 ± 2.5 | 7.0 ± 6.0 | 73, 48 |
| St. Jude | Not reported | 22 ± 12.0 | 12.0 ± 7.0 | 71 |
| | Not reported | 27 ± 9 | 16 ± 6 | 16 |
| | Not reported | 15.5 ± 8.2 | 6.0 ± 2.5 | 90 |
| | Not reported | 30 ± 9.0 | 16 ± 5.6 | 48 |
| | 19 | 31 ± 17 | 22 ± 11 | 16, 71, 48 |
| | 21 | 30 ± 5.7 | 14.4 ± 5.0 | 16, 71, 48, 19 |
| | 23 | | 10.8 ± 6.3 | 16, 71, 48 |
| | 25 | 19.8 ± 8.2 | 11.0 ± 6.0 | 16, 71 |
| **Bioprosthetic** | | | | |
| Hancock | Not reported | 22 ± 10 | | 93 |
| | Not reported | 30 | | 79 |
| | Not reported | 26 ± 4.7 | | 73 |
| | Not reported | 16.0 ± 3.0 | 11.0 ± 2.3 | 81 |
| | Not reported | 16–25 | | Personal experience, 16 cases |
| | 23 | 23 ± 4.6 | 12.0 ± 2.0 | 81, 73 |
| Hancock | 25 | 21 ± 4.6 | 11.0 ± 2.0 | 81, 73 |
| | 27 | 21 ± 5.7 | 10.0 ± 3.0 | 81, 73 |
| | 29 | 20 ± 7 | 10.0 ± 3 | 73 |
| Carpentier-Edwards | Not reported | 24 ± 9 | | 28 |
| | Not reported | 19 ± 9 | | 73 |
| | Not reported | 31 ± 15 | 18.0 ± 9.0 | 48 |
| | Not reported | 26.1 ± 4.8 | 15 ± 4.8 | 16 |
| | Not reported | 23.1 ± 8.2 | 12.3 ± 5.9 | 60 |
| | Not reported | 17–31 | | Personal experience, 5 cases |
| | 19 | 32 ± 14 | 17 ± 1.4 | 16, 60 |
| | 21 | 27.3 ± 10 | 14.5 ± 6.0 | 60 |
| | 23 | 27 ± 9 | 13 ± 5.7 | 16, 73, 60, 48 |
| | 25 | 25 ± 8 | 11 ± 2.3 | 16, 60, 48 |
| | 27 | 24 ± 7.2 | 10.4 ± 2.3 | 16, 60, 73, 48 |
| | 29 | 23 ± 8.4 | 12 | 48, 73 |
| | 31 | 23 ± 8 | 12 | 73 |
| Ionescu-Shiley | Not reported | 27 ± 9.1 | 16 ± 5 | 16 |
| | Not reported | 22 ± 6 | 12 ± 3 | 60 |
| | Not reported | 22–31 | | Personal experience, 11 cases |

# References

1. Abbasi AS, Allen MW, DeCristofaro D, et al. Detection and estimation of the degree of mitral regurgitation by range-gated pulsed Doppler echocardiography. Circulation. 1980; 61:143–147.

2. Alam M, Goldstein S. Echocardiographic features of a stenotic porcine aortic valve. Am Heart J. 1980; 100:517–519.

3. Alam M, Goldstein S, Lakier JB. Echocardiographic changes in the thickness of porcine valves with time. Chest. 1981; 6:663–668.

4. Alam M, Lakier JB, Pickard SD, et al. Echocardiographic evaluation of porcine bioprosthetic valves: Experience with 309 normal and 59 dysfunctioning valves. Am J Cardiol. 1983; 52:309–315.

5. Alam M, Madrazo AC, Magilligan DJ, et al. M-mode and two-dimensional echocardiographic features of porcine valve dysfunction. Am J Cardiol. 1979; 43:502–509.

6. Belenkie I, Carr M, Schlant RC, et al. Malfunction of the Cutter-Smeloff mitral ball valve prosthesis: Diagnosis by phonocardiography and echocardiography. Am Heart J. 1973; 86:339–346.

7. Ben-Zvi J, Hilder FJ, Chandraratna PA, et al. Thrombosis on Bjork-Shiley aortic valve prosthesis. Am J Cardiol. 1974; 34:538–544.

8. Bjork VO, Henze A. More than six and one-half years experience with Bjork-Shiley heart valves in the aortic, mitral and tricuspid positions. In: Davila JC, ed. Second Henry Ford Hospital International Symposium on Cardiac Surgery. New York: Appleton-Century-Crofts; 1977; 454–466.

9. Bjork VO, Olin C. A hydrodynamic comparison between the new tilting disc aortic valve prosthesis (Bjork-Shiley) and the corresponding prostheses of Starr-Edwards, Kay-Shiley, Smeloff-Cutter in the pulse duplicator. Scand J Thorac Cardiovasc Surg. 1970; 4:31–36.

10. Bloch WN Jr, Felner JM, Schlant RC, et al. The echocardiogram of the porcine aortic bioprosthesis in the aortic position. Chest. 1977; 72:640–646.

11. Bloch WN Jr, Felner JM, Wickliffe C, et al. Echocardiogram of the porcine aortic bioprosthesis in the mitral position. Am J Cardiol. 1976; 38:292–298.

12. Chaitman BR, Bonan R, Lepage G, et al. Hemodynamic evaluation of the Carpentier-Edwards porcine xenograft. Circulation. 1979; 60:1170–1182.

13. Chandraratna P, San Pedro SB. Echocardiographic features of the normal and malfunctioning porcine xenograft valve. Am Heart J. 1978; 95:548–554.

14. Crexalls C, Aerichide N, Bonny U, et al. Factors influencing hemolysis in valve prosthesis. Am Heart J. 1972; 84:161–170.

15. Cruitus JM, Pawelzik H, Mittmann B, et al. Doppler echokardiographische normwerte fur verschiedene mitralprothesentypen. Z Kardiol. 1987; 76:25–29.

16. Cooper DM, Stewart WJ, Schiavone WA, et al. Evaluation of normal prosthetic valve function by Doppler echocardiography. Am Heart J. 1987; 114:576–582.

17. Dellsperger KC, Wieting DW, Baehr DA, et al. Regurgitation of prosthetic heart valves: Dependence on heart rate and cardiac output. Am J Cardiol. 1983; 51:321–328.

18. Denbow CE, Pluth JR, and Ciuliani ER. The role of echocardiography in the selection of mitral valve prosthesis. Am Heart J. 1980; 5:586–588.

19. Dubach-Reber PA, Vargus-Barron J. Velocidad maxima del flujo en la prosthesis mitrale de Bjork-Shiley normofuncionante. Arch Inst Cardiol Mex. 1986; 56:57–61.

20. Douglas JE, Willmans GD. Echocardiographic evaluation of the Bjork-Shiley prosthetic valve. Circulation. 1974; 50:52.

21. Effron MK, Popp RL. Two-dimensional echocardiographic assessment of bioprosthetic valve dysfunction and infective endocarditis. J Am Coll Cardiol. 1983; 2:597–606.

22. Emery R, Palmquist W, Arom K, et al. A new cardiac prosthesis: All pyrolyte carbon bileaflet central flow valve. Circulation. 1978; 58(Suppl. 2):83.

23. Escarous A. The Bjork-Shiley tilting disc valve prosthesis: Echocardiographic findings. Scand J Thorac Cardiovasc Surg. 1975; 9:192–196.

24. Fawzy ME, Halim M, Ziady G, et al. Hemodynamic evaluation of porcine bioprostheses in the mitral position by Doppler echocardiography. Am J Cardiol. 1987; 59:643–646.

25. Feigenbaum H. Echocardiography. 3rd ed. Philadelphia: Lea & Febiger; 1981; 298–315.

26. Fishbein MC, Gilssen SA, Collins, JJ Jr, et al. Pathologic findings after cardiac valve replacement with glutaraldehyde-fixed porcine valves. Am J Cardiol. 1977; 40:331–337.

27. Giancarlo C, Gibson D, Heart B, et al. Severe late failure of a porcine xenograft mitral valve: Clinical echocardiographic and pathological findings. Thorax. 1980; 35:210–212.

28. Gibbs JC, Wharton GA, Williams GJ. Doppler echocardiographic characteristics of the Carpentier-Edwards xenograft. Eur Heart J. 1986; 7:353–356.

29. Gibson TC, Starek JK, Moos S, et al. Echocardiographic and phonocardiographic characteristics of the Lillehei-Kaster mitral valve prosthesis. Circulation. 1974; 49:434–440.

30. Gimenez JL, Winters WL, Davila JC, et al. Dynamics of the Starr-Edwards ball valve prosthesis: A cinefluorographic and ultrasonic study in humans. Am J

Med Sci. 1965; 250:652–656.

31. Grenadier E, Sahn DJ, Roche AHG, et al. Detection of deterioration or infection of homograft and porcine xenograft bioprosthetic valves in mitral and aortic positions by two-dimensional echocardiographic examination. J Am Coll Cardiol. 1983; 2:452–459.

32. Griffiths BE, Charles R, Coulshed N. Echophonocardiography in diagnosis of mitral paravalvular regurgitation with Bjork-Shiley prosthetic valve. Br Heart J. 1980; 43:325–331.

33. Gross CM, Wann LS. Doppler echocardiographic diagnosis of porcine bioprosthetic cardiac valve malfunction. Am J Cardiol. 1984; 53:1203–1205.

34. Gross CM, Wann LS. Doppler echocardiography in the assessment of prosthetic cardiac valves. In: Nanda NC, ed. Doppler Echocardiography. Tokyo: Igaku-Shoin; 1985; 293.

35. Hatle L. Non-invasive assessment and differentiation of left ventricular outflow obstruction with Doppler ultrasound. Circulation. 1981; 64:381–387.

36. Hatle L, Angelsen B, Tromsdal A. Non-invasive assessment of aortic stenosis by Doppler ultrasound. Br Heart J. 1980; 43:284–292.

37. Hatle L, Angelsen B. Doppler Ultrasound in Cardiology: Physical Principles and Clinical Applications. 2nd ed. Philadelphia: Lea & Febiger; 1985; 102–105; 196–200.

38. Hehrlein FW, Gottwik M, Fraedrich G, et al. First clinical experience with a new all pyrolytic carbon bileaflet heart valve prosthesis. J Thorac Cardiovasc Surg. 1980; 79:632–636.

39. Holen J, Nitter-Hauge S. Evaluation of obstructive characteristics of mitral disc valve implants with ultrasound Doppler techniques. Acta Med Scand. 1977; 201:429–433.

40. Holen J, Hoie J, Semb B. Obstructive characteristics of Bjork-Shiley, Hancock, and Lillehei-Kaster prosthetic mitral valves in the immediate post-operative period. Acta Med Scand. 1978; 204:5–10.

41. Holen J, Simonsen S, Froysaker T. An ultrasound Doppler technique for the non-invasive determination of the pressure gradient in the Bjork-Shiley mitral valve. Circulation. 1979; 59:436–442.

42. Holen J, Simonsen S, Froysaker T. Determination of pressure gradient in the Hancock mitral valve from non-invasive ultrasound Doppler data. Scand J Clin Lab Invest. 1983; 41:177–183.

43. Horowitz MS, Goodman DJ, Popp RL. Echocardiographic diagnosis of calcific stenosis of a stented aortic homograft in the mitral position. J Clin Ultrasound. 1974; 2:179–185.

44. Horowitz MS, Tecklenberg PL, Goodman DJ, et al. Echocardiographic evaluation of the stent mounted aortic bioprosthetic valve in the mitral position in

vitro and in vivo studies. Circulation. 1976; 54: 91–96.

45. Ionescu MI, Tandon AP, Mary DAS, et al. Heart valve replacement with Ionescu-Shiley pericardial xenograft. Cardiol Digest. 1977; 73:31.

46. Johnson ML, Holmes JH, Paton BC. Echocardiographic determination of mitral disc valve excursion. Circulation. 1973; 47:1274–1280.

47. Johnson ML, Paton BC, Holmes JH. Ultrasonic evaluation of prosthetic valve motion. Circulation. 1970; 41:3.

48. Kawai N, Segal BL, Linhart JW. Delayed opening of Beall mitral prosthetic valve detected by echocardiography. Chest. 1975; 67:239–241.

49. Kisanuki A, Tei C, Arikawa K, et al. Continuous-wave Doppler assessment of prosthetic valves in the mitral position: Comparison of the St. Jude Medical mechanical valve and the porcine xenograft valve. J Cardiogr. 1985; 15:1119–1127.

50. Kisanuki A, Tei C, Arikawa K, et al. Continuous-wave Doppler echocardiographic assessment of prosthetic aortic valves. J Cardiogr. 1986; 16:121–132.

51. Lamberti JL, Wainer BH, Fisher KA, et al. Calcific stenosis of the porcine heterograft. Ann Thorac Surg. 1979; 28:28–32.

52. Lefrak E, Starr A. Cardiac Valve Prostheses. New York: Appleton-Century-Crofts; 1979; 167–179; 181–204; 215–244; 246–268; 330–339.

53. Lesbre JP, Chasset C, Lesperance J, et al. Evaluation des nouvelles bioprostheses pericardiques par Doppler pulsé et continu. Arch Mal Coeur. 1986; 79:1439–1448.

54. Levang OW, Nitter-Hauge S, Levorstad K, et al. Aortic valve replacement. A randomized study comparing the Bjork-Shiley and Lillehei-Kaster disc valves: Late hemodynamics related to clinical results. Scand J Thorac Cardiovasc Surg. 1979; 13:199–213.

55. Libanoff AJ, Rodbard S. Evaluation of the severity of mitral stenosis and regurgitation. Circulation. 1966; 33:218–226.

56. Libanoff AJ, Rodbard S. Atrioventricular pressure half-time: Measure of mitral valve orifice area. Circulation. 1968; 38:144–150.

57. Magilligan DJ, Fisher E, Alam M. Hemolytic anemia with porcine xenograft aortic and mitral valves. J Thorac Cardiovasc Surg. 1980; 79:628–631.

58. Martin RP, French JW, Popp RL. Clinical utility of two-dimensional echocardiography in patients with bioprosthetic valves. Adv Cardiol. 1980; 27:294–304.

59. Mary DAS, Pakrashi BC, Catchpole RW, et al. Echocardiographic studies of stented fascia lata grafts in the mitral position. Circulation. 1974; 49:237–245.

60. Nanda NC, Thomson K, Gramiak R. Late diastolic motion of the mitral prosthesis: Echocardiographic

studies. In: White DN, Ross AE, eds. Ultrasound in Medicine. New York: Plenum; 1977; 3:10.

61. Nanda NC, Gramiak R, Shah PM, et al. Echocardiographic assessment of left ventricular outflow width in the selection of mitral valve prosthesis. Circulation. 1973; 48:1208–1214.

62. Nevaril CG, Lynch EC, Alfred CP Jr, et al. Erythrocyte damage and destruction induced by shearing stress. J Lab Clin Med. 1968; 71:784–790.

63. Numura Y, Miyatake K, Okamoto M, et al. Assessment of tricuspid regurgitation by two-dimensional Doppler echocardiography. In: Spencer MP, ed. Cardiac Doppler Diagnosis. Boston: Nijhoff; 1983; 263–269.

64. Pandis IP, Ross J, Mintz GS. Normal and abnormal prosthetic valve function as assessed by Doppler echocardiography. J Am Coll Cardiol. 1986; 8:317–326.

65. Raizada W, Benchomol A, Desser KB, et al. Echocardiographic features of normal functioning Hancock porcine heterograft valve in the aortic position. Clin Res. 1977; 25:246 (abstr).

66. Ramirez ML, Wong M. Reproducibility of stand-alone CW Doppler recordings of aortic flow velocity across bioprosthetic valves. Am J Cardiol. 1986; 55:1197–1199.

67. Ramirez ML, Wong M, Sadler N, et al. Doppler evaluation of 106 bioprosthetic and mechanical aortic valves. J Am Coll Cardiol. 1985; 5:527 (abstr).

68. Reis RL, Glancy DL, O'Brien K, et al. Clinical and hemodynamic assessments of fabric-covered Starr-Edwards prosthetic valves. J Thorac Cardiovasc Surg. 1970; 59:84–91.

69. Reisner SA, Meltzer RS. Normal values of prosthetic valve Doppler echocardiographic parameters: A review. J Am Soc Echocardiogr. 1988; 1:201–225.

70. Roeser WH, Powell LW, O'Brien MF. Hemolysis after heterograft and prosthetic valve replacement. Am Heart J. 1970; 79:281–283.

71. Rogers BM, Sabiston DC Jr. Hemolytic anemia following prosthetic valve replacement. Circulation. 1969; 39(suppl I):155–161.

72. Rothbart RM, Smucker ML, Gibson RS. Pulsed and continuous Doppler examination of prosthetic valves: Correlation with clinical and cardiac catheterization data (abstr). Circulation. 1985; 72(suppl III):373.

73. Ryan T, Armstrong WF, Dillon JC, et al. Doppler echocardiographic evaluation of patients with porcine mitral valves. Am Heart J. 1986; 111:237–244.

74. Sagar KB, Wann LS, Paulsen WHJ, et al. Doppler echocardiographic evaluation of Hancock and Bjork-Shiley prosthetic valves. J Am Coll Cardiol. 1986; 7:681–687.

75. Schuchman H, Feigenbaum H, Dillon JC, et al. Intracavitary echoes in patients with mitral prosthetic valves. J Clin Ultrasound. 1975; 3:111–119.

76. Shapira JN, Martin RP, Fowles RE, et al. Two-dimensional echocardiographic assessment of patients with bioprosthetic valves. Am J Cardiol. 1979; 43:510–519.

77. Siggers DC, Srivongse SA, Deuchar D. Analysis of dynamics of mitral Starr-Edwards valve prosthesis using reflected ultrasound. Br Heart J. 1971; 33:401–408.

78. Strasberg B, Kanakis C, Echner F, et al. Echocardiographic demonstration of porcine mitral valve vegetation and dehiscence. Eur J Cardiol. 1980; 12:41–45.

79. Tandon AP, Smith DR, Ionescu MI. Hemodynamic evaluation of the Ionescu-Shiley xenograft in the mitral position. Am Heart J. 1978; 95:595–601.

80. Ubsgo JL, Figueroa A, Colman T, et al. Hemodynamic factors that affect calculated orifice areas in the mitral Hancock xenograft valve. Circulation. 1980; 61:388–394.

81. Vardan S, Warner R, Mookherjee S, et al. Echocardiographic and phonocardiographic studies in patients with Lillehei-Kaster aortic valve prosthesis. Jpn Heart J. 1979; 3:277–288.

82. Waggoner AD, Quinones MA, Young JB, et al. Echophonocardiographic evaluation of obstruction of prosthetic mitral valve. Chest. 1980; 78:60–68.

83. Weinstein IR, Marbarger JP, Perez JE. Ultrasonic assessment of the St. Jude prosthetic valve: M-mode, two-dimensional and Doppler echocardiography. Circulation. 1983; 68:897–905.

84. Wilkes HS, Berger M, Gallerstein PE, et al. Left ventricular outflow obstruction after aortic valve replacement: Detection with continuous wave Doppler ultrasound recording. J Am Coll Cardiol. 1983; 1:550–553.

85. Wilkins GT, Gillan LD, et al. Validation of continuous wave Doppler echocardiography measurements of mitral and tricuspid prosthetic valve gradients: A simultaneous Doppler-catheter study. Circulation. 1986;74:786–795.

86. Williams GA, Labovitz AJ. Doppler hemodynamic evaluation of prosthetic (Starr-Edwards and Bjork-Shiley) and bioprosthetic (Hancock and Carpentier-Edwards) cardiac valves. Am J Cardiol. 1985; 56:325–332.

87. Yacoub MH, Kothari M, Keeling D, et al. Red-cell survival after homograft replacement of the aortic valve. Thorax. 1969; 24:283–286.

88. Yuste P, Minguez I, Aza V, et al. Mitral valve prostheses and left ventricular function: An echocardiographic study. J Cardiovasc Surg. 1973; 421–424.

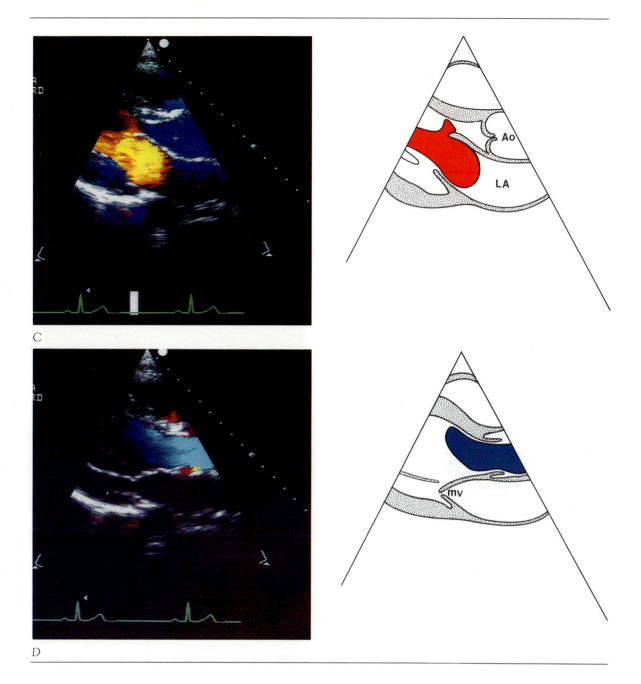

C

D

FIGURE 6-5. Color-flow map in diastole (C) and systole (D) from the parasternal long-axis perspective. Although the direction of flow relative to the acoustic beam is not optimal for qualitative assessments, qualitative judgments regarding the characteristics of flow can be made. Note the absence of turbulent flow behind the mitral valve in systole in this normal patient (Ao, aorta; LA, left atrium; MV, mitral valve).

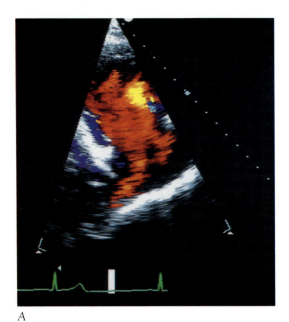

A

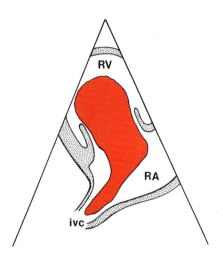

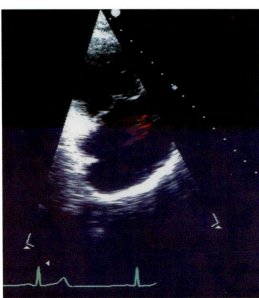

B

FIGURE 6-7. (A) Color-flow map applied to the right ventricular inflow tract view. In this diastolic frame, the flow across the tricuspid valve is encoded in red because its direction is toward the transducer. Also seen in this frame is flow entering the right atrium (RA) from the inferior vena cava (ivc). (B) Systole. In the absence of tricuspid regurgitation, no flow will be seen behind the coaptation point of the leaflets (RV, right ventricle).

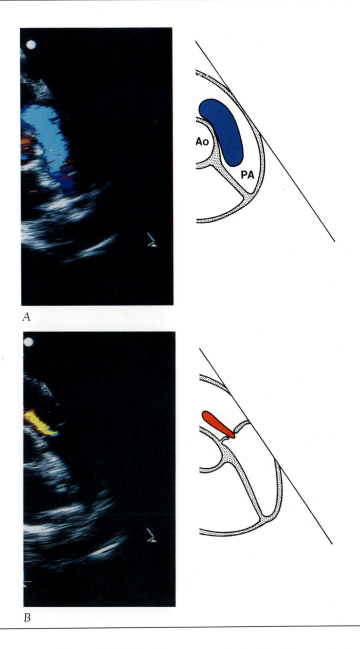

FIGURE 6-10. Color-flow map applied to the right ventricular outflow tract view. (A) Systolic view reveals flow across the pulmonary valve into the pulmonary artery (PA), which is encoded in shades of blue, because of its direction away from the transducer. (B) Diastolic frame demonstrates pulmonary regurgitation that is commonly seen in normal patients (Ao, aorta).

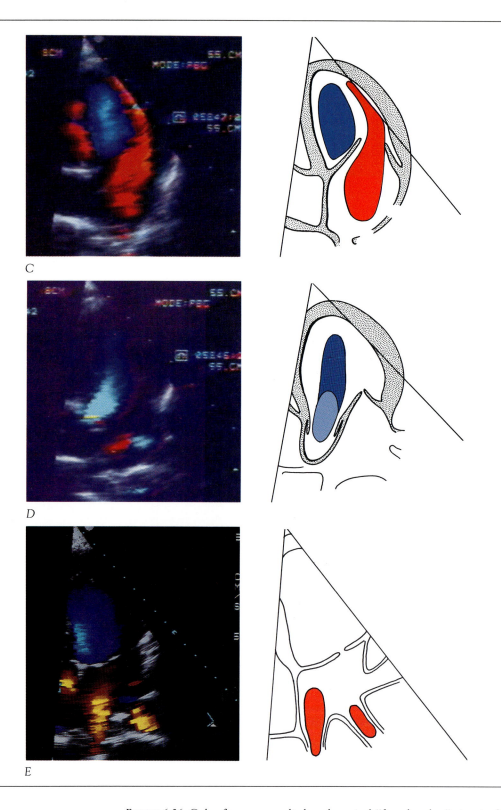

C

D

E

FIGURE 6-26. Color-flow map applied to the apical "five-chamber" view in diastole (C) and systole (D). Flow across the mitral valve into the left ventricle is toward the transducer in this orientation and, therefore, is encoded in red. Flow across the left ventricular outflow tract into the aorta (Ao) is moving away from the transducer and is encoded in blue. (E) Pulmonary venous inflow, encoded in red, is seen entering the left atrium (LA).

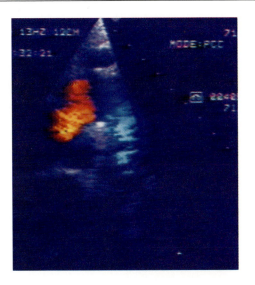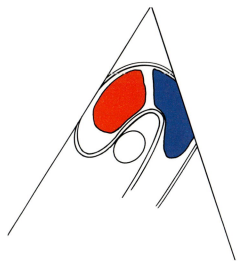

FIGURE 6-40. Color-flow map applied to image of the transverse arch. The ascending aortic flow is encoded in red as it flows toward the transducer and descending aortic flow is encoded in blue as it flows away from the transducer.

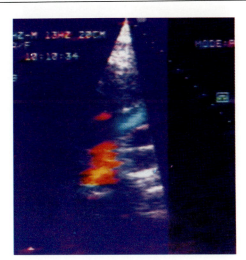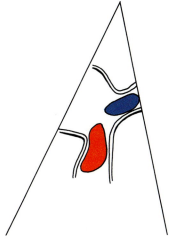

FIGURE 6-46. Color-flow map applied to the image of the venae cavae illustrated in Figure 6-45. The superior vena caval flow, moving away from the transducer, is encoded in blue. The inferior vena caval flow, moving toward the transducer, is encoded in red.

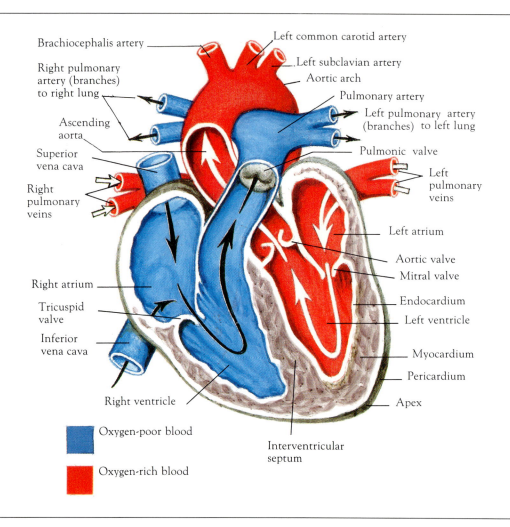

Brachiocephalis artery

Left common carotid artery

Left subclavian artery

Right pulmonary artery (branches) to right lung

Aortic arch

Pulmonary artery

Left pulmonary artery (branches) to left lung

Ascending aorta

Superior vena cava

Pulmonic valve

Left pulmonary veins

Right pulmonary veins

Left atrium

Aortic valve

Right atrium

Mitral valve

Tricuspid valve

Endocardium

Left ventricle

Inferior vena cava

Myocardium

Pericardium

Right ventricle

Apex

Oxygen-poor blood

Oxygen-rich blood

Interventricular septum

FIGURE 9-2. (A) Anatomy of the heart.

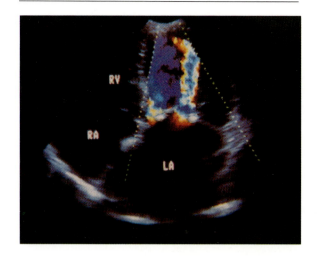

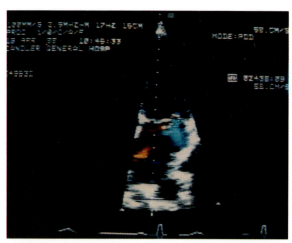

FIGURE 9-8. Doppler color-flow map demonstrates mitral stenosis. Note the flow jet showing increased velocity and turbulence.

FIGURE 9-9. Doppler color-flow map demonstrates mitral regurgitation.

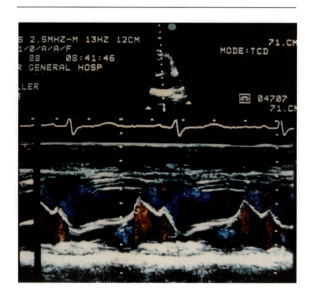

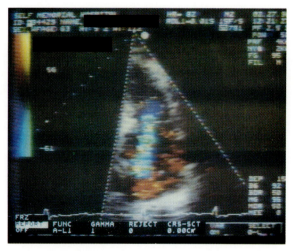

FIGURE 9-32. Color-flow scan of tricuspid insufficiency.

FIGURE 9-10. Color M-mode image demonstrates mitral regurgitation.

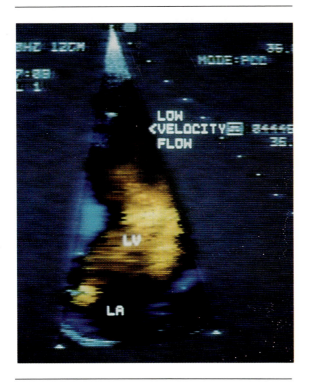

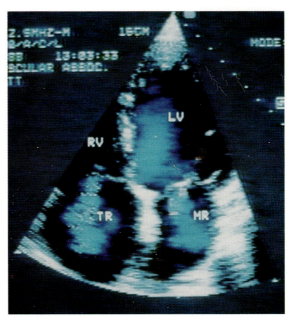

FIGURE 11-14. Apical four-chamber 2-D echocardiogram with color-flow Doppler mapping. The patient has mitral (MR) and tricuspid (TR) valve regurgitation. (RV, right ventricle; LV, left ventricle.)

FIGURE 11-13. Color-flow Doppler tracing of a patient with congestive cardiomyopathy. Note the low-velocity flow in the middle to distal left ventricle (LV). See arrow. (LA, left atrium.)

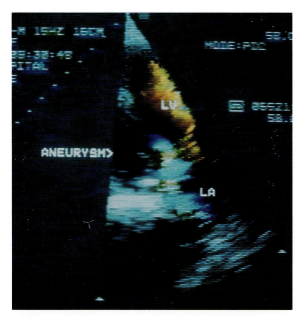

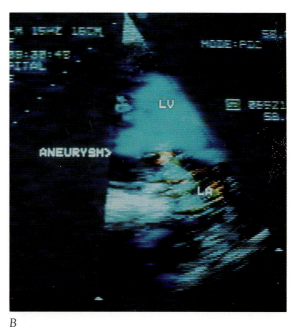

*A*                                    *B*

FIGURE 12-11. (*A*) Parasternal long-axis view and (*B*) color-flow Doppler shows posteroinferior wall aneurysm. The abnormal flow into the aneurysm is displayed in blue. (LV, left ventricle; MV, mitral valve; LA, left atrium.)

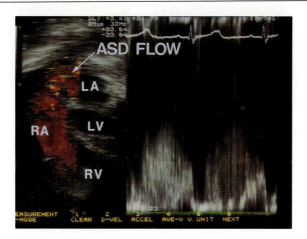

FIGURE 19-3. Echocardiographic findings of atrial septal defect (ASD). (*B*) Split-screen frozen frame showing flow through a secundum ASD by color-flow Doppler (apical four-chamber view), with the PW Doppler spectral tracing of the shunt flow shown to the right. (LA, RA, left and right atria; LV, RV, left and right ventricles; SVC, superior vena cava.)

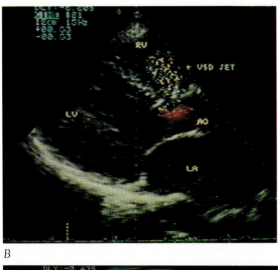

B

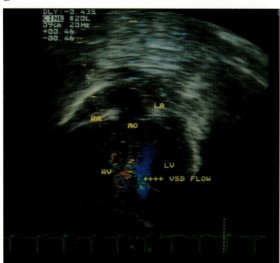

C

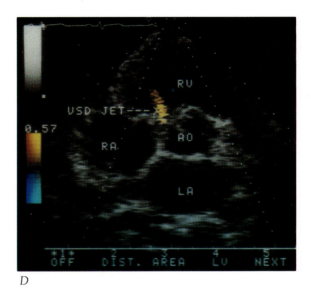

D

FIGURE 19-4. Echocardiographic findings of ventricular septal defect (VSD).
(B) Color-flow Doppler image illustrates the turbulent, high-velocity left-to-right
shunt through the perimembranous VSD as a speckled, mosaic pattern of flow
within the VSD and coursing into the right ventricle (parasternal long-axis view).
(C) Color-flow Doppler image illustrates a left-to-right shunt through a muscular
VSD (apical four-chamber view). (D) Color-flow Doppler image illustrating a left-
to-right shunt through a perimembranous VSD (parasternal short-axis view). (LV,
RV, left and right ventricles; LA, RA, left and right atria; AO, aorta.)

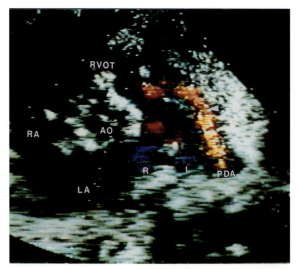

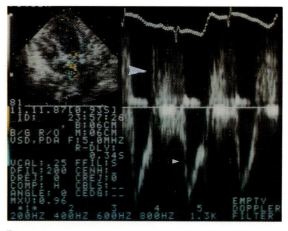

*C*

*D*

FIGURE 19-6. Echocardiographic findings of patent ductus arteriosus (PDA). (C) Color-flow Doppler was added to *B* to visualize lateral jet of flow from the PDA into the main pulmonary artery (MPA). (D) PW Doppler spectral tracing obtained from the MPA shows normal, laminar pulmonic flow away from the transducer in systole (small arrow), and harsh, turbulent flow toward the transducer in diastole. The diastolic flow (large arrow) represents the PDA shunt into the MPA. (RVOT, right ventricular outflow tract; AO, aorta; PA, pulmonary artery; RA, LA, right and left atria.)

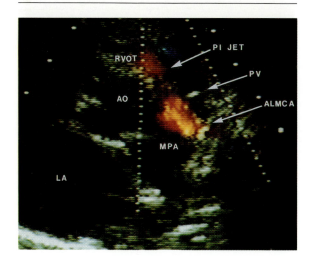

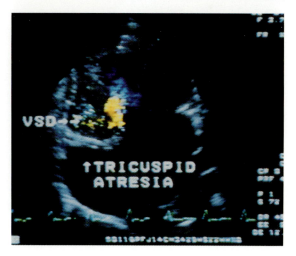

FIGURE 20-6. Anomalous origin of the left main coronary artery from the MPA. A cross-sectional color flow image of the great vessels reveals a flow jet from the left lateral wall of the MPA less than 1 cm from the pulmonary valve (PV). This diastolic jet emanates from the origin of the ALMCA. A small plume of pulmonary insufficiency (PI) is seen in the RVOT.

FIGURE 21-6. Two-dimensional echocardiogram, apical four-chamber view illustrates color flow through shunt. VSD, ventricular septal defect.

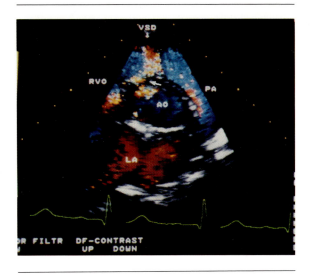

FIGURE 21-7. Two-dimensional echocardiogram, parasternal short-axis view. Note color through ventricular septal defect (VSD). LA, Left atrium; AO, aorta; RVO, right ventricular outflow; PA, pulmonary artery.

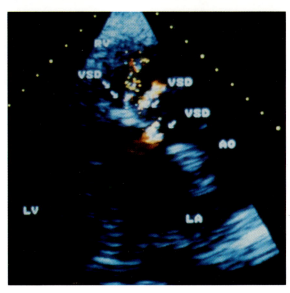

FIGURE 21-8. Two-dimensional echocardiogram, parasternal long-axis view (note color). VSD, ventricular septal defects; RV, right ventricle; LV, left ventricle; LA, left atrium; AO, aorta.

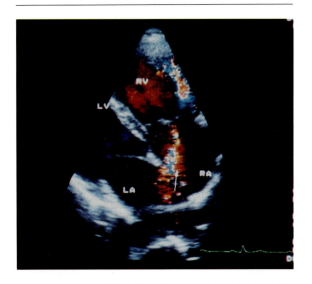

FIGURE 21-9. Two-dimensional echocardiogram, modified apical four-chamber view. Note color through left-to-right (L, R) shunt. RV, Right ventricle; RA, right atrium; LV, left ventricle; LA, left atrium.

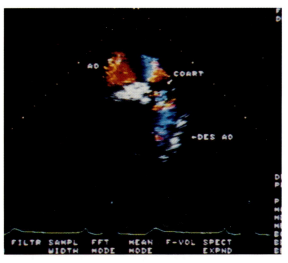

FIGURE 21-10. Two-dimensional subtraction 2-D echocardiogram, suprasternal notch view of ascending aorta, demonstrates coarctation of the aorta (COART).

# Special Echocardiographic Techniques

# CHAPTER 17

# Transesophageal and Intraoperative Echocardiography

## DAVID ADAMS

In this chapter I will describe the history, basic procedures, and clinical utility of transesophageal and intraoperative echocardiography. In many cases the two techniques complement each other, and both may be used to collect different diagnostic information about one patient. A transesophageal echocardiogram provides high-quality images, because interference from air in the lungs is minimal when a transducer is positioned in the esophagus. The study may be performed with the patient awake or anesthetized. Intraoperative echocardiography uses high-frequency transducers placed directly on the epicardial surface of the heart and also provides images of excellent quality compared to those produced with standard transthoracic approaches. I will discuss these techniques in terms of their role in defining anatomy, diagnosing cardiac pathology, assisting the planning of operative procedures, and evaluating surgical repair.

Transesophageal imaging allows direct observation of the movement of heart walls, valves, and great vessels before, during, and just after surgery. Transesophageal echocardiograms typically are performed for the following reasons: (1) to procure images that are better than transthoracic ones; (2) to evaluate aortic dissection or aneurysm; (3) to evaluate mitral, tricuspid, or aortic valve prostheses; (4) to identify tumors or other masses, particularly in the atria and atrial appendages; (5) to evaluate mitral, tricuspid, or aortic valve repair in-

traoperatively; and (6) to monitor left ventricular function or the presence of air during operative procedures. Positioning the transducer in the esophagus obviates the image-degrading effects of structures that are interposed when imaging from the chest wall—ribs, air in the lungs, and subcutaneous tissue.

Over the past few years there has been tremendous growth in the utilization of echocardiography in the operating room. Much of this interest is due to the diagnostic information now available through transesophageal echocardiography and by placing transducers directly on the epicardial surface during operative procedures. Intraoperative echocardiographic techniques, particularly Doppler color-flow imaging, have many applications. Preoperative diagnosis assists in planning the operative repair. Intraoperative evaluation demonstrates the results of repair. Ventricular function can be evaluated, which is especially important after cardiopulmonary bypass procedures. In some studies, echocardiography during surgical repair of congenital heart defects has revealed unsuspected anomalies that were not revealed by the preoperative echocardiogram or angiogram in up to 20% of patients.[10] An intraoperative scan immediately after repair may also help the patient's prognosis, and it provides a baseline measurement against which to judge future transthoracic echocardiographic findings.

## Transesophageal Echocardiography

### History

Although ultrasound has been used to evaluate cardiac structures since 1954, transesophageal echocardiography was not performed until 1976. Frazin and coworkers[4] placed an M-mode transducer on the end of a coaxial cable in order to obtain images from the esophagus. Because the transducer could not be controlled, the quality of images varied and structures of interest were not always visualized. The transducer became more manageable when an available gastroscope was rewired with an M-mode transducer at the tip.[7] Adaptation of a two-dimensional (2-D) mechanical transducer to a gastroscope was the next step. A high-speed, rotating, 2-D transducer was placed at the tip of the gastroscope in an oil-filled bag in order to reduce friction in the esophagus.[6] Some patients complained of an unusual sensation in the chest when these mechanical transducers were used. Since 1982, when Schulter and coworkers first reported 2-D imaging in 26 conscious patients, small phased-array transducers have been preferred over mechanical ones for transesophageal echocardiography.[9] Phased-array transducers afford utilization of M-mode, 2-D, pulsed-wave, and color-flow Doppler techniques for transesophageal examinations. In the future, smaller transesophageal transducers will be built and the techniques will be applicable to small children.

### The Transesophageal Transducer

At first it might seem that transesophageal echocardiography must be rather traumatic for the patient, but the techniques of inserting and manipulating the transducer are very similar to those of standard endoscopy employed by gastroenterologists many times each day to examine ambulatory patients. Extensive experience—in both conscious and anesthetized patients—has confirmed the safety of the technique. To date the only complications reported have been two cases of transient vocal cord paralysis in patients undergoing neurosurgical procedures that required extremé neck flexion.[2] Other potential complications of this approach are aspiration of gastric contents and esophageal perforation.

The transesophageal probe is typically a 5-MHz, short-focused, phased-array transducer mounted

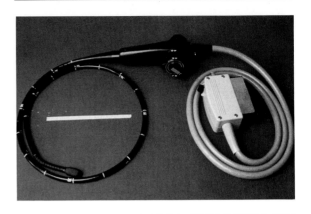

Figure 17-1. A Hewlett-Packard 64-element, 5-MHz transesophageal probe. The external diameter of the shaft is 9 mm. The external controls for flexion, extension, and lateral movement can be seen. (By permission from Kisslo JA, Adams DB, Belkin RN (eds.). Doppler Color-Flow Imaging. New York: Churchill Livingstone; 1988; 167–176.)

on the distal tip of a 100-cm gastroscope. A commercially available gastroscope from which the fiberoptics component has been removed and replaced with an ultrasound transducer is shown in Figure 17-1. This gastroscope has been rewired with a 64-element, 5-MHz transducer that measures 9 × 12 mm. External controls allow manipulation of the tip of the gastroscope: one controls lateral movement and the other antero-posterior movement, or flexion and extension. Once the transducer is in the desired position, the controls can be locked. Rotating the transducer is accomplished by simply twisting the cable. The manuevers possible with the transesophageal probe are shown in Figure 17-2. During the transesophageal examination lateral angulation is seldom used; most of the manipulation is rotation, flexion, and extension.

### Insertion of the Transducer

When transesophageal echocardiography is performed on a conscious patient the physician or cardiac sonographer must take the time to fully explain the reason for the study and the various steps, in order to obtain the patient's full cooperation. The coach, who stands opposite the physician

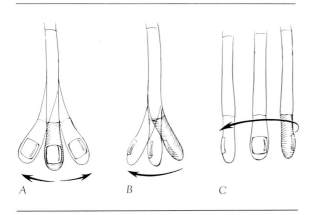

FIGURE 17-2. Range of transducer angulation under operator control: (A) lateral; (B) anteroposterior flexion and extension; and (C) rotation. (From deBriujn NP, Clements FM. Transesophageal Echocardiography. Boston: Martinus Nijhoff; 1987.)

during the insertion to encourage and "talk the patient through" the procedure, plays a vital role in the critical stages of the examination. Because introduction of the transducer may produce significant gagging in a conscious patient, a topical anesthetic is sprayed in the throat to facilitate passage of the probe. The anesthetic effect persists for 30 or 40 minutes. (It is important that the patient be given nothing by mouth until the anesthesia has worn off.) It is recommended that all patients fast for approximately 6 hours before undergoing transesophageal imaging, to minimize the risk of aspiration of vomitus. A mild sedative may be given prior to the examination, although many patients tolerate the procedure quite well without premedication. An agent that reduces the amount of saliva may also be given, but usually it is not necessary. Cardiologists learning this procedure will need to spend a number of hours with a gastroenterologist to master the technique of inserting and manipulating the endoscope.

Prior to the examination, all patients receive an intravenous line as a precaution against the event of a vagal reaction or in case venous access is required for another reason. In addition to the topical anesthetic, an emesis basin, towels, tongue depressors, and oxygen should be at the bedside. It is of utmost importance to have a suction machine readily available in case the patient aspirates vom-

itus. If the patient's history suggests esophageal pathology, a barium swallow study may be necessary to define anatomy. Possible contraindications to transesophageal echocardiography include a history of esophageal varices, upper gastrointestinal bleeding, dysphagia, and chest trauma of unknown extent.

Before it is inserted, the transesophageal transducer should be inspected for cracks and tested to ensure that the controls are working properly. In order for the transducer to pass easily through the pharynx into the esophagus the probe tip should be in the unlocked position.

After sufficient topical anesthetic is applied to deaden the gag reflex, a bite block is placed between the patient's teeth to prevent damage to the transesophageal probe. A light coating of lubricating gel is applied to the transesophageal transducer to facilitate its passage. With the patient in the right lateral decubitus position the transducer is inserted through the bite block to the back of the patient's throat. It is important for the patient to cooperate by swallowing repeatedly until the transducer passes into the esophagus. Once it has passed the glottis and is advanced approximately 30 to 40 cm, the worst part is over and the patient can usually relax. Transesophageal examination with the patient awake is performed to detect problems such as presence of thrombus, valve dysfunction, and interatrial septum anomalies; the examination usually lasts 5 to 10 minutes. Once the examination is completed extracting the transducer may cause transient discomfort.

Introducing a transesophageal transducer into an anesthetized patient is usually much easier. Their trachea is already intubated and the gag reflex is absent. As there is no danger of aspiration the patient is usually in a recumbent position; the neck should be slightly flexed. Other catheters in the esophagus (such as a temperature probe or nasogastric tube) should be removed so they do not interfere with the sonographic images. Insertion is accomplished simply by directing the tip into the posterior part of the pharynx and with gentle pressure directing the transducer to the opening of the esophagus.

Whether the patient is awake or asleep, the transducer should always slide easily. Any resistance indicates an obstruction, and in this case further manipulation should be avoided and the transducer removed.

## VIEWS

In the transesophageal examination, the heart is imaged from a posterior approach (Fig. 17-3). Different cross-sectional orientations of the heart can be obtained by advancing, rotating, and angulating the transducer.

In most cases the first cardiac chamber visualized is the left atrium, then the mitral and aortic valves are examined, and finally the left ventricle. It has been recommended that a standardized image orientation be used for the transesophageal approach. The four-chamber view should appear with the apex of the heart at the bottom and the left ventricle to the viewer's right (Fig. 17-4). All other views are to be displayed as they appear from the transducer orientation required to generate this four-chamber view. When the esophageal transducer is positioned behind the left atrium and directed toward the cardiac apex, the ultrasound beam is aligned in a plane parallel to blood flow through the mitral valve. This provides an excellent means for detecting mitral regurgitation and high-velocity flow through a stenotic mitral valve. It is important to realize that this view is usually not a true long-axis view of the left ventricle but a tangential one. So with this technique measurements such as ejection fraction, which require exact long-axis dimensions, are difficult to make with accuracy.

When the imaging plane is directed more anteriorly from the original position behind the left atrium, the great vessels and atria appear. The interatrial septum can also be well-defined, as it now lies at a right angle to the ultrasound beam. Likewise, the aortic valve is imaged in cross section, and the aortic root can be imaged. Coronary arteries frequently are seen by this transesophageal approach and with color-flow Doppler technique coronary arterial flow can be visualized.

Advancing the transducer farther down the esophagus usually affords a view of the heart in the short-axis view. By moving the transducer up and down the esophagus, short-axis images can be seen from the apex all the way up to the mitral valve leaflets. Figure 17-5 shows a transesophageal short-axis view at the level of the papillary muscles. The

posterior left ventricular wall is interrogated first; the anterior wall is farthest from the transducer. In this short-axis view, the midpapillary level usually affords the best image for intraoperative monitoring of left ventricular function.

Rotating the transducer 180 degrees after obtaining a four-chamber view provides images of the descending thoracic aorta. Slowly withdrawing the probe produces scans of the aorta from the level of the diaphragm up to the descending aorta.

## CLINICAL APPLICATIONS

Transesophageal echocardiography is a useful technique for cardiologists, anesthesiologists, and surgeons. A major benefit is the high resolution of the images. Even in obese, barrel-chested patients with chronic respiratory problems such as emphysema and asthma high-quality images can be obtained via the transesophageal approach.

For cardiologists, transesophageal echocardiography provides a clear, unobstructed view of the heart when results of precordial examination are inadequate. A principal application of the transesophageal technique is to image prosthetic valves,

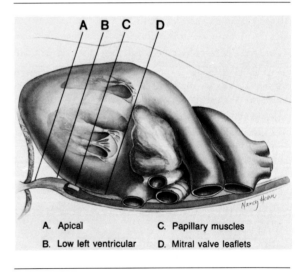

| A. | Apical | C. | Papillary muscles |
| B. | Low left ventricular | D. | Mitral valve leaflets |

FIGURE 17-3. Schematic diagram of the transesophageal ultrasound transducer in the esophagus. The transducer is positioned behind the left ventricle or left atrium. (From deBruijn NP, Clements FM. Transesophageal Echocardiography. Boston: Martinus Nijhoff; 1987.)

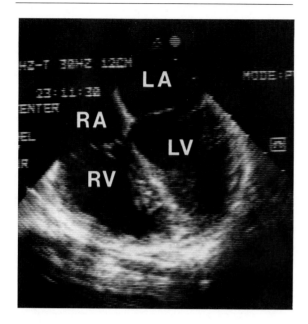

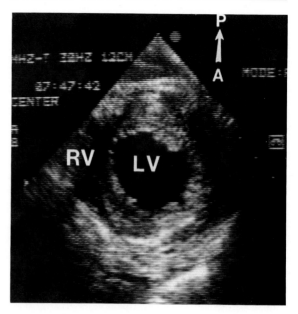

FIGURE 17-4. Transesophageal four-chamber view with the ultrasound transducer positioned behind the left atrium. The tip is "overextended," so that the beam is directed anteroinferiorly, producing a four-chamber view. (RA, right atrium; RV, right ventricle; LA, left atrium; LV, left ventricle.)

FIGURE 17-5. Two-dimensional view of the left ventricular (LV) short axis at the papillary muscle level. Anterior (A) and posterior (P) walls are well visualized. This view is useful for monitoring left ventricular function and the detection of regional wall motion abnormalities. (RV, right ventricle.)

particularly in the mitral position. From standard transthoracic approaches, the prosthesis may mask regurgitant flow in the left atrium by producing reverberation and attenuation. This makes detection and estimation of the severity of mitral regurgitation difficult, if not impossible. Viewed from the transesophageal approach the mitral valve prosthesis does not mask the left atrium, and the extent of mitral regurgitation can be assessed. On color-flow Doppler examination clinically significant mitral regurgitation appears as a wide, mosaic jet of blood flow extending far back into the left atrium. This is in sharp contrast to the small perivalvular leaks that are sometimes seen following mitral valve replacement, which are not clinically significant.

The proximity of the probe to the heart allows high-frequency transducers to be used. This is particularly useful for ruling out an embolic source within the left atrium or detecting valvular endocarditis or a vegetative mass lesion on the left atrial

wall. This technique is also useful for assessing the extent or point of attachment of intracardiac mass lesions. Because the interatrial septum lies perpendicular to the ultrasound beam, the transesophageal probe is excellent for detecting an atrial septal defect or an aneurysm of the interatrial septum.

Dissecting aortic aneurysms frequently are difficult to image with ultrasound from outside the chest wall. Except for a small area in the upper portion of the ascending aorta where the air-filled trachea is between the esophagus and the ascending aorta, the rest of the aorta is easily imaged with this technique, making aortic dissection easily detectable.[7] An intimal flap can usually be seen and the true lumen separated from the false lumen at the site of the intimal tear.

For the anesthesiologist, transesophageal echocardiography is an excellent monitoring device that provides instantaneous information about overall cardiac contractility. By using this technique to monitor global left ventricular function and any changes in regional wall motion due to ischemia, the anesthesiologist cannot only respond with proper drug interventions but can also monitor the effectiveness of the treatment on myocardial function. Direct visualization of left ventricular filling and performance can provide rapid, accurate assessment of critically ill patients, in the operating room or during the perioperative period. This technique may be particularly useful in cardiac patients at high risk who must undergo major abdominal, peripheral, or carotid vascular reconstructive procedures. Certainly the transesophageal echocardiogram is more sensitive than the electrocardiogram for detecting ischemia and may be the most sensitive technique for monitoring the contractility of the left ventricle.[1]

For cardiac surgeons, the transesophageal approach provides a monitoring and diagnostic tool for the assessment of valvuloplasty, interatrial septal repairs, aneurysmal repairs, and prosthetic valves, particularly mitral valve replacement. During open heart surgery this technique allows direct observation of the cardiac walls and valves, which is useful to the cardiac surgeon for assessing regional wall motion before and after cardiopulmonary bypass surgery. The high sensitivity of transesophageal Doppler color-flow imaging has led to its use in the operating room for making on-the-spot decisions about the necessity to repair or replace a mitral valve, primarily in patients with ischemic mitral regurgitation. Many of these patients with coronary artery disease had mitral regurgitation at the time of angiography. Often it is deemed to be catheter induced and not clinically significant.

Many patients show small perivalvular leaks immediately following mitral valve replacement. Small jets usually appear intermittently from the mitral valve annulus, adjacent to the prosthetic valve. Omoto has found that such leaks, apparent immediately after surgery, have disappeared 2 weeks later.[8] This suggests that small suture line leaks are obliterated during the healing process and are not an indication for revision of the new mitral valve prosthesis. Intracardiac air is always a concern during open heart surgery, and the transesophageal technique provides an excellent means of detecting microbubbles within the cardiac chambers. Of even greater importance may be the detection of intracavitary air emboli in patients undergoing neurologic surgery, which frequently is performed with the patient in an upright position.[2]

## Intraoperative Echocardiography

### HISTORY

The advantage of intraoperative echocardiography is the high-quality images that can be obtained by positioning a transducer directly on the heart. Intraoperative echocardiography has been a useful tool for assessing cardiac anatomy and function for many years. Since 1979, high-frequency ultrasound probes have been used to guide the extraction of intramyocardial foreign bodies.[5] With the recent advances in Doppler color-flow imaging, the use of echocardiography in the operating room has risen sharply.

### PROCEDURE

Because the transducer is applied directly on the epicardial surface of the heart, a high-frequency transducer can be used. A 5-MHz, short-focused, phased-array transducer is used for the majority of intraoperative examinations. When pulsed-wave Doppler examinations must be performed a 3.5-MHz transducer is easily brought into the operative field. Because the sample volume is usually positioned in the near field, the 3.5-MHz transducer is usually adequate for evaluating gradients across the pulmonic and aortic valve.

The results of intraoperative continuous-wave Doppler examination with a stand-alone transducer have been unsatisfactory. The movement of the heart against the transducer introduces an enormous amount of artifact in the spectral trace, making interpretation of the Doppler information impossible.

In order to maintain the sterility of the operative field the transducers are wiped down with a 2% glutaraldehyde solution (Cidex) and wrapped in a sterile towel for approximately 15 minutes before they are inserted into a sterile sheath. To sterilize the probe itself requires soaking it in the solution for at least 10 hours. Because of the protective coating on the transducer face, most probes cannot be steam- or gas autoclaved. Sterile gel is first placed in the plastic sheath to create an airtight seal within the transducer and the sterile bag. The transducer can then be passed over the ether screen into the plastic sheath held by the surgeon. Direct epicardial scanning requires that the heart be covered by blood or saline solution, in order to maintain a good, airtight interface. The echocardiography machine itself is positioned close to the ether screen in such a way that the surgeon or cardiologist performing the study has a clear view of the display. Since time is a critical factor, intraoperative echocardiography requires the participation of additional personnel who are skilled in adjusting the controls of the machine.

### Clinical Applications

In many instances, particularly with congenital heart disease, the preoperative diagnosis may be incomplete even though the patient may have undergone cardiac catheterization and had multiple transthoracic echocardiograms. Intraoperative echocardiography can confirm the preoperative diagnosis and may reveal new abnormalities, which is of great value to the cardiovascular surgeon.

While direct surgical inspection would have identified many unsuspected findings, the advantage of intraoperative echocardiography is that the cardiac surgeon may plan the operative approach better. Often this appreciably reduces the time the patient is supported by the cardiopulmonary bypass machine.

The number of operations for the repair of valves is increasing, and intraoperative echocardiography may enhance postoperative assessment of the valves, specifically in patients who undergo mitral valve repairs. In these patients postoperative mitral stenosis or significant mitral regurgitation is a potential complication and such findings may be corrected more easily when the patient is still on the operating table and a second thoracotomy is obviated.

## Summary

The clinical application of transesophageal and intraoperative echocardiography is still evolving. The field of cardiac ultrasonography is rapidly expanding as the technology provides a means to circumvent imaging problems when evaluating the heart. The techniques complement each other, particularly in the operating room. The capability of evaluating ventricular function and valve repairs at the time of surgery is new. Surgeons no longer have to wait for postoperative catheterization studies to evaluate the efficacy of repairs. As experience in these techniques increases new questions will be asked and patients ultimately will benefit as the quality of health care improves.

## References

1. Clements FM, de Bruijn NP. Perioperative evaluation of regional wall motion by two-dimensional echocardiography. Anesth Analg. 1987; 66:249–261.
2. Cucchiara RF, Nugent M, Seward JB, et al. Air embolism in upright neurosurgical patients: Detection and localization by two-dimensional transesophageal echocardiography. Anesthesiology. 1984; 60:353–355.
3. Erbel R, Borner N, Steller D, et al. Detection of aortic dissection by transesophageal echocardiography. Br Heart J. 1987; 58:45–50.
4. Frazin L, Talano JV, Stephanides L, et al. Esophageal echocardiography. Circulation. 1976; 54:102–108.
5. Harrison LH, Kisslo JA, Sabiston DC. Extraction of intramyocardial foreign body utilizing operative ultrasonography. J Thorac Cardiovasc Surg. 1981; 82:345–349.
6. Hisanaga K, Hisanaga A, Hibi N, et al. High-speed rotating scanner for transesophageal cross-sectional echocardiography. Am J Cardiol. 1980; 46:837–842.
7. Matsumoto M, Oka Y, Strom J, et al. Application of transesophageal echocardiography to continuous intraoperative monitoring of left ventricular performance. Am J Cardiol. 1980; 46:95–106.
8. Omoto R, ed. Color Atlas of Real-Time Two-Dimensional Doppler Echocardiography. 2nd ed. Tokyo: Shindan-to-Chiryo; 1987.
9. Schluter M, Langenstein BA, Polster J, et al. Transesophageal cross-sectional echocardiography with a phased-array transducer system: Technique and initial clinical results. Br Heart J. 1982; 48:67–78.
10. Ungerleider R, Greeley M, Sheikh K, et al. Routine intraoperative epicardial pre and post bypass color-flow imaging simplifies evaluation of repairs for congenital heart defects. Circulation. 1988; 78:649–660.

# PART FIVE

## Pediatric Echocardiography

# CHAPTER 18

# Cardiac Embryology

LORE TENCKHOFF, ANDREA C. SKELLY

The development of the heart in the human embryo begins very early. An early functioning circulatory system is needed to transport nutrients and waste products within the embryo and between the extraembryonic membranes and the maternal circulation. Although overall, knowledge of cardiac development is fairly well-established, many details remain unclear. The objective of our brief description of cardiac development is to help the sonographer correlate congenital cardiac defects with abnormalities in cardiac development. Those who desire more detailed information should consult the references.[1,2]

By the time the embryo is approximately 23 days old, the future heart is represented by a single straight tube lying within the pericardial cavity. The future left and right atria lie at the caudal end of the tube, outside the pericardial cavity. The cephalad end of the heart tube lies outside the pericardium and will be involved in the formation of the aortic arches (Fig. 18-1).

During the next stage of development, starting about the 23rd day after conception, the intrapericardial heart tube rapidly grows longer. Because the two ends of the tube are fixed—cephalad by the branchial arches and caudad by the septum transversum—the tube bends, usually to the right. This rightward bending is termed dextro looping (or *d* looping). While the heart tube grows, the primitive atrium also grows, dilates, and appears to move

more cephalad. The common atrium thus comes to lie posterior and somewhat cephalad to the heart tube. This common atrium is continuous with the proximal end of the heart tube, which is destined to become the left ventricle. With the rightward bending of the heart tube, the future left ventricle comes to lie on the left side of the heart and the more distal part of the heart tube (the future right ventricle and outflow tracts) comes to lie on the right side of the heart. At this stage of development the heart is still essentially a single tube with the ability to contract in a peristaltic fashion. On the inside of the heart tube is a layer of tissue, termed the cardiac jelly, which acts as a valve as blood is propelled from the atrial end of the heart tube to the distal end (Fig. 18-2).

Approximately 24 days after conception, the heart tube has grown so much that it occupies the entire pericardial cavity. The future left and right ventricles have expanded, and diverticula have developed in the cardiac jelly, the beginning of the ventricular cavities. Distal to the future right ventricle, the heart tube is called the conus cordis; this will form the future right and left ventricular outflow tracts. Distal to the conus cordis the tube is termed the truncus arteriosus; it will divide to form the aorta and pulmonary artery. The conus cordis and truncus arteriosus together are called the conotruncal region. The conotruncal region together with the right ventricle are termed the bulbus cor-

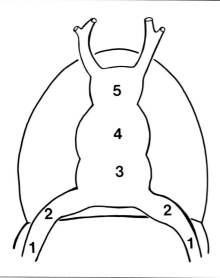

FIGURE 18-1. Primitive heart tube. Right and left sinus venosus (1); right and left atria (2); ventricle (3); bulbus cordis (4, 5).

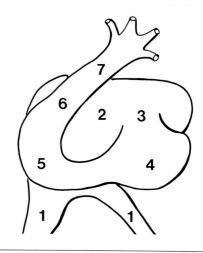

FIGURE 18-2. Rightward or dextro (d) looping of the heart tube. Right and left sinus venosum (1); common atrium (2); atrioventricular canal (3); primitive left ventricle (4); primitive right ventricle (5); conus cordis (6); truncus arteriosus (7).

dis. Further growth of the heart tube causes the conotruncal region to shift more centrally (Fig. 18-3). With this leftward movement, torsion and twisting of the conotruncal region occurs, which may in part contribute to the way the aorta and pulmonary artery curve around each other in the fully developed normal heart. During the time that the conotruncal region is shifting, septation of the heart tube is also taking place. It will be completed by about 37 days' gestational age. It is easier to describe septation of different portions of the heart tube separately, even though septation is taking place at approximately the same time in each part.

## Congenital Abnormalities of Early Cardiac Development

### ABNORMALITIES OF CARDIAC LOOPING

It is thought that if the heart tube loops to the left (levo or "l" looping) rather than rightward (dextro or "d" looping) as it normally does, malposition of the ventricles and the great vessels will result. Such abnormalities may take many forms (Table 18-1). The best known is the entity called congenitally corrected transposition (Fig. 18-4).

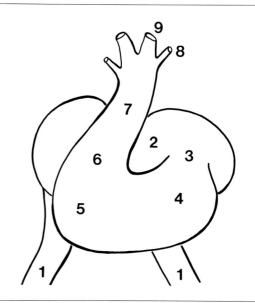

FIGURE 18-3. Medial shift of the conotruncal region. Right and left sinus venosus (1); common atrium (2); atrioventricular canal (3); primitive left ventricle (4); primitive right ventricle (5); conus cordis (6); truncus arteriosus (7); second aortic arches (8); first aortic arches (9).

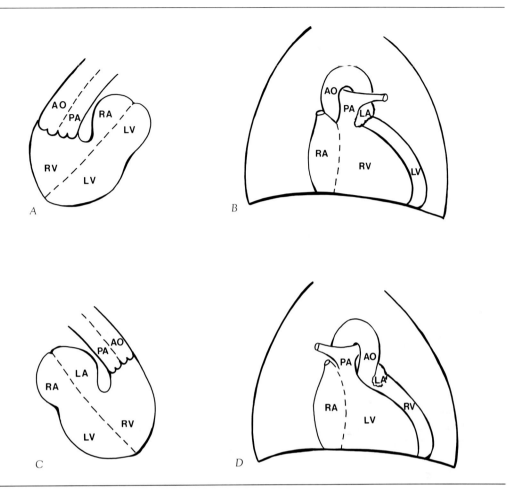

FIGURE 18-4. (A) Rightward or dextro (d) looping of the heart tube. Future normal septation is indicated by the broken line. (B) Normal or dextro (d) bulboventricular looping. Normal heart in the left chest. (C) Normally positioned atria with levo (l) looping of the remainder of the heart tube. (D) Congenitally corrected transposition. Normally positioned atria, levo (l) bulboventricular looping and transposed great arteries. The right-sided atrium empties into the right-sided, anatomic left ventricle, which empties into the pulmonary artery. The hemodynamic connections are correct; the anatomic connections are not.

## SINGLE VENTRICLE

The congenital cardiac defect known as single ventricle, or doublet-inlet left ventricle, is the result of an error in early embryonic cardiac development, at the time when the common atrium enters the beginning of the primitive heart tube. Usually, but not always, the common atrium does divide into right and left atria and the opening between the atrium (or atria) and the beginning of the heart tube is divided into two atrioventricular orifices. Both atrioventricular orifices then enter the proximal part of the heart tube, which normally is destined to be the left ventricle. Frequently the ventricular portion of the cardiac tube differentiates

Table 18-1. Schematic timetable of normal and abnormal cardiac development

| Approximate Gestational Age (days) | Normal Development | Appearance of Cardiac Defects |
|---|---|---|
| 23–26 | Bulboventricular looping | Congenitally corrected transposition |
| 26–29 | 1. Enlargement of AV canal to right | Double inlet left ventricle |
| | 2. Development of truncus and conus cushions | Persistent truncus arteriosus |
| | 3. Development of muscular septum | Muscular ventricular septal defects |
| | 4. Appearance of septum primum | |
| 30–32 | Fusion of truncus swellings | Transposition of great arteries |
| 33–36 | 1. Development of intercalated swellings and semilunar valve cusps | Pulmonary and aortic stenosis |
| | 2. Fusion of conus cushions with one another and with truncus cushions | Supracristal ventricular septal defects; tetralogy of Fallot |
| | 3. Fusion of endocardial cushions | Atrioventricular canal defects |
| | 4. Development of septum secundum and fusion of septum primum fuses with endocardial cushions | Atrial septal defects |
| 37–42 | 1. Completion of fusion of conus cushions with endocardial cushions and muscular septum | Perimembraneous ventricular septal defects |
| | 2. Formation of atrioventricular valve cusps | Stenosis or atresia of mitral and tricuspid valves |

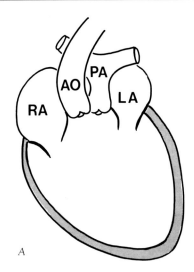
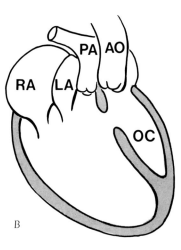

Figure 18-5. Double-inlet or single ventricle. (A) Single ventricle with dextro (d) transposed great arteries. (B) Single ventricle with levo (l) transposed great arteries and a primitive outflow chamber (OC).

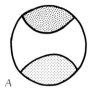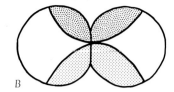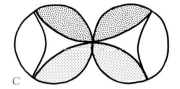

FIGURE 18-6. Formation of the semilunar valve cusps. (A, B) Division of the truncus by two truncus cushions, which are also the precursors of four of the semilunar valve cusps. (C) Formation of the semilunar valve cusps. The third cusp of each valve is formed from the intercalated swelling.

no further, in which case both atrioventricular valves enter a single ventricular chamber, which in turn gives rise to both great arteries, hence the name single ventricle or double-inlet left ventricle. Sometimes a small right ventricular outflow chamber is formed, which, however, is not a true right ventricle, as no atrioventricular valve is related to it. The development of the great arteries usually also is abnormal, the great arteries usually being transposed with respect to one another (Fig. 18-5).

A single ventricle can occur whether the cardiac looping is dextro or levo. Single ventricles are therefore usually classified as (1) "d" or "l" loops; (2) with or without a primitive outflow chamber; and (3) with or without transposed great arteries. Normally related great arteries are rarely associated with a single ventricle. A single ventricle with normally related great arteries is also known as an Holmes' heart.

## Division of the Truncus Arteriosus

The division of the truncus arteriosus starts around the 28th day of development. Two swellings (truncus swellings) arise from the wall of the common trunk (Fig. 18-8). These grow rapidly and fuse, dividing the truncus into the future aortic and pulmonary channels. Division starts at the distal end of the truncus arteriosus and progresses toward the conus cordis. At the level adjacent to the conus cordis, the truncus swellings develop into valve cusps and form two of the three cusps in each vessel. A third swelling, the intercalated swelling, forms the third cusp (Fig. 18-6).

## CONGENITAL ABNORMALITIES OF TRUNCAL DEVELOPMENT

*Stenosis and Atresia of the Semilunar Valves.* Interference with development at the time of aortic and pulmonary valve cusp formation may result in valve abnormalities, which usually lead to stenosis. One or more of the valve cusps may be thickened. Two of the cusps may fuse, creating a bicuspid valve, which may be stenotic. All three cusps may fuse, producing a narrow stenotic orifice (Fig. 18-7). Complete fusion of all three cusps results in aortic or pulmonary atresia. Aortic and pulmonary ste-

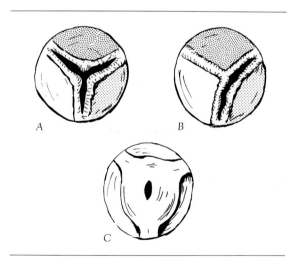

FIGURE 18-7. Stenotic semilunar valves. (A) Stenotic tricuspid valve. (B) Stenotic bicuspid valve. (C) Stenotic unicuspid valve.

nosis can occur together, but more often they are isolated lesions. Frequently they are associated with other congenital cardiac malformations.

*Persistent Truncus Arteriosus.* Interference with the division of the truncus may result in the cardiac abnormality termed persistent truncus arteriosus. Under these circumstances the truncus swellings and the intercalated swelling continue to form valve cusps, usually three or four. Rarely the truncus valve is bicuspid or has six cusps. The cusps often are thickened, producing regurgitation and, less frequently, regurgitation combined with stenosis.

During cardiac development, the truncus arteriosus initially arises from the future right ventricle (see Fig. 18-2). If development goes awry early, before the truncus has had time to shift more medially, the persistent truncus arteriosus continues to originate from the right ventricle. More often, the truncus either "straddles" the interventricular septum (overrides it) or originates entirely from the left ventricle. With persistent truncus arteriosus the conus cushions are thought not to develop or to remain hypoplastic; the result is a ventricular septal defect immediately below the truncus arteriosus. This defect may be medium-sized or large, depending on the extent to which it extends into the muscular septum (Fig. 18-13B). (See the discussion of the ventricular outflow tract division.) The truncus arteriosus is continuous with the aortic arch. The pulmonary artery branches are derived from the pulmonary plexus and grow to join the truncus arteriosus directly.

## Formation of the Interventricular Septum

### THE MUSCULAR INTERVENTRICULAR SEPTUM

The formation of the muscular interventricular septum begins around 27 days' gestational age. At this time the ventricular cavities are still quite small and the future ventricles communicate by a somewhat narrow channel (see Fig. 18-2). The ventricles themselves begin to grow and enlarge rather rapidly, whereas the narrow joining communicating grows much more slowly. As a result, the inferior opposing walls of the ventricles give the appearance of an invagination between the ventricular chambers (Fig. 18-8). The opposing ventricular walls fuse and form what is termed the muscular interventricular septum.

The cardiac tube is initially filled with cardiac jelly, which acts as a primitive valve system. It is transformed gradually into a mass of spongy tissue, from which the papillary muscles, chordae tendineae, and ventricular trabeculae are formed by differential cell growth and cell death.

### Congenital Abnormalities of Development of the Muscular Septum

*Muscular ventricular septal defects.* Remnants of spongy tissue (embryonic mesenchyme) may persist after birth, filling the left ventricular apex. Both the embryonic mesenchyme and muscular ventricular septal defects at the apex or septum are probably the result of inappropriate cell growth and cell death. Apical septal defects are usually multiple, whereas septal defects elsewhere in the muscular septum are more often single.

*Left ventricular false tendons.* Remnants of the embryonic mesenchyme may persist as strands stretching across the left ventricular cavity and are referred to as left ventricular false tendons.

### THE INFLOW SEPTUM AND DIVISION OF THE ATRIOVENTRICULAR CANAL

The primitive atrium initially empties only into the primitive left ventricle through an opening known as the atrioventricular canal. As development progresses, this opening enlarges to allow atrial blood to flow into both primitive ventricles (Fig. 18-8). Around the edges of the atrioventricular orifice mesenchymal swellings appear called endocardial cushions. There are two lateral and two endocardial cushions. These endocardial cushions serve as precursors of the atrioventricular valves and act as primitive valves.

The endocardial cushions grow toward one another and fuse, dividing the common atrioventricular canal into two openings, the future tricuspid and mitral valve orifices (Fig. 18-9). This division begins at approximately the same time as the formation of the muscular septum, around 27 days' gestation.

The endocardial cushions are the precursors of the septal leaflet of the tricuspid valve and the an-

Key to the embryonic cushions involved in septation

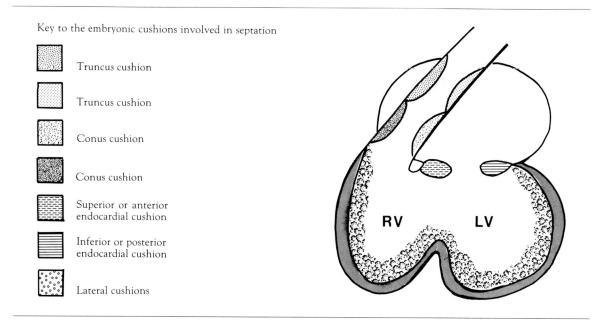

- Truncus cushion
- Truncus cushion
- Conus cushion
- Conus cushion
- Superior or anterior endocardial cushion
- Inferior or posterior endocardial cushion
- Lateral cushions

FIGURE 18-8. Division of the conotruncal region and the formation of the muscular septum. See key for identification of the truncus cushions, the conus cushions, and the endocardial cushions. Note the invagination between the primitive right and left ventricles and early formation of the muscular septum. Embryonic mesenchyme fills much of the ventricular cavities at this stage and is indicated here only for clarity.

terior leaflet of the mitral valve. The lateral cushions are the forerunners of the anterior and posterior leaflets of the tricuspid valve and the posterior leaflet of the mitral valve. Further valve differentiation is thought to occur by undermining of the ventricular musculature covered by the endocardial and lateral cushion tissue. The undermining of the ventricular septum and free wall, as well as the sculpting, thinning, and shaping of the leaflet tissue, the chordae, and the papillary muscles, is accomplished by differential cell growth and death. In addition to their role in the development of the mitral and tricuspid valves, the endocardial cushions are thought to contribute the portion of the ventricular septum that lies between the mitral and tricuspid leaflets (the inflow portion of the ventricular septum). The most anterior portion of interventricular septum, derived from the endocardial cushions, becomes thinned and is termed the membranous septum (Fig. 18-13A).

*Congenital Abnormalities of Endocardial and Lateral Cushion Development*
*Membranous ventricular septal defects.* These are small defects of the membranous septum. Often the membranous septum is present as an aneurysm with one or more openings that allow shunting of blood between the ventricles. More often the membranous defect extends to involve the muscular septum or the conus cushions or both, forming a so-called perimembranous ventricular septal defect, which may be quite large.

*Atrioventricular Canal Defects.* Should there be early interference in the development of the endocardial cushions the superior and inferior endocardial cushions may not meet, leaving the atrioventricular opening or canal undivided. This results in the abnormality termed complete persistent atrioventricular canal (Fig. 18-9A). If such interference in development occurs slightly later, the superior and inferior endocardial cushions may

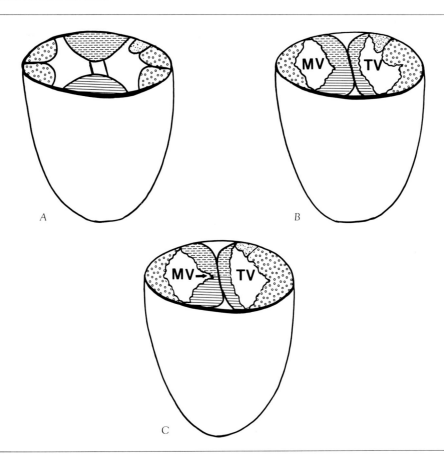

FIGURE 18-9. Division of the atrioventricular canal. (A) Early developmental stage showing the endocardial cushions, the lateral cushions, and the conus cushion contribution. The free edge of the muscular septum is visible between the endocardial cushions. (B) Normal development. Mitral and tricuspid valve leaflets and their embryological precursors. (C) Abnormal development. Cleft mitral valve (*arrow*) results from lack of fusion of the endocardial cushions.

meet without fusing completely, leading to a so-called cleft in the anterior leaflet of the mitral valve (Fig. 18-9C).

*Ebstein's anomaly.* Ebstein's anomaly is the result of interference in the normal undermining, free-ing, and shaping of the tricuspid valve leaflets. The septal leaflet may be freed to varying degrees. The site at which the freeing process is arrested creates a hinge, where the free portion of the leaflet meets that portion that is still adherent to the septal wall. This gives the illusion of the valve ring being dis-placed into the right ventricular cavity both ana-tomically, that is, on gross inspection, and echo-cardiographically. This led to the expression "atrialization of the right ventricle." The motion of this leaflet is often restricted by short chordae. The anterior leaflet of the tricuspid valve is usually freed up to the true annulus. The shaping of the leaflet, however, is abnormal, resulting in a large, saillike anterior leaflet with short, often thickened chordae and papillary muscles that usually mark-edly restrict the mobility of the leaflet (Fig. 18-10).

*Other abnormalities of the mitral and tricuspid valves.* Other atrioventricular valve abnormalities result-

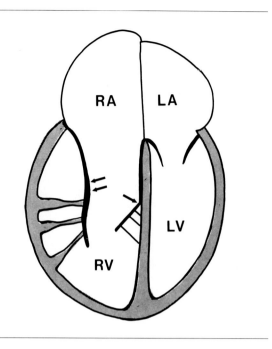

FIGURE 18-10. Ebstein's anomaly of the tricuspid valve. Note the lack of freeing of the septal leaflet (*single arrow*) and the long anterior leaflet (*double arrow*).

ing from abnormal lateral and endocardial development include mitral stenosis in its various forms, tricuspid stenosis, and mitral or tricuspid atresia.

## THE OUTFLOW SEPTUM AND FORMATION OF THE VENTRICULAR OUTFLOW TRACTS

The outflow region of the left and right ventricles is divided by another set of swellings, the conus cushions. At the same time as the division of the truncus arteriosus via the truncus cushions begins, the division of the outflow tract also starts with the formation of the conus cushions. The truncus cushions grow faster than the conus cushions. Only after the truncus cushions have fused, dividing the truncus arteriosus into pulmonary and aortic channels, do the conus cushions begin to grow more rapidly. The right-sided truncus and conus cushions are in continuity, as are the left-sided ones. The conus cushions grow and eventually fuse, to divide the conus cordis into the right and left ventricular outflow tracts (see Figs. 18-8, 18-11). The right conus cushion fuses with the right lateral cushion of the tricuspid orifice. It contributes to the formation of the most anterior portion of the

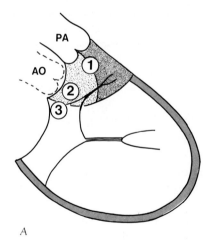

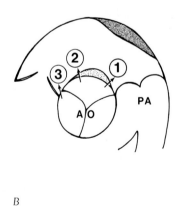

*A*                                                    *B*

FIGURE 18-11(A) The interventricular septum viewed from the right side. It is readily apparent that the papillary muscle of the conus is derived from one conus cushion. (B) Echocardiographic location of supracristal and retrocristal ventricular septal defects. Short axis view. Note, in the normal heart the conus cushions (crista supraventricularis) do not protrude into the right ventricular outflow tract as portrayed here. See key for identification of the conus cushions. Supracristal ventricular septal defect (1); retrocristal subaortic ventricular septal defect (2); retrocristal defect of the membranous septum (3).

anterior leaflet of the tricuspid valve. The left conus cushion also contributes to this area in the form of the papillary muscle attached to this portion of the anterior tricuspid leaflet (the papillary muscle of the conus; Fig. 18-11). Sometimes this papillary muscle is represented by chordae only. The tissue derived from the conus cushions, the crista supraventricularis, constitutes that portion of the septum that divides the outflow tracts. It is readily recognized anatomically on the right side of the heart as the muscular area separating the tricuspid valve from the pulmonary valve. On the left ventricular aspect this area tends to blend in with the rest of the interventricular septum.

### Congenital Abnormalities of Conus Cushion Development

*Supracristal and retrocristal septal defects.* Maldevelopment of the conus cushions may result in ventricular septal defects of the crista supraventricularis. Defects that lie adjacent to the pulmonary valve are termed supracristal ventricular septal defects. Those that lie more inferior or posterior with respect to the crista are termed retrocristal defects and are typically subaortic. These often extend to involve both the muscular and membranous septum. Isolated defects of the membranous septum from their anatomic location are also retrocristal defects although not derived from the conus cushions. When using the term retrocristal ventricular defects it is important to recognize that this indicates anatomic position and not embryologic origin (Fig. 18-11).

*Tetralogy of Fallot.* In tetralogy of Fallot the conus septum divides the outflow tract unequally, and the crista supraventricularis can be thought of as being displaced anteriorly. Depending on the degree of displacement, the right ventricular outflow tract is more or less narrowed. Because the conus septum is displaced, a gap, or septal defect, is present posterior to the crista. Usually development of the membranous septum and part of the muscular septum is also defective and a large ventricular septal defect remains. The division of the truncus (which occurs about the same time) is also unequal, so that the main pulmonary artery typically is small and the ascending aorta large. It should be remembered that while the truncus and conus portions of the cardiac tube are dividing the truncus is

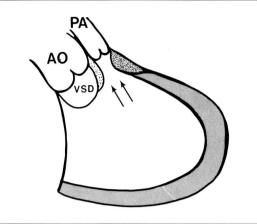

FIGURE 18-12. Tetralogy of Fallot viewed from the right ventricle. The main pulmonary artery and right ventricular outflow tract are narrow (*arrows*). There is a large ventricular septal defect below the large aortic root.

moving more medially. An error in embryonic development at this time can arrest medially movement of the conotruncal region, leaving the aortic root originating partially from the right ventricle and "straddling" or overriding the ventricular septum (Fig. 18-12). While in tetralogy of Fallot the pulmonary valve is always hypoplastic; it is frequently stenotic, but not always. The findings of tetralogy of Fallot include (1) narrowed right ventricular outflow tract; (2) ventricular septal defect posterior to the crista supraventricularis; (3) overriding of the aorta; and (4) right ventricular hypertrophy as a result of the right ventricle having to pump against the high systemic pressure and the right ventricular outflow obstruction. Valvular pulmonic stenosis is a frequent association, as is a right aortic arch.

### NOMENCLATURE OF THE INTERVENTRICULAR SYSTEM

The interventricular septum is derived from three embryonic components: the endocardial cushions, the conus cushions, and the muscular septum (Fig. 18-13A). The endocardiographic division (Fig. 18-13B) of the interventricular septum bears no relationship to the embryonic derivatives, and it is important to recognize this distinction.

The endocardiographic classification is useful to

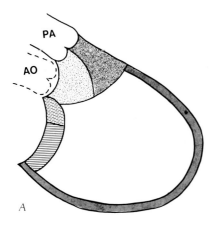 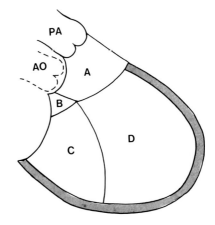

Figure 18-13. (A) Embryonic derivatives of the interventricular septum. See key for identification of the conus cusions and the endocardial cushions. The muscular septum is the large unshaded area. (B) Echocardiographic division of the interventricular septum: outlet septum (A); membranous septum (B); inlet septum (C); trabecular septum (D).

convey the anatomic site of a defect. A knowledge of the embryonic components of the ventricular septum serves as a reminder that other cardiac structures developing at the same time as the ventricular septum may also exhibit abnormal development.

For instance, a ventricular septal defect with an overriding great artery is indicative of a developmental interference at the time that the conotruncal region shifts medially and divides. This finding should prompt careful evaluation of the conotruncal region for such abnormalities as truncus arteriosus, transposition of the great arteries, and tetralogy of Fallot.

A ventricular septal defect of the membranous septum should prompt a search for other abnormal developments of the endocardial cushions, such as a cleft mitral valve or other atrioventricular valve abnormalities as well as defects of septum primum (see below).

*Summary.* To simplify some of the foregoing concepts, it is helpful to remember that endocardial cushions divide the inflow to the ventricles, the conus cushions divide the outflow region of the ventricles, and the truncus cushions divide the truncus into the aorta and the main pulmonary artery.

## Formation of the Interatrial Septum

The interatrial septum forms between the 27th and 37th day of embryonic development concurrent with the development of the ventricular septum and the division of the truncus arteriosus. The atrial cavity divides into right and left atria as changes in the sinus venosum are occurring. The sinus venosum initially is paired (Fig. 18-14). It receives blood from the yolk sac via the vitelline veins and blood from the chorionic villi (which later becomes the placenta) via the umbilical veins. It also receives blood from the embryo via the anterior and posterior cardinal veins, which drain, respectively, the cranial region of the embryo, and the body. The communication between the right and left sinus horns initially is quite wide; however, a fold develops between the left side of the atrium and the left side of the sinus venosus, obliterating the left umbilical and then the left vitelline vein. Subsequently the common cardinal vein is also obliterated, and at this point the left sinus horn re-

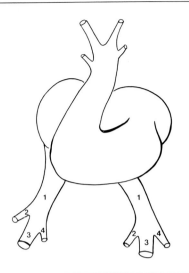

FIGURE 18-14. Early cardiac development: sinus venosum (1); vitelline veins (2); umbilical veins (3); posterior cardinal veins (4).

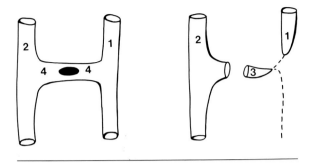

FIGURE 18-15. Development of coronary sinus: left common cardinal vein (1); right common cardinal vein (2); coronary sinus (3); sinus venosum (4).

mains only as the coronary sinus; the previous connections are obliterated. Ultimately all that is left of the left sinus horn is the coronary sinus. The right sinus horn gradually is incorporated into the right atrium and enlarges (Fig. 18-15).

At the junction of the right side of the sinus venosus and the atrium, the wall of the atrium folds inward to form the right venous or sinus valve. This is quite large in the embryo and helps to direct blood from the inferior vena cava across the interatrial septum. The valve extends inferiorly to also cover the coronary sinus. In newborns, the right venous valve may be quite prominent and readily recognizable echocardiographically as a large valve of the inferior vena cava (also called the eustachian valve). In older infants this venous valve is usually present only as a network of tissue strands known as Chiari's network. The eustachian valve may persist into adult life.

In Figure 18-3 the common atrium is seen to have expanded cephalad so as to lie superior and posterior to the heart tube. The truncus arteriosus causes a depression in the roof of the common atrium, as described previously. This creates a septum, the septum primum, which has its free edge directed toward the endocardial cushions (Fig. 18-16). This septum enlarges downward. The endocar-

dial cushions grow along the free edge of the septum, and proliferation of the endocardial cushion tissue closes the opening between the future right and left atrium.

As closure of the ostium primum is occurring, multiple perforations appear on the middle to upper aspect of septum primum and coalesce, forming the ostium secundum (Fig. 18-17). This ensures that there is continued communication between the primitive right and left atrium allowing blood—particularly that from the inferior vena cava—to flow into the left atrium.

As the right atrium expands, the right horn of the sinus venosus is incorporated into the roof of the atrium. At the junction of the right atrium and sinus venosum, a fold is formed, resulting in another septum, the septum secundum. The septum secundum remains quite small (see Fig. 18-17) and extends downward only a short way to overlap the ostium secundum. The septum secundum acts as a type of flap valve, covering the ostium secundum. This area of the ostium secundum is then called the foramen ovale. As long as the pressure in the right atrium is higher than in the left, blood can pass from the right atrium into the left atrium via the foramen ovale. After birth pressure decreases in the right atrium and increases in the left atrium; as a result the septum primum is pressed against the septum secundum, closing it. In the first weeks to months of life the two septa fuse in about 80% of all infants. In 20%, the foramen ovale remains patent and can open if right atrial pressure exceeds left atrial pressure.

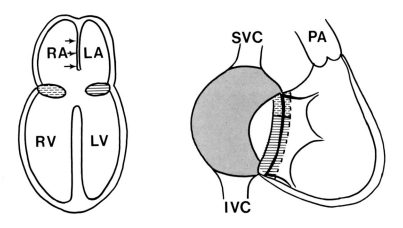

FIGURE 18-16. Development of interatrial septum (septum primum, *arrows*).

### Congenital Defects of the Atrial Septum and Related Structures

*Ostium Primum Atrial Septal Defects.* Should the downward growth of the septum primum be arrested, an opening between the right and the left atrium persists. This ostium primum defect lies just above the atrioventricular valves and is a low defect of the interatrial septum. It is called an ostium primum atrial septal defect. As the endocardial cushions help to close this opening, it is not sur-prising that the cardiac abnormality most commonly associated with ostium primum septal defect is some type of atrioventricular valve anomaly, in particular a cleft mitral valve.

*Ostium Secundum Atrial Septal Defects.* If for some reason the septum secundum is not formed or is incomplete, it will not cover the ostium secundum and an opening will remain between the right and left atria that is called an ostium secundum atrial

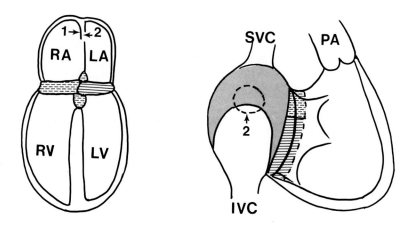

FIGURE 18-17. Development of interatrial septum: septum secundum (1); foramen ovale (2).

septal defect. If the foramen secundum becomes abnormally large as a result of coalescence of many perforations in the septum primum into one large opening, septum secundum will only partially cover the opening. Again, the result is an ostium secundum defect. Sometimes multiple perforations of varying sizes in the septum primum result in multiple ostium secundum defects. From an echocardiographic point of view, septum primum defects are those that are immediately above the atrioventricular valves and extend down to the valves. Secundum atrial defects almost always have a recognizable spur of interatrial tissue just above the atrioventricular valves. Most frequently they lie in the middle or upper third of the interatrial septum, that is, in the area of the ostium secundum normally covered by septum secundum.

*Persistent Left Superior Vena Cava.* Occasionally the connection between the coronary sinus (or the remnant of the left sinus horn) is maintained, so that connection with the common cardinal vein and the anterior cardinal vein persists. This entity is known as a persistent left superior vena cava. The persistent left superior vena cava drains into the coronary sinus; this is a frequent finding in congenital heart disease.

## References

1. Henry WL. Suggested Nomenclature for Cardiac Septa. Raleigh, NC: American Society of Echocardiography; 1986.
2. Moore KL. The Developing Human. Philadelphia: WB Saunders; 1988; 4.
3. Netter FH. The Ciba Collection of Medical Illustrations. Heart. Rochester, NY: Case-Hoyt Corporation; 1969; 5.

# CHAPTER 19

# Simple Congenital Heart Disease

DIANA KAWAI YANKOWITZ

The evaluation of congenital heart disease presents a challenge to echocardiographers. When congenital defects are suspected, it cannot be assumed the chambers and vessels are related properly. A segmental approach to the examination is imperative. This entails delineation of the situs, ventricular looping, and great vessel relationship. Documentation of anatomic landmarks for each chamber and great vessel facilitates the identification of their embryologic origins.[53] Anatomic landmarks for the right atrium include the entrances of the inferior and superior venae cavae. The left atrium receives the pulmonary veins. The ventricles are identified by the atrioventricular valves leading into them. The tri-leaflet tricuspid valve appears to open as a camera shutter does on short-axis views and inserts slightly more apically than the bi-leaflet mitral valve, which opens as a fish mouth does on short-axis views.

A standard protocol should be followed to ensure against missed diagnoses or repeat examination to seek additional suspected defects. A complete examination should include two-dimensional (2-D) echocardiography, M-mode, pulsed-wave (PW) Doppler, color-flow Doppler, and, if a high-velocity jet is suspected, continuous-wave (CW) Doppler studies. High–pulse repetition frequency (high–PRF) Doppler has been reported to be as accurate as CW Doppler for evaluation of congenital heart disease and, so, may be used in its place.[57]

Each septum must be examined exhaustively for evidence of defects. Each valve must be evaluated for structural or flow abnormalities. Because multiple defects are common, particularly with left ventricular outflow obstructions, the discovery of a single lesion does not rule out additional malformations.

Chapters 19 and 20 are intended as an introduction to the specialty of pediatric echocardiography. A comprehensive discussion of the variety and range of congenital heart diseases would require several hundred pages. The purpose of the following chapters is to give the reader an introductory level understanding of the anatomic malformations and their effects on cardiovascular hemodynamics. The discussion is limited to isolated lesions. Simple congenital heart defects, classified as shunt lesions or obstructive lesions, are discussed in this chapter. Valvular insufficiency occurs in children as isolated lesions, in conjunction with congenital malformations or as acquired lesions. The hemodynamic sequelae and echocardiographic evaluation of insufficiency are the same as for acquired heart disease in adults, so they are not discussed again here. Complex congenital heart disease is discussed in Chapter 20.

Each disease entity is introduced with a brief description of the anatomic anomaly. The hemodynamic effects of the defect are also discussed. To evaluate congenital heart disease effectively, the hemodynamics of each patient must be considered individually. Interpretation of Doppler data must take into account the effects of flow volumes and cardiac function. The severity of each lesion, and the effect of each lesion on any coexisting lesions must be carefully considered.

Echocardiographic findings are presented in outline form. Primary findings (those which characterize a particular malformation) are designated with an asterisk, secondary findings (abnormalities which develop as a result of the malformation) with a minus sign, and quantitative or semiquantitative findings with a plus sign. Transducer positions or imaging planes are noted in parentheses. Echocardiographic images and diagrams present the apical and subxiphoid views in either the apex up or apex down orientation. (Pediatric echocardiography groups display them in either orientation.) A discussion of specific echocardiographic techniques and quantification follows. Finally, a brief discussion of the treatment of each disease is presented. Many patients who have undergone palliative or corrective surgery are surviving into adulthood and require periodic follow-up. They may also present for cardiac evaluation because of symptoms unrelated to their congenital defect. A cursory understanding of the surgical procedure enables the echocardiographer to begin to interpret an "abnormal" finding as an expected one, given the patient's surgical history.

Table 19-1 is a list of common abbreviations. Table 19-2 sets forth the respective prevalence of various congenital heart defects, as reported in the literature. Statistically uncommon malformations are discussed briefly in the text.

## Simple Shunt Lesions

A shunt lesion is an abnormal communication between chambers or great vessels. Some shunt lesions are remnants of fetal circulation that should close within the first few days of life. Others may result from incomplete development of a cardiac structure. Blood flows across a communication from a high-pressure source to an area of lower pressure. This may result in a volume or pressure overload in the receiving chamber or vessel. The degree of volume or pressure overload is influenced by the anatomic resistance offered by the defect

TABLE 19-1. Common abbreviations in pediatric echocardiography

| | |
|---|---|
| 2-D. | Two-dimensional echocardiography |
| Ao. | Aorta |
| ASD. | Atrial septal defect |
| ASH. | Asymmetric septal hypertrophy |
| AT. | Acceleration time |
| AV. | Aortic valve |
| AVC. | Atrioventricular canal defect |
| AV valve. | Atrioventricular valve |
| BAS. | Balloon atrial septostomy |
| CHF. | Congestive heart failure |
| CW Doppler. | Continuous-wave Doppler |
| DOLV. | Double-outlet left ventricle |
| DORV. | Double-outlet right ventricle |
| D-TGA. | Dextro transposition of the great arteries |
| ET. | Ejection time |
| HOCM. | Hypertrophic obstructive cardiomyopathy |
| IHSS. | Idiopathic hypertrophic subaortic stenosis |
| IVC. | Inferior vena cava |
| IVS. | Interventricular septum |
| LA. | Left atrium |
| LMCA. | Left main coronary artery |
| LPA. | Left pulmonary artery |
| L-TGA. | Levo transposition of the great arteries |
| LV. | Left ventricle |
| LVOT. | Left ventricular outflow tract |
| mm Hg. | Millimeters of mercury (pressure gradient or difference) |
| M-mode. | Time-motion echocardiography |
| MPA. | Main pulmonary artery |
| PA. | Pulmonary artery |
| PAPVR. | Partial anomalous pulmonary venous return |
| PBF. | Pulmonary blood flow |
| PEP. | Preejection period |
| PTA. | Persistent truncus arteriosus |
| PW Doppler. | Pulsed-wave Doppler echocardiography |
| Qp : Qs. | Ratio of pulmonary blood flow to systemic blood flow |
| RA. | Right atrium |
| RPA. | Right pulmonary artery |
| RV. | Right ventricle |
| RVOT. | Right ventricular outflow tract |
| SV. | Single ventricle |
| SVAS. | Supravalvular aortic stenosis |
| SVC. | Superior vena cava |
| TAPVR. | Total anomalous pulmonary venous return |
| TOF. | Tetralogy of Fallot |
| VSD. | Ventricular septal defect |

TABLE 19-2. Incidence of various congenital cardiac
anomalies*

| CARDIAC MALFORMATION | INCIDENCE (%) |
| --- | --- |
| Ventricular septal defect | 16–35 |
| Atrial septal defect | 8–11 |
| Coarctation of the aorta | 7–8 |
| Dextro transposition of great arteries | 5–10 |
| Atrioventricular canal defect | 4–9 |
| Hypoplastic left heart syndrome | 6–7 |
| Pulmonic valve stenosis | 3–7 |
| Tetralogy of Fallot | 4–9 |
| Patent ductus arteriosus | 3–6 |
| Aortic stenosis | 2–3 |
| Pulmonary atresia | 2–3 |
| TAPVR | 2–3 |
| Single ventricle | 2–3 |
| Double outlet right ventricle | 2–3 |
| Tricuspid atresia | 1–3 |
| Ebstein's anomaly | 1 |
| Truncus arteriosus | 1 |
| Levo transposition of great arteries | <1 |
| Interrupted aortic arch | <1 |

*Composite of frequency of each major type of congenital heart
malformation as a percentage of congenital heart disease. Statistics were combined from the Baltimore-Washington Infant
Study,[12] New England Regional Study,[22] and the Alberta Heri-
tage Pediatric Cardiology Program.[26]

and by vascular resistance to flow. Included in this
category of congenital heart defects are the predominantly left-to-right shunts: atrial septal defects (ASD), ventricular septal defects (VSD), atrioventricular malformations, and persistent patent
ductus arteriosus (PDA).

### ATRIAL SEPTAL DEFECTS

An ASD is a communication between the atria
which allows blood to flow from the higher-pressure left atrium to the lower-pressure right atrium.
ASDs occur in various locations (Fig. 19-1), the
most common being the area of the foramen ovale,
where they are called ostium *secundum ASDs* (see
Fig. 19-1).[51,53] Ostium secundum ASDs occur in females twice as often as in males. An ostium secundum ASD should not be confused with a *patent foramen ovale*, which is considered to be a normal
anatomic variant and generally is not repaired. In
approximately 5% of the adult population, the foramen flap does not fuse completely and an intra-

cardiac shunt may develop if the interatrial septum
is stretched due to atrial dilatation or if the right
atrial pressure is abnormally high.[16]

Ostium *primum ASDs* are much less common
than ostium secundum defects, and they are located low in the interatrial septum near the atrioventricular valves (Fig. 19-1A).[11,51,53] No atrial septal tissue exists between the crux of the
atrioventricular valves and the defect. Ostium primum ASD is a form of atrioventricular canal defect and may occur with an inlet VSD, "cleft" mitral valve, or as part of a more complex
malformation.[38] In some cases, the ventricular component of the atrioventricular canal defect may be
very small and totally occluded by the chordal attachments of the atrioventricular valves.[53] In this
case, the VSD may not be appreciated prior to surgery.

The least common type of ASD is the *sinus venosus ASD*. It is located at the entrance of the superior vena cava into the right atrium (Fig. 19-
1B).[11,53] Sinus venosus ASDs often are associated
with anomalous return of the right pulmonary
veins into the right atrium.[11,13,51,53]

Multiple holes or fenestrations may also be seen
in the center of the atrial septum. Multiple ASDs
should be distinguished from a *Chiari network*,
which is a freely mobile meshwork or netlike membrane occasionally found in the right atrium near
the orifice of the coronary sinus. The Chiari network is thought to be an embryonic remnant, similar to the eustachian valve[1,53,68] (Fig. 19-2).

Finally, in cases of atrioventricular canal defects
or complex congenital heart disease, the atrial septum may be entirely absent, resulting in a *common
atrium*.[53] This malformation is not an ASD, since
no septal tissue exists. A common atrium may on
occasion have muscle bands coursing through it,
which may be mistaken echocardiographically for
portions of the atrial septum, leading to misdiagnosis as an ASD.[11]

*Hemodynamics.* Blood always flows from an area
of higher pressure to one of lower pressure. Because
pressure in the left atrium is usually higher than in
the right atrium, the flow of blood through an
ASD is generally from left to right, with some degree of variation with respiration.[56] The shunting
of blood from the left to the right atrium results in
a volume increase or overload to the right side of

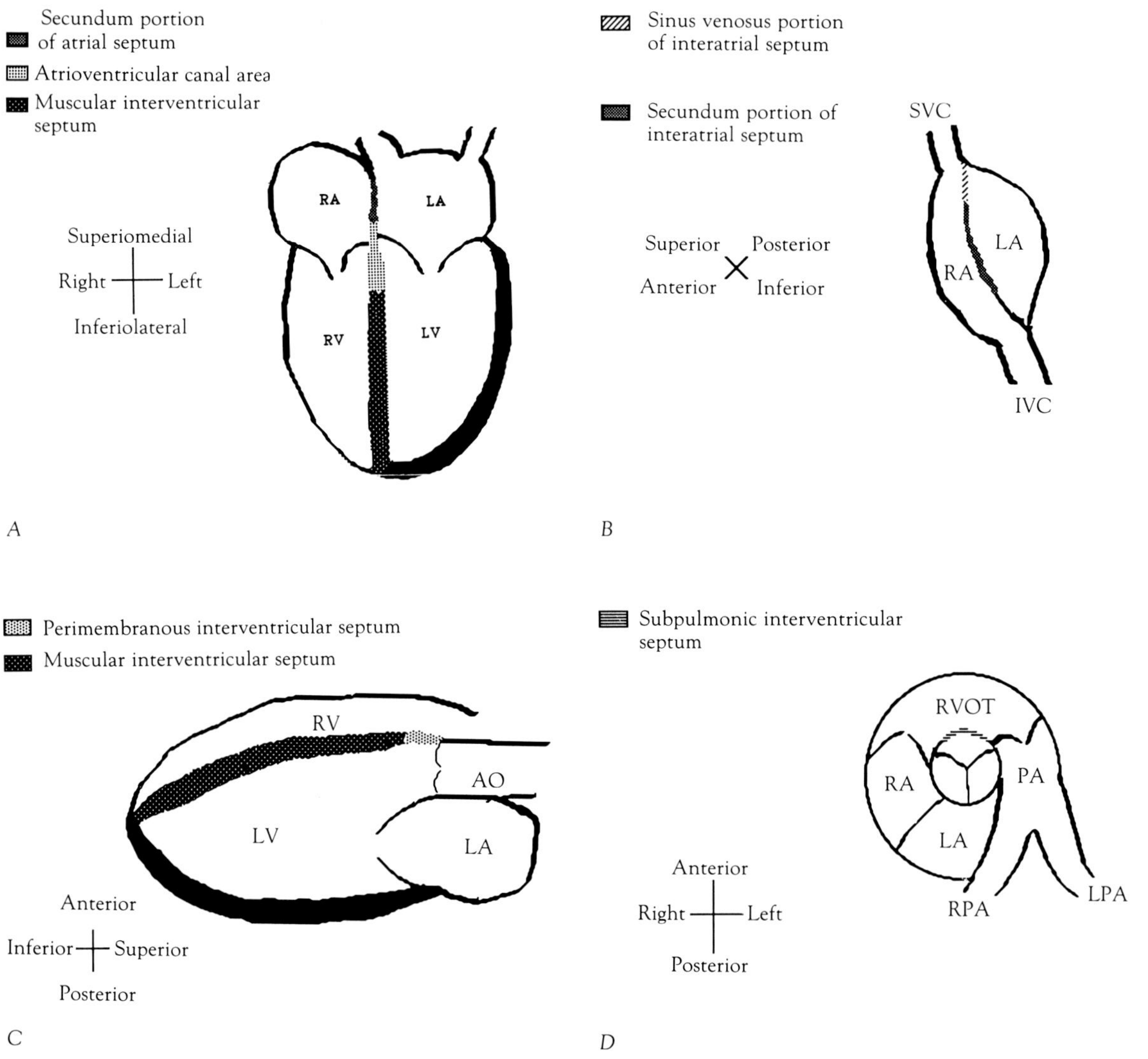

Secundum portion
of atrial septum

Atrioventricular canal area

Muscular interventricular
septum

Superiomedial

Right ──┼── Left

Inferiolateral

RA    LA

RV    LV

A

Sinus venosus portion
of interatrial septum

Secundum portion of
interatrial septum

Superior   Posterior
         X
Anterior   Inferior

SVC

LA
RA

IVC

B

Perimembranous interventricular septum

Muscular interventricular septum

RV

AO

LV    LA

Anterior

Inferior ──┼── Superior

Posterior

C

Subpulmonic interventricular
septum

RVOT

RA    PA

LA

Anterior

Right ──┼── Left

Posterior

RPA    LPA

D

FIGURE 19-1. Schematic illustrations delineating areas of the interatrial and interventricular septum as visualized on echocardiographic views. (A) Schematic drawing of the apical four-chamber view illustrating the location of the ostium secundum and -primum areas of the interatrial septum, and the inflow and muscular areas of the interventricular septum. (RA, right atrium; LA, left atrium; RV, right ventricle; LV, left ventricle.) (B) Schematic drawing of the subxiphoid short-axis view illustrating the location of the ostium secundum and sinus venosus areas of the interatrial septum. (SVC, superior vena cava; IVC, inferior vena cava.) (C) Schematic drawing of the parasternal long-axis view illustrating the perimembranous and muscular regions of the interventricular septum. (Ao, aorta.) (D) Schematic of the parasternal short-axis view illustrating the subpulmonic region of the interventricular septum. (RVOT, right ventricular outflow tract; PA, pulmonary artery; RPA, right pulmonary artery branch; LPA, left pulmonary artery branch.)

the heart. Flow velocities through the right-sided heart valves increase, and the right heart chambers dilate.

The hemodynamic significance of an ASD is determined by the volume of the shunt, which is a function of the physical size of the defect and the relative compliance of the left and right ventricles.[11] Increased flow volume through the pulmonary artery and pulmonary vasculature causes an increase in pulmonary arterial pressure. By early adulthood, increased blood flow through the pulmonary arterioles will cause hypertrophy of the intimal and medial layers. This will result in an increase in pulmonary vascular resistance referred to as pulmonary hypertension.[13,39] Pulmonary hypertension resulting from an ASD is often reversible by surgical closure of the ASD. Pulmonary hypertension may progress to pulmonary vascular obstructive disease if a large shunt is not closed.

*Echocardiographic findings and quantification.*[*]

TWO-DIMENSIONAL ECHOCARDIOGRAPHY

*Localization of the defect as a break in the continuity of the echogenic line representing the atrial septum (subxiphoid short-axis, subxiphoid long-axis,[4] parasternal short-axis views[53,58]) (Fig. 19-3A)
—Dilated right ventricle and right atrium
—Dilated pulmonary artery
*Negative contrast effect on contrast echocardiography[14,53,64]
*Positive contrast effect on contrast echocardiography[14,53,64]
—Visualization of septal aneurysm formation in the area of the fossa ovalis in unusual cases[41,51,53]

M-MODE ECHOCARDIOGRAPHY

—Dilated right ventricle[53]
—Paradoxical motion of the interventricular septum[53]

DOPPLER ECHOCARDIOGRAPHY

*Mildly turbulent, low-velocity left-to-right shunt across the atrial septum (parasternal or subxiphoid position; Fig. 19-3B) on PW examination
*Blood flow visualized crossing the atrial septum from left to right by color-flow Doppler (subxi-

*Primary findings are designated by an asterisk; secondary findings with a minus sign; and quantitative or semiquantitative findings with a plus sign.

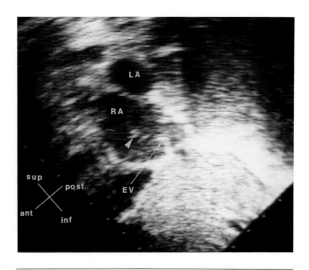

FIGURE 19-2. Two-dimensional visualization of a Chiari membrane (subxiphoid short-axis view of the interatrial septum). The small arrow points to the eustacian valve (EV) and the large arrowhead points to the Chiari membrane. (RA, LA, right and left atria.)

phoid short-axis,[31] subxiphoid long-axis,[31] apical four-chamber,[31] parasternal short-axis,[41] right parasternal short-axis views; see Fig. 19-3B)
—Mildly turbulent, increased velocity flow detected through tricuspid and pulmonic valves by PW Doppler[28,58]
+Quantification of shunt size by comparison of estimated blood flow through the pulmonary artery and the aorta (estimation of pulmonary blood flow/systemic blood flow or Qp/Qs)[28,49,58,59]
+Estimation of shunt size by determination of mean transatrial septal flow velocity, using angle correction if necessary[25]
+Semiquantification of shunt size by visualization of shunt flow area on color-flow Doppler images[31,40,58]

*Scanning techniques and interpretation of findings.* Atrial septal defects generally may be most effectively evaluated by 2-D echocardiography from the subxiphoid position.[53] From this approach, the sound beam is perpendicular to the atrial septum, utilizing the superior axial resolution of the transducer. In the apical four-chamber view, the atrial

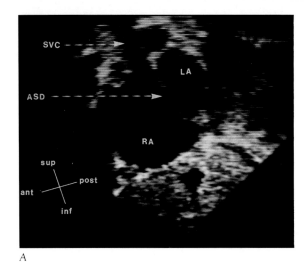

A

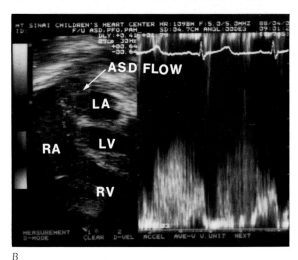

B

FIGURE 19-3. (See color insert for B.) Echocardiographic findings of atrial septal defect (ASD). (A) Two-dimensional visualization of an ostium secundum ASD (subxiphoid short-axis view). (B) Split-screen frozen frame showing flow through a secundum ASD by color-flow Doppler (apical four-chamber view), with the PW Doppler spectral tracing of the shunt flow shown to the right. (LA, RA, left and right atria; LV, RV, left and right ventricles; SVC, superior vena cava.)

septum lies parallel to the sound beam, making it difficult to differentiate spurious midseptal echo dropout from a true ostium secundum ASD. The apical four-chamber, subxiphoid long-axis, and parasternal short-axis views are the most helpful in the evaluation of ostium primum ASDs (see Fig. 19-1A).[51,53] The subxiphoid short-axis view is the only one in which the area of the atrial septum adjacent to the entrance of the superior vena cava may be visualized, so it is the view of choice when evaluating a sinus venosus ASD (Fig. 19-1B).[53] Sinus venosus ASD is the most difficult type of ASD to localize by 2-D echocardiography.[51] A sinus venosus ASD is suspected when an ASD cannot be localized in a patient with secondary findings of a right-sided heart volume overload.

The characteristic PW Doppler spectral tracing of an ASD shunt begins in midsystole, peaks to about 1.3 m/sec in late systole, and continues into diastole, often with slight augmentation during atrial systole.[28,53,56] The shunt is toward the transducer from any approach, as the blood flows from the posterior left atrium into the anterior right atrium, unless the right atrial pressure is elevated, resulting in a right-to-left shunt.[53]

Shunting may be visualized by color-flow Doppler imaging, a PW Doppler technique in which the direction of blood flow is color coded (flow toward the transducer is displayed in shades of red and flow away from the transducer, in shades of blue). A lighter shade of color represents relatively higher velocity flow, a deeper or darker shade, relatively low velocity. The color-flow "map" is superimposed on the traditional black-and-white 2-D image, creating a "color angiogram."[71] Color-flow Doppler is particularly useful in delineating the location of the ASD and in detecting multiple communications within the interatrial septum[40,58]

Contrast echocardiography is an older technique that is useful in demonstrating an ASD when the quality of the color-flow Doppler examination is suboptimal. A bolus of agitated normal saline solution or echocardiographic contrast injected into a peripheral vein may be visualized filling the right atrium and ventricle with microbubbles on 2-D echocardiography. The left-to-right shunt is appreciated as an area of non-contrast-enhanced blood entering the right atrium through the interatrial septum. This is referred to as the negative contrast effect. Minimal right-to-left shunting occurs during some portions of the cardiac cycle, so a few microbubbles may be visualized crossing the interatrial septum into the left atrium and ventricle by 2-D or M-mode echocardiography. The visualization of microbubbles in the left heart is referred to as the positive contrast effect.[14,51,53,64]

Shunt volume may be semiquantified by the degree of dilatation of the right side of the heart[53,58] or calculated by comparing pulmonary blood flow (Qp) with systemic blood flow (Qs). This is referred to as the Qp-Qs ratio (Qp/Qs). Since flow volume is equal to flow velocity multiplied by flow area,[58] Qp/Qs may be estimated by using PW Doppler to determine flow velocity and M-mode or 2-D echocardiography to determine flow area through the valve orifice or vessel lumen.[49,58,59] Pulmonary flow may be estimated using the pulmonary artery or tricuspid valve, and systemic flow may be estimated using the aorta or mitral valve.[48,49,59] In the normal heart these volumes are equal, so the ratio is 1:1. Determination of this ratio is not accurate in the presence of outflow obstruction, regurgitation, or systemic-to-pulmonary circulation shunts.[48]

*Treatment.* Large defects detected during infancy or early childhood rarely close spontaneously. Very small defects may occasionally close spontaneously during the first few years of life. When detected early, ASDs are usually repaired by age 5 years, before the child starts school. Surgical repair involves sewing the edges of the defect together or sewing a patch onto the right side of the atrial septum to occlude the shunt.[11]

## VENTRICULAR SEPTAL DEFECTS

VSDs are communications located within the interventricular septum that allow blood to shunt from the higher-pressure left ventricle to the lower-pressure right ventricle. Because the ventricular septum is curvilinear and the defect is often small, detection and localization may be facilitated by PW or CW Doppler. The advent of color-flow Doppler mapping has made detection even easier.[40,42,43] VSDs occur frequently as isolated lesions. They are also common in patients with chromosomal abnormalities[27] and as a component of com-

plex congenital heart disease. A patient may have multiple VSDs in various locations.[58]

Like ASDs, VSDs are described by their location. Various classifications use different divisions of the interventricular septum. The following is one of the most common classifications (see Fig. 19-1A,C,D). The most common location (75%[17]) is in or around the membranous portion of the interventricular septum, near the aortic valve; such VSDs are *perimembranous* or *infracristal* (see Fig. 19-1C).[27,52,53] In a subset of perimembranous VSDs referred to as *malalignment* defects, a great artery (aorta or pulmonary artery) may be visualized overriding the interventricular septum.[52,53] Malalignment VSDs are discussed in Chapter 20. VSDs located in the posterior portion of the interventricular septum at the level of the atrioventricular valves are called *inflow*,[11,27] *atrioventricular canal*,[52] or *endocardial cushion type*[31,58] VSDs (see Fig. 19-1A). *Muscular VSDs* may be located anywhere in the body of the muscular interventricular septum[27,52,53] (see Fig. 19-1A, C) and are most commonly seen in the newborn period. Multiple muscular VSDs are referred to as Swiss cheese defects.[17] Occasionally, *subpulmonic*[52] (*supracristal, outlet,*[53] *conal*[17]) VSDs may be seen in the right ventricular outflow tract. They are located distal to the crista supraventricularis, near the pulmonic valve[13,17,27] (see Fig. 19-1D). Subpulmonic and perimembranous VSDs may have associated aortic cusp herniation into the defect, which may cause aortic insufficiency.[27,53]

*Hemodynamics.* Blood flows through a VSD from the left ventricle to the right ventricle unless the right ventricular pressure is elevated to systemic levels due to pulmonary hypertension, severe pulmonary stenosis, or pulmonary atresia. In large, nonrestrictive VSDs, bidirectional shunting occurs as a result of equalization of pressure between the right and left ventricles. With bidirectional shunting, blood flows from left to right during some parts of the cardiac cycle and from right to left during other parts of the cycle, as the relative pressures of the ventricles vary slightly. Ventricular septal defects are considered to be nonrestrictive if they are equal to or larger than the diameter of the aortic annulus.[21] Evaluation of a VSD during the newborn period may reveal little shunting through even a large VSD, since the right and left ventricles face similar resistances prior to the decrease in pul-

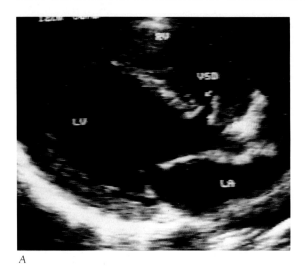

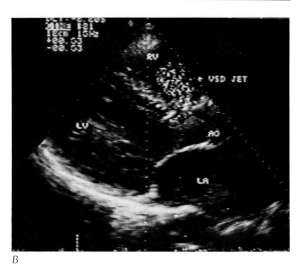

A

B

FIGURE 19-4. (See color insert for *B, C,* and *D.*) Echocardiographic findings of ventricular septal defect (VSD). (*A*) Two-dimensional visualization of a perimembranous VSD (parasternal long-axis view). Note brightness of echoes at edges of the defect, known as T artifact. A membrane appears to be forming from the superior aspect of the defect but does not appear to effectively close the defect. (*B*) Color-flow Doppler image illustrates the turbulent, high-velocity left-to-right shunt through the perimembranous VSD as a speckled, mosaic pattern of flow within the VSD and coursing into the right ventricle (parasternal long-axis view).

monary vascular resistance and increase in ventricular compliance. Poor left ventricular function decreases the degree of shunting through a VSD.[59]

The significance of a VSD is related to its size, as the size of the defect determines the shunt volume.[27] The shunt volume may cause varying degrees of volume overload to the pulmonary artery, pulmonary bed, and left side of the heart. In VSDs of moderate shunt size, the systolic timing of the shunt results in an additional pressure overload. As the left ventricle contracts, blood is forced through the VSD, through the right ventricle, and directly into the pulmonary vascular bed through the open pulmonic valve. Because the jet courses almost directly into the pulmonary bed, the effect on the pulmonary vasculature is generally greater than the effect on the right ventricle. Eventually, the combined volume and pressure overload induces pulmonary vascular obstructive disease[13] by causing the hypertrophy and scarring of the medial and intimal layers of the pulmonary arterioles.[39] As pulmonary vascular obstructive disease progresses,

the degree of left-to-right shunting at the VSD decreases, until the pulmonary resistance exceeds systemic resistance. In this case, the right ventricular pressure exceeds left ventricular pressure, and blood is shunted from right to left, causing the patient to become cyanotic. Cyanosis due to pulmonary vascular obstructive disease secondary to a systemic-to-pulmonary shunt is called Eisenmenger's syndrome.[13,17,27]

*Echocardiographic findings and quantification.*
TWO-DIMENSIONAL ECHOCARDIOGRAPHY
*Localization of the VSD (parasternal long- and short-axis, apical four-chamber, subxiphoid long- and short-axis views[27,53]; Fig. 19-4A)
—Dilated left atrium and left ventricle
*Negative contrast effect at level of VSD[52,53]
—"Aneurysm" formation of a secondarily malformed tricuspid valve septal leaflet visualized bulging into the right ventricle, covering the VSD (parasternal long-axis and apical four-chamber views)[27,52,53]

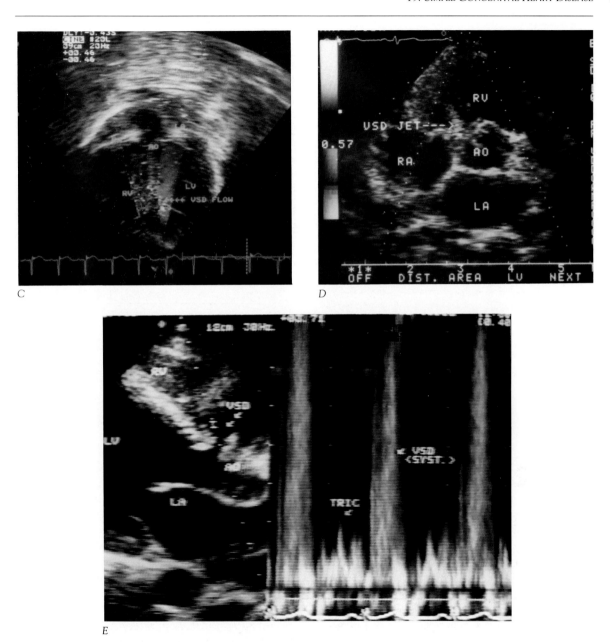

FIGURE 19-4 *(continued)*. (C) Color-flow Doppler image illustrates a left-to-right shunt through a muscular VSD (apical four-chamber view). (D) Color-flow Doppler image illustrating a left-to-right shunt through a perimembranous VSD (parasternal short-axis view). (E) PW Doppler tracing of the perimembranous VSD illustrating positive, turbulent, high-velocity flow through the VSD during systole (syst). Tricuspid valve flow (TRIC) is seen as a positive, low-velocity flow during diastole. (LV, RV, left and right ventricles; LA, RA, left and right atria; AO, aorta.)

M-MODE ECHOCARDIOGRAPHY

— Atrioventricular valve leaflets appear to cross the interventricular septum into the other ventricle in cases of atrioventricular canal VSDs
— Dilated left atrium and left ventricle[17]
— Evaluate pulmonic valve for evidence of pulmonary hypertension

DOPPLER ECHOCARDIOGRAPHY

*Blood flow through the interventricular septum visualized by color-flow Doppler[31,40] (parasternal long- and short-axis, apical four-chamber, subxiphoid long- and short-axis views; Fig. 19-4B–D)
*Localization of the defect by PW detection of a turbulent, high-velocity systolic jet on the right side traced through the interventricular septum, indicating a left-to-right shunt (parasternal, apical, subxiphoid positions[28,52,53,58,60,61]; Fig. 19-4E)
— Increased velocity and turbulence through the pulmonic valve on PW examination[53,56,58]
— Associated aortic insufficiency[53]
— PW and color-flow Doppler evidence of pulmonary hypertension[28,31,40]
+ Estimation of right ventricular (and therefore pulmonary artery) pressure by determination of peak instantaneous gradient through the VSD on CW Doppler[28,35,44]

*Discussion of echocardiographic findings and quantification techniques.* On 2-D echocardiography, ventricular septal defects measuring greater than 2 mm in diameter[52] may be visualized as areas of echo drop-out in the interventricular septum. A distinct, bright echo, known as a **T** artifact may demarcate the margins of the defect at the interventricular septal tissue–blood interface.[1,7] Because the interventricular septum is a curvilinear structure, the most effective way to visualize defects is to record sweeps produced when the imaging plane is swept through the heart so that the entire septum is visualized on real-time display. In this way, defects that do not appear in the standard views are not overlooked. Color-flow Doppler has been reported to be particularly useful in the localization of multiple defects, which may not all occur in the same area.[31,58]

Pulmonic valve M-mode findings suggestive of pulmonary hypertension are absence of the a wave and midsystolic notching[69] (flying **W** sign). PW

Doppler findings suggestive of increased pulmonary vascular resistance include midsystolic notching of pulmonary flow, ratio of acceleration time to right ventricular ejection time less than 0.36, and a ratio of right ventricular preejection period to right ventricular ejection time greater than 0.34.[28] If pressure in the right ventricle is similar to that in the left ventricle, bidirectional shunting may be seen on color-flow Doppler as alternating red and blue flashes through the VSD.[31]

Right ventricular pressure, and by inference, pulmonary artery pressure, may be estimated by placing the CW Doppler beam through the VSD jet to determine the maximum velocity of flow[28,34,35,54] by the following equation[28]:

Maximum velocity of flow =

$$\frac{\text{Change in frequency} \times \text{Speed of sound in tissue}}{2 \times \text{transducer frequency} \times \cos \Theta}$$

in which angle $\Theta$ is the incident angle of the sound beam to the blood flow. The acoustic beam should be kept as nearly parallel to blood flow as possible to optimize the accuracy of the estimate.[28] The peak instantaneous pressure gradient through the VSD is calculated using the modified Bernoulli equation[28]:

$$\text{Pressure gradient} = 4 \times \text{Maximum velocity}^2$$

In the absence of aortic valve disease or aortic arch anomalies, the systolic blood pressure measured from the patient's arm is equal to the systolic left ventricular pressure. The peak instantaneous gradient through the VSD may be subtracted from the left ventricular pressure to estimate right ventricular pressure. In the absence of right ventricular outflow obstruction, right ventricular pressure should equal pulmonary artery pressure.[28,34,35] The success of this calculation depends on the accurate assessment of the maximum velocity. Angle correction may decrease the accuracy of the velocity determination, so it is recommended that every effort be made to aim the Doppler beam as directly through the center of the jet as possible. Color-flow Doppler technique has been reported to improve alignment of the CW Doppler beam with the VSD jet, particularly when the jet is eccentrically oriented.[40,44] Underestimation of the maximum velocity (and therefore pressure gradient) will result in an erroneously high pulmonary artery pressure estimate. If elevated pulmonary artery pressure is suspected, further evaluation is warranted[59] by determination of a tricuspid insufficiency gradient[28] or catheterization.

The peak instantaneous gradient of tricuspid insufficiency may be added to a clinical estimation of right atrial pressure to estimate the right ventricular pressure (expressed in millimeters of mercury).[56,70] Again, in the absence of right ventricular outflow obstruction, the right ventricular pressure should equal the pulmonary artery pressure.

The Qp/Qs may be estimated by calculating flow through the ascending aorta as systemic flow (Qs), and flow through the pulmonary artery as pulmonary flow (Qp). Since flow across the mitral valve is that of pulmonary venous return, mitral flow equals pulmonary flow and may be used when pulmonary artery flow is turbulent due to the VSD[48] or a coexisting PDA.[49] Similarly, tricuspid flow (systemic venous return) equals aortic flow in the absence of a systemic-to-pulmonary shunt and may be used to determine Qs.[49]

*Treatment.* Many VSDs close spontaneously. Frequency of spontaneous closure varies with the size of the defect and its location. As many as 60 to 80% of small VSDs close spontaneously, usually within the first 2 years of life.[17] Persistent small VSDs are followed clinically and do not require surgical closure, as they appear to have no detrimental long-term effects. To prevent the development of bacterial endocarditis, patients are given prophylactic antibiotics whenever they undergo a surgical procedure or dental work that may expose the blood to bacterial infection.[27] Perimembranous VSDs may close spontaneously through the formation of a membrane or aneurysm of the septal tricuspid valve leaflet.[27,52,53]

In the absence of clinical complications, a moderate size VSD with a Qp/Qs of 1.5:1 or greater is usually surgically closed before the child begins school.[17] Surgery may be performed earlier if a child develops significant pulmonary hypertension, suffers from repeated respiratory infections or growth retardation, or develops clinical signs of heart failure.[27]

Large, nonrestrictive VSDs are least likely to close spontaneously. If the infant does not respond to medical treatment for left ventricular failure, the VSD is surgically corrected within the first year of life.[27] If the infant is responsive to medical treatment, closure is scheduled during the second year of life, when the operative risk is not as great as in the first year. There is evidence that increased pulmonary resistance is less likely to regress, and in some cases it continues to progress after surgical correction if closure is delayed beyond the second year of life.[17,39] In the infrequent case of a VSD that causes aortic insufficiency, surgical closure of the defect and repair of the aortic valve is performed to obviate progression of the insufficiency.[27]

Surgical correction involves sewing a patch onto the right side of the interventricular septum, closing the VSD. Residual leaks (shunting) around the patch may be visualized by color-flow Doppler and confirmed by PW Doppler during the first few weeks of the postoperative period.[17,31] Small residual leaks are not hemodynamically significant and usually disappear in time. It is estimated that 25% of children who have undergone surgical closure have persistent residual VSDs that are of no hemodynamic significance.[17] Residual VSDs must be differentiated from patches that come loose and result in significant shunts.

### ATRIOVENTRICULAR CANAL DEFECTS

Atrioventricular canal (AVC) defects, also referred to as *atrioventricular septal defects* (AVSD) or *endocardial cushion defects*, occur when the atrial and ventricular components of the cardiac septum fail to develop properly.[10] This results in a communication between the atria, the ventricles, or both. There are several anatomic components to this entity, and a particular patient may have any number of them. The components include *ostium primum ASD*, *inlet VSD*, *common atrioventricular valve*, and *cleft mitral valve*. Ostium primum ASD and inlet VSD have been described above.

A *common atrioventricular valve* is a single, often four- or five-leaflet valve that is displaced inferiorly and straddles the interventricular septum. The chordae of the leaflets may attach to papillary muscles in either ventricle or to the interventricular septum.[11,52] Common atrioventricular valves are accompanied by inlet VSDs. The VSDs of AVC are generally large and nonrestrictive. On occasion, restrictive inlet VSDs may be seen and a pressure gradient can be appreciated between the ventricles.[52] Straddling tricuspid valves may also be seen with inlet VSDs. The right ventricle is usually hypoplastic, and chordal attachments are to both sides of the interventricular septum or to the left and right ventricular papillary muscles.[52]

If an ostium primum ASD coexists with an inlet VSD and common atrioventricular valve, the defect is referred to as a *complete AVC* or *complete endocardial cushion defect.* Complete AVC is most often found in patients with Down's syndrome.[11] In the classic form of complete AVC, the right and left ventricles are similar in size,[53] but unbalanced types also exist in which one ventricle is small. Complete AVC may be a feature of complex congenital heart disease.[11]

Mitral insufficiency is a common complication of AVC defects. The anterior leaflet of the mitral valve often develops abnormally into two components that do not coapt well during systole, resulting in varying degrees of mitral insufficiency. This condition is called *cleft mitral valve.*[11,52] Although cleft mitral valves usually are associated with AVC defects, they are occasionally seen as isolated lesions.[52] Isolated cleft mitral valves result from a different embryonic malformation[38] but have similar echocardiographic characteristics.[53]

*Hemodynamics.* Since the septal defects usually are quite large, the degree of shunting through the ASD or VSD of an AVC is generally determined by the relative pulmonary and systemic resistance and the compliance of the ventricles. The combined pressure and volume overload to the pulmonary bed causes patients to develop pulmonary vascular disease at an early age.[13] Elevated pulmonary artery pressures (and therefore right ventricular pressures) result in a pattern of shunting in which blood flows from left to right when left-sided pressures are higher, and from right to left when right-sided pressures are higher. This process is referred to as bidirectional shunting, as the pattern reverses several times during a single cardiac cycle as instantaneous pressures change in the respective ventricles.

*Echocardiographic findings and quantification.*
TWO-DIMENSIONAL ECHOCARDIOGRAPHY
*Visualization of the ostium primum ASD or inlet VSD (apical four-chamber and subxiphoid long-axis views[51-53]; Fig. 19-5A,B)

*Visualization of the common atrioventricular valve (apical four-chamber, subxiphoid long- and short-axis, and parasternal short-axis views[32,52,53]; see Fig. 19-5A,B)
*Delineation of chordal insertions of atrioventricular valve leaflets (apical four-chamber, subxiphoid long-axis views[10,32,52,53,58]; see Fig. 19-5A,B)
*Visualization of the cleft mitral valve as two anterior components opening peripherally in place of the usual appearance of the anterior mitral valve leaflet (parasternal short-axis view[51-53]; Fig. 19-5C)
—Dilated right atrium[53]
—Dilated right ventricle[53]
—Dilated pulmonary artery

M-MODE ECHOCARDIOGRAPHY
*"Mitral valve" leaflet appears to cross the interventricular septum into the right ventricle[10,11]
—Evaluate pulmonic valve tracing for evidence of pulmonary hypertension

DOPPLER ECHOCARDIOGRAPHY
*Shunt flow through ostium primum ASD on PW or color-flow Doppler examination[31]
+Assess severity of atrioventricular valve regurgitation[11,32,58] by PW or color-flow Doppler[31]
+Evaluate bidirectional shunting or quantitate pressure gradient through VSD[11] by PW, CW, and color-flow Doppler (parasternal position)
+Evaluate pulmonary artery PW Doppler tracing for evidence of pulmonary hypertension[11]
+Estimate of pulmonary vascular resistance by CW Doppler determination of pulmonary insufficiency gradient[58]

*Treatment.* Complete AVD is treated surgically during the first year of life, when medical management of congestive heart failure is unsuccessful, or before the risk of developing irreversible pulmonary vascular obstructive disease becomes unacceptable.[11] There are two options for surgical treatment: palliation by pulmonary artery banding or definitive repair. Definitive repair is preferred. This involves closure of the ASD and VSD, reconstruction of the atrioventricular valve into competent mitral and tricuspid valves, and repair of associated malformations.[11] Pulmonary artery banding may be the only surgical option if there is chordal in-

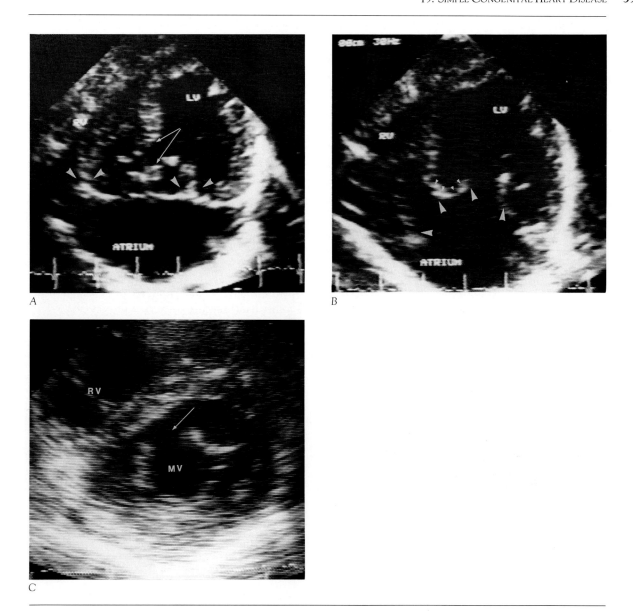

Figure 19-5. Echocardiographic findings of atrioventricular canal (AVC) defects. (A) Two-dimensional visualization of complete AVC during systole (apical four-chamber view). The small arrow points to the VSD component, and the large arrowheads point to the closed common atrioventricular valve. This patient has a single atrium. (B) Two-dimensional visualization of the AVC shown in A open during diastole. Note the VSD may not be appreciated when the common atrioventricular valve is open. Small arrowheads point to the bridging leaflet of the single atrioventricular valve. Large arrowheads point to common atrioventricular valve leaflets. (C) Two-dimensional visualization of an open cleft mitral valve (MV) during diastole (parasternal short-axis view). The arrow points to the cleft in the anterior mitral valve leaflet. (RV, LV, right and left ventricles.)

sertion into the ipsilateral ventricle. In such a case, closure of the inlet VSD may result in severe atrioventricular valve regurgitation.[46] Pulmonary artery banding is the surgical creation of a pulmonary artery stenosis by tying a band around the main pulmonary artery to limit flow to the pulmonary vascular bed.

### PATENT DUCTUS ARTERIOSUS

The ductus arteriosus connects the left or main pulmonary artery to the descending aorta obliquely, immediately distal to the left subclavian artery. During fetal life, 55 to 60% of the combined ventricular output is shunted from the pulmonary artery to the descending aorta through the ductus arteriosus, thus bypassing the lungs.[29] Within the first day of life, the ductus arteriosus should begin to close,[13,29] becoming a strand called the ligamentum arteriosum by around 3 weeks of age.[29] When this process does not occur and the ductus arteriosus remains open, it is referred to as a *patent ductus arteriosus* (PDA). Spontaneous PDA closure is often delayed in premature newborns, particularly in infants with lower birth weights.[29] In general, isolated PDAs are more common in females than in males.[13] The incidence of PDAs has been reported to be 30 times greater in areas of high altitude (>4500 m) over that in populations at sea level, and is thought to be due to arterial hypoxemia. PDA is frequently associated with pulmonary artery stenosis in infants with rubella syndrome, and may be familial.[29]

*Hemodynamics.* During fetal life, pulmonary resistance is greater than systemic resistance, so blood flows from the main pulmonary artery, through the ductus arteriosus to the descending aorta (i.e., right to left). Within the first few days of life, pulmonary vascular resistance—and therefore pulmonary artery pressure—decreases to below aortic pressure, causing blood flow through the PDA to shunt from left to right. The volume of blood shunted is determined by the size of the PDA and the pulmonary-systemic pressure gradient which in turn is determined by the difference between pulmonary and systemic resistance.[29] A left-to-right shunt results in increased flow volume through the lungs, and consequently the left side of the heart. The left atrium and later the left ventricle dilate in response to the increased blood volume. A large volume overload may induce left ventricular failure.[29] In time, the volume overload to the pulmonary bed may result in pulmonary hypertension.[13] With elevated pulmonary artery pressure or interrupted aortic arch, the shunting through the ductus will be from right to left. In these cases, 2-D visualization of the duct and Doppler detection of flow through the duct from the pulmonary artery to the descending aorta should be documented.

*Echocardiographic findings and quantification.*

TWO-DIMENSIONAL ECHOCARDIOGRAPHY

*A large PDA may be visualized coming from the left or main pulmonary artery (high parasternal long-axis view of the right ventricular outflow tract[47,53]; Fig. 19-6A,B)

*A large PDA may be visualized entering the descending aorta at the level of the subclavian ar-

---

▶

FIGURE 19-6. (See color insert for C and D.) Echocardiographic findings of patent ductus arteriosus (PDA). (A) Two-dimensional visualization of a PDA connecting the PA and descending aorta (DAO) (parasternal short-axis view). (B) Two-dimensional visualization of large PDA opening into the main pulmonary artery (MPA) to the left of the left pulmonary artery branch (L). Right pulmonary artery branch (R). (C) Color-flow Doppler was added to B to visualize lateral jet of flow from the PDA into the MPA. (D) PW Doppler spectral tracing obtained from the MPA shows normal, laminar pulmonic flow away from the transducer in systole (small arrow), and harsh, turbulent flow toward the transducer in diastole. The diastolic flow (large arrow) represents the PDA shunt into the MPA. (E) PW Doppler spectral tracing of the descending aorta just above the diaphragm (subxiphoid transducer position). Normal aortic flow is seen as laminar flow coming toward the transducer in systole. The reversal of flow seen in diastole represents retrograde aortic flow to fill a large PDA. (RVOT, right ventricular outflow tract; AO, aorta; PA, pulmonary artery; RA, LA, right and left atria.)

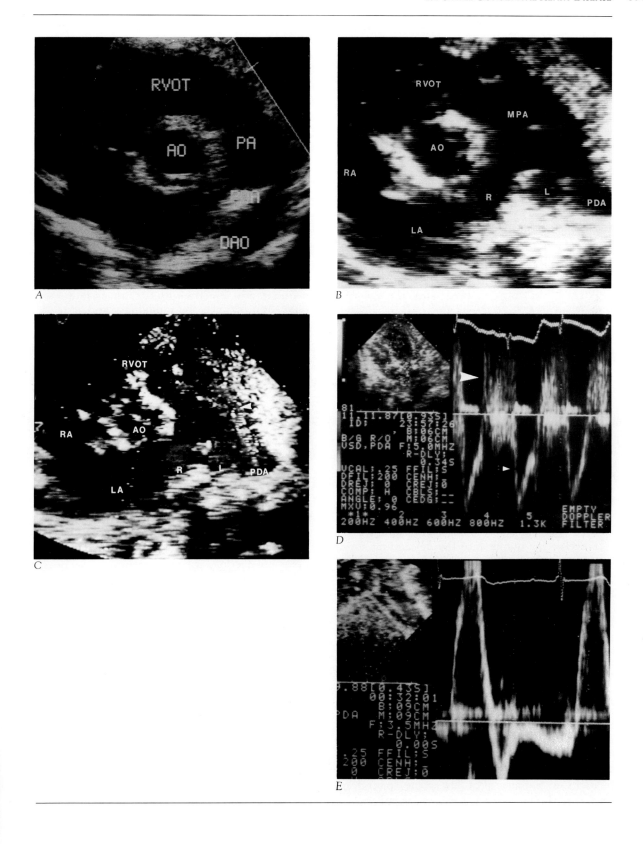

tery (suprasternal notch, left subclavicular or high parasternal position)[30]

*The entire length of a large PDA may be visualized (subxiphoid short-axis, suprasternal notch, or left subclavicular view)[55]

—Dilated left atrium
—Dilated left ventricle
—Dilated main pulmonary artery

M-MODE ECHOCARDIOGRAPHY

—Dilated left atrium[47]
—Increased ratio of diameter of left atrium to aorta (diameter measurements from the parasternal position)
—Dilated left ventricle[47]

DOPPLER ECHOCARDIOGRAPHY

*Color-flow Doppler visualization of ductal flow into the main or left pulmonary artery as a red, mosaic diastolic jet along the lateral superior border of the vessel (parasternal short-axis or parasternal long-axis views[31,40]; Fig. 19-6C)

*PW Doppler detection of diastolic flow in the pulmonary artery toward and/or away from the transducer, depending on the entry angle of the duct relative to the Doppler sample volume (parasternal position[56]; Fig. 19-6D)

*PW or color-flow Doppler detection of reversal of flow throughout diastole in the descending aorta distal to takeoff of the subclavian artery[40] (suprasternal notch, left subclavicular, or subxiphoid position; Fig. 19-6E)

*Normal aortic flow pattern detected by PW Doppler proximal to the subclavian artery and the entrance of the ductus into the descending aorta (suprasternal notch, left subclavicular, or subxiphoid position)

—Increased flow detected through the mitral and aortic valve by PW Doppler (apical position)

—Left-to-right shunt may be appreciated through a patent foramen ovale, which may become stretched secondary to left atrial dilatation[29]

*Discussion of Doppler findings.* Reversal of flow in the descending aorta, and continuous flow in the pulmonary artery may be seen in any type of systemic-to-pulmonary shunt. The most common systemic-to-pulmonary shunt is PDA. Others include aortic-to-pulmonary artery window, and surgically created shunts. Reversal of flow in the descending aorta may also be due to severe aortic insufficiency,

and continuous flow in the pulmonary artery may be due to pulmonary insufficiency.

*Treatment.* In the preterm infant, PDAs often close successfully in response to administration of indomethacin, but indomethacin is ineffective in the treatment of term infants.[29] In older patients and patients in whom indomethacin treatment fails, PDAs may be corrected by interventional catheterization or by surgery. Interventional catheterization techniques involve transcatheter placement of a foam plastic plug[29] or an umbrella device[37,40] within the ductus to occlude the lumen. Surgical correction involves ligation with transection. (Ligation alone carries risks of recanalization and tearing.)[29]

PDA frequently is associated with complex congenital heart disease. Often, the infant relies on the patency of the ductus arteriosus to maintain communication between the pulmonary and systemic circulation.[18] In such a case, the congenital heart defect is said to be duct dependent and the PDA is kept patent medically by administration of prostaglandin $E_1$ until a pulmonary-systemic shunt can be created surgically.[29] One of the important uses of echocardiography is to rule out the presence of a duct-dependent lesion when PDA is diagnosed clinically.

## Primary Obstructive Lesions

Obstructive lesions in children usually are due to congenital malformations of the inflow or outflow tracts. As with acquired obstructive lesions, the primary hemodynamic problem is increased afterload or pressure overload to the chamber or vessel proximal to the obstruction. Because left-sided obstruction may occur at multiple levels in one patient's heart, the discovery of a left-sided obstruction should prompt a thorough search for additional sites of obstruction.

The severity of an obstruction is estimated by calculating the instantaneous pressure gradient across it. The highest instantaneous velocity across the obstruction as determined by CW Doppler is converted into an estimated pressure gradient by applying the modified Bernoulli equation, as discussed above. When estimating the severity of obstruction by the use of Doppler echocardiography, cardiac output[28] and flow volume must be considered. Significant variations in cardiac output may generate misleading pressure gradients and lead to an inaccurate estimate of obstructive severity. The volume of flow through an obstruction may be affected by intracardiac shunts, extracardiac shunts, and regurgitation. The echocardiographer must consider the effect of flow volume on the pressure gradient. For example, if the volume of flow is reduced due to an intracardiac shunt out of the chamber or vessel proximal to the obstruction, then the detected pressure gradient will be low and the severity of the obstruction will be underestimated.[56]

### LEFT VENTRICULAR OUTFLOW OBSTRUCTION

Left ventricular outflow may be obstructed proximally (in the left ventricular outflow tract), at the level of the aortic valve, or distally (in the aorta). Valvular obstruction accounts for 90% of cases of left ventricular outflow obstruction.[20] The hemodynamic consequences of outflow obstruction are similar to those seen with acquired valvular aortic stenosis, principally, thickening of the left ventricular wall.

*Bicuspid Aortic Valve.* Bicuspid aortic valve is the most common congenital heart defect[15] and is thought to be present in 1% of the general population.[18] The aortic valve develops two cusps instead of the usual three. The third commissure is fused and may often be visualized as a raphe, or ridge, on the larger of the two aortic cusps.[53] Bicuspid aortic valves have a tendency to become stenotic during adulthood.[20] Valvular aortic stenosis is four times as common in males as in females. Associated cardiac anomalies occur in 20% of cases, usually coarctation of the aorta.[15]

*Hemodynamics.* The hemodynamics of bicuspid aortic valve range from virtually no obstruction or insufficiency to severe degrees of either. Obstruction to outflow results in increased pressure within the left ventricle, which causes the muscle of the left ventricle to become hypertrophic. If aortic valve insufficiency coexists, the left ventricle may be dilated.

*Echocardiographic findings and quantification.*
TWO-DIMENSIONAL ECHOCARDIOGRAPHY
*Visualization of an oval orifice during systole (parasternal short-axis view; Fig. 19-7)
*Visualization of only two functioning cusps (para-

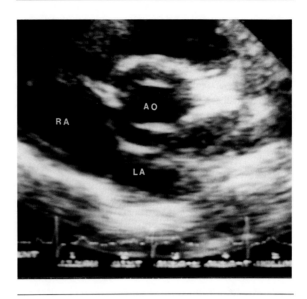

FIGURE 19-7. Two-dimensional visualization of a bicuspid aortic valve (parasternal short-axis view) during systole. (RA, LA, right and left atria; Ao, aorta.)

sternal short-axis view; Fig. 19-7)
—Cusps may appear pliant and move well or may appear stenotic
—Doming of the aortic valve cusps (parasternal long-axis view)[15]

M-MODE ECHOCARDIOGRAPHY
—Aortic eccentricity index greater than 1.5 in some cases
—Reduced aortic valve excursion[15]
+Estimated LV pressure = 225

$$\times \frac{\text{LV posterior wall thickness at end systole}^{5,15}}{\text{LV end-systolic diameter}}$$

DOPPLER ECHOCARDIOGRAPHY
*Turbulent, high-velocity systolic flow detected distal to the aortic valve by PW or color-flow Doppler[31]
+Estimation of pressure gradient by CW Doppler (apical, suprasternal notch, high right parasternal positions)[28,53,56]
—Prolonged time to peak velocity[28]
+Calculation of AT/LVET ratio[28]
—Associated aortic insufficiency may be detected by PW, CW, or color-flow Doppler

*Discussion of echocardiographic findings and quantification.* The aortic eccentricity index is a measure of the degree of eccentricity of the aortic valve closure line within the aortic root on an M-mode tracing of the valve. The calculation is done by multiplying the aortic root diameter by 0.5 then dividing by the distance between closure line of aortic valve and wall of aortic root during diastole.[15]

The time required to reach peak systolic velocity through the aortic valve increases as the severity of obstruction increases. The ratio of acceleration time (AT), defined as the time to peak velocity of flow, to left ventricular ejection time (LVET) greater than 0.30, as determined from a maximum velocity CW Doppler tracing, has been reported by Hatle and coworkers[28] to suggest a pressure gradient greater than 50 mm Hg. A ratio of 0.55 or greater is considered an indication for surgery. Severe mitral regurgitation or left ventricular failure may create a false positive result by shortening left ventricular ejection time. Severe aortic insufficiency may create a false negative result by increasing left ventricular ejection time.[28]

*Treatment.* Prophylaxis against subacute bacterial endocarditis is recommended for all patients with bicuspid aortic valve.[20] Medical and surgical treatments for bicuspid aortic valve are reserved for patients with severe stenosis. Surgical commissurotomy or valve replacement is offered when the peak systolic pressure gradient is higher than 75 mm Hg[15,20] or when the orifice is estimated to be smaller than 0.5 cm$^2$/m$^2$ body surface area, at which time aortic stenosis is considered to be critical.[15] Currently, percutaneous balloon valvuloplasty of the aortic valve is being utilized as well to relieve isolated valve obstruction.[15,34]

*Unicuspid Aortic Valve.* A unicuspid aortic valve is virtually a membrane or dome with an orifice.[15] In this rare malformation, only one commissure is not fused. The restricted orifice results in varying degrees of stenosis,[53] usually severe. Usually there is also some degree of insufficiency, as the orifice courses from the annulus to the center of the valve and coaptation of the edges is inadequate during diastole.

*Aortic Hypoplasia.* Aortic hypoplasia is part of the spectrum of hypoplastic left heart syndrome.[15] The aortic annulus is small. The cusps may be relatively normal or dysplastic. Secondary findings on echocardiography are similar to severe or critical valvular aortic stenosis.

*Aortic Atresia.* In aortic atresia, an imperforate membrane exists where the aortic valve leaflets should have differentiated. There may be a hypoplastic or interrupted aortic arch.[1]

*Hypoplastic Left Heart Syndrome.* In hemodynamically complex cases of hypoplastic left heart syndrome, the entire left heart is hypoplastic, stenotic, or atretic. The left atrium, mitral valve, left ventricle, aortic valve, and aorta are involved with various degrees of underdevelopment. An ASD may shunt pulmonary venous return to the right side of the heart, and a large PDA supplies the descending aorta, as the ascending aorta is hypoplastic.[53]

*Treatment.* Treatment for hypoplastic left heart syndrome is cardiac transplantation or a two-stage surgical procedure known as the Norwood procedure.[2]

*Coarctation of the Aorta.* Coarctation of the aorta is a constrictive malformation of the aortic arch, usually located just distal to the origin of the left subclavian artery from the aortic arch. This anomaly is slightly more common in males than in females.[24] In the classic case, a ridge of tissue protrudes into the lumen of the posterior aspect of the aorta, immediately distal to the left subclavian artery, opposite the entrance of the ductus arteriosus. This area often is narrowed. In severe cases, a segment of the arch may be hypoplastic.[24]

Coarctation of the aorta creates a pressure increase proximally and a pressure decrease distally. This malformation is suspected when hypertension is noted in an infant, child, or adolescent. Upon further evaluation, decreased pulse pressure may be appreciated in the lower extremities and a significant systolic pressure difference between the right arm and the lower extremities.[19]

Coarctation of the aorta is associated with other cardiac and noncardiac anomalies. The most frequent association (40 to 80% of cases) is with bicuspid aortic valve,[19,24,36] but because subaortic stenosis and other forms of left-sided heart obstruction may coexist systematic investigation is required.[24] Isolated coarctation may present clinically any time from the neonatal period through adulthood, depending on the severity of the obstruction. When associated with major intracardiac abnormalities, the coarctation is generally preductal in location and symptoms appear during infancy.[19] Coarctation of the aorta may be associated with VSD,[36] transposition of the great arteries, mitral valve disease,[19] Taussig-Bing double-outlet right ventricle, and other abnormalities that do not have a component of severe right-sided heart obstruction.[24] Coarctation of the aorta and other left-sided heart obstructions are common in females with Turner's syndrome. Some patients have associated cerebral aneurysms. The elevated systolic blood pressure in these vessels in the presence of a significant coarctation increases their risk for cerebrovascular accidents.[17,24]

*Hemodynamics.* In coarctation of the aorta, blood pressure builds proximal to the site of obstruction. Pressures are elevated in the arm and head vessels and in the arch, ascending aorta, and left ventricle. Patients often develop collateral circulation to compensate for the decrease in blood flow distal to the obstruction.[19] Beyond the obstruction, pulsatility is damped; therefore the Doppler waveform also is damped and often it does not return to baseline during diastole. Poststenotic dilatation of the descending aorta may occur distal to the obstruction.

*Echocardiographic findings and quantification.*
TWO-DIMENSIONAL ECHOCARDIOGRAPHY
*Narrowing of the juxtaductal portion of the aortic arch (suprasternal notch, high parasternal,[30] supraclavicular[53] views)
*Discrete membrane or ridge appreciated in the juxtaductal area of the aortic arch (suprasternal notch, high parasternal, and subxiphoid views[23,30,36]; Fig. 19-7A,B)
—Poststenotic dilatation of the descending aorta distal to the obstruction (Fig. 19-8A,B)
—Proximal portion of the arch may be small
—Secondary findings similar to those of aortic valve stenosis

DOPPLER ECHOCARDIOGRAPHY
*Normal PW Doppler waveform in the aortic arch, proximal to the subclavian artery[53]

*Low-velocity waveform with prolonged acceleration and deceleration times[23,36,56] and spectral broadening detected in the abdominal aorta by PW Doppler (subxiphoid position; Fig. 19-8C)
*High-velocity jet detected in the descending thoracic aorta by PW or CW Doppler (suprasternal notch position)[23,36,53,56,58]
+Estimation of instantaneous pressure gradient across the coarctation site by CW Doppler (suprasternal notch position); color-flow Doppler may facilitate alignment of the CW Doppler beam with the stenotic jet[31,53,58]

*Discussion of echocardiographic findings and quantification.* When attempting to determine the pressure gradient through the coarctation site by continuous-wave Doppler from the suprasternal notch position, the flow velocity distal to the obstruction may be superimposed on the tracing. Estimation of the instantaneous pressure should take into account a high velocity of flow distal to the coarctation site.[36,58] With severe coarctation there may be little detectable flow through the coarctation site, due to the development of collateral circulation.[56,58] A coexisting PDA also complicates gradient estimates.[58]

*Treatment.* The mortality rate for uncorrected coarctation of the aorta is reported to be 20% during the first and second decades of life and 80% by the fifth decade, so correction during childhood is recommended.[24] Surgical correction may involve resection of the coarctation site and end-to-end reanastamosis of the aorta. Alternative surgical procedures include excising the membranous shelf of the coarctation, then widening the aortic lumen with a patch or turning down the proximal portion of a divided left subclavian artery (the subclavian flap procedure). In cases of diffuse narrowing or interruption, a conduit may be placed.[19,24]

*Discrete Membranous Subaortic Stenosis.* Discrete membranous subaortic stenosis accounts for about 10% of congenital forms of aortic stenosis and is twice as common in males as in females. A ring of tissue develops within the left ventricular outflow tract, creating an obstruction proximal to the aortic valve. This fibromuscular ring may be concentric or eccentric.[15] When discrete membranous subaortic stenosis, coarctation of the aorta, supra-

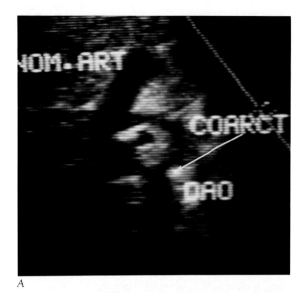

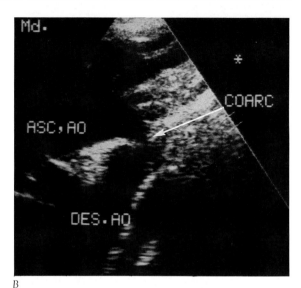

A

B

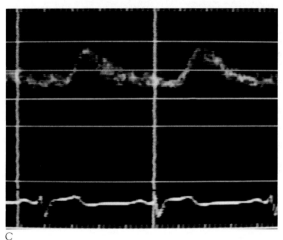

C

Figure 19-8. Echocardiographic findings of coarctation of the aorta (COARC). (A) Two-dimensional visualization of coarctation shelf (suprasternal notch view). Note poststenotic dilatation of the aorta distal to the obstruction. (B) Two-dimensional visualization of coarctation membrane (suprasternal notch view). Note poststenotic dilatation of the aorta distal to the obstruction. (ASC, AO, ascending aorta; DES, AO, descending aorta.) (C) PW Doppler spectral tracing of descending aortic flow (subxiphoid transducer position). Note blunted waveform indicating decreased pulsatility and slow deceleration rate.

valvular mitral ring, and parachute mitral valve all occur in the patient, this is described as Shone syndrome.[53]

*Hemodynamics.* The hemodynamic sequelae of membranous subaortic stenosis are generally similar to those of aortic valve stenosis. A unique finding in subaortic stenosis is that the high-velocity jet created by the membrane may damage the aortic cusps, causing aortic insufficiency.[20] In some cases, the abnormal tissue of the membrane is actually adherent to the aortic cusps and may contribute to the development of aortic insufficiency.[15]

*Echocardiographic findings and quantification.*

TWO-DIMENSIONAL ECHOCARDIOGRAPHY

*Bright, linear echo visualized throughout the cardiac cycle in the left ventricular outflow tract immediately proximal and parallel to the aortic valve (parasternal long-axis, apical five-chamber, and apical two-chamber views[15,53]; Fig. 19-9A)

*Bright, distinct echoes visualized on the anterior aspect of the anterior mitral valve leaflet, near the mitral annulus[15,53]

—Secondary findings similar to aortic valve stenosis

FIGURE 19-9. Echocardiographic findings of discrete subaortic membrane. (A) Two-dimensional visualization of discrete subaortic membrane (MEMB; parasternal long-axis view). (B) M-mode example of early systolic closure of the aortic valve (*small arrow*). The arrowhead points to the subaortic membrane in the 2-D image. (RV, LV, right and left ventricles; AO, aorta; LA, left atrium; AV, aortic valve.)

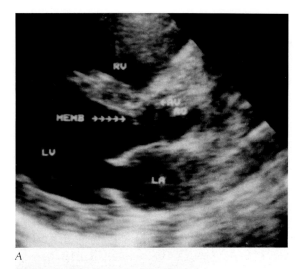

*A*

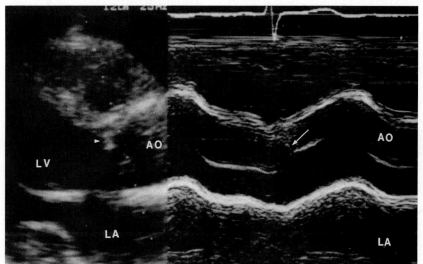

*B*

M-MODE ECHOCARDIOGRAPHY
—Coarse systolic fluttering of the aortic cusps
—Early systolic closure of the aortic valve[15,53] (Fig. 19-9B)
—Secondary findings similar to aortic valve stenosis

DOPPLER ECHOCARDIOGRAPHY
*Increased velocity and turbulence of systolic flow proximal to the aortic valve by PW Doppler[15,28]
+Estimation of pressure gradient by CW Doppler[53]
+Quantification of associated aortic insufficiency by PW or color-flow Doppler[53]

*Treatment.* In most cases, the membrane is excised surgically to relieve the obstruction and avoid the development or progression of aortic insufficiency.[15]

*Idiopathic Hypertrophic Subaortic Stenosis.* Idiopathic hypertrophic subaortic stenosis (IHSS) is a form of hypertrophic cardiomyopathy. Other names for IHSS are asymmetric septal hypertrophy (ASH) and hypertrophic obstructive cardiomyopathy (HOCM). The hallmark of this type of cardiomyopathy is asymmetric thickening of the interventricular septum, which then acts as a dynamic left ventricular outflow obstruction. IHSS is thought to be transmitted genetically and is more common in males than in females.[20] This disease process is described in greater detail in Chapter 11.

*Tunnel Subaortic Stenosis.* Tunnel subaortic stenosis is a rare, diffuse form of obstruction in which the entire left ventricular outflow tract is narrowed. There is valvular as well as subvalvular obstruction.

*Echocardiographic findings and quantification.*

TWO-DIMENSIONAL ECHOCARDIOGRAPHY

*Diffusely narrowed left ventricular outflow tract[53] (Fig. 19-10)
—Thick aortic valve cusps[15,53]
—Hypoplastic ascending aorta and aortic annulus[15,53]
—Secondary findings similar to those of aortic valve stenosis

M-MODE ECHOCARDIOGRAPHY

*Diffusely narrowed left ventricular outflow tract
—Secondary findings similar to those of aortic valve stenosis

DOPPLER ECHOCARDIOGRAPHY

+Estimation of pressure gradients by CW Doppler

*Treatment.* In severe cases, the pressure in the left ventricle may be relieved by providing a second outflow tract to the ventricle by surgically placing a valved conduit from the left ventricle to the aorta. One end of the conduit is sewn into the apex of the heart; the other end is connected to the descending aorta below the diaphragm. The valve in the conduit is located superficially at the lateral aspect of the abdomen, to enable the surgeon to replace the valve if it becomes insufficient.[50,63] Competency of the valve may be evaluated by two-dimensional and Doppler echocardiography. An-

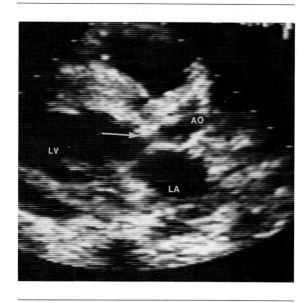

FIGURE 19-10. Two-dimensional visualization of tunnel subaortic stenosis *(arrow)* on parasternal long-axis view. Note thickness of left ventricular (LV) walls. (LA, left atrium; Ao, aorta.)

other surgical procedure to relieve the pressure in the left ventricle is Konno's procedure, in which the aortic annulus and left ventricular outflow tract are widened.[15]

*Supravalvular Aortic Stenosis.* Supravalvular aortic stenosis occurs directly superior to the exit of the coronary arteries from the ascending aorta. The stenosis may be a discrete hourglass constriction of the ascending aortic lumen, a discrete fibromuscular membrane, or diffuse hypoplasia of the aortic root.[15,20] Associated lesions include valvular aortic stenosis, valvular pulmonic stenosis, and mitral valve anomalies. Supravalvular aortic stenosis may be familial or sporadic; often it is found in patients with William's syndrome.[15] Surgical treatment involves resection of the membrane, widening of the aortic root, or aortic root replacement. Surgery is recommended when the systolic pressure gradient by catheterization surpasses 50 mm Hg.[15]

LEFT VENTRICULAR INFLOW OBSTRUCTION

Several types of obstruction to left ventricular inflow occur as a result of congenital anomalies. As with acquired mitral stenosis, the hemodynamic result is rising pulmonary pressures, leading to increased pulmonary vascular resistance, and eventually, pulmonary hypertension. Congenital heart lesions associated with mitral valve stenosis include other left heart obstruction, ostium secundum and primum ASD, transposition of the great vessels, and double-outlet right ventricle.[3]

*Echocardiographic evaluation.*
TWO-DIMENSIONAL ECHOCARDIOGRAPHY
*Delineation of left atrial, mitral valve, chordae, papillary muscle, and left ventricular anatomy (parasternal long-axis and short-axis and apical four-chamber views)[3,52]
−Dilated left atrium
−Small left ventricle

M-MODE ECHOCARDIOGRAPHY
−Measurement of left atrium and left ventricle
−Evaluation of mitral valve leaflet motion

DOPPLER ECHOCARDIOGRAPHY
+Estimation of pressure gradient by CW Doppler (apical position)[56]
+Derivation of orifice size by pressure half-time calculation[3,52] (see Chapter 9)

*Mitral Valve Stenosis.* Congenital mitral valve stenosis is rare. Abnormal embryonic development of the mitral valve apparatus may result in dysplastic valves with thickened, lobular leaflets, abnormal commissure development, fused or shortened chordae, and closely spaced, hypertrophic papillary muscles.[51−53] The left ventricle is often small. Echocardiographic findings are similar to those of acquired mitral stenosis, except that there is no calcification.

*Mitral Valve Hypoplasia.* A hypoplastic mitral valve has a small but normally developed annulus and small but normally formed leaflets. The left ventricle is also small, and associated left ventricular outflow obstruction is common.[3] Differentiation from mitral atresia depends on 2-D visualization of leaflet separation in the parasternal and apical views[52] and Doppler evidence of flow through the valve. This malformation often is part of hypoplastic left heart syndrome.[1,3,52] Survival beyond the neonatal

period is unusual if the left ventricle is smaller than 70% of normal size.[3]

*Mitral Atresia.* In mitral atresia, the mitral leaflets fail to develop normally. A dense tissue membrane covers the mitral annulus. The membrane is imperforate.[52] Mitral valve atresia is usually part of hypoplastic left heart syndrome, although it may also be seen as part of a single ventricle malformation. Rarely, in the presence of a large VSD, mitral atresia may be found with a normal left ventricle and a normal aortic valve. This form of mitral atresia may be surgically palliated.[3] Straddling tricuspid valve and double-outlet right ventricle may be associated findings.[52]

*Parachute Mitral Valve.* Parachute mitral valve is a malformation in which the chordae of both leaflets of the mitral valve converge onto a single prominent papillary muscle (usually the posteromedial one) or onto a group of fused papillary muscles within the left ventricle.[53] Papillary muscle anatomy is variable; there may be two papillary muscles, only one of which receives chordae.[3,52] Associated findings include supramitral ring, subvalvular aortic stenosis, valvular aortic stenosis, coarctation of the aorta, and right ventricular outflow obstruction.[3,52]

*Echocardiographic findings and quantification.*
TWO-DIMENSIONAL ECHOCARDIOGRAPHY
−Thin, pliant mitral valve leaflets and chordae (all views)[53]
−Mitral leaflet motion restricted so that valve opens in a funnel shape or domes (all views)[53]
−Single prominent papillary muscle or two partially fused muscles visualized in the left ventricle[53]
*All mitral valve chordae may be traced to insert onto a single papillary muscle
−Thick and short chordae
−Dilated left atrium

M-MODE ECHOCARDIOGRAPHY
−Decreased excursion of thin mitral valve leaflets[53]
−Movement of posterior mitral leaflet parallels that of anterior leaflet[53]
−Dilated left atrium

DOPPLER ECHOCARDIOGRAPHY

*Turbulent flow detected distal to the mitral valve by PW and color-flow Doppler

*Increased velocity of flow detected through the mitral valve by PW and color-flow Doppler

+Quantification of transmitral flow gradient by CW Doppler[53]

*Cor Triatriatum.* Cor triatriatum is a rare[53] malformation in which the membrane that results from the fusion of the common pulmonary veins and the embryonic left atrium does not regress completely. A fibrous membrane remains which divides the left atrium into upper and lower chambers. The membrane is located immediately superior to the left atrial appendage and the fossa ovalis[51,53,62] All of the pulmonary veins drain into the upper chamber. The lower chamber communicates with the mitral valve. The size and location of the communication(s) in the membrane vary and often are not appreciated by 2-D echocardiography.

*Hemodynamics.* The degree of obstruction to mitral inflow is a function of the size and number of communications.

*Echocardiographic findings and quantifications.*
TWO-DIMENSIONAL ECHOCARDIOGRAPHY

*Thin membrane visualized coursing anterior to posterior in the left atrium (apical four-chamber, parasternal long-axis, or subxiphoid long-axis view[51]; Fig. 19-11)

—Membrane appears to move toward the mitral valve during diastole (when the valve is open) and away from the valve during systole[51,62]

—Dilated left atrium[62]

—Normal-sized left ventricle

—Normal appearance of mitral valve leaflets, chordae, and papillary muscles

—Dilated right ventricle[67]

M-MODE ECHOCARDIOGRAPHY

—Reduced E to F slope of mitral valve[1]

—Fluttering of posterior mitral valve leaflet[1]

DOPPLER ECHOCARDIOGRAPHY

*Turbulent, high-velocity flow detected proximal to the mitral valve by PW or color-flow Doppler (apical or parasternal positions)

+Quantification of stenotic gradient by CW Doppler (apical position)

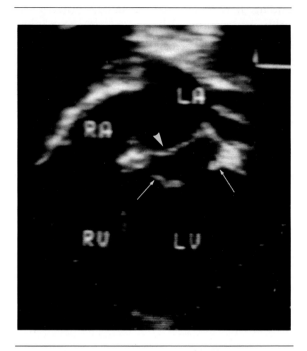

FIGURE 19-11. Two-dimensional visualization of cortriatriatum (apical four-chamber view). Small arrows point to the mitral valve leaflets; large arrowhead points to the membrane. (RA, LA, right and left atria; RV, LV, right and left ventricles.)

*Treatment.* The membrane is surgically excised to reverse or prevent the development of pulmonary hypertension secondary to increased resistance to left atrial filling.[3]

*Supravalvular Mitral Ring.* The ring of connective tissue referred to as a supravalvular mitral ring is located immediately superior to the mitral valve annulus—and therefore inferior to the left atrial appendage and fossa ovalis.[51–53] Supravalvular mitral ring presents with echocardiographic findings similar to cor triatriatum and differs only in placement within the atrium. Supravalvular mitral ring is more common than cor triatriatum.[53] The ring of tissue may be very close and actually adherent to the mitral valve apparatus. Meticulous investigation from the subxiphoid and parasternal views is required, as the proximity of the membrane to the valve often may be appreciated only on diastolic stop frames.[62] Isolated supramitral ring is a rare finding. It is usually associated with other mitral valve abnormalities.[3,52,53]

*Arcade Mitral Valve.* In this extremely rare congenital malformation, short, fused chordae from thickened mitral valve leaflets attach to multiple small papillary muscles of the left ventricle,[1] or to a bar of fibrous tissue connecting the two major papillary muscles of the left ventricle.[52] As would be expected, M-mode criteria used to assess severity of acquired mitral stenosis are not useful in these cases.[1] Since the coaptation of the mitral leaflets often is affected, there is usually some degree of mitral insufficiency.[3]

*Double-Orifice Mitral Valve.* In this rare congenital malformation, a fibrous tissue bridge divides the mitral valve into two halves, with the chordae from each attaching to their own papillary muscles. Occasionally, the second orifice is in one of the mitral valve leaflets. Double-orifice mitral valve usually is associated with atrioventricular canal defects,[32] and may result in mitral stenosis or regurgitation.[52] This anomaly is best appreciated on 2-D echocardiography from the parasternal short-axis view as what appear to be two side-by-side mitral valve orifices at the tips of the mitral valve leaflets.[53]

### RIGHT VENTRICULAR OUTFLOW OBSTRUCTION
An obstruction to right ventricular outflow may occur proximal to, distal to, or at the level of the pulmonic valve. The right ventricular muscle thickens in response to the pressure overload. Increased muscle mass enables the right ventricle to generate the increased pressure required to push the blood out into the pulmonary artery in systole against the increased resistance caused by the obstruction. Since the free wall of the right ventricle is thinner than that of the left ventricle, the right ventricle may dilate as well as thicken in response to increased pressure.

*Pulmonic Valve Stenosis.* Pulmonic valve stenosis appears similar on echocardiograph to stenosis of any of the other heart valves. The pulmonary cusps may be thickened or dysplastic, and movement is restricted. This form of pulmonic stenosis is found more commonly in males than in females.[13]

*Hemodynamics.* Blood flow through the pulmonic valve is turbulent and accelerated. High-velocity eddy currents produced distal to the valve may cause poststenotic dilatation of the pulmonary artery.[53] The degree of poststenotic dilatation is not predictive of the severity of the obstruction.

*Echocardiographic findings and quantification.*
TWO-DIMENSIONAL ECHOCARDIOGRAPHY
*Thickened pulmonic valve cusps (parasternal short-axis and long-axis views[31,53]; Fig. 19-12A and B)
*Restricted opening or doming of the pulmonic valve cusps (parasternal short-axis and long-axis views[31,53]; Fig. 19-12B)
—Thickened and possibly dilated right ventricle
—Poststenotic dilatation of the main pulmonary artery (parasternal long-axis view)[53]

M-MODE ECHOCARDIOGRAPHY
*Thickened pulmonic valve cusps[1]
—Accentuated a wave on pulmonic valve tracing[1]
—Thickened and possibly dilated right ventricle
—Dilated main pulmonary artery

DOPPLER ECHOCARDIOGRAPHY
—Normal flow velocity in right ventricular outflow tract
*Detection of increased velocity and turbulence of systolic flow distal to the pulmonic valve by PW or color-flow Doppler[31,40]
+Quantification of peak instantaneous gradient by CW Doppler—accuracy increases with proper alignment to flow using color-flow imaging[31,40] (parasternal or subxiphoid position[56])

*Treatment.* Treatment for pulmonic valve stenosis is recommended when the patient has symptoms or a gradient greater than 50 mm Hg.[21] Traditionally, surgical commissurotomy has been the treatment of choice for correcting pulmonic stenosis. In recent years, percutaneous balloon valvuloplasty has become the method of choice,[33] since this procedure may be done in the catheterization laboratory and has been successful in reducing the peak instantaneous gradient[37] while causing minor pulmonary insufficiency in only a few cases. Percutaneous balloon valvuloplasty involves repeatedly inflating a balloon catheter placed at the level of the pulmonic valve for short periods until the cusps of the valve rupture, usually along the fused commissures.

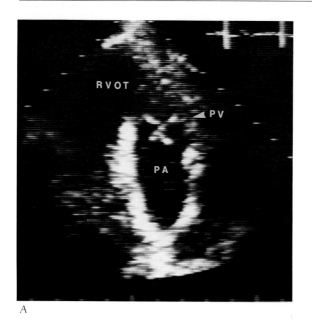
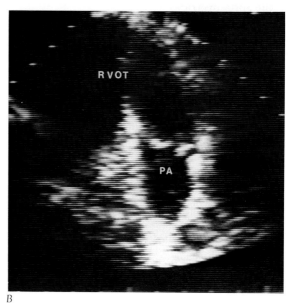

A

B

FIGURE 19-12. Echocardiographic findings of valvular pulmonic stenosis. (A) Two-dimensional visualization of pulmonic valve (PV) during diastole (parasternal short-axis view). Note abnormal appearance of valve. (B) Two-dimensional visualization of pulmonic valve in A in systole. Note doming of PV. (PA, pulmonary artery; RVOT, right ventricular outflow tract.)

*Critical Pulmonic Stenosis.* Critical pulmonic stenosis is a term used to describe severe pulmonic valve stenosis, which may severely restrict flow to the lungs. Patients with this degree of pulmonary stenosis are very ill, and require emergency relief of the obstruction.

*Pulmonary Atresia.* Pulmonary atresia may occur in several forms.[6,8] The first is as an imperforate membrane between the right ventricular outflow tract and the main pulmonary artery. The second is a thick band of tissue between the right ventricular outflow tract and the main pulmonary artery. In the third form, the main pulmonary artery has an atretic section, therefore the pulmonary artery is located at a variable distance from the right ventricular outflow tract. In some cases, a main pulmonary artery fails to form, and branch pulmonary arteries may be located at quite a distance from the right ventricular outflow tract.[6]

*Hemodynamics.* Patients with pulmonary atresia are dependent on a PDA or collateral vessels for blood oxygenation.[6,8,53] Blood is shunted from the descending aorta to the pulmonary artery (left to right). An intracardiac shunt, usually a VSD, is required to permit systemic venous blood to be circulated through the left side of the heart, mixed with pulmonary venous return (resulting in cyanosis), and ejected back out to the systemic circulation through a large aortic root.[8]

*Echocardiographic findings and quantification.*
TWO-DIMENSIONAL ECHOCARDIOGRAPHY
*Right ventricular outflow tract ends blindly and may be hypoplastic (parasternal short-axis view)[31,53]
*Main pulmonary artery may or may not be identified (all views)
—Visualization of PDA[31]
—Large aortic root[53]

—May have a large subaortic VSD, in which case the aorta overrides[53]
—Small right ventricle[31]

—Evaluation of interatrial communication and PDA by PW and color-flow Doppler[31]
—Evaluate severity of tricuspid regurgitation[31]

*Treatment.* An imperforate membrane may be opened surgically. Infants may require palliation in the form of a systemic-to-pulmonary shunt.[6] Older patients may be candidates for definitive repair. Surgical correction of a thick band of tissue replacing a native pulmonic valve may require reconstruction of the area, and possibly a prosthetic valve. The most complicated correction is required if there is a hypoplastic right ventricular outflow tract and an interrupted main pulmonary artery.[8]

*Infundibular Pulmonic Stenosis.* Hypertrophy of infundibular muscle or a fibrous ring within the right ventricular outflow tract may result in infundibular pulmonic stenosis.[13,53] Infundibular stenosis is generally caused by a VSD or pulmonic valve stenosis and rarely occurs as an isolated lesion.[20] The echocardiographic findings are similar to those of pulmonic valve stenosis, except that the pulmonary valve itself is thin and pliable, unless there is concomitant pulmonary valve stenosis. Doppler evaluation is most accurate from the subxiphoid position.

*Pulmonary Artery Stenosis.* The pulmonary artery may be stenotic anywhere along its length and branches, at one or several sites, as localized or diffuse narrowing.[6] The main pulmonary artery and the initial portions of the right and left branches may be evaluated by 2-D echocardiography from the parasternal long- and short-axis, anteriorly angled apical five-chamber, and high parasternal views.[53] More distal sections of the pulmonary arterial tree may not be evaluated by echocardiography, except to determine whether or not there is increased resistance to flow (findings similar to those of pulmonary hypertension). Pulmonary artery stenosis is classified by location as pulmonary artery stenosis, branch stenosis, or peripheral pulmonic stenosis. Patients with rubella syndrome often have some degree of pulmonary artery stenosis.[6,13]

*Anomalous Muscle Bundles.* Anomalous muscle bundles may occur at a variety of locations between the inflow and outflow portions of the right ventricle, dividing it into two chambers.[13] This condition is often referred to as *double-chamber right ventricle.*[52] The walls of the proximal portion of the right ventricle may be thickened to varying degrees depending on the severity of the obstruction. This abnormality is very difficult to diagnose by echocardiography but has been detected from the apical four-chamber and subxiphoid short-axis and long-axis views.[52] Occasionally, color-flow Doppler may detect a small area of disturbed flow within what appears to be a band of muscle in the right ventricle. PW or CW Doppler findings are very similar to those of VSD, with which this lesion may be confused. Angiography is the study of choice to diagnose this anomaly.[52] Anomalous muscle bundles often are associated with perimembranous VSD and subaortic stenosis.[52]

RIGHT VENTRICULAR INFLOW OBSTRUCTION
*Tricuspid Atresia.* In this anomaly, the tricuspid valve leaflets fail to develop during fetal life. In place of valve leaflets there is a band of dense fibrous tissue. Tricuspid atresia may occur with an intact interventricular septum and pulmonary atresia or a VSD of variable size with pulmonary stenosis. Associated congenital heart disease is common.[45]

*Hemodynamics.* Since the normal route of blood flow into the right ventricle is completely obstructed, an obligatory right-to-left shunt occurs at the level of the atria, mixing venous and arterial blood and resulting in cyanosis. The shunt may be through a patent foramen ovale (80%) or an ostium secundum ASD.[45,52]

*Echocardiographic findings and quantification.*
TWO-DIMENSIONAL ECHOCARDIOGRAPHY (SEE FIG. 19-13)
*Dense fibrous band visualized across area of tricuspid annulus (apical four-chamber or subxiphoid long-axis views)
*Absence of tricuspid valve leaflets (apical four-chamber and subxiphoid long-axis views)

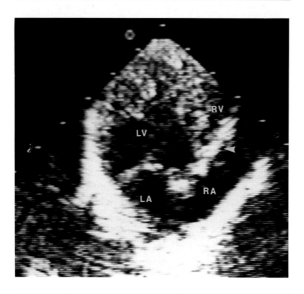

FIGURE 19-13. Two-dimensional visualization of tricuspid atresia (*large arrowhead*) using an apical four-chamber view. (LA, RA, left and right atria; LV, RV, left and right ventricles.) (Image is reversed left to right.)

—Dilated right atrium[52]
—Visualization of ASD[9] (apical four-chamber and subxiphoid long-axis views)
—Small right ventricle[45] or infundibular chamber[52] (apical four-chamber and subxiphoid long-axis views)
—Size of great vessel coming from right ventricle or infundibular chamber corresponds to the size of the VSD[52] (parasternal views)
—Visualization of VSD[9]
—Contrast injection may be seen to cross into the left atrium, fill the left ventricle, and then fill the right ventricle[1]
—Assess ventricular function[9]

DOPPLER ECHOCARDIOGRAPHY
—Right-to-left shunt at the level of the atria by PW or color-flow Doppler (subxiphoid position)
—Left-to-right shunt at the level of the VSD by PW or color-flow Doppler (subxiphoid position)
—Quantification of mitral regurgitation by PW or color-flow Doppler[9] (apical position)
+ Quantification of pulmonary stenosis by CW Doppler (parasternal or apical positions)

*Treatment.* Palliative surgery may be performed to regulate blood flow to the pulmonary bed. Blood flow to the pulmonary vasculature may be decreased by pulmonary artery banding or increased by creating a systemic-to-pulmonary shunt. Balloon atrial septostomy or Park blade septostomy may be carried out to increase shunting at the atrial level should the interatrial communication become restrictive. The surgical procedure that creates a physiologic correction is the Fontan procedure, in which the interatrial communication is closed, the systemic-to-pulmonary shunt is ligated, and the right atrium is connected to the pulmonary artery by use of a patch or conduit. The best candidates for this procedure are between 4 and 15 years of age and have normal pulmonary vascular resistance, mean pulmonary artery pressure of less than 20 mm Hg, pulmonary artery-to-aortic diameter ratio greater than 0.75, good left ventricular function, and normal sinus rhythm.[45]

*Tricuspid Hypoplasia or Stenosis.* In tricuspid stenosis, the diameter of the annulus is small. Rarely seen as an isolated lesion, tricuspid stenosis is often associated with pulmonary atresia with intact interventricular septum, critical pulmonic stenosis, or Ebstein's anomaly of the tricuspid valve.[52] Although attempts have been made to differentiate tricuspid stenosis from imperforate tricuspid valve by contrast echocardiography[52] and various Doppler techniques, the results have not always been successful. This lesion is best evaluated from the apical or subxiphoid four-chamber view.

*Imperforate Tricuspid Valve.* If the leaflets form but fail to separate during embryonic development, the tricuspid valve is imperforate. The tricuspid valve membrane may be visualized by 2-D echocardiography from the apical and subxiphoid four-chamber views.[52] Differentiation from tricuspid atresia is important, as imperforate valves may be treated surgically.

MALFORMATION OF THE TRICUSPID VALVE
*Ebstein's Anomaly.* Ebstein's anomaly of the tricuspid valve is a malformation in which the leaflets of the tricuspid valve do not separate completely from the myocardium of the right ventricle during embryonic development.[52] Although the tricuspid valve annulus is in the proper location, the leaflets

are large and adherent to the walls of the right ventricle, so that the orifice of the valve is displaced apically, into the right ventricular cavity. The portion of the right ventricle that contains the adherent tricuspid valve leaflets is considered to be "atrialized," as it functions as part of the right atrium.[52,53,66] The abnormally large valve leaflets do not coapt well, so there is some degree of tricuspid regurgitation and right atrial dilatation.[31,52,58] As pulmonary vascular resistance decreases during the newborn period, the severity of the tricuspid regurgitation decreases. The severity of this malformation is determined by the size of the functional right ventricular chamber. Patients with a larger functional right ventricular chamber have a better prognosis. Associated congenital heart disease includes patent foramen ovale, ASD, VSD, pulmonary stenosis, and pulmonary atresia.[66] Familial occurrence and association with maternal lithium ingestion during pregnancy have been recognized.[66] This malformation is discussed further in Chapter 9.

## Miscellaneous Malformations

### VENOUS MALFORMATIONS

*Total Anomalous Pulmonary Venous Return (TAPVR).* In this anomaly, the pulmonary veins fail to coalesce into the back of the left atrium during embryonic development. Instead of emptying into the posterior aspect of the left atrium, they drain into a common vein, which may empty into a variety of structures. The common vein may empty directly into the coronary sinus or right atrium. In other cases, the common vein may drain into a vertical vein, which in turn empties superiorly into the innominate vein or inferiorly below the diaphragm.[13,65] If the vertical vein courses below the diaphragm, it courses between the inferior vena cava (IVC) and the descending aorta and then empties into the inferior vena cava or portal vein.[51] Pulmonary venous return into the portal vein reaches the IVC by way of the ductus venosus.[13] On occasion, there may be multiple drainage sites in a single patient.[51]

*Hemodynamics.* In the absence of pulmonary venous obstruction, all of the returning pulmonary venous volume empties into the right atrium instead of the left atrium. The right side of the heart and the pulmonary bed, therefore, receive an increased volume of flow. This increase in blood flow through the pulmonary vasculature eventually leads to pulmonary hypertension.[13] Because the left atrium does not receive any pulmonary venous flow, there is an obligatory right-to-left shunt at the foramen ovale or ASD. The blood flowing into the left atrium from the right atrium consists of a mixture of deoxygenated systemic venous return and oxygenated pulmonary venous return. As a result, the systemic blood is somewhat desaturated (deoxygenated) and the patient is mildly cyanotic.[13]

If an obstruction occurs in the common pulmonary vein or vertical channel, pulmonary venous pressure will rise, which in turn causes pulmonary artery and right heart pressures to rise. Pulmonary edema usually ensues, and the patient presents with right-sided heart failure.[13] Although obstruction may occur with any of the described configurations of anomalous pulmonary venous return, it is most commonly seen when the vertical vein courses below the diaphragm.[13]

*Echocardiographic findings and quantification.*
TWO-DIMENSIONAL ECHOCARDIOGRAPHY
—Dilated coronary sinus (parasternal long-axis view)[51]
—Dilated right atrium and right ventricle
—Small left atrium and small to normal-sized left ventricle[51]
—ASD
*Visualization of the pulmonary venous channel posterior to but separate from the left atrium (subxiphoid, apical, parasternal and suprasternal notch transducer positions); the channel, which may be traced inferiorly or superiorly to where it empties into the superior vena cava or inferior vena cava, is called the ascending or descending vein.[51]
—Peripheral venous contrast injection opacifies the right atrium[51]

M-MODE ECHOCARDIOGRAPHY
—Dilated right ventricle
—Echogenic line visualized within the "left atrium"[51]
—Small to normal-sized left ventricle
—Paradoxical septal motion

DOPPLER ECHOCARDIOGRAPHY

*Turbulent, continuous flow detected in a vessel by PW or color-flow Doppler[31,41,51]

—Right-to-left shunt through the patent foramen ovale or ASD by PW or color-flow Doppler

—Decreased flow through the mitral and aortic valves by PW Doppler

—Laminar increased flow through the tricuspid and pulmonic valves by PW Doppler

*Increased flow detected at the entrance of the SVC, IVC, or coronary sinus into the right atrium by PW or color-flow Doppler[12,31,41]

*Increased flow detected at site of anastamosis of venous channel and SVC, IVC, or coronary sinus by PW or color-flow Doppler (subxiphoid and suprasternal positions)[12,31,41]

*Discussion of echocardiographic findings and quantification.* Color-flow Doppler imaging greatly facilitates localization of the common vein and evaluation of drainage sites. The presence and localization of pulmonary venous obstruction is also readily assessed with this modality and may assist in placement of the PW Doppler sample volume for quantification of the degree of obstruction.[12,41]

*Treatment.* Surgical correction involves closure of the interatrial communication and anastamosis of the venous channel to the left atrium.[12]

*Partial Anomalous Pulmonary Venous Return.* Partial anomalous pulmonary venous return, in which one or more of the pulmonary veins empties into something other than the left atrium, is not reliably diagnosed or evaluated by echocardiography.[51] Anomalous drainage of one or more pulmonary veins would result in increased volume to the right heart, so secondary findings of a right heart volume overload may be seen by 2-D echocardiography.

*Persistence of the Left Superior Vena Cava.* Sometimes the left superior vena cava, which formed during embryonic development, does not regress. This abnormality may be an isolated finding, but it often is associated with other congenital heart lesions.

*Hemodynamics.* The persistent left superior vena cava drains into the coronary sinus, causing it to dilate.

*Echocardiographic findings.*

TWO-DIMENSIONAL ECHOCARDIOGRAPHY

—Dilated coronary sinus (parasternal long-axis and short-axis or subxiphoid long-axis views)[51]

—Visualization of the left superior vena cava along the left side of the descending aorta (subxiphoid short-axis view)[51]

—Opacification of the coronary sinus, and subsequently the right atrium, by contrast echocardiography[51]

## Acknowledgments

Thanks to the Pediatric Cardiology Department of Mount Sinai Hospital in New York City and the Pediatric Cardiology Department of University of Maryland Hospital for contribution of echocardiographic images to be included in the text. A special thanks to Kathleen Baker, B.S., R.D.M.S., and Joel Brenner, M.D. for reviewing the text and making invaluable suggestions to improve it.

## References

1. Armstrong WF. Congenital heart disease. In: Feigenbaum H, ed. Echocardiography, 4th ed. Philadelphia: Lea & Febiger, 1986.

2. Bash SE, Huhta JC, Vick GW, et al. Hypoplastic left heart syndrome: Is echocardiography accurate enough to guide surgical palliation? J Am Coll Cardiol. 1986; 7:610–616.

3. Baylen BG, Waldhausen JA. Diseases of the mitral valve. In: Adams FH, Emmanoulides GC, Riemenschneider TA, eds. Moss' Heart Disease in Infants, Children and Adolescents, 4th ed. Baltimore: Williams & Wilkins; 1989.

4. Bierman FZ, Williams RG. Subxiphoid two-dimensional imaging of the interatrial septum in infants and neonates with congenital heart disease. Circulation. 1979; 60(1):80–90.

5. Brenner JI, Baker KR, Berman MA. Prediction of left ventricular pressure in infants with aortic stenosis. Br Heart J. 1980; 44:406–410.

6. Burrows PE, Freedom RM, Rabinovitch M, et al. The investigation of abnormal pulmonary arteries in congenital heart disease. Radio Clin North Am. 1985; 23(4):689–717.

7. Canale JM, Sahn DJ, Allen HD, et al. Factors affecting real-time, cross-sectional echocardiographic imaging of perimembranous ventricular septal defects. Circulation. 1981; 63(3):689–697.

8. Driscoll DJ, McGoon DC. Congenital heart disease

in adolescents and adults: Pulmonary atresia with ventricular septal defect. In: Brandenburg RO, Fuster V, Giulani ER, et al., eds. Cardiology: Fundamentals and Practice. Chicago: Year Book Medical Publishers, 1987.

9. Driscoll DJ, McGoon DC. Congenital heart disease in adolescents and adults: Tricuspid atresia. In: Brandenburg RO, Fuster V, Giulani ER, et al., eds. Cardiology: Fundamentals and Practice. Chicago: Year Book Medical Publishers; 1987.

10. Driscoll DJ, Fuster V, McGoon DC. Congenital heart disease in adolescents and adults: Atrioventricular canal defect. In: Brandenburg RO, Fuster V, Giulani ER, et al., eds. Cardiology: Fundamentals and Practice. Chicago: Year Book Medical Publishers, 1987.

11. Feldt RH, Porter CJ, Edwards WD, et al. Defects of the atrial septum and the atrioventricular canal. In: Adams FH, Emmanouilides GC, Riemenschneider TA, et al., eds. Moss' Heart Disease in Infants, Children and Adolescents, 4th ed. Baltimore: Williams & Wilkins; 1989.

12. Ferencz C, Rubin JD, McCarter RJ, et al. Cardiac and noncardiac malformations: Observations in a population-based study. Teratology. 1987; 35:367–378.

13. Fink BW. Congenital Heart Disease: A Deductive Approach to Its Diagnosis, 2nd ed. Chicago: Year Book Medical Publishers; 1985.

14. Fraker TD, Harris PJ, Behar VS, et al. Detection and exclusions of interatrial shunts by two-dimensional echocardiography and peripheral venous injection. Circulation. 1979; 59(2):379–384.

15. Friedman WF. Aortic stenosis. In: Adams FH, Emmanouilides GC, Riemenschneider TA, eds. Moss' Heart Disease in Infants, Children and Adolescents, 4th ed. Baltimore: Williams & Wilkins; 1989.

16. Fuster V, Driscoll DJ, McGoon DC. Congenital heart disease in adolescents and adults: Atrial septal defect. In: Brandenburg RO, Fuster V, Giulani ER, et al., eds. Cardiology: Fundamentals and Practice. Chicago: Year Book Medical Publishers; 1987.

17. Fuster V, Driscoll DJ, McGoon DC. Congenital heart disease in adolescents and adults: Ventricular septal defects. In: Brandenburg RO, Fuster V, Giulani ER, et al., eds. Cardiology: Fundamentals and Practice. Chicago: Year Book Medical Publishers; 1987.

18. Fuster V, Driscoll DJ, McGoon DC. Congenital heart disease in adolescents and adults: Patent ductus arteriosus and other aortico-pulmonary communications. In: Brandenburg RO, Fuster V, Giulani ER, et al., eds. Cardiology: Fundamentals and Practice. Chicago: Year Book Medical Publishers; 1987.

19. Fuster V, McGoon DC. Congenital heart disease in adolescents and adults: Coarctation of the aorta. In:

Brandenburg RO, Fuster V, Giulani ER, et al., eds. Cardiology: Fundamentals and Practice. Chicago: Year Book Medical Publishers; 1987.

20. Fuster V, Driscoll DJ, McGoon DC. Congenital heart disease in adolescents and adults: Congenital left sided outflow obstruction. In: Brandenburg RO, Fuster V, Giulani ER, et al., eds. Cardiology: Fundamentals and Practice. Chicago: Year Book Medical Publishers; 1987.

21. Fuster V, McGoon DC. Congenital heart disease in adolescents and adults: Pulmonary stenosis with intact ventricular septum. In: Brandenburg RO, Fuster V, Giulani ER, et al., eds. Cardiology: Fundamentals and Practice. Chicago: Year Book Medical Publishers; 1987.

22. Fyler DC, Buckley LP, Hellenbrand WE, et al. Report of the New England Regional Infant Cardiac Program. Pediatrics. 1980; 65(2):388, 392–403.

23. George B, DiSessa TG, Williams R, et al. Coarctation repair without cardiac catheterization in infants. Am Heart J. 1987; 114(6):1421–1425.

24. Gersony WM. Coarctation of the aorta. In: Adams FH, Emmanouilides GC, Riemenschneider TA, eds. Moss' Heart Disease in Infants, Children and Adolescents, 4th ed. Baltimore: Williams & Wilkins; 1989.

25. Goldberg SJ, Allen HD, Marx GR, et al. Doppler Echocardiography. Philadelphia: Lea & Febiger; 1985.

26. Grabitz RG, Joffres MR, Collins-Nakai RL. Congenital heart disease: Incidence in the first year of life. Am J Epidemiol. 1988; 128(2):381–388.

27. Graham TP, Bender HW, Spach MS. Ventricular septal defect. In: Adams FH, Emmanouilides GC, Riemenschneider TA, eds. Moss' Heart Disease in Infants, Children and Adolescents, 4th ed. Baltimore: Williams & Wilkins; 1989.

28. Hatle L, Angelsen B. Doppler Ultrasound in Cardiology: Physical Principles and Clinical Applications. 2d ed. Philadelphia: Lea & Febiger; 1985.

29. Heymann MA. Patent ductus arteriosus. In: Adams FH, Emmanouilides GC, Riemenschneider TA, eds. Moss' Heart Disease in Infants, Children and Adolescents, 4th ed. Baltimore: Williams & Wilkins; 1989.

30. Huhta JC, Gutgesell HP, Latson LA, et al. Two-dimensional echocardiographic assessment of the aorta in infants and children with congenital heart disease. Circulation. 1984; 70(3):417–424.

31. Kyo S. Congenital heart disease. In: Omoto R, ed. Color Atlas of Real-Time Two-Dimensional Doppler Echocardiography, 2nd ed. Philadelphia: Lea & Febiger; 1987.

32. Lipshultz SE, Sanders SP, Mayer JE, et al. Are routine preoperative cardiac catheterization and angiography necessary before repair of ostium primum atrial septal defect? J Am Coll Cardiol. 1988; 11(2):373–378.

33. McKay RG. Balloon valvuloplasty for treating pulmonic, mitral and aortic valve stenosis. Am J Cardiol. 1988; 61:102G–108G.

34. Marx GR, Allen HD, Goldberg SJ. Doppler echocardiographic estimation of systolic pulmonary artery pressure in pediatric patients with interventricular communications. J Am Coll Cardiol. 1985; 6(5):1132–1137.

35. Murphy DJ, Ludomirsky A, Huhta JC. Continuous-wave Doppler in children with ventricular septal defect: Noninvasive estimation of interventricular pressure gradient. Am J Cardiol. 1986; 57:428–432.

36. Nihoyannopoulos P, Karas S, Sapsford RN, et al. Accuracy of two-dimensional echocardiography in the diagnosis of aortic arch obstruction. J Am Coll Cardiol. 1987; 10(5):1072–1077.

37. Perry SB, Keane JF, Lock JE. Interventional catheterization in pediatric congenital and acquired heart disease. Am J Cardiol. 1988; 61:109G–117G.

38. Pillai R, Yen S, Anderson RH, et al. Ostium primum atrioventricular septal defect: An anatomical and surgical review. Ann Thorac Surg. 1986; 41:458–461.

39. Rabinovitch M. Pulmonary hypertension. In: Adams FH, Emmanouilides GC, Riemenschneider TA, eds. Moss' Heart Disease in Infants, Children and Adolescents. 4th ed. Baltimore: Williams & Wilkins; 1989.

40. Ritter SB. Application of Doppler color-flow mapping in the assessment and the evaluation of congenital heart disease. Echocardiography. 1987; 4(6):543–556.

41. Ritter SB, Arnon R, Steinfeld L, et al. Anomalous venous drainage: Identification by Doppler color-flow mapping (abstr). Circulation. 1986; 74:37.

42. Ritter SB, Rothe W, Kawai D, et al. Identification of ventricular septal defects by Doppler color-flow mapping: A study in enhanced sensitivity (abstr). J Ultrasound Med. 1988; 7(10):S69.

43. Ritter S, Rothe W, Kawai D, et al. Identification of ventricular septal defects by Doppler color-flow mapping (abstr). Clin Res. 1988; 36(3):311A.

44. Ritter SB, Segal K, Kawai D, et al. Estimation of pulmonary artery pressure in children with ventricular septal defect: Real-time color-flow/continuous-wave Doppler application (abstr). J Ultrasound Med. 1988; 7(10):S69.

45. Rosenthal A, Dick M. Tricuspid atresia. In: Adams FH, Emmanouilides GC, Riemenschneider TA, eds.

Moss' Heart Disease in Infants, Children and Adolescents, 4th ed. Baltimore: Williams & Wilkins;1989.

46. Rowley KM, Kopf GS, Hellenbrand W, et al. Atrioventricular canal with intact atrial septum. Am Heart J. 1988; 115(4):902–906.

47. Sahn DJ, Allen HD. Real-time cross-sectional echocardiographic imaging and measurement of the patent ductus arteriosus in infants and children. Circulation. 1978; 58(2):343–354.

48. Sahn DJ, Valdes-Cruz LM. New advances in two-dimensional Doppler echocardiography. Prog Cardiovasc Dis. 1986; 28(5):367–382.

49. Sahn DJ, Valdes-Cruz LM. Ultrasound Doppler methods for calculating cardiac volume flows, cardiac output and cardiac shunts. In: Kotler MN, Steiner RM, eds. Cardiac Imaging: New Technologies and Clinical Applications. Philadelphia: FA Davis, 1986.

50. Salter DR, Wechsler AS. Apicoaortic shunts for left ventricular outflow obstruction. Ann Thorac Surg. 1986; 42:607.

51. Sanders SP. Echocardiography and related techniques in the diagnosis of congenital heart defects. I. Veins, atria and interatrial septum. Echocardiography. 1984; 1(2):185–217.

52. Sanders SP. Echocardiography and related techniques in the diagnosis of congenital heart defects: II. Atrioventricular valves and ventricles. Echocardiography. 1984; 1(3):333–391.

53. Seward JB, Tajik AJ, Edwards WD, et al. Two Dimensional Echocardiographic Atlas. Congenital Heart Disease. New York: Springer-Verlag; 1987; 1.

54. Silbert DR, Brunson SC, Schiff R, et al. Determination of right ventricular pressure in the presence of ventricular septal defect using continuous-wave Doppler ultrasound. J Am Coll Cardiol. 1986; 8(2):379–384.

55. Smallhorn JF. Patent ductus arteriosus: Evaluation by echocardiography. Echocardiography. 1987; 101–118.

56. Snider AR. Doppler echocardiography in congenital heart disease. In: Berger M, ed. Doppler Echocardiography in Heart Disease. New York: Marcel Dekker; 1987.

57. Snider R, Stevenson JG, French JW, et al. Comparison of high pulse repetition frequency and continuous-wave Doppler echocardiography for velocity measurement and gradient prediction in children with valvular and congenital heart disease. J Am Coll Cardiol. 1986; 7(4):873–879.

58. Stevenson JG. Doppler evaluation of atrial septal defect, ventricular septal defect, and complex malformations. Acta Paediatr Scand. 1986; 329 (Suppl):21–43.

59. Stevenson JG. The use of Doppler echocardiography for detection and estimation of severity of patent ductus arteriosus, ventricular septal defect, and atrial septal defect. Echocardiography. 1987; 4(4):321–346.

60. Stevenson JG, Kawabori I, Guntheroth WG. Differentiation of ventricular septal defects from mitral regurgitation by pulsed Doppler echocardiography. Circulation. 1977; 56(1):14–18.

61. Stevenson JG, Kawabori I, Dooley T, et al. Diagnosis of ventricular septal defects by pulsed Doppler echocardiography. Circualtion. 1978; 58(2):322–326.

62. Sullivan ID, Robinson PJ, DeLeval M, et al. Membranous supravalvular mitral stenosis: A treatable form of congenital heart disease. J Am Coll Cardiol. 1986; 8(1):159–164.

63. Sweeney MS, Walker WE, Cooley DA, et al. Apicoaortic conduits for complex left ventricular outflow obstruction: 10-year experience. Ann Thorac Surg. 1986; 42:609–611.

64. Valdez-Cruz LM, Sahn DJ. Ultrasonic contrast studies for the detection of cardiac shunts. J Am Coll Cardiol. 1984; 3(4):978–985.

65. VanHare GF, Schmidt KG, Cassidy SC, et al. Color Doppler flow mapping in the ultrasound diagnosis of total anomalous pulmonary venous connection. J Am Soc Echocardiogr. 1988; 1(5):341–347.

66. VanMierop LHS, Kutsche LM, Victorica BE. Ebstein anomaly. In: Adams FH, Emmanouilides GC, Riemenschneider TA, eds. Moss' Heart Disease in Infants, Children and Adolescents, 4th ed. Baltimore: Williams & Wilkins; 1989.

67. Vick GW, Murphy DJ, Ludomirsky A, et al. Pulmonary venous and systemic ventricular inflow obstruction in patients with congenital heart disease: Detection by combined two-dimensional and Doppler echocardiography. J Am Coll Cardiol. 1987; 9(3):580–587.

68. Werner JA, Cheitlin MD, Gross BW, et al. Echocardiographic appearance of the Chiari network: Differentiation from right-heart pathology. Circulation. 1981; 63:1104.

69. Weyman AE, Dillon JC, Feigenbaum H, et al. Echocardiographic patterns of pulmonic valve motion with pulmonary hypertension. Circulation. 1974; 50:905–910.

70. Yock PG, Popp RL. Noninvasive estimation of right ventricular systolic pressure by Doppler ultrasound in patients with tricuspid regurgitation. Circulation. 1984; 70(4):657–662.

71. Yoshikawa Y, Koyano A. Equipment. In: Omoto R, ed. Color Atlas of Real-Time Two-Dimensional Doppler Echocardiography, 2nd ed. Philadelphia: Lea & Febiger; 1987.

CHAPTER **20**

# Complex Congenital Heart Disease

KATHLEEN R. BAKER

In this chapter a wide range of complex cardiac anomalies are presented. These diseases are considered to be complex not only because of the severity of the variation from normal anatomy, but also because the hemodynamic effects are more complicated. This chapter will address the practical needs of an adult echocardiographer who occasionally will be called on to screen for congenital cardiac disease, or the sonographer who is just beginning in the specialty practice of pediatric echo. None of the anomalies presented could be accurately described as common; they are, however, among those most frequently encountered by the novice practitioner and considered to be among the most confusing.

The first three sections cover a variety of congenital lesions which involve abnormal connections between the ventricles and the great vessels (ventriculoarterial discordance). All of these diseases may be thought of as related steps off the normal pathways of conotruncal rotation, septation, and alignment. Therefore, a review of conotruncal embryology is included in the first section on transposition of the great arteries (TGA). Single ventricle (SV) is presented in the second section. SV and TGA are commonly found in association with each other and with other congenital cardiac defects. The third section presents a series of defects which share a primary common diagnostic finding: a great vessel overriding a ventricular septum through a ventricular septal defect (VSD). These defects represent the possible differential diagnosis when override is encountered. The last section presents three interesting, uncommon lesions, one of which is an acquired disease, Kawasaki's disease, which has recently become more prevalent in this country.

Many more diseases exist which were not covered for this text. It is not possible to present a complete compendium of pediatric echocardiography in a single chapter. However, a solid foundation has been provided for beginning the study of the complex congenital heart diseases.

## Transposition of the Great Arteries

The mechanism of the embryonic development of TGA is not absolutely clear. In some fashion the normal separation and alignment processes of the outflow tracts and great vessels is disrupted. (See Chapter 18 for a review of cardiac embryology.) During normal embryonic development the great vessels undergo a spiraling septation process, producing a configuration in which the great vessels are "wrapped around" each other. The ascending aorta (AAo) normally originates posteriorly and leftward. It then courses anteriorly and rightward, crossing behind the right ventricular outflow tract (RVOT) and over the right pulmonary artery (RPA). Finally it curves posteriorly as the transverse aortic arch (TAA) and into the descending aorta (DAO).

The rightward RVOT passing anterior to the aortic valve gives rise to the main pulmonary artery (MPA). The MPA then dives posteriorly, bifurcating into the left and right branches. If during development the process of spiraling is disrupted, parallel nonspiraling great vessels result which may have any of several possible variations of spatial relationships.

A similarly complex process of division and alignment occurs for the ventricles and outlet chambers. Normal rightward looping (dextro or d-looping) of the primitive heart tube places the morphologic right ventricle on the right side of the heart. When the direction of looping is diverted a leftward (levo) placement of the morphologic right ventricle results (levo- or l-looping). Additional important structures referred to as conal tissue, or conus, develop as part of the outflow tracts. Conotruncal development determines the relationships of both great vessels to the left and right outflow tracts as well as the relationships of the outflow tracts and atrioventricular (AV) valves. In the development of the normal heart the subaortic conus is absorbed, producing direct fibrous continuity of both the interventricular septum anteriorly and mitral valve (MV) ring posteriorly with the aorta. On the right an intervening conus prevents fibrous continuity of the tricuspid valve (TV) and pulmonary valve (PV) rings. Transposition and other complex anomalies are thought to involve abnormal placement of the conus, producing both an abnormal relationship of the great vessels and ventricles and discontinuity between the mitral valve and aorta. In some abnormalities no conal absorption occurs and bilateral conus is present.

TGA falls within a wide spectrum of diseases reported in the literature that involve abnormal positioning of the great vessels. Only the two most common classifications are described here, simple physiologically uncorrected dextrotransposition (DTGA) and physiologically corrected levotransposition (LTGA).[17,20–25]

The diagnosis of TGA relies on (1) clear identification of the aortic and pulmonary arteries, (2) an accurate description of their spatial relationship, (3) identification of the ventricular morphology and positions, and (4) the parallel connections of venous return (cavae and pulmonary veins) to atrium, atrium to ventricle, and ventricle to great vessel.[9–19] The first echocardiographic indication of TGA usually is seen in the long-axis view when parallel, "unwrapped" great arteries are discovered (Fig. 20-1). Even when transposed vessels lie more nearly side by side, this presentation is easily identified.

The next step is to confirm that the anterior great vessel is the aorta by identifying the origin of the coronary arteries, the transverse aortic arch (TAA), the vessels emanating from the TAA (innominate, left carotid, left subclavian), and the descending aorta (see Fig. 20-1A). Cross-sectional views are used to clarify whether the aorta is to the right of the MPA, producing DTGA (see Fig. 20-1B), or to the left of the MPA (LTGA). Then, a combination of cross-sectional, apical, and subcostal views can be utilized to establish the atrial-ventricular-arterial connections. With a careful examination of the atrioventricular (AV) valves, the ventricular shapes, and the patterns of trabeculation, the morphologic identity of the ventricles can be determined.[33,37]

The variety of forms of transposition and the multiple systems of nomenclature in use can cause severe problems in communicating about TGA. Using a descriptive approach, in which structural continuity and spatial relationships are clearly outlined, is more productive for the examining sonographer than trying to apply a precise diagnostic label. Each structure is labeled as to identity, position, and continuity. For example: *In patient A, a morphologic right ventricle in a leftward position is connected to an anterior leftward aorta.* Such a system of description allows all sonographers and physicians to clearly understand the anatomy and implied physiology, regardless of what form of transposition (in this case LTGA) is involved or what system of labels they are accustomed to using.

Over 50% of all TGAs have associated anomalies such as single ventricle (SV), ventricular septal defect (VSD), patent ductus arteriosus (PDA), or valvular and outflow tract abnormalities.

Echocardiographic Findings in
Dextrotransposition of the Great Arteries*
*Two-Dimensional Study*
+ Both great vessels course superiorly together and then posteriorly together without crossing (i.e., they can be imaged simultaneously on parasternal long-axis views)

---

*Primary findings are designated by a plus sign; secondary findings with a minus sign.

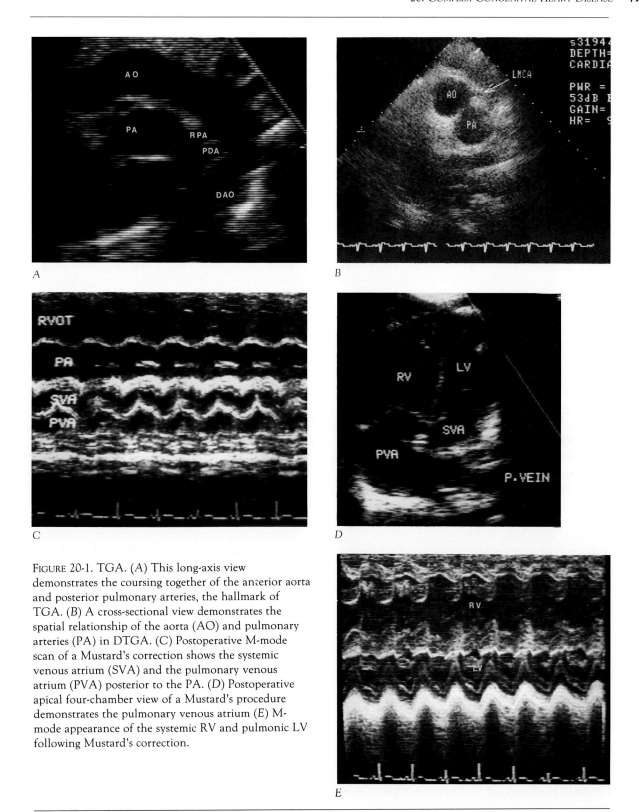

FIGURE 20-1. TGA. (*A*) This long-axis view demonstrates the coursing together of the anterior aorta and posterior pulmonary arteries, the hallmark of TGA. (*B*) A cross-sectional view demonstrates the spatial relationship of the aorta (AO) and pulmonary arteries (PA) in DTGA. (*C*) Postoperative M-mode scan of a Mustard's correction shows the systemic venous atrium (SVA) and the pulmonary venous atrium (PVA) posterior to the PA. (*D*) Postoperative apical four-chamber view of a Mustard's procedure demonstrates the pulmonary venous atrium (*E*) M-mode appearance of the systemic RV and pulmonic LV following Mustard's correction.

+ Anterior rightward aorta
+ Posterior leftward PA
+ Rightward morphologic right ventricle continuous with the aorta
+ Leftward morphologic left ventricle continuous with the posterior PA
+ RA-TV-RV-AO connections on the right
+ LA-MV-LV-PA connections on the left
− Associated anomalies such as pulmonary stenosis

### M-Mode Study

+ An anterior rightward semilunar valve/great vessel
+ A posterior leftward semilunar valve/great vessel
+ Reversed anterior (right) and posterior (left) preejection period/ventricular ejection time (PEP-VET) ratios

### Doppler Study

− Principally used to assess flow in associated lesions such as ASD, VSD, PDA pulmonary stenosis, or flow through a balloon atrial septostomy (BAS)

### ECHOCARDIOGRAPHIC FINDINGS IN LEVOTRANSPOSITION OF THE GREAT ARTERIES

#### Two-Dimensional Study

+ Both great vessels course superiorly together and then posteriorly together without crossing (i.e., they can be imaged simultaneously on parasternal long-axis views)
+ Leftward anterior aorta
+ Rightward posterior PA
+ Leftward morphologic right ventricle with TV in continuity with the leftward anterior aorta
+ Rightward morphologic LV with MV in continuity with the posterior rightward PA
+ RA-MV-LV-PA connections on the right (physiologically corrected)
+ LA-TV-RV-AO connections on the left (physiologically corrected)
− Associated anomalies such as VSD, pulmonary stenosis (PS) at various levels, single ventricle, Ebstein's anomaly

### M-Mode Study

+ Anterior leftward and posterior rightward great vessels/semilunar valves
+ Normal left-right PEP-VET ratios

### Doppler Study

− Principally used to assess associated lesions

### HEMODYNAMICS

In DTGA systemic venous return through the right side of the heart is directed to the aorta, returning desaturated blood (low oxygen content) to the systemic circulation. Pulmonary venous return to the left heart is directed through the MPA back to the pulmonary vasculature. This produces two parallel circulatory loops. There is no outlet to the systemic circulation for oxygenated blood. Patients with DTGA usually present as newborns with severe cyanosis. The patent ductus arteriosus and/or the foramen ovale allows some oxygenated blood to reach the systemic bed as long as these structures remain patent. Associated lesions such as ASD or VSD can relieve the cyanosis if they are large enough to allow significant mixing of blood from both sides of the heart.

In LTGA the serial circulation is physiologically correct, as systemic return to the right side of the heart is then directed to the PA and pulmonary return flows into the left heart and out the aorta. This lesion is frequently undetected through childhood unless an associated lesion such as Ebstein's or single ventricle occurs, resulting in an extensive cardiac exam.

### TREATMENT

Balloon atrial septostomy (BAS), which allows atrial flow mixing, has been used as a palliative procedure. A large, stiff balloon catheter is inserted from the vena cava into the right atrium, and then through the atrial septum into the left atrium. The balloon is inflated with radiopaque liquid and withdrawn abruptly through the septum, producing a hole.[29,30,35] This allows the atrial flows to mix through the tear and may provide adequate oxygenation for many months of growth. Administration of prostaglandins can also be used to reopen the ductus arteriosus to improve an infant's severe cyanosis until septostomy or early corrective surgery can be performed.

The preferred form of surgical correction for DTGA has changed over the last several years. In the Mustard procedure the atrial septum is excised and a synthetic patch is placed so as to keep separate and redirect systemic and pulmonary venous return through the physiologically appropriate AV valves.[32,33] A variation of the Mustard procedure, the Senning procedure, uses pericardium as patch material to construct the two channels.[36] The newly created posterior pathway is called the pulmonary venous atrium (PVA), through which pulmonary vein flow crosses to the right-sided AV valve. The new systemic venous atrium (SVA) directs systemic venous return to the left-sided AV valve. Figure 20-1C demonstrates both channels posterior to the PA on an M-mode tracing. Figure 20-1D shows a PVA on an apical four-chamber view.[28,37,38]

The principal concerns with these procedures are (1) development of stenosis involving the patch, (2) inability of the morphologic right ventricle to maintain adequate function as a systemic pumping chamber over a normal life span (Fig. 20-1E), and (3) surgery may damage the conduction system causing dysrhythmias that may later result in sudden death.[37,38]

Recently, many centers have had vastly better results with the arterial switch (Jantene) operation for early correction of simple isolated DTGA.[31,34] Swapping the vessels, and moving the coronary arteries at the same time, restores the normal physiologic functions of the ventricles. One of the keys seems to be early operation, before the left ventricle becomes conditioned to functioning as the pulmonary outflow ventricle. When the anatomic configuration allows, this procedure is the treatment of choice.

## Single Ventricle

Single ventricle (SV) is diagnosed by the presence of a single large ventricular chamber into which enter two AV valves (Fig. 20-2). (Many other configurations can be thought of as functionally similar to SV despite different anatomy or embryonic development. For instance, common AV valve with a single ventricle or atresia of one AV valve with single ventricle will have similar hemodynamic characteristics.) Most single ventricles contain a small "outlet chamber" positioned in a subpulmonary or subaortic location. Flow enters the outlet chamber through a VSD and then goes to the related great vessel. Infrequently, small chambers or pouches may be found that are unrelated to a great vessel. The large, single ventricular chamber may be identifiable morphologically as a left or

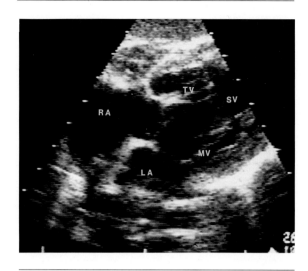

FIGURE 20-2. SV demonstrated in a subcostal four-chamber view. Two AV valves are demonstrated within a single large ventricular chamber.

right ventricular type. Other terms for this entity are "univentricular heart" and "common ventricle."[39,40,44–51]

A "stump" of tissue is sometimes present in any of several locations. It resembles a rudimentary septum but has no hemodynamic significance. A large papillary muscle can also resemble a ventricular septum and must be examined closely to detect the attached AV valve apparatus. The majority of SVs are associated with some variety of TGA. SV is also associated with tricuspid atresia. Additionally, there may be abnormal situs of the abdominal organs.

Echocardiography is extremely useful for delineating SV anatomy. The configuration of AV valves is often more clearly defined by 2-D echocardiography than by angiography. The AV valves may be side by side, be directly anterior and posterior to each other ("upstairs-downstairs"), share common attachments, or have a crisscrossing orientation.[1,3,7,40,44,48] They may be unbalanced in size or have many other anatomic variations. Morphologic identity of the ventricle can be defined by 2-D studies. Color flow and Doppler interrogation can detect obstruction through the outlet chamber or VSD and obstructions or insufficiencies of any of the valves. This is particularly important because SV is so often associated with other anomalies, such as pulmonary stenosis and transposition, and less often with a range of other defects. SV and TGA often are seen in constellations of multiple anomalies, such as SV with TGA and pulmonary obstruction. Contractility should also be assessed by evaluation of LV size in multiple planes on each cross-sectional view.

## Echocardiographic Findings in Single Ventricle

### 2-D Study
+ Large single ventricular chamber
+ Outlet chamber in a subpulmonary or subaortic position (or pouch unrelated to a great vessel)
+ AV valve anomalies: number, relative size and position, configuration, and attachment of valves
− Relationship of the great vessels (often transposed)
− Contractility of the ventricle

### M-Mode Study
+ Large single chamber
+ AV valves, number and position

## Hemodynamics
SV allows essentially unrestricted mixing of systemic and pulmonary return within the ventricle. Relative positions, size, and orientation of outlet and inlet structures all play a role in determining pulmonary blood flow, ventricular mixing, and therefore the level of desaturation of systemic outflow. Normal pulmonary resistance in the absence of obstruction to pulmonary outflow allows unrestricted (and therefore increased) pulmonary blood flow. This situation usually produces congestive heart failure early in life.

Associated defects such as restrictive subpulmonary VSD or valvular, subvalvular, or supravalvular pulmonary stenosis produce various degrees of obstruction to pulmonary blood flow. In these instances the patient is protected from the pulmonary vascular damage that can occur in unrestricted shunting. If the obstruction is severe enough, cyanosis will result, and treatment may be required to augment pulmonary blood flow.

The common association of TGA with SV usually is not significant hemodynamically, owing to the free mixing of systemic and pulmonary return in the single ventricular chamber. In the absence of obstruction, outflow is controlled by the relative resistances of the systemic and pulmonary beds, regardless of great vessel orientation.

Tricuspid atresia in association with SV allows no direct systemic return to the ventricle. If no ASD or patent foramen large enough to allow unrestricted flow from right to left atrium exists, atrial septostomy can be performed as a palliative step.

## Treatment
Rarely is definitive repair by septation possible because the apparatus of the AV valves often cannot be divided surgically. Common sites of insertion, crisscrossing, shared papillary muscle, and intermingling of structures make it impossible to septate SV and preserve adequate ventricular and AV valve function. When a significant septal remnant exists in conjunction with cleanly separated AV valves, septation may be feasible.

More often septation is not feasible and the Fontan procedure is performed. The tricuspid valve is sewn closed and the right atrium is connected directly to the pulmonary artery, producing separate pulmonary and systemic flow circuits. Low pulmonary resistance allows flow into the pulmonary system with the lower atrial pumping force. A modified Fontan operation may also be performed, which connects the superior vena cava (SVC) to the right pulmonary artery (RPA) and the inferior vena cava (IVC) to the left pulmonary artery (LPA). Surgical intervention by Fontan or septation often must wait until the patient reaches a minimum size.[1,3,6,8,41,43]

SV without significant pulmonary obstruction may allow excessive pulmonary blood flow, necessitating early intervention. Usually PA banding is performed. As the patients grow and require increased pulmonary blood flow, procedures such as the Blalock-Taussig shunt may be done to provide controlled additional pulmonary blood flow.[1,3,8]

## Congenital Heart Defects with Overriding Great Vessels
Many complex forms of congenital heart disease are actually constellations of simpler lesions that often appear in certain patterns. The group of de-

fects to be discussed next has one predominant common diagnostic feature—a posterior great vessel that overrides or straddles the ventricular septum through a moderate-sized to large VSD. In the vast majority of cases the overriding vessel is the aorta (Fig. 20-3).

These particular lesions are discussed as a group in order to demonstrate a functional approach to the diagnosis of several lesions that have a common primary diagnostic feature, VSD with aortic override. The idea is to illustrate the possible range of the differential diagnosis when aortic override is visualized.

These defects all have hemodynamic consequences beyond those of the simple shunt lesions. This is because the VSDs tend to be large and aortic override facilitates bidirectional shunting. As other anatomic defects are added to the increasingly complex diseases, the hemodynamic consequences are more variable and more thorough study is required to assess them accurately. These

diseases can now be assessed and defined extensively through echocardiographic techniques, which reduce the number of invasive studies required.

MALALIGNMENT VENTRICULAR SEPTAL DEFECT
Isolated malalignment VSD involves aortic override of less than 50%. The anatomic communication between the right ventricle and aorta due to the override may allow some degree of right-to-left shunting, depending on the size and orientation of the defect and the degree of override. The PA is normal. The predominant shunt is still left to right as long as the normally lower resistance of the pulmonary vascular bed (PBF) is preserved. Eventually the increased PBF may cause pulmonary vascular damage resulting in increased pulmonary vascular resistance and changes in shunt flow. The diagnostic criteria and hemodynamic consequence are similar to those already described in the section on VSDs, with the following added considerations.

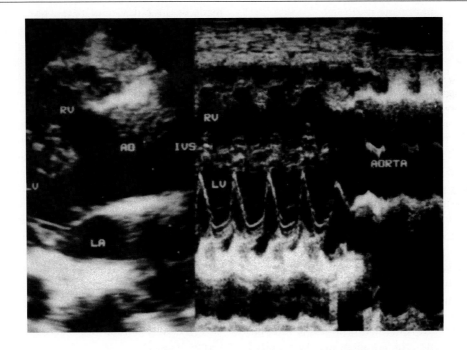

FIGURE 20-3. Simultaneous M-mode and two-dimensional presentations of an aorta overriding an IVS through a VSD.

## Echocardiographic Findings
### Two-Dimensional Study
+ Moderate-sized to large VSD
+ Override of ventricular septum by the aorta of less than 50% multiple approaches (parasternal, apical and subxyphoid long-axis; apical and subxyphoid) must be used to ensure appreciation of the full extent of the override.
− Enlarged PA
− Enlarged LA
− Enlarged RV in some cases

### M-Mode Study
+ Septal-aortic discontinuity
+ Aortic override of less than 50%

### Doppler Study
+ Predominant left-to-right shunting in the absence of pulmonary vascular disease
− Bidirectional shunting more easily appreciated by color-flow imaging
− Increased pulmonary-to-system flow ratio (Qp-Qs)

## Hemodynamics
The hemodynamics are similar to those discussed in the section on VSDs (see pp. 385–386).[1,29,44,76] Turbulent shunt flow may cause damage to the aortic valve leaflets.

## Treatment
Malalignment VSDs do not close spontaneously. Management depends on the shunt volume and pressure communicated to the right side of the heart, as in isolated, moderate-sized to large VSDs. Surgical closure often is feasible at 1 year of age and usually is performed early in life, because the risk of irreversible pulmonary hypertension increases with age. Primary surgical repair is now-possible at increasingly early ages, so palliative pulmonary artery banding rarely is required. Infrequently, left ventricular outflow tract obstruction or aortic valve damage may result from surgical correction. This can be prevented by enlarging the VSD at surgery to remove potentially obstructive conal tissue.

## Double-Outlet Right Ventricle
According to Kirklin[1,57] double-outlet right (DORV) or left (DOLV) ventricle occurs when more than one-and-one-half great arteries arise from one ventricle. (Because both DOLV[1,3,52,74] and DORV without VSD[71] are exceedingly rare, only DORV with VSD is considered here.) The spatial orientation of the great vessels varies, as does their relationship to the VSD. In the vast majority of cases of DORV a large VSD is related to an overriding posterior great vessel. If the great vessels are normally related the VSD is subaortic.[69] When DTGA is present, the defect is related to the pulmonary artery (subpulmonic), a configuration called the Taussig-Bing malformation.[57,87]

Since ultrasound beam angulation and subjective judgment may affect the echocardiographic assessment of the degree of override, the dividing line between the simplest form of DORV and malalignment VSD is not always clear by this criterion. Detection of an intervening band of tissue (conus) disrupting fibrous mitral valve-aortic continuity is an important diagnostic feature of DORV, but it may not be appreciated by sonographers who are inexperienced with congenital lesions.[1,6,7,53,56,70] Bilateral conus may be visualized in many cases.[69,70] DORV also often is seen with pulmonary stenosis (DORV/PS), and in this association it may be difficult to differentiate from Tetralogy of Fallot (TOF; see below). The functional hemodynamic features of TOF and DORV/PS are similar in most instances. Problems in surgical correction differ, owing to the presence and position of intervening conus tissues; hence the need for clear differentiation to avoid surgical creation of LVOT obstruction.[61,67]

## Echocardiopgraphic Findings
### Two-Dimensional Study
+ Large VSD
+ Overriding aorta, usually 50% or more
+ Subaortic or bilateral conus
− Enlarged RV
− Narrowed LVOT
− Associated defects

### M-Mode Study
+ Aortic-mitral discontinuity (conus)
+ Aortic-septal discontinuity (override or conus)

— Enlarged RV
— Narrowed LVOT

*Doppler Study*
+ Predominant left-to-right shunting detected by PW and color-flow Doppler studies
+ Bidirectional shunting
— LVOT flow disturbance or obstruction

HEMODYNAMICS
The hemodynamic concerns are related to the large VSDs and possible LVOT obstruction.[1,3,54,69] Pulmonary blood flow usually is excessive in the absence of PS. Some flow mixing (bidirectional shunting) may occur, producing mild desaturation, which usually is insignificant. The ventricular pressures are equal. Pulmonary hypertension is the principal risk. When PS is associated, shunting will be limited, according to the severity of obstruction. This type of shunt dependency is described more fully under both Tetralogy of Fallot and single ventricle.

*Treatment.* Surgical correction is possible quite early in life for infants who develop ventricular failure or pulmonary hypertension. The VSD is patched from the right ventricular side, and particular care is taken to minimize LVOT narrowing. Conal tissue may be excised to prevent LVOT obstruction. Pulmonary artery banding is an option as a palliative procedure for those who do not qualify for primary repair.

TAUSSIG-BING MALFORMATION
DORV is often associated with dextrotransposition of the great arteries (DTGA), and the combination is called the Taussig-Bing malformation.[1,7,57,87] The "unwrapped" great vessels travel straight up and then posteriorly without wrapping around each other. They may lie anterior-posterior or side by side or be diagonally related. Both great vessels "arise" from the right ventricle and the pulmonary artery overrides the ventricular septum. The VSD is then described as being subpulmonic. The AV valves usually lie side by side at the same depth. Bilateral conus is usually present. Pulmonary stenosis and AV valve malformations are associated with this anomaly.[1,6,8,53,57,70]

ECHOCARDIOGRAPHIC FINDINGS
*Two-Dimensional Study*
+ Large VSD
+ Features of DTGA
+ Overriding PA
— Side-by-side AV valves
— Large right ventricle
— Bilateral conus

*M-Mode Study*
+ Features similar to those of DORV
+ Spatial orientation of dextro TGA
+ Side-by-side AV valves

*Doppler Study*
+ Features similar to those of DORV

HEMODYNAMICS
Owing to lower pulmonary resistance and pulmonary override the predominant direction of shunting is still systemic-to-pulmonary with the usual risk of increased pulmonary blood flow causing irreversible pulmonary hypertension. In the absence of pulmonary vascular disease or other lesions, pressures in both great vessels are the same.

TREATMENT
Surgical correction has been performed in two ways: (1) direction of the VSD flow to the aorta by intraventricular tunnel and (2) closure of the VSD to the pulmonary artery with atrial baffle, as in the Mustard procedure.[57,61,75,82]

TETRALOGY OF FALLOT
TOF has four principal components; moderate to large VSD, override of the aorta, obstruction to pulmonary blood flow at any or all of a variety of levels, and right ventricular hypertrophy (Fig. 20-4A). A variety of clinical presentations occurs owing to the wide ranges of type and severity of the pulmonary outflow tract obstruction. Infants with severely obstructive forms of this disease have been called blue babies, because of the marked cyanosis that is often present in this lesion. Occasionally TOF is seen later in life, if the obstruction is not

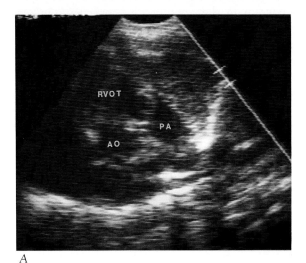
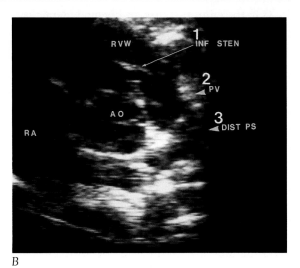

FIGURE 20-4. Tetralogy of Fallot. (A) A cross-sectional view of the great vessels shows a single level of obstruction, a domed stenotic pulmonary valve. (B) A cross-sectional view demonstrates multiple sites of obstruction in another patient (1) infundibular muscular impingement, (2) narrowed pulmonary annulus (AO, 1.9 cm; PA, 1.0 cm), (3) tortuous distal pulmonary artery.

severe and the patient has not received regular medical care. These "pink tets" may be able to pursue a normally active lifestyle until the obstruction progresses farther.

The anterior displacement of the aorta that contributes to override is often accompanied by muscular impingement of the RVOT, referred to as infundibular stenosis. Often multiple levels of obstruction are present (Fig. 20-4B). Severe tunnel-like stenosis (hypoplasia) of the pulmonary artery may also be seen. Pulmonary atresia with VSD is often thought of as a severe form of TOF. Multiple 2-D approaches as well as rigorous Doppler investigation are required to assess the types and severity of obstruction in each patient.

ECHOCARDIOGRAPHIC FINDINGS

*Two-Dimensional Study*
+ Override of the aorta
+ Moderate to large VSD
+ RV hypertrophy
+ Right outflow obstruction in any single or com-

bined form at the infundibulum, pulmonary valve, or distal pulmonary artery
− Enlarged RV
− LV is normal size though it may appear small relative to the RV

*M-Mode Study*
+ Aortic override
+ VSD (discontinuity on LV-Ao sweep)
+ RV outflow obstruction

*Doppler Study*
+ Color-flow demonstration of turbulent flow to localize obstruction
+ Severity of the obstruction (CW Doppler assessment) (*Warning:* Estimation of pressure gradients by the modified Bernoulli's equation is unreliable in the presence of multiple levels of obstruction.)
− Shunt patterns (color-flow assessment); some bidirectional shunting through the VSD is seen in most cases

## HEMODYNAMICS

In TOF the clinical course and hemodynamic patterns depend primarily on the degree of obstruction to pulmonary blood flow.[1,3,6,8,65] Usually, even mild obstruction is enough to protect the lungs from the severe overcirculation that can occur in isolated large VSD. The predominant direction of shunting is left to right until obstruction becomes moderate to severe. As the obstruction increases, a point of equilibrium between pulmonary and systemic flow is reached at which resistances (and therefore flow volumes) are equal. Some mixing of flows may occur producing mild systemic desaturation. Balanced TOF with predominant left-to-right shunting or equal flows may not produce overt clinical symptoms.

As the muscular infundibular obstruction continues to increase, shunting becomes predominantly right to left. As right-to-left shunting increases and pulmonary blood flow decreases, cyanosis becomes more severe. Patients with long-standing significant cyanosis may develop clubbed fingers.[8] In some patients, intermittent muscular outflow tract contractions occur, producing transient, severe obstruction to pulmonary blood flow ("tet spells"). Ambulatory patients experiencing one of these intermittent spells instinctively squat in an attempt to increase systemic return.[1,3,8]

## TREATMENT

TOF was one of the first congenital heart defects to be treated surgically. Before the advent of open heart correction, the Blalock-Taussig shunt operation afforded many patients a more normal lifestyle. The left subclavian artery was ligated distally, and the end of the proximal segment was anastomosed to the pulmonary artery, thereby supplementing pulmonary flow in a controlled fashion. This operation and other modified versions are still used as palliative procedures for patients whose hearts are not yet large enough to allow definitive repair. Final repair is accomplished by closing the VSD with a patch, resecting infundibular obstruction, pulmonary valvotomy, and reconstructing the RVOT or MPA as necessary.[1,3,6,8]

## TRUNCUS ARTERIOSUS

During development the embryonic truncus arteriosus undergoes a spiraling septation process to fi-

nally produce the normal PA and aorta; these then hook up to the appropriate ventricular outflow tracts. When this process fails, the single large vessel may persist in various stages of division, all called persistent truncus arteriosus (PTA).[1,3,7,8] In all varieties there is a blind pouch instead of an RVOT-PA connection. There is a single, large, complex, semilunar valve that allows egress of flow from both ventricles. The valve leaflets are abnormal, thick, and redundant in appearance, usually numbering four or more, and often producing stenosis or insufficiency.[1,3,5,6,8,60,62]

PTA usually is categorized in four groups or types. In type I an MPA segment of some sort usually arises from the left lateral or back wall of the ascending trunk (Fig. 20-5). Type II has no discernible MPA segment, but both PA orifices emanate in close proximity to each other from the back wall of the truncal root. In type III the pulmonary arteries arise from separate sides of the trunk, and in type IV the vessels arise not from the trunk but from other systemic thoracic vessels.[1,5,77,85,88] Other variations of pulmonary vessel anatomy may be seen that do not fit easily into this classification. Echocardiography must be performed in a range of parasternal, apical, subcostal, and suprasternal views to adequately define the configuration of the pulmonary vessel or vessels. Other associated anomalies, such as mitral valve stenosis and coarctation, must also be assessed.[1,3,73,88] As for many congenital lesions, standard views may be inadequate, and inventive imaging techniques often are necessary.[6,63,77,78,88]

## ECHOCARDIOGRAPHIC FINDINGS

*Two-Dimensional Study*
+ Single overriding great vessel
+ Large VSD
+ Complex abnormal semilunar valve
+ Configuration of the pulmonary vessels
− Any associated anomalies

*M-Mode Study*
+ IVS-truncus discontinuity with override
+ One large great vessel with complex valve. (Truncal valves usually appear markedly abnormal on M-mode studies, with thick multiple closure lines and/or marked eccentricity.

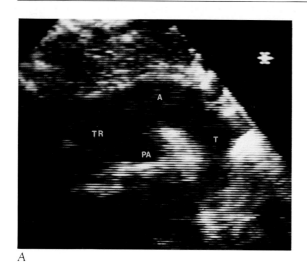
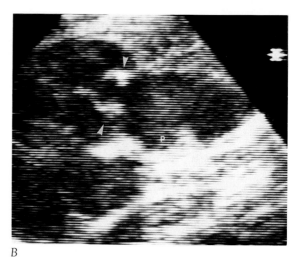

FIGURE 20-5. Truncus arteriosus in a long-axis view. (A) A large truncal root (TR) gives rise to a posterior pulmonary artery (PA) and anterior aorta (A). (T, transverse aortic arch.) (B) The arrowheads indicate the open leaflets of a complex truncal valve. (P, posterior pulmonary artery.)

*Doppler Study*

+ Color-flow demonstration of flow from both ventricles into the truncus
+ Color-flow demonstration of the takeoff of pulmonary vessels (may be very helpful when origin of these vessels is difficult to visualize by 2-D alone)
+ Pulmonary stenosis or increased pulmonary flow
+ Truncal insufficiency or stenosis when present

HEMODYNAMICS

The hemodynamic status of truncus arteriosus hinges on whether the pulmonary artery configuration allows adequate, insufficient, or excessive pulmonary blood flow. Regardless of the volume of pulmonary blood flow, systemic flow is desaturated from flow mixing within the truncus.[1,3]

TREATMENT

Surgical correction of PTA usually is performed by inserting a conduit to connect the right ventricle with the pulmonary vasculature. The VSD is closed with a patch.[1,3,64,76,85] Infrequently, surgical treatment of PTA may be required to control pulmonary blood flow (PBF) before correction is possible. When large pulmonary vessels allow unrestricted PBF, pulmonary artery banding may be performed to prevent irreversible pulmonary hypertension and/or failure. When pulmonary anatomy restricts PBF too severely, a shunt procedure may be necessary to augment PBF.[1,3]

## Some Unusual Cases

ANOMALOUS ORIGIN OF THE LEFT MAIN CORONARY ARTERY

The usual sites of origin of the coronary arteries are the right and left sinuses of Valsalva.[1,8] Fully oxygenated blood is perfused through both coronaries to the myocardium under systemic diastolic pressure. In rare instances a coronary artery originates elsewhere.[1,2,3,6] Anomalous origin of the left main coronary artery (ALMCA) from the MPA has been difficult to identify echocardiographically.[92,96,99] ALMCA usually presents early in life because it produces symptoms of congestive heart failure (CHF) mimicking myocarditis.[1,7,92] Inability

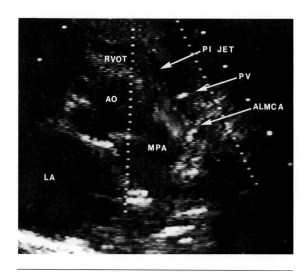

FIGURE 20-6. (See color insert.) Anomalous origin of the left main coronary artery from the MPA. A cross-sectional color flow image of the great vessels reveals a flow jet from the left lateral wall of the MPA less than 1 cm from the pulmonary valve (PV). This diastolic jet emanates from the origin of the ALMCA. A small plume of pulmonary insufficiency (PI) is seen in the RVOT.

to image an LMCA arising from the aorta in a patient with CHF has often necessitated cardiac catheterization for definitive diagnosis. The availability of color-flow Doppler imaging enhances the ability to diagnose this lesion noninvasively.[93,94]

Figure 20-6 demonstrates color-flow visualization of reflux into the MPA from a vessel arising from the left margin very close to the pulmonary valve. This flow jet was not distinguishable from a PDA by PW or CW Doppler technique alone. The localization of the flow source by color-flow technique, in such close proximity to the valve, along with the direction of the flow jet being across rather than along the length of the MPA allowed the diagnosis of ALMCA with much greater certainty.[91-94]

## KAWASAKI DISEASE
Kawasaki's disease is characterized by a febrile illness of 5 days or longer, with a characteristic rash,

changes in the oral mucosa, and redness and edema of the palms of the hands and soles of the feet followed by skin peeling around fingers and toes. Few cases have been reported in adults. The incidence of the disease has been rising rapidly in the United States over the last few years.[89,95] Kawasaki's disease is diagnosed clinically, not echocardiographically, but one sequela is an arteritis that causes aneurysms in a variety of locations such as the kidneys, brain, and coronary arteries. These aneurysms begin to form about 2 weeks into the illness; the most common location is the coronary arteries.[1,2,89] Echocardiography is now being used to rule out coronary aneurysms in suspected cases of Kawasaki's disease. Aneurysms may occur anywhere along the length of the coronary arteries. The use of aspirin, and more recently intravenous gamma globulin, to treat the arteritis can prevent or minimize aneurysm formation.[89,95]

Significant lengths of normal coronary arteries may be readily visualized[91,93,94] with practice. Figure 20-7A shows a normal LMCA in a 7.5-kg patient. An image of an unusual case of Kawasaki's (Fig. 20-7B) reveals a large RCA aneurysm that is sonolucent. Figure 20-7C demonstrates an even larger LMCA aneurysm filled in with thrombus in the same patient, whose cardiac function was normal.

## SUPRAVALVULAR AORTIC STENOSIS
Supravalvular aortic stenosis (SVAS) may be found beginning at or beyond the margin of the sinus of Valsalva.[1,6,8] It may occur as a discrete hourglass-shaped constriction, as a fibromuscular ring, or as a diffuse tubular or even hypoplastic structure.[90,99] This anomaly is most often present as a clinical component of Williams' syndrome, which is characterized by elfin facies, growth retardation, and deep voice.[1,3] Abnormalities of the aortic, pulmonary, or mitral valve may be associated.

Figure 20-8 shows a case of a short tunnel segment of the ascending aorta beginning at the margin of the sinus and extending 1.5 cm along the ascending aorta. The lumen at the aortic valve is 1.47 cm and the valve is thickened. The ascending aorta measures 1.37 cm, and the tunnel lumen, 0.7 cm. The aortic valve was bicuspid. This patient did not have Williams' syndrome.

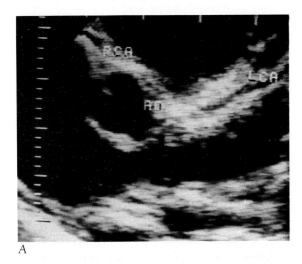

A

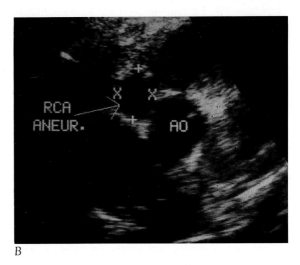

B

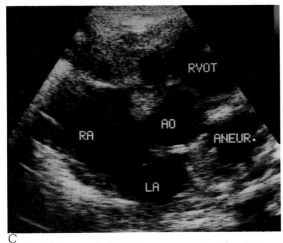

C

FIGURE 20-7. Kawasaki's disease. (A) A cross-sectional view of the aorta and LCA demonstrates a long segment of a normal LCA. (B) A cross-sectional view angled to visualize the RCA shows a large proximal aneurysm. (C) A similarly angled view of the LCA shows a massive proximal aneurysm with thrombus deposition.

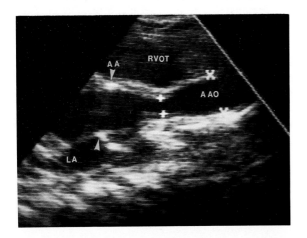

FIGURE 20-8. Supravalvular aortic stenosis. This long-axis view shows an aortic annulus (AA) of 1.47 cm, a distal ascending aorta (AAO) of 1.37 cm, and a tunnel segment beginning at the superior margin of the sinus of Valsalva with a lumen of 0.83 cm.

# References

1. Adams FH, Emmanouilides GC, Riemenschneider TA. Moss' Heart Disease in Infants, Children and Adolescents. 4th ed. Baltimore: Williams & Wilkins; 1989.

2. Allan LD, Leanage R, Wainwright R, et al. Balloon atrial septostomy under two-dimensional echocardiographic control. Br Heart J. 1982; 47(1):41–43.

3. Allwork SP, Bentall HH, Becker AE, et al. Congenitally corrected transposition of the great arteries: Morphologic study of 32 cases. Am J Cardiol. 1976; 38(7):910–923.

4. Anderson RH, Becker AE, Tynan M, et al. The univentricular atrioventricular connection: Getting to the root of a thorny problem. Am J Cardiol. 1984; 54(7):822–828.

5. Anderson RH, Becker AE, Wilcox BR, et al. Surgical anatomy of double-outlet right ventricle—A reappraisal. Am J Cardiol. 1983; 52(5):555–559.

6. Anderson RH, Macartney FJ, Shinebourne EA, et al. Definitions of cardiac chambers. In: Anderson RH, Shinebourne EA, eds: Paediatric Cardiology 1977. Edinburgh: Churchill-Livingstone; 1978:5.

7. Assad-Morell JL, Seward JB, Tajik AJ, et al. Echophonocardiographic and contrast studies in conditions associated with systemic arterial trunk overriding the ventricular septum: Truncus arteriosus, tetralogy of Fallot, and pulmonary atresia with ventricular septal defect. Circulation. 1976; 53(4):663–673.

8. Aziz KU, Paul MH, Bharati S, et al. Two-dimensional echocardiographic evaluation of Mustard operation for d-transposition of the great arteries. Am J Cardiol. 1981; 47(3):654–664.

9. Baker EJ, Allan LD, Tynan MJ, et al. Balloon atrial septostomy in the neonatal intensive care unit. Br Heart J. 1984; 51(4):377–378.

10. Bharati S, Lev M. The relationship between single ventricle and small outlet chamber and straddling and displaced tricuspid orifice and valve. Herz. 1979; 4(2):176–183.

11. Bharati S, McAllister H, Rosenquist G, et al. The surgical anatomy of truncus arteriosus communis. J Thorac Cardiovasc Surg. 1974; 67:501.

12. Bierman FZ. M-mode and two-dimensional echocardiography—Contributions and limitations in management of interatrial and interventricular septal defects and conotruncal anomalies. Ultrasound Med Biol. 1984; 10(6):721–734.

13. Bierman FZ, Gersony WM. Kawasaki disease: Clinical perspective. J Pediatr. 1987, 111:789–793.

14. Bierman FZ, Williams RG. Prospective diagnosis of d-transposition of the great arteries in neonates by subxiphoid, two-dimensional echocardiography. Circulation 1979; 60(7):1496–1502.

15. Bolen JL, Popp RL, French JW. Echocardiographic features of supravalvular aortic stenosis. Circulation 1975; 52:817.

16. Burke EC, Kirklin JW, Edwards JE. Sites of obstruction to pulmonary blood flow in tetralogy of Fallot. Proc Mayo Clin. 1951; 26:498.

17. Caldwell RL, Ensing GJ. Coronary artery abnormalities in children. J Am Soc Echocardiogr. 1989; 2:259–268.

18. Caldwell RL, Weyman AE, Hurwitz RA, et al. Right ventricular outflow tract assessment by cross-sectional echocardiography in tetralogy of Fallot. Circulation. 1979; 59:395.

19. Caldwell RL, et al. Cross-sectional echocardiographic evaluation of coronary artery abnormalities in children. Am J Cardiol. 1980; 45:467 (abstr).

20. Caldwell RL, et al. Two-dimensional echocardiographic differentiation of anomalous left coronary artery from congestive cardiomyopathy. Am Heart J. 1983; 106:710.

21. Chin AJ, et al. Accuracy of prospective two-dimensional echocardiographic evaluation of left-ventricular outflow tract in complete transposition of the great arteries. Am J Cardiol. 1985; 55:759.

22. Coto EO, Jimenez MQ, Castaneda AR, et al. Double outlet from chambers of left ventricular morphology. Br Heart J. 1979; 42(1):15-21.

23. Daskalopoulos DA, Edwards WD, Driscoll DJ, et al. Correlation of two-dimensional echocardiographic and autopsy findings in complete transposition of the great arteries. J Am Coll Cardiol. 1983; 2(6):1151–1157.

24. Deal BJ, Chin AJ, Sanders SP, et al. Subxiphoid two-dimensional echocardiographic identification of tricuspid valve abnormalities in transposition of the great arteries with ventricular septal defect. Am J Cardiol. 1985; 55(9):1146–1151.

25. DiSessa TG, Child JS, Perloff JK, et al. Systemic venous and pulmonary arterial flow patterns after Fontan's procedure for tricuspid atresia for single ventricle. Circulation. 1984; 70(5):898–902.

26. DiSessa TG, Hagan AD, Pope C, et al. Two-dimensional echocardiographic characteristics of double-outlet right ventricle. Am J Cardiol. 1979; 44(6):1146–1154.

27. Duncan WJ, Freedom RM, Rowe RD, et al. Echocardiographic features before and after the Jatene procedure (anatomical correction) for transposition of the great vessels. Am Heart J. 1981; 102(2):227–232.

28. Feigenbaum H. Echocardiography. 4th ed. Philadelphia: Lea & Febiger; 1986.

29. Fisher EA, et al. Two-dimensional echocardiographic visualization of the left coronary artery in anomalous origin of the left coronary artery from the pulmonary artery. Circulation. 1981; 63:698.

30. Foale R, Stefanini L, Rickards A, et al. Left and right ventricular morphology in complex congenital heart disease defined by two-dimensional echocardiography. Am J Cardiol. 1982; 49:93.

31. Freedom RM, Picchio F, Duncan WJ, et al. The atrioventricular junction in the univentricular heart: A two-dimensional echocardiographic analysis. Pediatr Cardiol. 1982; 3(2):105–117.

32. George L, Waldman JD, Mathewson JW, et al. Two-dimensional echocardiographic discrimination of normal from abnormal great artery relationships. Clin Cardiol. 1983; 6(7):327–332.

33. Goor DA, Edwards JE. The spectrum of transposition of the great arteries with specific reference to developmental anatomy of the conus. Circulation. 1968; 48:406.

34. Guo DW, Lin ML, Gu ZQ, et al. Double-outlet right ventricle: A clinical-roentgenologic-pathologic study of 28 consecutive patients. Chest. 1984; 85(4):526–532.

35. Hagler DJ, Seward JB, Tajik AJ, et al. Functional assessment of the Fontan operation: Combined M-mode two-dimensional and Doppler echocardiographic studies. J Am Coll Cardiol. 1984; 4:756–764.

36. Hagler DJ, Tajik AJ, Seward JB, et al. Wide-angle two-dimensional echocardiographic profiles of conotruncal abnormalities. Mayo Clin Proc. 1980; 55(2):73–82.

37. Hagler DJ, Tajik AJ, Seward JB, et al. Atrioventricular and ventriculo-arterial discordance (corrected transposition of the great arteries): Wide-angle two-dimensional echocardiographic assessment of ventricular morphology. Mayo Clin Proc. 1981; 56(10):591–600.

38. Hagler DJ, Tajik AJ, Seward JB, et al. Double-outlet right ventricle: Wide-angle two-dimensional echocardiographic observations. Circulation. 1981; 63(2):419–428.

39. Hightower BM, Barcia A, Bargeron LM, et al. Double-outlet right ventricle with transposed great arteries and subpulmonary ventricular septal defect: The Taussig-Bing malformation. Circulation. 1969; 39–40(suppl. I):207.

40. Houston AB, Gregory NL, Murtagh E, et al. Two-dimensional echocardiography in infants with persistent truncus arteriosus. Br Heart J. 1981; 46(5):492–497.

41. Huhta JC, Gutgesell HP, Latson LA, et al. Two-dimensional echocardiographic assessment of the aorta in infants and children with congenital heart disease. Circulation. 1984; 70:417.

42. Huhta JC, Seward JB, Tajik AJ, et al. Two-dimensional echocardiographic spectrum of univentricular atrioventricular connection. J Am Coll Cardiol. 1985; 5(1):149–157.

43. Keeton BR, Macartney FJ, Hunter S, et al. Univentricular heart of right ventricular type with double or common inlet. Circulation. 1979; 59:403.

44. Keith JD, Rowe R, Vlad P. Heart Disease in Infancy and Childhood. 3rd ed. New York: Macmillan; 1978.

45. Lavoie R, Sestier F, Gilbert G, et al. Double-outlet right ventricle with left ventricular outflow tract obstruction due to small ventricular septal defect. Am Heart J. 1971; 82:290.

46. Lev M, Bharati S. Double-outlet right ventricle, association with other cardiovascular anomalies. Arch Pathol. 1973; 95:117.

47. Lev M, Bharati S, Meng CCL, et al. A concept of double-outlet right ventricle. J Thorac Cardiovasc Surg. 1972; 64:271.

48. Macartney FJ, Rigby ML, Anderson RH, et al. Double-outlet right ventricle: Cross-sectional echocardiographic findings, their anatomical explanation, and surgical relevance. Br Heart J. 1984; 52(2):164–177.

49. MacMahon HE, Lipa M. Double-outlet right ventricle with intact interventricular septum. Circulation. 1964; 30:745.

50. Mar'in-Garc'ia J, Tonkin IL. Two-dimensional echocardiographic evaluation of persistent truncus arteriosus. Am J Cardiol. 1982; 50(6):1376–1379.

51. Mason DT, Morrow AG, Elkins RC, et al. Origin of both great vessels from the right ventricle associated with severe obstruction to left ventricular outflow. Am J Cardiol. 1969; 24:118.

52. Meyer R. Echocardiography in Kawasaki disease. J Am Soc Echocardiogr. 1989; 2:269–275.

53. Mustard WT. Successful two-stage correction of transposition of the great vessels. Pediatr Surg. 1964; 55:469.

54. Mustard WT, Keith JD, Trusler GA, et al. The surgical management of transposition of the great vessels. J Thorac Cardiovasc Surg. 1964; 48:953.

55. Newburger JW, et al. The treatment of Kawasaki syndrome with intravenous gamma globulin. N Engl J Med. 1986; 315:345–347.

56. Omoto R. Color Atlas of Real-Time Two-Dimensional Doppler Echocardiography. Philadelphia: Lea & Febiger; 1984.

57. Pasquini L, Sanders SP, Parness IA, et al. Diagnosis of coronary artery anatomy by two-dimensional echocardiography in patients with transposition of the great arteries. Circulation. 1987; 75:557–564.

58. Patrick DL, McGoon DC. An operation for double-outlet right ventricle with transposition of the great arteries. J Cardiovasc Surg. 1968; 9:537.

59. Paul MH, Sinha SN, Muster AJ, et al. Double-outlet left ventricle: Report of an autopsy case with an intact ventricular septum and consideration of its developmental implications. Circulation. 1970; 41:129–139.

60. Quaegebeur JM, Rohmer J, Ottenkamp J, et al. The arterial switch operation: An eight-year experience. J Thorac Cardiovasc Surg. 1986; 92:361–384.

61. Rashkind WJ, Miller WM. Creation of an atrial septal defect without thoracotomy: A palliative approach to complete transposition of the great arteries. JAMA. 1966; 196:992.

62. Reeder GS, Currie PJ, Fyfe DA, et al. Extracardiac conduit obstruction: Initial experience in the use of Doppler echocardiography for noninvasive estimation of pressure gradient. J Am Coll Cardiol. 1984; 4(5):1006–1011.

63. Rice MJ, Seward JB, Hagler DJ, et al. Definitive diagnosis of truncus arteriosus by two-dimensional echocardiography. Mayo Clin Proc. 1982; 57(8):476–481.

64. Rigby ML, Anderson RH, Gibson D, et al. Two-dimensional echocardiographic categorisation of the univentricular heart. Br Heart J. 1981; 46:603.

65. Riggs TW, Paul MH. Two-dimensional echocardiographic prospective diagnosis of common truncus arteriosus in infants. Am J Cardiol. 1982; 50(6):1380–1384.

66. Ritter DG, Seward JB, Moodie D, et al. Univentricular heart (common ventricle): Preoperative diagnosis. Hemodynamic, angiocardiographic and echocardiographic features. Herz. 1979; 4(2):198–205.

67. Rupprath G, Vogt J, de Vivie ER, et al. Conduit repair for complex congenital heart disease with pulmonary atresia or right ventricular outflow tract obstruction: II. Early and late hemodynamic and echocardiographic findings. Thorac Cardiovasc Surg. 1981; 29(6):337–344.

68. Sahn DJ, Anderson F. Two-Dimensional Anatomy of the Heart. New York: John Wiley; 1982.

69. Sahn DJ, Harder JR, Freedom RM, et al. Cross-sectional echocardiographic diagnosis and subclassification of univentricular hearts: Imaging studies of atrioventricular valves, septal structures and rudimentary outflow chambers. Circulation. 1982; 66(5):1070–1077.

70. Sahn DJ, Terry R, O'Rourke R, et al. Multiple crystal cross-sectional echocardiography in the diagnosis of cyanotic congenital heart disease. Circulation. 1974; 50:230.

71. Senning A. Surgical correction of transposition of the great arteries. Surgery. 1959; 45:966.

72. Seward JB, Tajik AJ, Hagler DJ. Two-dimensional echocardiographic features of univentricular heart. In: Lundstrom NR, ed. Pediatric Echocardiography—Cross-Sectional, M-Mode and Doppler. Amsterdam: Elsevier/North Holland; 1980: 157–169.

73. Seward JB, Tajik AJ, Edwards WD, et al. Two-Dimensional Echocardiography Atlas. Congenital Heart Disease. New York: Springer-Verlag; 1987.

74. Silove ED, DeGiovanni JV, Shiu MF, et al. Diagnosis of right ventricular outflow obstruction in infants by cross-sectional echocardiography. Br Heart J. 1983; 50:416.

75. Smallhorn JF, Gow R, Freedom RM, et al. Pulsed Doppler echocardiographic assessment of the pulmonary venous pathway after the Mustard or Senning procedure for transposition of the great arteries. Circulation. 1986; 73(4):765–774.

76. Sondheimer HM, Freedom RM, Olley PM. Double-outlet right ventricle: Clinical spectrum and prognosis. Am J Cardiol. 1977; 39(5):709–714.

77. Stevenson JG, Kawabori I, Bailey WW. Noninvasive evaluation of Blalock-Taussig shunts: Determination of patency and differentiation from patent ductus arteriosus by Doppler echocardiography. Am Heart J. 1983; 106:1121.

78. Terai M, Nagai Y, and Toba T. Cross-sectional echocardiographic findings of anomalous origin of left coronary artery from pulmonary artery. Br Heart J. 1983; 50:104.

79. Thompson K, Serwer GA. Echocardiographic features of patients with and without residual defects after Mustard's procedure for transposition of the great vessels. Circulation. 1981; 64(5):1032–1041.

80. Van Mierop LHS. Diseases: Congenital anomalies. In Netter FH, Yonkman FF, eds. The Ciba Collection of Medical Illustrations: The Heart. Rochester, NY: Case-Hoyt Corporation; 1969; 5:112–130.

81. Van Mierop LHS. Transposition of the great arteries: I. Clarification or further confusion? Am J Cardiol. 1971; 28:735.

82. Van Mierop LHS, Wiglesworth FW. Pathogenesis of transposition complexes: II. Anomalies due to faulty transfer of the posterior great artery. Am J Cardiol. 1963; 12:226–232.

83. Van Mierop LHS, Wiglesworth FW. Pathogenesis of transposition complexes: III. True transposition of the great vessels. Am J Cardiol. 1963; 12:233–239.

84. Van Mierop LHS, Alley RD, Kausell HW, et al. Pathogenesis of transposition complexes: I. Embryology of the ventricles and great arteries. Am J Cardiol. 1963; 12:216–225.

85. Van Praagh R. What is the Taussig-Bing malformation? Circulation. 1968; 38:445–449.

86. Van Praagh R. Classification of truncus arteriosus communis (TAC). Am Heart J. 1976; 92:129.

87. Van Praagh R, Takao A. Etiology and Morphogenesis of Congenital Heart Disease. New York: Futura; 1980.

88. Van Praagh R, Van Praagh S. Isolated ventricular inversion: A consideration of the morphogenesis, definition and diagnosis of nontransposed and transposed great arteries. Am J Cardiol. 1966; 17:395.

89. Van Praagh R, Vlad P. Dextrocardia, mesocardia, and levocardia: The segmental approach to diagnosis in congenital heart disease. In: Keith JD, Rowe RD, Vlad P, eds. Heart Disease in Infancy and Childhood. 3rd ed. New York: Macmillan; 1978; 638.

90. Van Praagh R, Ongley PA, Swan HJC. Anatomic types of single or common ventricle in man: Morphologic and geometric aspects of sixty autopsied cases. Am J Cardiol. 1964; 13:367.

91. Van Praagh R, Weinberg PM, Van Praagh S. Malposition of the heart. In: Moss AJ, Adams FH, Emmanouilides GC, eds. Heart Disease in Infants, Children and Adolescents. 2d ed. Baltimore: Williams & Wilkins; 1977: 394.

92. Van Praagh R, Weinberg PM, Calder AL, et al. The transposition complexes: How many are there? In: Davila, JC ed. Second Henry Ford Hospital International Symposium on Cardiac Surgery. New York: Appleton-Century-Crofts; 1977; 207–213.

93. Van Praagh R, Van Praagh S, Nebesar RA, et al. Tetralogy of Fallot: Underdevelopment of the pulmonary infundibulum and its sequelae. Am J Cardiol. 1970; 26:25.

94. Vargas BJ, Sahn DJ, Attie F, et al. Two-dimensional echocardiographic study of right ventricular outflow and great artery anatomy in pulmonary atresia with ventricular septal defects and in truncus arteriosus. Am Heart J. 1983; 105(2):281–286.

95. Vitarelli A, Gheorghiade M, Gentile R, et al. Echocardiographic features of truncal abnormalities: Special emphasis to the evaluation of pulmonary arteries. G Ital Cardiol. 1984; 14(4):245–252.

96. Vogt J, Rupprath G, Grimm T, et al. Qualitative and quantitative evaluation of supravalvular aortic stenosis by cross-sectional echocardiography. Pediatr Cardiol. 1982; 3:13.

97. Weyman AE, Caldwell RL, Hurwitz RA, et al. Cross-sectional echocardiographic characterization of aortic obstruction: I. Supravalvular aortic stenosis and aortic hypoplasia. Circulation. 1978; 57:491.

98. Worsham C, Sanders SP, Burger BM. Origin of the right coronary artery from the pulmonary trunk: Diagnosis by two-dimensional echocardiography. Am J Cardiol. 1985; 55:232.

# CHAPTER 21

# A Systematic Approach to Evaluating Congenital Heart Disease with Echocardiography

BARBARA STERNLIGHT

A common scenario in a pediatric echocardiography laboratory: An infant is scheduled for an examination, and the referring physician's request is *Rule out heart disease*. When a definitive clinical diagnosis has not been agreed upon, the challenge to the sonographer is, first, to determine whether heart disease is present and, second, to document any anomalies thoroughly and comprehensively.

Entire textbooks have been written on the anatomy and pathophysiology of congenital heart disease (CHD). The purpose of this chapter is not to duplicate them or present a condensed version. Rather, the objective is to offer sonographers a logical approach to the evaluation of CHD, an efficient method that makes the process of data collection less arbitrary and more systematic.

The approach used to identify cardiac lesions in neonates is somewhat different from that employed to scan adults with known heart disease. Needless to say, young infants may not be as cooperative as adults during the scanning procedure. Toys, music, and other distractions are useful to calm young patients; many laboratories prefer to sedate pediatric patients to ensure collection of accurate data.

Some scanning techniques are unique to pediatrics. Supplementing the standard, accepted views used in adult echocardiography are views sometimes omitted from an adult examination. The *subcostal window*, in particular, is frequently difficult to use in a large adult, but the view is quite accessible in an infant, and in most instances it illustrates complete intracardiac anatomy.

A sonographer scanning an infant's heart with ultrasound should never assume anything. The cardiac anatomy of a child with CHD can be very different from that of a typical normal adult. Extremely complex forms of CHD can be characterized by missing valves and chambers, holes between chambers, or malposition of vessels or chambers. The heart may even be on the "wrong" side of the body. The sonographer's role is to identify all cardiac structures and document their relationships to one another. The best approach to take in examining a patient with CHD is a logical, systematic one. It is good to start with a segmental approach. (See Table 21-1.)

There are three segments of the heart that must be identified: the atrial, ventricular, and great artery location. *Situs solitus* is the term for a normal anatomic configuration. The liver and inferior vena cava (IVC) lie to the right of the spine, and the descending aorta lies to the left. From the subcostal window, a transverse cross-sectional view demonstrates this relationship. *Situs inversus* is usually a mirror image of situs solitus. *Situs ambiguus* is the term applied when a scan from the subcostal window demonstrates the liver occupying a transverse position in the abdominal cavity, with the IVC and descending aorta both lying on the same side of the spine. The term is also applied when the

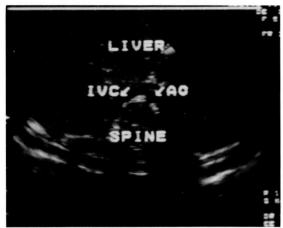

FIGURE 21-1

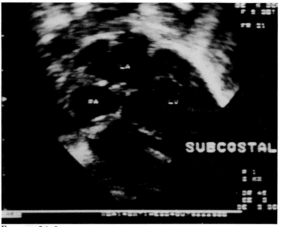

FIGURE 21-2

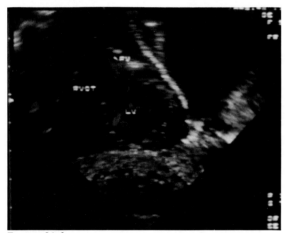

FIGURE 21-3

FIGURE 21-1. Two-dimensional echocardiogram, subcostal view, transverse (cross-section) view: IVC, inferior vena cava; AO, aorta.

FIGURE 21-2. Two-dimensional echocardiogram, subcostal four-chamber view, anterioposterior sweep: RA, Right atrium; LA, left atrium; LV, left ventricle.

FIGURE 21-3. Two-dimensional echocardiogram, subcostal four-chamber view, more posterior sweep than in Figure 21-2. RVOT, Right ventricular outflow tract; RV, right ventricle; LV, left ventricle.

positions of the other abdominal viscera, the atria, the IVC, and the descending aorta remain uncertain (ambiguous). Often in this instance the IVC is interrupted with hemiazygous continuation (Fig. 21-1).

A scan sweeping from the abdomen to the heart documents which chamber receives the IVC flow. This atrium is usually the anatomic right atrium. Once atrial situs (position) is established, the next segment to be assessed is ventricular position. Each ventricle has its own morphologic characteristics, which can be identified by echocardiography (Figs. 21-2–21-4).

The *right ventricle* contains a three-leaflet inlet valve, is shaped like a pyramid, and is thickly trabeculated. The moderator band can be seen in the anterior portion of the body of the ventricle, separating the inflow and outflow portions of the chamber. The outflow tract has an infundibulum, so the tricuspid valve annulus and the pulmonary valve annulus are discontinuous. The medial papillary muscle of the tricuspid valve (the papillary muscle of the conus) attaches to the interventricular septum.

The *left ventricle* contains a two-leaflet inlet valve and is shaped like a prolate ellipse. The annulus of the mitral valve is in fibrous continuity with the annulus of the aortic valve, because there is no infundibulum. In the left ventricle are two papillary muscles—one anterior and lateral, one posterior

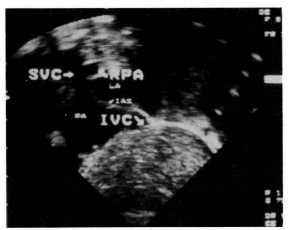

FIGURE 21-4

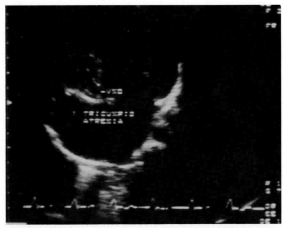

FIGURE 21-5

FIGURE 21-4. Two-dimensional echocardiogram, subcostal view, sagittal (short axis): SVC, Superior vena cava; RPA, right pulmonary artery; IVC, inferior vena cava; IAS, interatrial septum; RA, right atrium; LA, left atrium.

FIGURE 21-5. Two-dimensional echocardiogram, apical four-chamber view: VSD, ventricular septal defect.

FIGURE 21-6. (See color insert.) Two-dimensional echocardiogram, apical four-chamber view illustrates color flow through shunt. VSD, ventricular septal defect.

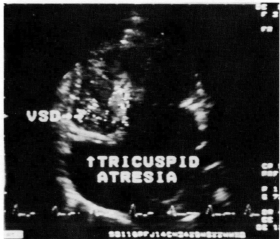

FIGURE 21-6

and medial. Unlike the papillary muscle in the tricuspid valve, neither attaches to the interventricular septum.

Ventricular morphology is evaluated from several anatomic planes (echocardiographic views). For example, the apical four-chamber view best illustrates the tricuspid valve, which can be seen in a more apical position than the mitral valve. It is helpful to keep in mind that an atrioventricular valve is always concordant with its corresponding ventricle. Therefore, the mitral valve will always be found in the morphologic left ventricle, and the tricuspid valve will be in the morphologic right ventricle.

The next segment to assess is great artery orientation. Normally, the aorta arises from the anatomic left ventricle and the pulmonary artery arises from the anatomic right ventricle. (Again, for a more complete understanding of the many possible anatomic variations, the reader can consult a comprehensive textbook.) In the process of establishing the anatomic placement of the chambers, valves, and vessels, the number of each must be ascertained. All available imaging modalities should be used. Valve tissue may appear to exist and move normally, but the addition of color-flow imaging may demonstrate no flow across an atretic valve (Figs. 21-5 and 21-6).

Table 21-1. A clinical classification of congenital heart disease

General

Innocent or normal murmurs
The cardiac malpositions
Congenitally corrected transposition of the great arteries
Congenital complete heart block

Acyanotic Without a Shunt

*Malformations Originating in the Left Side of the Heart (from Most Proximal to Most Distal)*
1. Obstruction to left atrial inflow
    a. Pulmonary vein stenosis
    b. Mitral stenosis
    c. Cor triatriatum
2. Mitral regurgitation
    a. Endocardial cushion defect
    b. Congenitally corrected transposition of the great arteries
    c. Anomalous origin of the left coronary artery from the pulmonary trunk
    d. Miscellaneous (congenital perforations, accessory commissures with anomalous chordal insertion, congenitally short or absent chordae, cleft posterior leaflet, and so on*
3. Primary dilated endocardial fibroelastosis
4. Aortic stenosis
    a. Discrete subvalvular
    b. Valvular
    c. Supravalvular
5. Aortic valve regurgitation
6. Coarctation of the aorta

*Malformations Originating in the Right Side of the Heart (from Most Proximal to Most Distal)*
1. Acyanotic Ebstein's anomaly of the tricuspid valve
2. Pulmonic stenosis
    a. Subinfundibular
    b. Infundibular
    c. Valvular
    d. Supravalvular (stenosis of pulmonary artery and its branches)
3. Congenital pulmonary valve regurgitation
4. Idiopathic dilatation of the pulmonary trunk
5. Primary pulmonary hypertension

Acyanotic with a Shunt (Left to Right)

*Shunt at Atrial Level*
1. Atrial septal defect
    a. Ostium secundum
    b. Ostium primum
    c. Sinus venosus
2. Partial anomalous pulmonary venous connection
3. Atrial septal defect with mitral stenosis (Lutembacher's syndrome)

*Shunt at Ventricular Level*
1. Ventricular septal defect
    a. Inlet septum
    b. Trabecular septum
    c. Perimembranous septum
    d. Infundibular septum
2. Ventricular septal defect with aortic regurgitation
3. Ventricular septal defect with left ventricular to right atrial shunt

*Shunt Between Aortic Root and Right Side of Heart*
1. Coronary arteriovenous fistula
2. Ruptured sinus of Valsalva aneurysm
3. Anomalous origin of left coronary artery from pulmonary trunk

*Shunt at Aortopulmonary Level*
1. Aortopulmonary window
2. Patent ductus arteriosus

*Shunts at More Than One Level*
Complete common atrioventricular canal

Cyanotic

*Increased Pulmonary Arterial Blood Flow*
1. Complete transposition of the great arteries
2. Taussig-Bing anomaly
3. Truncus arteriosus
4. Total anomalous pulmonary venous connection
5. Univentricular heart with low pulmonary vascular resistance and no pulmonic stenosis
6. Common atrium
7. Fallot's tetralogy with pulmonary atresia and increased collateral arterial flow
8. Tricuspid atresia with nonrestrictive ventricular septal defect

*Normal or Decreased Pulmonary Arterial Blood Flow*
1. Dominant left ventricle
   a. Tricuspid atresia
   b. Pulmonary atresia with intact ventricular septum
   c. Ebstein's anomaly of the tricuspid valve
   d. Single morphologic left ventricle with pulmonic stenosis
   e. Congenital vena caval to left atrial communication
2. Dominant right ventricle

*No Pulmonary Hypertension*
   a. Pulmonic stenosis or atresia with ventricular septal defect (Fallot's tetralogy)
   b. Pulmonic stenosis with intact ventricular septum and right to left interatrial shunt
   c. Pulmonic stenosis with complete transposition of the great arteries
   d. Double outlet right ventricle with pulmonic stenosis

*Pulmonary Hypertension*
   a. Atrial septal defect with reversed shunt
   b. Ventricular septal defect with reversed shunt (Eisenmenger's complex)
   c. Patent ductus arteriosus or aortopulmonary window with reversed shunt
   d. Double outlet right ventricle with high pulmonary vascular resistance
   e. Complete transposition of the great arteries with high pulmonary vascular resistance
   f. Total anomalous pulmonary venous connection with high pulmonary vascular resistance
   g. Hypoplastic left side of heart (aortic atresia, mitral atresia)
3. Normal or nearly normal ventricles
   a. Pulmonary arteriovenous fistula
   b. Vena caval to left atrial communication

(From Perloff JK. Clinical Recognition of Congenital Heart Disease. Philadelphia: WB Saunders; 1987; 3:4–5.)

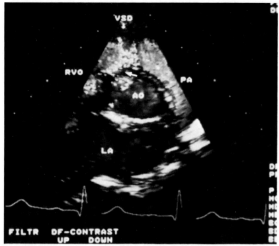

FIGURE 21-7

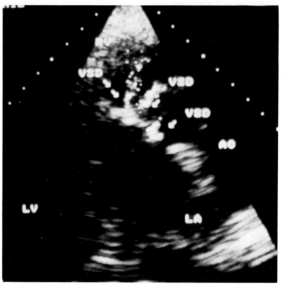

FIGURE 21-8

FIGURE 21-7. (See color insert.) Two-dimensional echocardiogram, parasternal short-axis view. Note color through ventricular septal defect (VSD). LA, Left atrium; AO, aorta; RVO, right ventricular outflow; PA, pulmonary artery.

FIGURE 21-8. (See color insert.) Two-dimensional echocardiogram, parasternal long-axis view (note color). VSD, ventricular septal defects. RV, right ventricle; LV, left ventricle; LA, left atrium; AO, aorta.

FIGURE 21-9. (See color insert.) Two-dimensional echocardiogram, modified apical four-chamber view. Note color through left-to-right (L, R) shunt. RV, Right ventricle; RA, right atrium; LV, left ventricle; LA, left atrium.

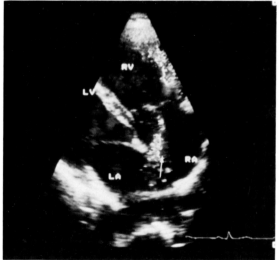

FIGURE 21-9

It is imperative that a sonographer study and understand the physiology and hemodynamics of the heart in order to evaluate complex CHD. Interrogation of the heart must be systematic. No lesion exists by itself without affecting the hemodynamics of the entire cardiopulmonary system, so chambers proximal and distal to a malformed or malfunctioning valve must be examined, as must the size of the left atrium if a shunt occurs at the level of the ventricles or great arteries. The resultant hemodynamics of flow in these chambers must be documented. (See Figs. 21-7–21-10.)

A sonographer should utilize an approach of anticipation and supposition[2] in evaluating a heart with diagnostic ultrasound and should consider, when an abnormality exists in one location, what else might be happening as a result. This approach guides the search. Also, lesions are documented in more than one view to demonstrate their presence conclusively and to illustrate their extent.

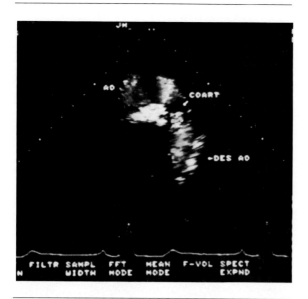

FIGURE 21-10. (See color insert.) Two-dimensional subtraction 2-D echocardiogram, suprasternal notch view of ascending aorta, demonstrates coarctation of the aorta (COART).

Patients should always be examined from all established echocardiographic planes and views. Only then can a sonographer be satisfied that all important anatomic and physiologic features have been correctly documented. The whole heart should be evaluated as the sum of all of its parts. (See Table 21-1.)

## Summary

A segmental approach ensures sequential evaluation of the heart. The number, position, and placement of chambers, valves, and vessels must be determined. The relationship of the anatomic parts to the heart as a whole should be established. An approach of anticipation and supposition is helpful. The anatomy proximal and distal to all lesions must be identified.

Flow patterns must be documented by conventional Doppler (pulsed-wave and continuous-wave) and color-flow imaging to assess jet direction, size, and velocity.

All modalities of echocardiography have applications. A combination of data derived from M-mode (helpful for making measurements), two-dimensional echocardiography (for a more global spatial assessment of the heart), Doppler, and color-flow imaging (imperative for evaluating flow dynamics) will provide a comprehensive picture of cardiac anatomy and pathophysiology. The sonographer's objective is to document the characteristics of all of the patient's anatomy, even if the name of the disease is not known or recognized. Thorough collection of data will provide the physician with the information needed to render a diagnosis.

## References

1. Hagan A, DeMaria A. Congenital heart disease. In: DiSessa TG, ed. Clinical Applications of Two-Dimensional Echocardiography and Cardiac Doppler. Boston: Little, Brown; 1989; 2.
2. Perloff JK. Introduction: Formulation of the problem. In: Perloff JK. Clinical Recognition of Congenital Heart Disease. Philadelphia: WB Saunders; 1987; 3.
3. Sahn DJ. Applications of color-coded Doppler flow imaging in the evaluation of children with congenital heart disease. Tokyo: Toshiba Med Rev.; 1988.
4. Sahn DJ, Anderson F. Two-Dimensional Anatomy of the Heart. New York: John Wiley; 1982.
5. Snider AR, Serwer GA. Echocardiography in Pediatric Heart Disease. Chicago: Year Book Medical Publishers; 1989.

# PART SIX

# The Profession of Diagnostic Cardiac Sonography

CHAPTER **22**

# Essentials of Cardiac Sonography

MARVEEN CRAIG

In the United States most echocardiography is performed by cardiac sonographers. The exceptional level of skill, knowledge, and experience required of them is unique among diagnostic procedures not performed by physicians. There is no question that the results of such studies are sonographer dependent.[4]

Because the cardiac sonographer is the initial examiner, it is critical that there be an interpretive interchange between sonographer and interpreting physician. The value of such a colleagial relationship is that it helps foster learning and reinforces the understanding of cardiac principles. Such an effort can only be beneficial to all involved (particularly the patient), as it allows for critical assessment of the techniques of each individual study and helps to achieve and maintain even higher standards.[3]

It is equally important for physicians who interpret echocardiograms to be skilled in examination techniques, to ensure that the technical quality of studies is optimal.

Cardiac sonographers must possess a keen understanding of ultrasound physics and instrumentation plus the manual dexterity to manipulate a transducer. To produce diagnostically adequate documentation of all the anatomic malformations that go with heart disease, cardiac sonographers must be familiar with cardiac anatomy and physiology and with the clinical aspects of cardiology.[3]

The recognition of diagnostic cardiac sonography as a special field of sonography has been a major milestone for the profession. Unlike members of other allied health professions, practitioners of sonography are not required to be certified or licensed[2]; rather, "credentialing" is voluntary. Credentials enhance professional status, ultimately improving the quality of patient care. Credentials not only constitute visible proof of a cardiac sonographer's abilities but they may also enhance remuneration and career benefits.[1]

In addition to credentialing organizations, cardiac sonographers are fortunate to have the special resources offered by professional organizations devoted to establishing and maintaining high professional standards, to bridging gaps between physicians and sonographers, alerting sonographers to proposed legislation and lobbying on their behalf.

The purpose of this chapter is to set forth the minimum educational requirements for cardiac sonographers, cardiovascular technologists, and physicians. The generous cooperation of the following organizations has enabled us to present this information:

American Cardiology Technologists Association (ACTA)
American College of Cardiology (ACC)
American College of Chest Physicians (ACCP)
American College of Radiology (ACR)

American Institute of Ultrasound in Medicine (AIUM)

American Medical Association (AMA)

American Registry of Diagnostic Medical Sonographers (ARDMS)

American Society of Echocardiography (ASE)

American Society of Radiologic Technologists (ASRT)

Canadian Society of Diagnostic Medical Sonographers (CSDMS)

Cardiovascular Credentialing International (CCI)

Joint Review Committee on Education in Cardiovascular Technology (JRC CVT)

Joint Review Committee on Education in Diagnostic Medical Sonography (JRC DMS)

National Alliance of Cardiovascular Technologists (NACT)

National Society of Cardiovascular Technologists (NSCT)

Society of Diagnostic Medical Sonographers (SDMS)

Society of Non-Invasive Vascular Technology (SNIVT)

Society for Vascular Surgery/International Society for Cardiovascular Surgery (SVS/ISCS)

## Diagnostic Cardiac Sonographer*

*General Competencies.*

1. Use oral and written medical communications;
   *Oral communication*
   *English composition*
   *Medical terminology*
2. Perform appropriate mathematical and algebraic functions;
   *Fundamental mathematical operations*
   *Exponential, logarithmic, and geometric functions*
   *Principles of graphing*
3. Anticipate and provide basic care and comfort;
   *Patient transport and handling*
   *Pertinent patient care procedures*
   *Principles of psychological support*
   *Principles of personal health*

*(Reprinted with permission from Essentials and Guidelines of an Accredited Educational Program for the Diagnostic Medical Sonographer (revised 1987). Provided by the Joint Review Committee on Education in Diagnostic Medical Sonography: Chicago, IL)

4. Recognize emergency patient conditions, initiate first aid and basic life support procedures;
   *Symptoms of pertinent emergency conditions*
   *Emergency procedures*
   *First aid and resuscitation techniques*
5. Demonstrate knowledge of human systemic and sectional anatomy;
   *Structure, organ, and system relationships*
   *Sectional anatomy*
6. Integrate patient history and physical findings to determine appropriate area(s) of interest for obtaining diagnostic examinations;
   *Patient interview and examination techniques*
   *Chart and referral evaluation*
   *Sonographic scan protocols related to specific disease conditions*
7. Demonstrate knowledge of ultrasound instrumentation;
   *Instrument options*
   *Principles of ultrasound instruments and modes of operation*
   *Operator control options*
8. Demonstrate knowledge and skills necessary to design and implement quality assurance programs, protocols, policies, and procedures for general function and operation of the ultrasound department;
   *Patient rights*
   *Equipment standards*
   *Applicable regulations*
   *Quality control*
   *Record maintenance, coding, indexing, and accounting*
   *Personnel and fiscal management*
   *Patient information resources*
   *Scheduling*
   *Support resources*
9. Demonstrate understanding of acoustical physics, Doppler ultrasound principles, and medical ultrasound imaging principles and instrumentation;
   *Acoustical physics*
   *Sound production and propagation*
   *Interactions of sound and matter*
   *Physics of Doppler*
   *Principles of Doppler techniques*
   *Methods of Doppler flow analysis*
10. Demonstrate knowledge and proficiency in optimal recording and analysis of data;

*Techniques for recording dynamic images*
*Techniques for optimal recordings of audible data*
*Techniques for quantifying data*

11. Demonstrate knowledge and understanding of the interactions between ultrasound and tissue;
    *Biological effects*
    *Image production*
    *Artifacts*

12. Demonstrate current knowledge related to biological effects;
    *In-vitro studies*
    *Animal studies*
    *Human studies*
    *Epidemiological investigation*

13. Exercise professional judgment and discretion in obtaining diagnostic information and correlating findings with supervising physicians;
    *Medical ethics*
    *Pertinent legal principles*
    *Teamwork principles*
    *Professional interaction skills*

14. Exercise professional judgment and discretion in communication with patients, coworkers, and the public concerning sonography;

15. Demonstrate knowledge that contributes to the development of diagnostic medical sonography;
    *Educational psychology and techniques*
    *Computer literacy*
    *Health administration*
    *Research statistics and design*
    *Trends in health care delivery systems*
    *Professional organizations and resources*
    *Continuing professional development*

*Specific Competencies.* Competencies specific to cardiac sonography shall include but not be limited to the following areas of proficiency:

1. Demonstrate knowledge of normal and abnormal cardiac and circulatory physiology and pathophysiology;
   *Normal and abnormal hemodynamics*
   *Descriptors of normal cardiac performance*
   *Descriptors of altered cardiac performance*
   *Congenital and acquired cardiovascular disease*

2. Demonstrate knowledge and understanding of clinical medicine as it relates to cardiac sonography;

*History and physical examination*
*Differential diagnostic considerations*
*Cardiovascular surgical procedures*

3. Demonstrate knowledge and understanding of the relationships of cardiac procedures;
   *Electrocardiography*
   *Phonocardiography and external pulse recording*
   *Holter monitoring*
   *Exercise testing*
   *Radionuclide procedures*
   *Cardiac catheterization and angiography*

4. Demonstrate proficiency in the performance of cardiac ultrasound diagnostic procedures and understanding of the applications and limitations of each of their relationships;
   *M-mode and two-dimensional (2-D) cardiac-sonography*
   *Doppler cardiac sonography—pulsed-wave, continuous-wave, color-flow*
   *Exercise cardiac sonography*
   *Contrast cardiac sonography*
   *Cardiac sonography–assisted pericardiocentesis*
   *Intraoperative cardiac sonography*
   *Transesophageal cardiac sonography*

5. Demonstrate knowledge and understanding of the role of cardiac sonography as it relates to clinical pharmacology and provocative maneuvers.

## Cardiovascular Technologist*

Cardiovascular technology is a multidisciplinary science requiring the student to be suitably trained and educated in the basic and applied principles of several diagnostic and/or therapeutic modalities. Upon completion of an educational program, each student must have acquired clinical skills and knowledge consistent with specific clinical performance objectives in one or more of the following areas of expertise: invasive cardiology, noninvasive cardiology, noninvasive peripheral vascular studies.

*(Reprinted with permission from Essentials and Guidelines of an Accredited Educational Program for the Cardiovascular Technologist (adopted 1985). Provided by the Joint Review Committee on Education in Cardiovascular Technology: Chicago, IL)

*Basic Instruction.* Students should acquire a clear understanding of the basic sciences and how basic scientific principles relate to clinical applications in the cardiovascular technology field. Suggested areas of instruction include:

*Introduction to the field of cardiovascular technology— including patient care techniques and the hospital environment*

*General and/or Applied Sciences—including biology, basic chemistry, physical principles of medicine, basic statistics and general mathematics at a level approaching that of intermediate algebra*

*Human Anatomy and Physiology—with emphasis on cardiac and vascular systems*

*Basic Pharmacology—pertaining to cardiovascular drugs*

*Basic Medical Electronics and Medical Instrumentation*

*Cardiac and Vascular Instruction.* The cardiac units of instruction should include two major areas: invasive and noninvasive cardiology. The vascular units of instruction should include subject matter relating to noninvasive peripheral vascular studies.

Clinical Instruction should include:

*Cardiac and Vascular Pathophysiology*
*Patient History and Physical Examination*
*Patient Psychology, Care and Communications*
*Cardiopulmonary Resuscitation*
*Therapeutic Measures*
*Clinical Cardiac and Vascular Medicine*
*Statistics, Management of Data, Physics*
*Medical-Legal Ethics*

The Curriculum shall be sufficient to provide:

1. Knowledge of the technical skills necessary to perform appropriate diagnostic cardiac or vascular testing;
2. An understanding of other diagnostic and interventional procedures as they relate to the clinical evaluation and treatment of cardiovascular disease;
3. Comprehension of the methodologies required to obtain correct data pertinent to the diagnostic procedures being performed;
4. An understanding of pertinent pharmacological effects that affect the cardiovascular status; and

5. A knowledge of the attendant risks to the patient of any of the procedures performed.

*Invasive Cardiology Instruction.* Recording and performing preliminary analysis of invasive cardiovascular data in procedures such as:

1. Measuring cardiovascular parameters such as cardiac output, blood flow and velocity, cardiopulmonary hemodynamics, cardiac electrophysiology, shunts, valve areas, and heart sounds with appropriate diagnostic procedures.
2. Conducting quantitative and qualitative analysis of arterial and venous blood gases.
3. Preparing, calibrating, and operating monitoring instrumentation utilized for determining the presence and extent of cardiovascular abnormalities in diagnostic laboratory or operating room settings.
4. Collecting and preparing diagnostic test data for review by a physician.

*Noninvasive Cardiology Instruction.* Recording and performing preliminary analysis of noninvasive cardiovascular data in procedures such as:

1. Echocardiography (M-mode, two-dimensional, and Doppler studies).
2. Other noninvasive modalities including vectorcardiography, electrocardiography, exercise stress testing, ambulatory monitoring (Holter), phonocardiography, external pulse tracings, and apexcardiography.

*Noninvasive Peripheral Vascular Instruction.* Recording and performing preliminary analysis of noninvasive peripheral vascular data in procedures such as:

1. The use of quantitative and qualitative methods of assessing arterial obstruction in the upper and lower extremities including the use of Doppler ultrasound, pneumoplethysmographic tracings, segmental pressure measurement, photoplethysmographic and strain gauge plethysmographic assessment of digits.
2. Quantitative and qualitative methods of detecting venous obstruction, venous reflux including use of Doppler ultrasound, impedance outflow plethysmography (electrical, strain gauge, and

TABLE 22-1. Levels of physician training in echocardiography

| OBJECTIVES | | DURATION (MONTHS) | EXAMINATIONS (NO.) |
|---|---|---|---|
| Physicians in a Cardiology Training Program | | | |
| Level 1 | Introductory experience | 3 | 150 2-D/M-mode<br>75 Doppler |
| Level 2 | Sufficient experience to take independent responsibility for echocardiographic studies | 3 beyond level 1 | 150 2-D/M-mode<br>150 Doppler |
| Level 3 | Sufficient expertise to direct an echocardiography lab | 6 beyond level 1 | 450 using both imaging and Doppler |
| Physicians Who Have Completed Cardiology Training | | | |
| | Responsibility for performance and interpretation of echocardiograms | Variable level of achievement equivalent to level 2 above | 250–300 2-D/M-mode and Doppler |
| | Direct echocardiography laboratory in hospital or large group practice | Variable level of expertise equivalent to level 3 above | 450 2-D/M-mode and Doppler |

(From Pearlman AS, Gardin JM, Martin RP, et al. Guidelines for optimal physician training in echocardiography. Am J Cardiol. 1987; 60:158–163.)

pneumoplethysmographic), and photoplethysmography (for reflux).

3. Quantitative and qualitative methods of determining the presence of cerebrovascular disease, including Doppler ultrasound of periorbital arterial signals, ocularplethysmography, carotid phonoangiography, continuous and pulsed Doppler ultrasound for audible assessment of the carotid artery, sound spectrum analysis of continuous and pulsed waveforms, A-mode imaging, and B-mode imaging.

The cardiovascular technologist is trained to perform the aforementioned tasks in various patient care settings. Each technologist is also trained in life support techniques.

## Physician Training in Echocardiography

In the rapidly evolving field of echocardiography much emphasis has been placed on the minimum standards of education for cardiac sonographers and cardiovascular technologists. Less emphasis was placed on developing optimal guidelines for physician training in echocardiography until the

Committee for Physician Training in Echocardiography was formed by the American Society of Echocardiography (Table 22-1).

The Committee acknowledged that the optimal use of echocardiographic techniques for diagnosis and clinical decision making is based on a great deal of theoretical knowledge, important technical abilities, and significant clinical experience with echocardiographic applications. They also acknowledged that proper development of such skills requires substantial training, which optimally should be carried out under the guidance of an experienced physician-echocardiographer.[4]

The American Society of Echocardiographers recommends three levels of training in echocardiography for cardiology fellows: introductory, intermediate, and advanced.

The guidelines also contain valuable information about background knowledge and the type of sites that are optimal for training physicians who take responsibility for conducting or interpreting echocardiographic examinations. It also recommends that physicians who have already completed their fellowship training attain equivalent levels of expertise appropriate to their needs.[4]

*Conclusion.* I have focused here on the tangible elements of education and training, but there is much more to the creation of a good sonographer. Patience, tenacity, intellectual curiosity, enthusiasm, and warmth are only a few of the intangible qualities that cannot be taught. These traits are the mark of a true professional.

## References

1. Adams D, Kisslo KB, Kisslo J. Credentialing of the cardiac sonographer: The need for unification. J Am Soc Echocardiogr. 1988; 1:100–102.

2. Kisslo J, Millman DS, Adams DB, et al. Interpretation of echocardiographic data: Are physicians and sonographers violating the law? J Am Soc Echocardiogr. 1988; 1:95–99.

3. Mazer MS. What constitutes a good cardiac echo lab: The "team" approach (guest editorial). J Diagn Med Sonogr. 1985; 1(2):47.

4. Pearlman AS, Gardin JM, Martin RP, et al. Guidelines for optimal physician training in echocardiography: Recommendations of the American Society of Echocardiography Committee for Physician Training in Echocardiography. Am J Cardiol. 1987; 60:158–163.

# Index

447

ISBN 0-397-50953-7

90000

780397 509539